PHYSICAL MEDICINE AND REHABILITATION

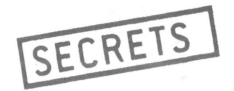

PHYSICAL MEDICINE AND REHABILITATION

SECRETS

Third Edition

Bryan J. O'Young, MD

Medical Director, Department of International
 Rehabilitation Medicine
Clinical Associate Professor, Department of
 Rehabilitation Medicine
New York University School of Medicine
Attending Physician, Rusk Institute of
 Rehabilitation Medicine
New York University Medical Center
New York, New York, U.S.A.
Visiting Professor
Department of Rehabilitation Medicine
Peking University School of Medicine
Peking First Hospital
Beijing, China
Visiting Professor
Department of Rehabilitation Medicine
Capital Medical University
Xuan Wu Hospital
Beijing, China
Adjunct Professor
Department of Rehabilitation Medicine
University of the Philippines College of Medicine
Manila, Philippines

Mark A. Young, MD, MBA, FACP

Chair, Department of Physical Medicine &
 Rehabilitation
The Maryland Rehabilitation Center/
 The Workforce & Technology Center
State of Maryland, Division of Rehabilitation,
 Department of Education
Adjunct Clinical Associate Professor
Department of Rehabilitation Medicine
New York University School of Medicine
New York, New York
Faculty, Department of Neurology
University of Maryland School of Medicine
Baltimore, Maryland
Professor, Department of Orthopedic Sciences
New York College of Podiatric Medicine
New York, New York

Steven A. Stiens, MD, MS

Associate Professor
Director of Spinal Cord Medicine Clinical
 Fellowship
Department of Rehabilitation Medicine
University of Washington School of Medicine
Attending Physician, Spinal Cord Injury Unit
VA Puget Sound Health Care System
University Hospital Harborview Medical Center
Seattle, Washington

MOSBY

ELSEVIER

MOSBY
ELSEVIER

1600 John F. Kennedy Blvd. Ste 1800
Philadelphia, PA 19103–2899

Physical Medicine and Rehabilitation   ISBN-13: 978-1-4160-3205-2
Third Edition

NOTICE

Knowledge and best practice in this field are constantly changing. As new research and experience broaden our knowledge, changes in practice, treatment and drug therapy may become necessary or appropriate. Readers are advised to check the most current information provided (i) on procedures featured or (ii) by the manufacturer of each product to be administered, to verify the recommended dose or formula, the method and duration of administration, and contraindications. It is the responsibility of the practitioner, relying on his or her own experience and knowledge of the patient, to make diagnoses, to determine dosages and the best treatment for each individual patient, and to take all appropriate safety precautions. To the fullest extent of the law, neither the Publisher nor the Editor assumes any liability for any injury and/or damage to persons or property arising out or related to any use of the material contained in this book.

Library of Congress Cataloging-in-Publication Data
Physical medicine and rehabilitation secrets / [edited by] Bryan J.
O'Young, Mark A. Young, Steven A. Stiens. – 3rd ed.
     p. ; cm. – (Secrets series)
  Includes bibliographical references and index.
  ISBN-13: 978-1-4160-3205-2
  ISBN-10: 1-4160-3205-3
  1. Physical therapy–Examinations, questions, etc. 2. Medical
rehabilitation–Examinations, questions, etc. I. O'Young, Bryan, 1962-
II. Young, Mark A., 1960- III. Stiens, Steven A., 1959- IV. Series.
  [DNLM: 1. Physical Medicine–Examination Questions. 2.
Rehabilitation–Examination Questions. WB 18.2 P57786 2007]

RM701.6.P52 2007
615.8'2076–dc22
                                                    2006036054

Acquisitions Editor: Jim Merritt
Developmental Editor: Stan Ward
Project Manager: Mary Stermel
Marketing Manager: John Gore

Printed in China.

Last digit is the print number: 9   8   7   6   5   4   3   2

Working together to grow
libraries in developing countries

www.elsevier.com | www.bookaid.org | www.sabre.org

ELSEVIER   BOOK AID International   Sabre Foundation

DEDICATION

To my beloved parents, Te See and Merla, for their lifelong love and inspiration.

To my siblings, Andrew, Crosby, Dorene, and Eldred, for their support and encouragement.

To my mentor, Keith Sperling MD who instilled in me the valuable ethic: "Treat each patient as though he or she is the most important person in the world."

To my department chairman, Mathew Lee, MD, who cultivated my resilience, creativity, and adaptivity to embrace life's challenges.

BJO

This book is dedicated to my loving wife, Marlene Malka, a true "women of valor" whose caring, courage, and dedication nurtures our beautiful family.

To my dear children, Michelle, Michael, and Jennifer, who represent an ongoing source of pride and accomplishment.

To my colleagues in Medicine and in Rehabilitation who have offered invaluable friendship, mentorship, and inspiration.

To my residents and students who have taught me how to ask the right questions.

In fond memory of my late parents, Michael and Rowena, whose glowing example has instilled in me an unwavering dedication to quality, compassionate care, education, and leadership.

MAY

To my lovely wife Beth (the teacher), and my children Hanna (the film maker), Duffy (the guitarist), and the twins: Olivia (the artist) and Luke (the scientist) for the joy of discovery, creative work, and love that they keep in our "nest."

To my parents who continually develop me with their love, understanding and direction, Jean (the psychiatrist, 1937–2005) and Bill (the building builder) for their devotion to meaningful work and their lifelong nurturing of me and our family.

To my brothers Scott (the world builder with the US State Dept.) and Doug (the building designer, builder, and restorationist) for their insights, visions, and implementation, and humor.

To a few of my mentors from my home state, Ohio: Randall Braddom, MD, MS, who teaches all of us that the hallmark of a successful physiatrist and a person is the demonstrated capability to very successfully **adapt** (see Epilogue) and teach these skills to your patients and protégés; Ernie Johnson, MD at Ohio State University, who taught me that leadership begins with self direction; Carl Rogers, PhD, also from Ohio State University, who taught me to listen to the patient as the person at the center of the rehabilitation process; George Engel, MD, once from the University of Cincinnati, who explained to me that the systems surrounding the patient as well as those within successfully respond to treatment; and Gustav Eckstein, MD from the University of Cincinnati, who reminded me as I grew up that "the body does have a head."

SAS

REFERENCES:

1. Pease WS, Lew HL, Johnson EW: Johnson's Practical Electromyography. Philadelphia, Lippincott, Williams & Wilkins, 2006.
2. Rogers C: On becoming a person: A therapist's view of psychotherapy. London, Constable, 1961.
3. Engel GL: The need for a new medical model: A challenge for biomedicine. Science 196:129–136, 1978.
4. Eckstein G: The Body Has a Head. New York, Harper & Row, 1970.

A portion of the proceeds from this textbook is donated to Whirlwind Wheelchair International, which works to make it possible for every person in the developing world who needs a wheelchair to obtain one that will lead to maximum personal independence and integration into society. Go to www.whirlwindwheelchair.org.

DEDICATION TO DR. MATHEW LEE

People are like stained-glass windows. They sparkle and shine when the sun is out, but when the darkness sets in, their true beauty is revealed only if there is a light from within.

Elizabeth Kubler Ross (1926–2004)

This 3rd edition of PM&R Secrets, the product of 4 years of painstaking editing, research, and literary revisions by the editors, is dedicated to a very special person: Dr. Mathew Lee, whose "light from within" perpetually shines. Dr. Lee is a caring, kind, compassionate, and brilliantly effective leader who has chaired the Department of Rehabilitation Medicine of the New York University Rusk Institute since 1989. Internationally known and revered, Dr. Lee is the embodiment of the PM&R Secrets spirit; an individual deeply committed to teaching, philanthropy, and international outreach. Throughout his tenure as Chair of NYU's legendary department of PM&R, Dr. Lee has introduced unique innovations, built bridges, and touched the lives of many.

An inveterate musician and music buff, Dr. Lee skillfully directs his department like a true maestro, offering a delicate balance of leadership, mentorship, academic stewardship, and, above all, a profound sense of sharing and caring. The symphony that he successfully orchestrates has made a global impact on the field of rehabilitation. His role model leadership style has spawned the careers of a new generation of emerging physiatric leaders. His passion for promoting the specialty of PM&R through grooming and shepharding of young physiatrists has left an indelible imprint on the field of rehabilitation medicine worldwide.

Always true to the roots and traditions of the department and institution that he serves, Dr. Lee frequently invokes the hallowed name of the man he has ultimately come to succeed: Dr. Howard Rusk, himself a legendary figurehead in rehabilitation. During simple times as well as challenging moments, Dr. Lee always maintains his aplomb and supreme sense of dignity and always finds time to chat with the residents or take a moment to congratulate young faculty for their achievements.

With the publication of this new edition of PM&R Secrets, we are constantly reminded of the gargantuan team effort in producing this work and are ever inspired by our role model physiatrist, leader, and above all friend, Dr. Mathew Lee. His compassion, his achievements, and his talents "sparkle and shine bright" like Kubler's proverbial "light from within."

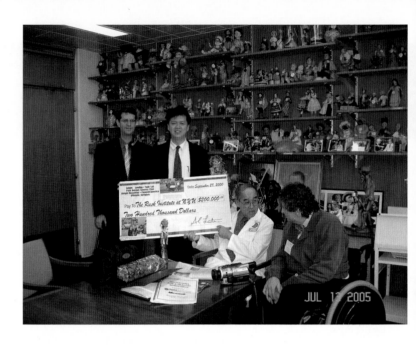

Pictured are Dr. Mathew Lee, and the three PM&R Secrets editors meeting in the "Doll Room" at the chairman's office suite for the New York University Department of Rehabilitation Medicine. From left to right are Mark Young MD, Bryan O'Young MD, Mathew Lee MD, and Steven Stiens MD. For over 50 years, travelers to the department from around the world have brought gifts of dolls. These dolls are displayed on all the walls of this conference room. Dr. Lee is reviewing the history of the department and is at this moment emphasizing the importance of philanthropic support of medical service, education, and research to meet the needs of all people who live with disabilities. The dark sculptured bust of Dr. Howard Rusk can be seen peering between Dr. Lee's and Dr. Stien's heads as a recent check of support for the international work of the Rusk Institute is displayed.

ACKNOWLEDGMENTS

"Feeling gratitude and not expressing it is like wrapping a present and not giving it."
William Arthur Ward (American scholar, author, editor, and teacher) (1921–1994)

The editors of this third edition of *PM&R Secrets* (Bryan, Mark, and Steve) wish to thank our dedicated students, residents, fellows, and colleagues for inspiring us to produce a "new and improved" version of this PM&R educational epic. Special gratitude is offered to the many chapter authors and readers of the first and second editions whose support has laid the foundation for this latest literary production. A dedicated and altruistic faculty of international authors embodying the fine academic spirit of teaching, research, and scholarship collaborated to create this third edition. In so doing, they have lived up to Helen Keller's hallowed philosophy: "Alone we can do so little, together so much!"

Special thanks are in order for the industrious and focused publishing staff at Elsevier, including Linda Belfus, Bill Lambsback, Stan Ward, and James Merritt, Senior Acquisitions Editor, and at SPi, including Trevor S. MacDougall, Project Manager, and Richard Hund, Senior Project Manager, for their steadfast dedication to excellence, attention to detail, commitment to success, and drive to innovate.

The editors of *PM&R Secrets* continue to prosper as clinicians, teachers, and scientists through our relationships and friendships with fellow faculty at our home institutions. Many of these connections enabled us to optimize content and style in this third edition. Again, gratitude is extended to our colleagues and residents at the New York University, University of Washington, Johns Hopkins University, the University of Maryland, the Veterans Administration, Sinai Hospital of Baltimore, and the Maryland Rehabilitation Center & The Workforce & Technology Center. A word of gratitude is due to cherished colleagues associated with the New York College of Podiatric Medicine including Louis Levine and Howard Rusk Jr.

Bestowing thanks and gratitude and paying homage to people who are no longer with us is the highest form of acknowledgment. Although this task poses a poignant challenge, the editors wish to offer our heartfelt memorial and kindest rememberance to our beloved colleagues who are dearly departed but whose spirit lovingly remains with us, including Mr. Norman Berger, Dr. David Berkin, Dr. Binyomin "Bradley" Bregin, Dr. Charles "Chuck" Cannizzarro, Dr. Scott Labaer, Dr. Justus Lehman, and Dr. Scott Nadler.

The many innovations that come with this third edition would never have been possible without the creative, congenial, collaborative, and diligent teamwork of many. Ms. Tammy Chan fashioned the structure of our outline in response to our design, and she enthusiastically maintained communication with all the authors as chapter concepts were defined and integrated into the textbook themes. Ms. Ivy Wang provided conscientious attention to detail and dedicated her continual support to the academic mission. Debra Walters, Linnea Preston, Makoto Edani, and Annie Liang provided clerical assistance in revising edited manuscripts to refine clarity and maximize educational content. Charles Goldmann as a certified nursing assistant and Mary Lou May as an experienced nurse and administrator sought out countless references and maintained our writing files to enable pertinent and contemporary literature to be cited. Mia Hannula provided clever searches of a variety of databases as an exploratory librarian and Scott

Campbell, library assistant, retrieved literature and various other learning media to provide a selective and rich array of resources for our readers.

The following medical media specialists are congratulated on their art and skills: Joseph Mathews, Alisa Holcomb, Christopher Pacheco, and Don Cabio. Over the years, they have collaborated to render custom diagrams, scan images, and generate posters, CD-ROMs, and movies to provide education that shares *PM&R Secrets'* core messages.

A unique word of thanks is due to IT (Information Technology) innovations such as Gmail of Google fame, which logistically enabled the editors to synchronously stay on top of the pile of daily authors' e-mail correspondence relating to book content. The novel storage and archiving capability of this program truly optimized the editors' efforts. Skype, a unique Internet-based telephonic service, also allowed the authors to maintain real-time contact with authors throughout the world.

In later production, manuscripts required review for educational impact, clarity, and correct grammatical style. Considering the variety of expression in this casual occasionally funny yet academic bridge textbook required discrimination and a sense of humor. These courageous test pilots provided hints about content, style, layout, and structure of the material for all readers. They relentlessly corrected typos and made suggestions for clarity throughout the text. Lisa Carey, Alexis Kruczek, Christina Hadzithedorou, Sarah Ritter, Elizabeth Bentzen, Hiwen Chen, Darryl Gray, and Anne Marie Mackey, as well as a few others, met these challenges with enthusiasm. THANKS!

The authors would like to express gratitude to the members of our arduous attending physician and resident peer review editorial panel who provided insights on the textbook as this edition was formulated. They include Dr. Michael Frey, Dr. Howard Choi, Dr. Tim Dillingham, Dr. Mathew Lee, Dr. Jennifer James, Dr. Ari Greis, Dr. Alfred Campbell, Dr. DJ Kennedy, Dr. Mohammed Yavari Rad, Dr. Maya Desai, Dr. Sheldon Rudin, Dr. Lee Gresser, Dr. Edwin Burstock, and a few others. Thanks to Dr. Stanley Kornhauser, Dr. Rhodora Tumanon, Dr. Margaret Hammond, Dr. Peter Esselman, and Dr. Larry Robinson for their support.

In closing, we wish to invoke the famous words of the world famous composer Lionel Hampton (1908–2002): "Gratitude is when memory is stored in the heart and not in the mind."

PREFACE

Mark A. Young, MD, MBA, Bryan J. O'Young, MD, Steven A. Stiens, MD, MS

"There are no impertinent questions—only impertinent answers"

—Oscar Wilde (1854–1900)

1. **What is evidence-based medicine and how does it relate to the art of rehabilitation learning in *PM&R Secrets*?**

   Evidence-based medicine (EBM) combines individual clinical expertise with external clinical evidence from systematic research in order to help clinicians make better decisions about patient care. The 3rd edition of *PM&R Secrets* continues to use the time honored "Question and Answer" (Q&A) format to share important evidence-based medical and rehabilitation information with readers. The list of frequently asked questions (FAQs) and answers that comprise each chapter are carefully prepared to assure the readers grasp and mastery of scientifically valid evidenced based information.

   The principles of EBM can similarly be extended to the process of medical education, rehabilitation learning and teaching. An evidence-based learning (EBL) approach champions "think out of the box" teaching methods that include some of the following key elements:

   - Providing an active, engaging curriculum
   - Enabling self-paced learning
   - Practicing continuous assessment and reassessment
   - Providing immediate feedback
   - Avoiding the widespread use of punitive or aversive teaching stratagem (e.g. "pimping," "rounding rage," or extra call duties)
   - *PM&R Secrets, 3rd Edition* skillfully employs many of these evidence-based learning tools, and in so doing has earned widespread recognition among international physiatrists.

   Sackett DL, Rosenberg WM, Gray JA, et al: Evidence-based medicine: What it is and what it isn't? BMJ 312:71–72, 1996.
   Davies P: Approaches to evidence-based teaching. Medical Teacher 22:14–21, 2000.

2. **Does didactic method matter? What is the evidence that Questions & Answers (Q&A) lead to better physiatric learning?**

   Using the Q&A approach, readers can dynamically acquire knowledge through an active learning process. Active or dynamic learning, as the name suggests, is a form of education which is used by progressive educators to dynamically involve the pupils during the learning process. Also known as "learning by doing," dynamic learning is different from less active modes of instruction like passively listening to lectures. (Wikipedia, Bonwell & Eison, 1991). The use of Q&A provides a unique, interactive and effective mode of active learning for the physiatrist. Pupils who actively interact and engage with the material are more likely to recall information later and to be able to apply that knowledge in different contexts (Bruner, 1961). The use of Q&A has been known throughout the ages as the "Socratic Approach" and is the direct, non-pretentious style of teaching employed by the preceding editions of *PM&R Secrets*.

   Bonwell C, Eison J: Active Learning: Creating Excitement in the Classroom. Washington, DC, AEHE-ERIC Higher Education Report No. 1, 1991.
   Bruner JS: The act of discovery. Harvard Educational Review 31(1):21–32, 1961.
   Wikipedia: http://en.wikipedia.org/wiki/Active_learning

3. **How is the 3rd edition of *PM&R Secrets* different from its preceding two editions?**
To quote the famous Australian songstress Olivia Newton John: "Let's make a good thing even better!"

The editors and contributors have made this objective a major priority by completely revamping content, updating references, reconfiguring format and even adding color to this 3rd edition. To maximize learning and emphasize dynamic education, many new visually attractive diagrams, pictures (sorry, none of Olivia!), and schematics have been added to illuminate the Q&A guided textual discussion. In order to keep up to date with current trends in physiatry, the editors have methodically reviewed curricular requirements, learning needs, and objectives of the 21st century physiatrists and have completely refreshed the 3rd edition with the inclusion of exciting, new, state-of-the-art material. While most chapters focus on traditional "bread, butter, and board" topics, brand new evidence-based chapters on pain management, interventional physiatry, and complementary medicine, to name a few, now have been included in the book. As a result of an ever growing global interest in rehabilitation as well as the editors' personal leadership roles in international PM&R affairs, a significant number of worldwide rehabilitation experts have joined our faculty of authors.

Distinguishing features of the 3rd edition are summarized here.

1. Expanded faculty of national and international expert contributors representing many countries
2. Enhanced Pain and Musculoskeletal Sections
3. New two color format
4. Optimization of tables, charts, and schematics to help elucidate topic matter
5. Concise, clear presentation of the latest scientific facts, models, and methods of practice.
6. Enhanced focus on fundamental practice as well as advanced concepts
7. Inclusion of key internet references
8. Clear and succinct summaries of key points and concepts
9. 100 top PM&R secrets revealed

4. **What is the mission of *PM&R Secrets, 3rd Edition*?**
Physical Medicine & Rehabilitation Secrets, 3rd Edition will serve as a portable international rehabilitation educational resource for students, interns, residents, attendings, physicians preparing for boards, faculty, and interdisciplinary rehabilitation professionals (physical therapists, occupational therapists, speech pathologists, nurses) by providing concise and accurate rehabilitation knowledge through an informative and engaging Q&A format. *PM&R Secrets*, bolstered by its expert editorial and authorship faculty, will continue to be recognized as a simple, straightforward, yet powerful and authoritative learning and educational tool for international rehabilitationists practicing in clinical settings as well as in academic environments. Through its novel format and one of a kind teaching style, *PM&R Secrets* will pay tribute to the roots and traditions of PM&R by helping to improve the quality of care and quality of life of all persons with disabilities.

5. **What is the logic behind the format of the 3rd edition?**
The chapter sequence of *PM&R Secrets, 3rd Edition* has been carefully configured to cluster similar categories of illness, disease, and disabilities in close proximity to enable easier learning. Chapters are designed to build on one another and questions have been sequenced to present fundamental concepts up front in the chapter before proceeding to more advanced subjects later on in the chapter.

Written in a plain, simple, straightforward fashion, the book covers all of the major topics in physiatry. Chapters are composed in a Q&A format. For every topic, clusters of carefully selected, clinically relevant, thought-provoking questions are accompanied by simple, straightforward, nonpretentious answers. *PM&R Secrets* has been called a "bridge-text" because it strategically links vital information culled from the literature, textbooks, and research.

Modeled after the acclaimed "Socratic Style" of medical education, *PM&R Secrets, 3rd Edition* offers readers a valuable learning advantage.

6. **How should the text be used?**

    PM&R Secrets strives to serve as a practical book of FAQs, providing its loyal readership with "just the facts". The book is intended to be a review text and can be effectively used as a learning tool and an adjunct to the classical textbooks in the field. The clinician can use the book in multiple ways:

    1. Keeping the text "close at hand" in clinic or during rounds for quick reference purposes
    2. To prepare for rounds by reviewing chapter content in problem based learning style
    3. To organize or craft a customized didactic session or lecture
    4. To inject a "journal club" discussion with some factual background learning matter
    5. To organizes tests and quizzes for residents and students

    This book is unique in that it offers the reader information suited to all stages of education and practice development. For the new student of rehabilitation, clear definitions and outlines of the rehabilitation process are offered. For the resident, specific practice pearls and pointers are generously provided. For the rehabilitation educator, tantalizing, thought-provoking questions are shared.

7. **What is the origin of *PM&R Secrets*?**

    It all began in 1993 when three maverick physicians (Bryan, Mark, and Steve) had a flash of inspiration. It was a vision to optimize the learning experience of their students, residents, and fellow physiatrists through creation of a "think out of a box" educational concept. On many an evening, the trio sat around the rehab ward munching on peanuts and studying with the residents. Posing questions and answers to one another helped to keep the discussions lively. What began as a casual get-together to share medical knowledge soon evolved into a comprehensive book of questions and answers, focusing on all dimensions of the field. By enlisting the collaborative efforts of leading physiatrists and rehabilitation experts, the editors have been able to present the very best teaching points in an attractive and engaging way. It has been translated into multiple languages and is a favorite due to its simplistic and straightforward format. Now 11 years since its debut, *PM&R Secrets* has found its way to libraries and call rooms throughout the world.

8. **Rehabilitation riddle: "How is reading *PM&R Secrets* like feasting at a banquet?"**

    PM&R Secrets can be viewed as a veritable smorgasbord of educational delicacies composed of 84 dishes (chapters) that you can sample at any hour, day or night. Depending on your desire, you, the reader, are able to indulge in these didactic delicacies and savor one or several at a time. Each chapter is composed of "juicy digestible morsels" that will hopefully leave readers with a good "educational" taste.

9. **Can this volume be used to enhance my practice of rehabilitation medicine?**

    Sure. By its design, this text is organized to provide rehabilitation knowledge that is relevant to the every day practice of medicine. Several weeks after this book was published, one of the editors received a grateful phone call from an internist in a remote town in the Midwest (where no physiatrists practice) who used *PM&R Secrets* to effectively manage a spinal cord patient with autonomic dysreflexia. This book can be used in the clinic, in the gym, or on the ward. It can be used for library research or for home study.

10. **How can "*PM&R Secrets* Readers" unite within the global rehabilitation community?**

    The unprecedented international success of *PM&R Secrets* since its humble launch in 1995 has been paralleled by another evolving phenomenon—the emergence and growth of the global information highway including the internet and the web. Web based technologies like e-mail, internet messaging, blogging, and internet teleconferencing (voice and video) have enabled closer communication between *PM&R Secrets* faculty and readers. The editors encourage our readers and faculty to become commuters on this global highway. Committed to uniting members of the *PM&R Secrets* community, the editors have created a website: www. pmrsecrets.com and e-mail address pmrsecrets@gmail.com where the authors can be contacted. A PM&R Secret blog also exists.

11. **What does the future hold for PM&R education?**
Throughout the history of medical education, the Q&A guided learning approach (AKA the Socratic approach) has held a hallowed and prominent place in the halls of academia. Questions, answers, memory strategies, and mnemonic devices are all fun, easy, and convenient way of learning. The future of PM&R education will see a growing dependence on online technologic learning tools. In fact, the contents of this edition of *PM&R Secrets* have broken ground through its complimentary availability online at the www.elsevier.com website. No matter what you do— go online or read the following printed pages—you are destined to learn. Have fun and carry forth the *PM&R Secrets* tradition!

FOREWORD

Professor Haim Ring, Professor Linamara Batistella, and Professor Chang-il Park

"Education is the Transmission of Civilization"
-*Will Durant (1885–1981)*

Throughout the ages, across multiple continents and beyond socioeconomic and geopolitical divides, education (especially rehabilitation medical education) remains a global priority—serving to strengthen and nurture society and helping to provide for a better tomorrow.

Physical Medicine and Rehabilitation (PM&R) Secrets, a monumental work now in its 3rd edition, is the embodiment of this noble philosophy. The volume—internationally recognized for its simplicity, its concise and thought-provoking question-and-answer format, and its authoritative coverage of the field of Physiatry—has been translated into multiple languages. In so doing, this book has made the rehabilitation world a smaller and a better place.

The editorial product of three caring and compassionate consummate academic educators—Bryan J. O' Young, Mark A. Young, and Steven A. Stiens—*PM&R Secrets,* 3rd edition continues its tradition of editorial excellence through its comprehensive overview of the field. It has garnered the acclaim of students of rehabilitation across the entire continuum of education, including physiotherapists, pre-medical students, medical students, interns, residents, fellows and attending faculty physicians. The editors have taken painstaking care to "give back" to the field of PM&R by contributing copies of their book to residents and students in many developing countries, through ISPRM-affiliated programs.

The core and substance of *PM&R Secrets* are the 84 comprehensive and fact-filled chapters each contributed by a distinguished international faculty of experts who have generously shared their knowledge and didactic skill. Without pomp, circumstance, or academic fanfare, each chapter presents a user-friendly FAQ (frequently asked question) synopsis of the field. The end product is a chapter that is destined to help promote a global knowledge of rehabilitation among the world's international community of rehabilitation.

Living up to the roots and traditions of the field of physiatry, *PM&R Secrets* reaches out to the masses—through education, through scholarship, and through charity.

The book is a living tribute to the good that can come of international scholarship and collaboration within the physical medicine and rehabilitation world. The editors are to be congratulated for their devoted work.

We are hopeful that education in PM&R as represented within the pages of this book can enhance the reader's ability to ask more pertinent questions in rehabilitation and motivate the rehabilitation professional to provide healing solutions that lead to a more functional tomorrow.

CONTENTS

III. THE REHABILITATION ASSESSMENT

IV. ELECTRODIAGNOSTIC FUNDAMENTALS

V. REHABILITATION AND WORK

VI. GENERAL THERAPEUTICS

VII. PHYSICAL MODALITIES

VIII. INTERVENTIONAL PHYSIATRIC TECHNIQUES

IX. ORTHOTICS, PROSTHETICS, AND WHEELCHAIRS

X. MUSCULOSKELETAL REHABILITATION

XIII. SELECTED REHABILITATION POPULATIONS

XIV. CHRONIC PAIN

CONTRIBUTORS

Mindy Aisen, MD
Director and CEO, United Cerebral Palsy Research and Educational Foundation, Washington, DC

Gulseren Akyuz, MD
Professor, Marmara University School of Medicine; Chief, Department of Physical Medicine and Rehabilitation, Istanbul, Turkey

Gad Alon, PhD, PT
Associate Professor, Department of Physical Therapy and Rehabilitation Sciences, University of Maryland School of Medicine, Baltimore, Maryland

Ronit Aloni, PhD
Certified Sexual Therapist, Sackler School of Medicine, Tel Aviv University; Private Practice, Tel Aviv, Israel

Dheera Ananthakrishnan, MD, MSE
Assistant Professor, Department of Orthopedics and Sports Medicine, University of Washington School of Medicine, Seattle, Washington

J. Michael Anderson, MD
Associate Professor of Rehabilitation Medicine, Division of Neurology, University of Maryland Medical School; Medical Director, Neurologic Rehabilitation, Sinai Hospital of Baltimore, Baltimore, Maryland

Charles E. Argoff, MD
Assistant Professor of Neurology, New York University School of Medicine; Director, Cohn Pain Management Center, North Shore University Hospital, Bethpage, New York, New York, New York

Rita N. Ayyangar, MD
Assistant Professor, Department of Physical Medicine and Rehabilitation, University of Michigan Health Systems, Ann Arbor, Michigan

John R. Bach, MD
Professor and Vice Chairman, Department of Physical Medicine and Rehabilitation; Professor of Neurosciences, University of Medicine and Dentistry of New Jersey, New Jersey Medical School, Newark, New Jersey

Karen Barr, MD
Assistant Professor, Department of Physical Medicine and Rehabilitation, University of Washington School of Medicine; Rehabilitation Physician, University of Washington Medical Center, Seattle, Washington

Jeffrey R. Basford, MD, PhD
Professor of Physical Medicine and Rehabilitation, Mayo Clinic, Rochester, Minnesota

Linamara Batistella, MD, PhD
Past President, International Society of Physical and Rehabilitation Medicine Chair, Physical Medicine & Rehabilitation University of Sao Paulo School of Medicine, Sao Paulo, Brazil

Kathleen R. Bell, MD
Professor, Department of Rehabilitation Medicine, University of Washington School of Medicine; Medical Director, Rehabilitation Medicine, Ambulatory Care and Brain Injury Rehabilitation Programs, University Hospital, Seattle, Washington

Scott E. Benjamin, MD
Department of Physical Medicine and Rehabilitation, Fletcher Allen Health Care, Colchester, Vermont

Leland Berkwits, MD
Mountain Neurological Center, Asheville, North Carolina

Peter E. Biglin, DO
Rehabilitation Physicians PC, Novi, Michigan

Valerie S. Bodeau, MD
Clinical Assistant Professor, Department of Rehabilitation Medicine, University of Washington School of Medicine, Attending Physician, Harborview Medical Center, Seattle, Washington

Elliot B. Bodofsky, MD
Associate Professor of Physical Medicine and Rehabilitation, UMDNJ-Robert Wood Johnson Medical School; Chief, Department of Physical Medicine and Rehabilitation, UMDNJ-Cooper University Hospital, Camden, New Jersey

Michael L. Boninger, MD
Assistant Dean for Medical Student Research, Professor and Vice Chair, Department of Physical Medicine and Rehabilitation, University of Pittsburgh; Medical Director, Human Engineering Research Laboratories; VA Pittsburgh Healthcare System, Pittsburgh, Pennsylvania

Joanne Borg-Stein, MD
Medical Director, Newton Wellesley Hospital Spine Center, Spaulding Newton-Wellesley Rehabilitation Center, Wellesley, Massachusetts

Randall L. Braddom, MD, MS
Clinical Professor, UMDNJ Medical School; Clinical Professor, Robert Wood Johnson Medical Schools, New Brunswick, New Jersey

Diane W. Braza, MD
Assistant Professor, Department of Physical Medicine and Rehabilitation, Medical College of Wisconsin, Milwaukee, Wisconsin

Scott E. Brown, MD
Chairman, The B. Stanley Cohen Department of Rehabilitation, Sinai Hospital, Baltimore, Maryland

Stephen P. Burns, MD
Associate Professor, Director of Advanced Spinal Cord Medicine Fellowship, Department of Rehabilitation Medicine, University of Washington School of Medicine; Attending Physician, Spinal Cord Injury Unit, VA Puget Sound Health Care System, Seattle, Washington

Ralph M. Buschbacher, MD
Professor and Chair, Department of Physical Medicine and Rehabilitation, Indiana University School of Medicine, Indianapolis, Indiana

Rene Cailliet, MD
Professor/Chairman Emeritus, Department of Medicine, Section of Physical Medicine and Rehabilitation, University of Southern California School of Medicine, Los Angeles, California

David A. Cassius, MD
Private Practice, Bellevue, Washington

Leighton Chan, MD, MPH
Chief, Rehabilitation Medicine Department, National Institutes of Health, Bethesda, Maryland

Tsai Chao, MD, FAAPMR
Clinical Assistant Professor, Department of Orthopaedic Surgery and Rehabilitation; Director, Department of Orthopaedic Surgery and Rehabilitation Medicine's Residency Program, State University of New York Downstate Medical Center, Brooklyn, New York

Howard Choi, MD, MPH
Assistant Professor, Department of Rehabilitation, Mount Sinai School of Medicine, New York, New York

James R. Christensen, MD
Associate Professor of Physical Medicine and Rehabilitation and Pediatrics, Johns Hopkins University School of Medicine/Kennedy Krieger Institute, Baltimore, Maryland

Jeffrey M. Cohen, MD
Clinical Associate Professor, Department of Rehabilitation Medicine, New York University School of Medicine; Co-Chief, the Jerry Lewis Neuromuscular Disease Center; Medical Director, Kathryn Walter Stein Chronic Pain Laboratory, Rusk Institute of Rehabilitation Medicine, New York University Medical Center, New York, New York

Neil B. Cohen, DC, DACRB
Director, Comprehensive Spine and Sports Center, Baltimore, Maryland

Jeffrey L. Cole, MD
Clinical Associate Professor of Rehabilitation Medicine, Department of Surgery, Weill Medical College of Cornell University, New York, New York; New York Hospital Center of Queens, Flushing, New York

Rory A. Cooper, PhD
FISA & Paralyzed Veterans of America (PVA) Chair and Distinguished Professor, Department of Rehabilitation Science and Technology, University of Pittsburgh, Pittsburgh, Pennsylvania

Tyler Childs Cymet, DO
Assistant Professor of Internal Medicine, Johns Hopkins School of Medicine; Section Head, Family Medicine and Medical Director, Outpatient Medicine, Sinai Hospital of Baltimore, Baltimore, Maryland

Joseph Czerniecki, MD
Professor, Department of Rehabilitation Medicine, University of Washington School of Medicine; Chief, Physical Medicine and Rehabilitation, VA Puget Sound Health Care System, Seattle, Washington

Shashank J. Dave, DO
Assistant Professor, Department of Physical Medicine and Rehabilitation, Indiana University School of Medicine, Indianapolis, Indiana

Ronald E. Delanois, MD
Attending Physician, Center for Joint Preservation and Reconstruction, Rubin Institute for Advanced Orthopedics Sinai Hospital of Baltimore, Baltimore, Maryland

Timothy R. Dillingham, MD
Professor and Chair, Department of Physical Medicine and Rehabilitation, Medical College of Wisconsin, Milwaukee, Wisconsin

Peter Daniel Donofrio, MD
Professor of Neurology, Wake Forest University Health Sciences Center, Winston-Salem, North Carolina

Hy Dubo, MD, FRCPC
Professor, Department of Medicine, Section of Physical Medicine and Rehabilitation, University of Manitoba and Health Sciences Centre; Pain Clinic, Segmental Neuromyotherapy Program, Winnipeg, Canada

Joan E. Edelstein, MA, PT, FISPO
Associate Professor of Clinical Physical Therapy and Director, Program in Physical Therapy, Columbia University, New York, New York

Nasser Eftekhari, MD
Clinical Associate Professor, Department of Rehabilitation Medicine, University of Miami School of Medicine, Miami, Florida

Arieh Eldad, MD
Professor of Plastic Surgery, Hadassah Ein Kerem University Hospital, Jerusalem, Israel

Maury R. Ellenberg, MD, FACP
Clinical Professor, Chief, Department of Physical Medicine and Rehabilitation, Wayne State University; Rehabilitation Physicians, Detroit, Michigan

Peter C. Esselman, MD
Professor and Chair, Department of Rehabilitation Medicine, University of Washington School of Medicine; Chief, Physical Medicine and Rehabilitation, Harborview Medical Center, Seattle, Washington

Frank J.E. Falco, MD
Clinical Assistant Professor, Temple University Medical School; Pain Medicine Fellowship Director, Physical Medicine & Rehabilitation Department, Temple University Hospital, Philadelphia, Pennsylvania; Medical Director, Mid-Atlantic Spine, P.A., Newark, Delaware

Gerald Felsenthal, MD
Clinical Professor, Department of Epidemiology and Preventive Medicine, University of Maryland School of Medicine; Chairman Emeritus, Department of Physical Medicine and Rehabilitation, Sinai Hospital of Baltimore, Baltimore, Maryland

Veronika Fialka-Moser, MD
Professor, Department of Physical Medicine and Rehabilitation, University Clinic for Physical Medicine and Rehabilitation, University of Vienna; General Hospital of the City of Vienna, Vienna, Austria

Andrew A. Fischer, MD, PhD
Associate Clinical Professor (retired), Department of Rehabilitation Medicine, Mount Sinai School of Medicine, City University of New York, New York; Medical Director, Pain Diagnostic and Rehabilitation Services, Great Neck, New York

Paul Fishman, MD, PhD
Professor of Neurology, University of Maryland School of Medicine, Baltimore, Maryland

Michael E. Frey, MD
Director of Interventional Physiatry, Advanced Pain Management and Spine Specialists, Fort Myers, Florida

Richard A. Frieden, MD
Assistant Professor, Department of Rehabilitation Medicine, Mount Sinai School of Medicine; Assistant Attending, Mount Sinai Medical Center; Director, Prosthetics and Orthotics Program; New York, New York

Alan Friedman, MD
Staff Physiatrist, Hadassah University Hospital, Jerusalem, Israel; Clinical Director, PM&R Barnert Hospital, Paterson, New Jersey

Michael B. Furman, MD, MS, FAAPMR
Clinical Assistant Professor, Temple University School of Medicine, Philadelphia, Pennsylvania; Attending Physiatrist, Orthopaedic and Spine Specialists, York, Pennsylvania; Fellowship Director, Pain Medicine and Interventional Spine Fellowship, Center for Pain Management and Rehabilitation; Special Consultant, Sinai Hospital of Baltimore, Baltimore, Maryland

Vincent Gabriel, MD
Assistant Professor, Department of Physical Medicine and Rehabilitation, University of Texas Southwestern Medical Center at Dallas, Dallas, Texas

Fae H. Garden, MD
Associate Professor, Department of Physical Medicine and Rehabilitation, Baylor College of Medicine; St. Luke's Episcopal Hospital, Houston, Texas

Susan J. Garrison, MD
Clinical Associate Professor of Rehabilitation Medicine, Weill Medical College of Cornell University, New York, New York

Robert J. Gatchel, PhD, ABPP
Nancy P. & John G. Penson Endowed Professorship in Clinical Health Psychology
Professor & Chairman Department of Psychology, College of Science,
The University of Texas at Arlington

Mouli Madhab Ghatak, MD
Assistant Professor, College of Physiotherapy, Nopany Institute; Director and Chief Consultant, Medical Rehabilitation Center, TRA General Hospital, Kolkata, India

William Gibbs, MD, DABPMR, DABPM
Director, Department of Rehabilitation Medicine, Queens Hospital Center; Medical Director, Center for Rehabilitation; Owner, William Gibbs, M.D., PLLC, Jamaica, New York

Theresa A. Gillis, MD
Clinical Associate Professor, Department of Rehabilitation Medicine, Jefferson Medical College, Philadelphia, Pennsylvania; Medical Director, Oncology Rehabilitation/Pain Services, Helen F. Graham Cancer Center, Christiana Care Health System, Newark, Delaware

Alessandro Giustini, MD
Professor of Physical and Rehabilitation Medicine, Florence Medical University, Florence, Italy; Professor of Physical and Rehabilitation Medicine, Rome Medical University, Rome, Italy; Scientific Director and Head of Severe Brain Injury Rehabilitation Department, Rehabilitation Center Auxilium Vitae, Volterra, Italy

John Giusto, MD
Plum Spring Clinic, Chapel Hill, North Carolina

Lance L. Goetz, MD
Associate Professor, University of Texas Southwestern; Attending Physician, Spinal Cord Injury Service, VA North Texas Health Care System, Dallas, Texas

Gary Goldberg, BASc, MD
Director, Acquired Brain Injury Rehabilitation Program, Mercy Center for Brain Injury Rehabilitation, Research and Training, Pittsburgh Mercy Health System, Pittsburgh, Pennsylvania

Stephen Goldberg, MD
Professor Emeritus, University of Miami School of Medicine, Miami, Florida. Partner, Medical Rehabilitation Inc.; Director, Acquired Brain Injury Rehabilitation Program/Mercy Center for Brain Injury Rehabilitation, Research and Training, Mercy Hospital of Pittsburgh, Pittsburgh, Pennsylvania

Barry Goldstein, MD, PhD
Professor, Department of Rehabilitation Medicine, University of Washington; Associate Chief Consultant, SCI/D Services (Department of Veterans Affairs); Attending Physician, Department of Rehabilitation Medicine, Harborview Medical Center, Seattle, Washington

Peter H. Gorman, MD, MS
Associate Professor, Department of Neurology and Rehabilitation Medicine, University of Maryland School of Medicine; Director, Spinal Cord Injury Service, Kernan Hospital; Attending Physician, Physical Medicine and Rehabilitation Service, Veterans Affairs Maryland Health Care System, Baltimore, Maryland

Patricia Graham, MD
Staff Physiatrist, University Medical Center of Princeton, Princeton, New Jersey

Christoph Gutenbrunner, MD, PhD
Department of Physical Medicine and Rehabilitation, Hannover Medical University, Hannover, Germany

Rochelle V. Habeck, PhD
Emeritus Professor, Department of Political Science; Office of Rehabilitation and Disability Studies, Michigan State University, East Lansing, Michigan

Harlan Hahn, PhD
Emeritus Professor, Department of Political Science, University of Southern California, Los Angeles, California

Kevin Hakimi, MD
Acting Assistant Professor, Department or Rehabilitation Medicine, University of Washington; Veterans Affairs Puget Sound Health Care System, Seattle, Washington

Eugen M. Halar, MD
Professor Emeritus, Department of Rehabilitation Medicine, University of Washington, Seattle, Washington

Margaret Hammond, MD
Chief Consultant SCI/D Services, Department of Veterans Affairs; Professor, Department of Rehabilitation Medicine, University of Washington School of Medicine; Chief Spinal Cord Injury Unit, VA Puget Sound Health Care System, Seattle, Washington

Robert L. Harmon, MD
Associate Clinical Professor, Departments of Medicine and Neurology, Medical College of Georgia, Augusta, Georgia

Mark Harrast, MD
Assistant Professor, Departments of Rehabilitation Medicine, Orthopaedics, and Sports Medicine, University of Washington, Seattle, Washington

Michael Hatzakis, Jr., MD
Assistant Professor, Department of Rehabilitation Medicine, University of Washington School of Medicine; Veterans Affairs Puget Sound Health Care System, Seattle, Washington

Joseph M. Helms, MD
President, Helms Medical Institute, Berkeley; Adjunct Clinical Professor, Division of Medical Acupuncture, Stanford University School of Medicine, Stanford, California

Rafi J. Heruti, MD
Certified Sexual Therapist, Head of Sexual Rehabilitation Clinic, Reuth Medical Center; Sackler School of Medicine, Tel-Aviv University, Tel-Aviv, Israel

Jeanne E. Hicks, MD
Department of Internal Medicine, George Washington University Medical Center, Department of Orthopedics, Georgetown University Medical Center, Washington, DC; Deputy Chief, Department of Rehabilitation Medicine, National Institutes of Health, Bethesda, Maryland

Steven R. Hinderer, MD, MS, PT
Associate Professor, Department of Physical Medicine and Rehabilitation, Wayne State University School of Medicine; Specialist-in-Chief, Department of Physical Medicine and Rehabilitation, Detroit Medical Center; Medical Director of the Center for Spinal Cord Injury Recovery, Rehabilitation Institute of Michigan, Detroit, Michigan

Howard J. Hoffberg, MD, MS
Associate Medical Director, Rosen-Hoffberg MD, Rehabilitation and Pain Management Associates, P.A., Towson, Maryland

Joseph C. Honet, MD, MS, FACP
Professor, Department of Physical Medicine, Wayne State University School of Medicine; Chief, Physical Medicine and Rehabilitation, Sinai Grace Hospital, Detroit, Michigan

Lawrence J. Horn, MD
Professor and Chairman, Department of Physical Medicine and Rehabilitation, Wayne State University; Director of Neuroscience and Traumatic Brain Injury Medicine, Rehabilitation Institute of Michigan, Detroit, Michigan

Edward A. Hurvitz, MD
Associate Professor, Department of Physical Medicine and Rehabilitation, Pediatric Rehabilitation Medicine, University of Michigan School of Medicine; University of Michigan Health Systems, Ann Arbor, Michigan

Marta Imamura, MD, PhD
Associate Professor of Physical Medicine and Rehabilitation, Division of Physical Medicine, Department of Orthopedics and Traumatology, University of Sao Paulo School of Medicine; Hospital das Clinicas of Brazil, Sao Paulo, Brazil

Tom Jackson, MD
Chief Resident, Department of Physical Medicine and Rehabilitation, Temple University School of Medicine, Philadelphia, Pennsylvania

Jennifer J. James, MD
Clinical Associate Professor, Department of Rehabilitation Medicine, University of Washington; Veterans Affairs Puget Sound Health Care System, Seattle, Washington

Galen O. Joe, MD
Senior Staff Physiatrist and Chief, Rehabilitation Medicine Consultation Service, Department of Rehabilitation Medicine, National Institutes of Health, Bethesda, Maryland

Kurt Johnson, PhD
Professor, Department of Rehabilitation Medicine, University of Washington School of Medicine, Seattle, Washington

Richard T. Katz, MD
Professor of Clinical Neurology, Washington University School of Medicine; Associate Clinical Professor of Internal Medicine and Associate Clinical Professor of Family and Community Medicine, Saint Louis University Medical School, St. Louis, Missouri; Associate Clinical Professor of Physical Medicine and Rehabilitation, University of Kansas Medical School, Kansas City, Kansas

David J. Kennedy, MD
Chief Resident, University Hospital, Department of Rehabilitation Medicine, University of Washington, Seattle, Washington

Ofer Keren, MD
Director, Department of Pediatric Rehabilitation, Alyn Rehabilitation Hospital, Jerusalem, Israel

D. Casey Kerrigan, MD, MS
Professor and Chair, Department of Physical Medicine and Rehabilitation, University of Virginia School of Medicine, Charlottesville, Virginia

Seema Khurana, DO
Assistant Professor, Department of Rehabilitation Medicine, University of Miami School of Medicine, Miami, Florida

Charles Kim, MD, CAc, FAAPMR
Assistant Professor, Departments of Anesthesiology and Rehabilitation Medicine, Mount Sinai School of Medicine, New York, New York

David Kim, MD
Assistant Professor of Medicine, Drexel University College of Medicine, Philadelphia, Pennsylvania; Medical Director, Pain Management Solutions, Inc., Moorestown, New Jersey

Heakyung Kim, MD
Assistant Professor, Physical Medicine and Rehabilitation and Pediatrics, University of Pennsylvania; Medical Director, Pediatric Rehabilitation Medicine, Children's Hospital of Philadelphia, Philadelphia, Pennsylvania

R. Lee Kirby, MD, FRCPC
Professor, Division of Physical Medicine and Rehabilitation, Department of Medicine Dalhouise University Faculty of Medicine, Queen Elizabeth II Health Sciences Centre, Halifax, Nova Scotia, Canada

Stanley H. Kornhauser, PhD
President, National Institute for Electromedical Information; Director of Planning, American Academy of Anti-Aging Medicine; Director of Institutional Advancement, New York College of Podiatric Medicine; Health and Sciences Editor, Queens Times, Queens, New York

Karen J. Kowalske, MD
Professor and Chair, Department of Physical Medicine and Rehabilitation, University of Texas Southwestern Medical Center at Dallas, Dallas, Texas

Ashley E. Kurz, BA
University of Pennsylvania, Philadelphia, Pennsylvania

Jorge Lains, MD
Physiatrist, Consultant; Servico Medicina Fisica Reabilitacao, Hospitais Universidade Coimbra; Medical Director, Clinica Medicina Fisica Reabilitacao, ABPG; President, Portuguese Society PRM; Assistant Secretary, ISPRM; Board of Directors, Mediterranean Forum PRM, Coimbra, Portugal

Mathew Lee, MD, MPH, FACP
Professor and Chairman, Department of Rehabilitation Medicine, New York University School of Medicine; Medical Director, Rusk Institute of Rehabilitation Medicine, New York University Medical Center, New York, New York

Peter Lee, MD
Professor and Chair, Department of Physical Medicine & Rehabilitation, Samsung University Hospital, Seoul, Korea

Yehoshua A. Lehman, MD
Rehabilitation Unit, Geriatric Center of Netanya; State of Israel, Ministry of Health, Netanya, Israel

James W. Leonard, DO, PT
Associate Professor and Chair, Rehabilitation Medicine Division, Department of Orthopedics and Rehabilitation, University of Wisconsin Hospital and Clinics, Madison, Wisconsin

Charles E. Levy, MD
Associate Professor, Department of Orthopaedics and Rehabilitation, University of Florida College of Medicine; Chief, Physical Medicine and Rehabilitation Service, North Florida–South Georgia Veterans Health System, Gainesville, Florida

Karen Y. Lew, PharmD
Clinical Pharmacist, Veterans Affairs Puget Sound Health Care System, Seattle, Washington

Jan Lexell, MD, PhD
Professor and Medical Director, Department of Health Sciences, Luleå University of Technology, Luleå, Sweden; Department of Rehabilitation, Lund University Hospital, Lund, Sweden

Janet C. Limke, MD
Clinical Instructor, Department of Physical Medicine and Rehabilitation, Harvard Medical School; Staff Physiatrist, The Spine Center, New England Baptist Hospital Boston, Massachusetts

Mark A. Lissens, MD, PhD
Professor, Physical Medicine and Rehabilitation, EMG and Clinical Neurophysiology, KHK University College; KU Leuven University Association; Vice President, ISPAPOFF; Board Member, International Society of Physical and Rehabilitation Medicine, Geel, Belgium

James Little, MD, PhD
Professor, Department of Rehabilitation Medicine, University of Washington School of Medicine; Assistant Chief, Spinal Cord Injury Unit, VA Puget Sound Health Care System, Seattle Washington

Ruth Torkelson Lynch, PhD
Professor and Chairperson, Department of Psychology and Special Education, Affiliate Faculty, Department of Rehabilitation Medicine, University of Wisconsin, Madison, Wisconsin

Ian B. Maitin, MD
Associate Professor, Department of Physical Medicine and Rehabilitation, Temple University School of Medicine, Philadelphia, Pennsylvania

German A. Marulanda, MD
Research Fellow, Center for Joint Preservation and Reconstruction, Rubin Institute for Advanced Orthopedics, Sinai Hospital of Baltimore, Baltimore, Maryland

Edward McFarland, MD
Consulting Team Physician, Baltimore Orioles; The Wayne H. Lewis Professor of Orthopedic and Shoulder Surgery; Vice-Chairman, Adult Reconstruction Co-Director, Division of Shoulder Surgery; The Department of Orthopedic Surgery, The Johns Hopkins University, Baltimore Maryland

Thomas McGunigal, MD
Attending Physician, Rehabilitation Hospital of Rhode Island, North Smithfield, Rhode Island

Gregg D. Meekins, MD
Assistant Professor, Department of Neurology, University of Washington School of Medicine, Seattle, Washington

Arun J. Mehta, MB, FRCPC
Associate Clinical Professor, Department of Medicine, University of California—Los Angeles, UCLA School of Medicine, Los Angeles, California

Jeffrey Meyers, MD, LAc
Medical Director, Delaware Curative Physical Therapy and Rehabilitation, Wilmington, Delaware

William F. Micheo-Martínez, MD
Professor and Chairman, Department of Physical Medicine, Rehabilitation, and Sports Medicine, University of Puerto Rico School of Medicine Instituto San Pablo, Bayamòn, Puerto Rico

Marc S. Micozzi, MD, PhD
National Center for Complementary and Alternative Medicine of the National Institutes of Health, Bethesda, Maryland

Michael A. Mont, MD
Director, Center for Joint Preservation and Reconstruction, Rubin Institute for Advanced Orthopedics, Sinai Hospital of Baltimore, Baltimore, Maryland

Stanley J. Myers, MD
A. David Gurewitsch Professor of Clinical Rehabilitation Medicine, Columbia University College of Physicians and Surgeons; New York Presbyterian Hospital; Columbia University Medical Center, New York, New York

Fred Newton, MD, MS
University of Virginia, Department of Physical Medicine and Rehabilitation, University of Virginia School of Medicine, Charlottesville, Virginia

Subhadra Lakshmi Nori, MD
Associate Professor, Clinical Physical Medicine and Rehabilitation; Chief, Department of Physical Medicine & Rehabilitation, Jacobi Medical Center, the Arthur S. Abramson Department of Physical Medicine and Rehabilitation, Bronx, New York

Rory J. O'Connor, MD, MRCP
Senior Lecturer in Rehabilitation Medicine, University of Leeds; Consultant Physician, Leeds Teaching Hospitals NHS Trust, Leeds, United Kingdom

Abna A. Ogle, MD
Clinical Associate Professor, Department of Rehabilitation Medicine, University of Kansas Medical Center; Staff Physician, Research Medical Center; Staff Physician, Baptist Medical Center; Kansas City Veterans Affairs Medical Center, Kansas City, Kansas

Bryan J. O'Young, MD
Medical Director, Department of International Rehabilitation Medicine, Clinical Associate Professor, Department of Rehabilitation Medicine, New York University School of Medicine, Attending Physician, Rusk Institute of Rehabilitation Medicine, New York University Medical Center, New York, New York; Visiting Professor, Department of Rehabilitation Medicine, Peking University School of Medicine, Peking First Hospital, Beijing, China; Visiting Professor, Department of Rehabilitation Medicine, Capital Medical University, Xuan Wu Hospital, Beijing, China; Adjunct Professor, Department of Rehabilitation Medicine, University of the Philippines College of Medicine, Manila, Philippines; Attending Physician, NY Downtown Hospital, New York,New York; Pain Consultant, International Center for the Disabled, New York, New York

Jeffrey B. Palmer, MD
Lawrence Cardinal Shehan Professor and Director, Department of Physical Medicine and Rehabilitation, Professor of Otolaryngology—Head and Neck Surgery and Functional Anatomy and Evolution, Johns Hopkins Hospital, Baltimore, Maryland

Atul T. Patel, MD
Kansas City Bone and Joint Clinic, Overland Park, Missouri

Jaywant J.P. Patil, MBBS, FRCP
Associate Professor (retired), Division of Physical Medicine, Department of Medicine, Dalhousie University Faculty of Medicine; Queen Elizabeth II Health Sciences Center, Halifax, Nova Scotia

Inder Perkash, MD, MS, FRCS, FACS
Professor of Urology and Functional Restoration (PM&R), Departments of Urology and Functional Restoration, Stanford University School of Medicine; Veterans Affairs, Palo Alto Health Care System, Palo Alto, California

Frank S. Pidcock, MD
Associate Professor of Physical Medicine and Rehabilitation and Pediatrics, Johns Hopkins University School of Medicine/Kennedy Krieger Institute, Baltimore, Maryland

James M. Plunkett, MD
Volunteer Assistant Professor, Department of Physical Medicine and Rehabilitation, University of Cincinnati, Cincinnati, Ohio

Russell K. Portenoy, MD
Professor of Neurology and Anesthesiology, The Albert Einstein School of Medicine; Chairman, Department of Pain Medicine and Palliative Care, Beth Israel Medical Center, New York, New York

Joel M. Press, MD
Department of Physical Medicine and Rehabilitation, Northwestern University Medical School; Rehabilitation Institute of Chicago, Chicago, Illinois

Michael M. Priebe, MD
Associate Professor, Department of Orthopedic Surgery and Rehabilitation, Loyola University Medical Center, Maywood, Illinois

Kristjan T. Ragnarsson, MD
Lucy G. Moses Professor and Chairman, Department of Rehabilitation Medicine, Mount Sinai School of Medicine, New York, New York

Mark Randall, PsyD, DrPH, MA
Adjunct Faculty, Indiana University School of Medicine; Community Hospital, Indianapolis, Indiana

Ira G. Rashbaum, MD
Clinical Associate Professor, Department of Rehabilitation Medicine, New York University School of Medicine; Chief, Stroke Rehabilitation, Rusk Institute of Rehabilitation Medicine, New York University Medical Center, New York, New York

Rajiv R. Ratan, MD, PhD
Burke Professor of Neurology, Rehabilitation Medicine, and Neuroscience, Weill Medical College of Cornell University, Ithaca; Executive Director, Burke Medical Research Institute, White Plains, New York

Albert C. Recio, MD, PT
Fellow, Spinal Cord Medicine, University of Washington School of Medicine, Seattle, Washington

John B. Redford, MD
Professor Emeritus, Department of Rehabilitation Medicine, University of Kansas Medical Center, Kansas City, Kansas

Rina Reyes, MD
Assistant Professor, Department of Rehabilitation Medicine, University of Washington School of Medicine; Attending Physician, University Hospital, Seattle, Washington

Mary Richardson, PhD, MHA
Professor Emeritus, Department of Health Services, School of Public Health and Community Medicine, University of Washington, Seattle, Washington

Haim Ring, MD, MSc PM&R
Professor and Chairman, Neurological Rehabilitation Department "C," Loewenstein Rehabilitation Center, Raanana; Sackler Faculty of Medicine, Tel Aviv University, Ramat Aviv; Chairman, National Rehabilitation Council, Ministry of Health, Jerusalem, Israel

Lawrence R. Robinson, MD
Vice Dean for Clinical Affairs, Professor, Department of Rehabilitation Medicine, University of Washington School of Medicine; Attending Physician, University Hospital, Seattle, Washington

Richard C. Robinson, MD
Assistant Professor, Department of Rehabilitation Medicine, University of Kansas Medical Center; Veterans Affairs Eastern Kansas Health Care System, Leavenworth, Kansas

Arthur A. Rodriquez, MD, MS
Associate Professor, Department of Rehabilitation Medicine, University of Washington School of Medicine; Attending Physician, Physical Medicine and Rehabilitation, VA Puget Sound Health Care System, Seattle, Washington

Richard A. Rogachefsky, MD
Good Samaritan Medical Center, West Islip, New York

Robert D. Rondinelli, MD, PhD
Director of Rehabilitation Services, Iowa Methodist Medical Center, Des Moines, Iowa

Barry Rosenblum, DPM
Assistant Clinical Professor of Surgery, Harvard Medical School, Boston, Massachusetts

Elliot J. Roth, MD
Paul B. Manguson Professor and Chair, Department of Physical Medicine and Rehabilitation, Northwestern University Medical School; Donelly Senior Vice President and Medical Director, Rehabilitation Institute of Chicago, Chicago, Illinois

Nathan J. Rudin, MD, MA
Associate Professor, Orthopedics and Rehabilitation, University of Wisconsin School of Medicine and Public Health, Madison, Wisconsin

Abner Salas, DC
Private Practice, Marietta, Georgia

Vivencio Salcedo, MD

Richard Salcido, MD
William Erdman Professor and Chair, Department of Physical Medicine and Rehabilitation; Director of Rehabilitation Services; Associate, Institute for Medical Bioengineering; Senior Fellow, Institute on Aging, University of Pennsylvania School of Medicine, Philadelphia, Pennsylvania

Francisco H. Santiago, MD
Attending Physician, Department of Physical Medicine and Rehabilitation, Bronx-Lebanon Hospital, Bronx, New York

Carson D. Schneck, MD, PhD
Professor of Anatomy and Diagnostic Imaging, Department of Anatomy and Cell Biology, Temple University School of Medicine, Philadelphia, Pennsylvania

Andrew Sears, PhD
Professor and Chair, Information Systems Department, University of Maryland, Baltimore County, Baltimore, Maryland

Thorsten M. Seyler, MD
Clinician Scientist Resident, Department of Orthopaedic Surgery, Wake Forest University, Winston-Salem, North Carolina

Tarek S. Shafshak, MD
Professor, Department of Physical Medicine, Rheumatology, and Rehabilitation, Faculty of Medicine, Alexandria University, Alexandria, Egypt

Jay P. Shah, MD
Senior Staff Physiatrist, Rehabilitation Medicine Department, Clinical Research Center, National Institutes of Health, Bethesda, Maryland

Aaron Shamberg, MLA
President, Landcare, Baltimore, Maryland

Shoshana Shamberg, OTR/L, MS
President and Clinical Director, Abilities O.T. Services, Inc., Baltimore, Maryland

Ki Y. Shin, MD
Associate Professor, Division of Cancer Medicine, Department of Palliative Care and Rehabilitation Medicine, The University of Texas M.D. Anderson Cancer Center, Houston, Texas

David A.N. Siegel, MD
Assistant Professor of Anesthesiology and Rehabilitation Medicine, The Albert Einstein School of Medicine; Director of Pain Medicine, Department of Rehabilitation Medicine, James J. Peters Veterans Affairs Medical Center, Bronx, New York

Kenneth H. Silver, MD
Associate Professor and Vice-Chair, Department of Physical Medicine and Rehabilitation; Medical Director, Rehabilitation Services, Johns Hopkins University at Good Samaritan Hospital, Baltimore, Maryland

Warren Slaten, MD
Staff Physiatrist, Rockland Orthopedics and Sports Medicine, Monsey, New York

Nachum Soroker, MD
Head, Department of Neurological Rehabilitation, Loewenstein Rehabilitation Hospital, Raanana; Sackler Faculty of Medicine, Tel-Aviv University, Tel-Aviv, Israel

Michelle Stern, MD
Assistant Professor of Clinical Rehabilitation Medicine, Columbia University College of Physicians and Surgeons; New York Presbyterian Hospital; Columbia University Medical Center, New York, New York

Ninad D. Sthalekar, MD
Pain Relief Center, Pinellas Park, Florida

Beth A. Stiens, MEd
Instructor, Early Childhood Education, North Seattle Community College, Shoreline, Washington

Steven A. Stiens, MD, MS
Associate Professor; Director of Spinal Cord Medicine Fellowship, Department of Rehabilitation Medicine, University of Washington School of Medicine; Spinal Cord Injury Unit, Veterans Affairs Puget Sound Health Care System, Seattle, Washington

Margaret G. Stineman, MD
Vice Chair and Director of Research, Department of Rehabilitation Medicine, University of Pennsylvania School of Medicine; Hospital of the University of Pennsylvania, Philadelphia, Pennsylvania

Nancy E. Strauss, MD
Associate Clinical Professor of Rehabilitation Medicine, Columbia University College of Physicians and Surgeons; Interim Chair, Vice Chair, and Residency Program Director, Department of Rehabilitation Medicine, New York Presbyterian Hospital—Columbia and Cornell; Associate Professor of Clinical Rehabilitation Medicine, Weill Medical College of Cornell University, New York, New York

Jonathan Strayer, MD
Associate Professor, Department of Physical Medicine and Rehabilitation; Chief, Physical Medicine and Rehabilitation, Cincinnati VA Medical Center, Cincinnati, Ohio

Gregory Strock, MD
Assistant Professor, Department of Physical Medicine and Rehabilitation, Indiana University School of Medicine, Indianapolis, Indiana

Gerold Stucki, MD, MS
Professor and Chair, Department of Physical Medicine and Rehabilitation, University Hospital Munich, Munich, Germany

Jelena N. Svircev, MD
Assistant Professor, Department of Rehabilitation Medicine, University of Washington School of Medicine; Attending Physician, Spinal Cord Injury Unit, VA Puget Sound Health Care System, Seattle, Washington

Atsushi Tasaki, MD
Research Fellow, Division of Sports Medicine and Shoulder Surgery, Department of Orthopaedic Surgery, Johns Hopkins University, Baltimore, Maryland

Mitch Tepper, PhD
Founder and President, The Sexual Health Network, Inc.; Assistant Director of the Center of Excellence for Sexual Health, Morehouse School of Medicine; National Center for Primary Care, Atlanta, Georgia

Donna C. Tippett, MPH, MA, CCC-SLP
Assistant Professor, Department of Otolaryngology—Head and Neck Surgery, Baltimore, Maryland

Melissa K. Trovato, MD
Assistant Professor, Department of Physical Medicine and Rehabilitation, Johns Hopkins University School of Medicine/Kennedy Krieger Institute, Baltimore, Maryland

Rhodora C. Tumanon, MD
Medical Director, Maryland Rehabilitation Center; Medical Advisor, Division of Rehabilitation Services, State of Maryland, Baltimore, Maryland

Gerard P. Varlotta, DO
Clinical Associate Professor, Department of Rehabilitation Medicine, New York University School of Medicine; Director of Sports Rehabilitation, Rusk Institute of Rehabilitation Medicine, New York University Medical Center, New York, New York

Richard Verville, JD
Power, Piles, Sutter, and Verville, Washington, DC

Stanley F. Wainapel, MD, MPH
Professor of Clinical Rehabilitation Medicine, Albert Einstein College of Medicine; Clinical Director, Rehabilitation Medicine, Montefiore Medical Center, Bronx, New York

Mao Bin Wang, MD
Professor and Chairman, Xuan Wu Hospital, Department of Rehabilitation Medicine, Capital Medical University; Chairman, Physiatrist Branch of Chinese Medical Doctor Association; Vice-Chairman, Chinese Association of Rehabilitation Medicine, Beijing, China

Ninghua Wang, MD, PhD
Associate Professor and Chair, Department of Physical and Rehabilitation Medicine, First Hospital, Peking University, Beijing, China

Ruth K. Westheimer, EdD
Professor, Department of Continuing Education, New York University, New York, New York

Olajide Williams, MD
Department of Neurology, Columbia University School of Medicine, New York, New York

Stuart Willick, MD
Associate Professor, Division of PM&R, Department of Orthopedics; Attending Physician, Orthopedic Center, Salt Lake City, Utah

Sam Wu, MD, MPH, MBA
Medical Director, Margaret Bogart Chair of Physical Medicine and Rehabilitation;, Assistant Clinical Professor, Columbia College of Physicians and Surgeons; Adjunct Clinical Assistant Professor, New York University School of Medicine, New York, New York; Visiting Assistant Professor, Albert Einstein College of Medicine of Yeshiva University, Bronx, New York

Eva Young, MD
Orthopedic Physician Associates, Seattle, Washington

Mark A. Young, MD, MBA, FACP
Chair, Department of Physical Medicine & Rehabilitation, The Maryland Rehabilitation Center/
The Workforce & Technology Center; State of Maryland, Division of Rehabilitation, Department
of Education; Adjunct Clinical Associate Professor, Department of Rehabilitation Medicine, New
York University; School of Medicine, New York, New York; University of Maryland School of
Medicine, Baltimore, Maryland; Professor, Department of Orthopedic Sciences, New York
College of Podiatric Medicine, New York, New York; Chair, ISPRM Faculty-Student Exchange
Committee, The International Society of Physical & Rehabilitation Medicine

Marlene M. Young, MA
Maryland Rehabilitation Center, Baltimore, Maryland

Gabi Zeilig, MD
Head, Department of Neurological Rehabilitation, Chaim Sheba Medical Center, Tel Hashomer;
Sackler Faculty of Medicine, Tel-Aviv University, Tel-Aviv, Israel

INTRODUCTION: METHODS AND MODELS FOR MASTERING PM&R

Steven A. Stiens, MD, MS, Bryan J. O'Young, MD, Mark A. Young, MD, MBA

"A physician is obligated to consider more than a diseased organ, more even than the whole person; the physician must view patients in their world."

–Harvey Cushing (1869–1939)

1. What is the Socratic method of learning and how does it relate to the study of physical medicine and rehabilitation?

Socrates, a famous Greek philosopher and moralist, once said: "I cannot teach anybody anything; I can only make a person think." Socrates deeply believed in the importance of didactic techniques that stimulate knowledge and learning through the artful use of tantalizing and thought-provoking questions.

By emphasizing "knowing and problem formulation" rather than blind memorization of raw knowledge, Socrates' legendary teaching style encourages dynamic, reason-based learning and has truly proven to be a time-honored tradition of medical education.

To this day, Socrates unique didactic style continues to play an essential role in contemporary PM&R education. Confronted with bedside clinical challenges and problems, the attending physician often poses questions to rounding PM&R physicians, which triggers an engaging and lively debate and dialogue. These discussions between the mentor and the protégé "bring the learner from a state of complacent dogmatic slumber of an unexamined opinion to a state of humility and perplexity." "It is this process of debunking pretensions that utilizes ignorance as a pedagogically useful device." (In plain English, we can learn a lot from what we don't know!)

Pekarsky D: Socratic teaching: A critical assessment. J Moral Educ 23:119–134, 1994.
Sherman RS: Is it possible to teach socratically? Thinking 6:28–36, 1986.

2. What is pimping? Is it legal?

Pimping is the ancient academic game played by a "teacher" who riddles the trainee with a series of difficult and obscure questions. Sir William Osler was reported to fire such questions at residents like a Gatling gun on the wards of Johns Hopkins Hospital at the turn of the century. The tradition is celebrated to this day and staged in clinics, on wards, and in treatment rooms worldwide. Wide-eyed novice clinicians are asked to recite the intricate details of history, physical findings, impairments, limitations to activity, barriers to participation, environmental characteristics, and a patient's life goals while under the scrutiny of the teacher. Besides the obvious mundane questions posed, such as a recitation of "Mr. Smith's" electrolytes or the results of his manual muscle test, PM&R trainees may also be queried about a variety of obscure factoids, including the number of steps into the patient's home, door widths to the bathroom, the height of carpet pile, and the personality of the patient's spouse. When pimping is performed by an attending physician on rounds, the event can be nerve-wracking and sometimes gut wrenching, yet educationally lively and humorous if orchestrated sensitively, nonhumiliatingly, and received without pretension. Often, the examined house staff or student emerges from the experience with a supreme feeling of deliverance and educational accomplishment. Pimping's purpose is not to reveal knowledge deficits but to promote the acquisition of knowledge and "thinking on your feet" wisdom.

A word of caution (black box warning): Pimping when performed chronically and in a disparaging way can induce sleep disturbance, anxiety, and decreased productivity.

Brancati FL: The art of pimping. JAMA 262:89–90, 1989.

3. **How can the reader interactively learn from this book?**
   One meaningful way for the readers to benefit from this text is to read the questions, close the book, take a deep breath and attempt to answer the questions independently **before** proceeding to look at the printed answers. ("Peeking" is ill advised.)

4. **What are the levels of learning required to maximize one's ability to practice physical medicine and rehabilitation?**
   The **levels of learning** include: knowledge, understanding, application, analysis, synthesis, and evaluation.
      Knowledge refers to basic definitions including anatomy and function.
      Understanding requires the appreciation of the impact of diseases and treatments that in turn allows the prediction of targeted outcomes.
      Application refers to the clinician's capability to prescribe therapeutic intervention to achieve a successful clinical outcome.
      Analysis is the ability to choose proper assessment methods and recognize proper patterns and trends embedded in the assessment results.
      Synthesis is the process of collecting and addressing all aspects of the treatment plan to achieve the optimal outcome for an individual in his/her unique setting.
      Evaluation is the ability to relate a patient's outcome to the literature.

5. **How can the questions and answers in a little paperback develop and expand a clinician's ability to transform patients' lives?**
   The questions and answers in PM&R Secrets enable the reader by presenting challenges that require a variety of clinical skills to achieve solutions.
      In each chapter, questions are arranged to represent a hierarchy of clinical complexity, starting from basic facts to advanced clinical conditions, with the aim of developing the learner's proficiency in clinical situations. The first few questions in each chapter present fundamental *knowledge*.
      Later in the chapter, the learners' *understanding* can be assessed by using a case presentation requiring the reader to respond with diagnoses, clinical treatments, or predicted outcomes. For example, the manual muscle testing findings from a case might be presented in a question that not only requires the reader to determine the appropriate spinal cord injury (SCI) level but also requires predictions of medical complications and functional outcomes such as transfer, wheelchair propulsion, and self care.
      Knowledge and comprehension of mechanisms further enable the learner to formulate hypothetical *applications* in response to clinical scenarios presented in the questions. For example, a question may provide a description of the patients' gait and may require the learner to provide an essential differential diagnosis and a proper prescription for an appropriate brace.
      To make a proper diagnosis and follow clinical progress, *analysis* is necessary to recognize patterns from the assessment methods. References and websites cited in the chapters guide the clinicians to appropriate sources to use in the scholarly exercise of *synthesis*. The learners' *evaluation* of all of this occurs in conversations with fellow clinicians and mentors. In this way, diagnostic and treatment options can be prepared, and research can be proposed. Clinicians and academic scholars can all benefit from this text by using it for discussions and presentations and as a springboard for topic review. *PM&R Secrets* is known as a bridge text because it links levels of learning with many dynamic resources beyond the confines of these pages.

6. **What is context and how does the application of this word lead to better learning?**
   Context refers to the environment surrounding a patient and the circumstances surrounding a patient in his/her environment.
      Learning in context is the method our authors use to embed the reader in actual clinical situations, and in the process, the reader is required to assess and respond. Many of the

questions in this book are clinical simulations. These questions are designed to evoke essential facts, formulate definitions, construct clinically pertinent taxonomies, and synthesize disparate information to allow the reader to make proper diagnoses and sound interdisciplinary solutions. To get the best learning experience, the reader should imagine a clinical situation for each question and envision the steps necessary to obtain further history and examination, make functional assessments, seek interdisciplinary consultations, and provide new interventions.

7. **What is connectile dysfunction, and how does it relate to good rehabilitation learning?**
   Connectile dysfunction is not a sexual impairment. Arguably, it is a recently described form of rehabilitation education learning disability (hopefully temporary) that arises when the physiatry trainee becomes disconnected with the material and encounters feelings of insecurity and isolation. The clinician may become so focused on insignificant parts of the case that proper analysis and synthesis is lost. Successful learning most optimally occurs when pupils are aroused by the material and are stimulated to seek new learning repertoires. Ideally, the successful learner becomes connected to the material by getting unique and pertinent history, discovering key findings on examination, and leading to life changing treatments. Designing a treatment plan that integrates patient-centered goals and interdisciplinary perspectives will set the patient and family up for delightful accomplishments. This provides a sense of deep gratification for all!

8. **How does the clinician organize patient information in the best way to plan interventions and guide learning?**
   The practice of rehabilitation is an extension beyond the medical model to interdisciplinary achievement of person-centered enablement. Rehabilitation practice requires simultaneous recognition of injury and pathology along with assessment of the patient's unique assets that will compensate for disablement. The application of the Biopsychosocial Model, which addresses not only the cause but also the secondary effects of injury and illness, and the World Health Organization Model of Disablement, which addresses impairment, activity limitation, and barriers to participation, is essential in formulating a comprehensive plan.

   A patient's overall clinical and functional condition can best be understood with a microscopic to macroscopic perspective like biopsychosocial levels as outlined in the Hierarchy of Natural Systems. These Natural System levels ascend through atoms, molecules, organelles, cells, tissues, organ systems, nervous systems, one-person, two-person, family, community, culture–subculture, society, nation, and biosphere systems. A detailed assessment of patient function at each system level and a comprehensive evaluation of all the system levels provide the best foundation for each intervention. Measurable outcome parameters provide a practical method of quantification to assess the effectiveness of the intervention.

   Learning through the practice of rehabilitation requires an ongoing commitment to understanding each patient's personal goals and tailoring interventions to achieve these goals. Rehabilitation is therefore learned one patient at a time as unique combinations of interventions are orchestrated to produce unique solutions for each individual. Thus, the practitioner becomes increasingly astute with each encounter and refines his/her ability to enable each patient. Patients are teachers. Each success is a lesson to guide future practice.

   Cohen J, Krackov SK, Black ER, Holyst M: Introduction to human health and illness: A series of patient-centered conferences based on the Biopsychosocial Model. Acad Med 75:390–396, 2000.

9. **What is a rehabilitation problem list, and how is it best used?**
   The **rehabilitation problem list** is a sequence of diagnoses, impairments, activity limitations, and participation barriers that guide goal setting. It is organized as a spectrum starting from active injuries and diagnoses through the domains of disablement, which are organized to include all specific diagnoses listed first. Thereafter, all significant impairments are listed in groups by organ

or systems (e.g., neurogenic bowel, neurogenic bladder). These are followed by activity limitations (e.g., mobility, activities of daily living). Finally, barriers to participation categories are listed: psychological adaptation, social role function, architectural adaptations, community reintegration, education/vocational development, and spirituality, as is most applicable to the case. Each problem list is unique to the patient and will evolve as progress is made.

A useful approach to a patient's problem list is to visualize the patient in his/her surroundings and to anticipate his or her outcome for each intervention. Individual problems, if specifically defined, are useful topics for focused research and study. When a clinician identifies a problem and discovers a solution, the skills for recognition of the diagnosis and implementation of a treatment plan are more easily remembered.

10. **What is a "model," and how can it help PM&R clinicians better understand the relationship(s) between patient care methods and outcome goals?**
A **model,** in engineering lingo, is defined as a theoretical account or framework consisting of a lattice of accepted definitions and theorem for the mechanism of a system's process. By examining models, we can learn much about rehabilitation. Since models present pictures of essential components and how they work together in a coordinated and synergistic fashion, various complex rehabilitation subjects can be more easily understood. For example, the rehabilitation team might be represented as a model along with its constituent components, including the various team members (physical therapist [PT], occupational therapist [OT], nurse, speech language pathologist [SLP]), the sum total of which "make things tick." A **definition** is a term to describe the individual parts, or components, of a system. A **theoretical account** is a document or diagram that shows how parts interact with one another. The **mechanism** is the parts of a system working together. Using models as guides for learning, the rehabilitation student and teacher can rapidly share the understanding of the complex relationships between the parts of systems.

11. **How can learning models and models of the patient care process provide structure to help navigate the context of patient problems and PM&R practice?**
There is a variety of learning process models that are key to successful PM&R education. Three will be discussed here:
   1. Situated Learning
   2. Experiential Learning
   3. Model Centered Instruction

Situated Learning, also known as contextual learning, is a model learning process that includes the student within or directly in contact with the actual system under study (e.g., an OT who spends time in the greenhouse learning about horticultural therapy or a student clinician in the ADL suite on the rehabilitation unit not only observing, but also immersing himself in the unique situation of the patient, such as mimicking a hemiplegic stroke patient who is doing laundry utilizing a one-handed technique [contextual learning]). The student observes the parts the system as they actually interact within the environment. During residency training in PM&R, at least one of the authors participated in a situated learning, gait analysis workshop. Residents were all assigned a particular pathological gait pattern and asked to simulate it. Often, the benefit of situated learning strategies for physiatrists is that it bolsters compassion and empathy and strengthens the interdisciplinary team's treatment plan development and delivery. This form of contextual study is valuable and unduplicated in any formal lecture or classroom setting.

Situated learning is a potent model of learning that allows "cognitive apprenticeships" in which the learner directly experiences patients' challenges, mentor clinicians at work, and the development of his/her own clinical skills through supervised practice. Examples of situated learning are as varied as places and people.

What are some examples of how a rehabilitation educator can promote situated learning, and what impact can this have on education?

- Rehabilitation teachers might require medical student and resident participation in house calls to patients with tetraplegia, since this real life didactic experience inculcates the student with knowledge about living with SCI in the context of a patient's own home.
- Situating a resident "on the field" as a team physician during the musculoskeletal rotation provides the resident with a "front row seat" to observe mechanisms of injury, impairments in strength and coordination, and the effectiveness of patients' performance after rehabilitation.
- Assigning a physical therapy student the role of "advisor" as staff on an adapted camping trip for patients with various disabilities demonstrates the challenges patients with different impairments have with activity in the natural environment and allows for discovery of adaptive solutions as the student works with the recreation therapist directing the expedition. Plainly put, the spirit and essence of situated learning is best summarized by a revered attending physician's proud proclamation, "Your patients are your best textbook."

Experiential Learning, described by Carl Rogers, is a model of learning that views the student as a self-directed learner who decides what skills need to be mastered and self-initiates his/her own education by seeking the most relevant subject matter. The roles of the teacher are to establish a positive learning climate, clarify the educational goals, organize and display educational resources, balance intellectual and emotional components, and share thoughts with the learner without dominating. To facilitate the search process for a subject matter, *PM&R* Secrets' table of contents is organized with related topics grouped together and provides an index for terms that may be addressed from varied perspectives in multiple chapters. Many references and websites complement the text as bridges to further student-directed learning.

Model-Centered Instruction promotes learning by teaching the student examples of models of patient care and rehabilitation and preparing them for clinical work by building their skills in observation and cause-and-effect prediction. Learning the models first gives them a working framework and teaches them how the system is expected to work before they start seeing patients or seeking out resources. Model-centered instruction can be used by students and educators to initiate the process of in-context learning. For example, detailed model-centered instruction in person-centered care, the Biopsychosocial Model, the Disablement Model, and interdisciplinary team processes provide a structure for students to use as they start a rotation on an inpatient rehabilitation unit or continuity clinic.

Models of patient care and rehabilitation therefore provide a structure to develop an understanding of patient care and rehabilitation processes. Model-centered instruction also includes the advanced technique of **Design Layering**, which teaches the student to refer to particular models to aid his/her understanding of the different layers or parts of medical care and rehabilitation of patients. Design layering allows a student to construct his/her own framework by linking together models for exploration of the effect of interventions in all processes in patient care. Students apply the test models they have learned. They leave the rotation having constructed their own models of the treatment process and their roles!

Gibbons AS: Model-Centered Instruction. Journal of Structural Learning and Intelligent Systems 14:511–540, 2001.

Rogers CR, Frieberg HJ: Freedom to Learn, 3rd ed. Columbus, OH, Merrill/Macmillan, 1994.

www.infed.org/biblio/b-learn.htm

12. **What are the major categories of resources that can enhance the reader's learning experience with PM&R Secrets?**
  - Access to the internet
  - The Academy of Physical Medicine and Rehabilitation Study Guide
  - General textbooks of PM&R
  - PM&R Clinics of North America
  - Atlas of Orthotics and Prosthetics

> "Knowing is not enough; we must apply. Willing is not enough; we must do."
>
> Johann Wolfgang von Goethe (1749–1842)

www.aapmr.org/education/studygd.htm

Albanese MA, Mitchell S: Problem-based learning: A review of literature on its outcomes and implementation issues. Acad Med 68:52–81, 1993.

Engel GL: The clinical application of the biopsychosocial model. Am J Psych 137:535–544, 1980.

TOP 100 SECRETS

These secrets are 100 of the top board alerts. They summarize the concepts, principles, and most salient details of physical medicine and rehabilitation.

1. Known in many countries as physical and rehabilitation medicine (P&RM), physiatry is a medical specialty that assesses patients' functional capabilities, evokes patients' life goals, designs interdisciplinary treatment plans, and coordinates rehabilitation interventions to maximize outcomes.

2. Eccentric or lengthening contraction occurs when muscle force is less than the load. This normally occurs when gravity is the prime mover. To control the effect of gravity, eccentric contraction occurs in muscle(s) that oppose(s) the direction that gravity tends to move the joint.

3. The gastrocnemius and soleus are the most active muscles in the lower limb during standing to resist the line of gravity's tendency to extend the knee and dorsiflex the ankle.

4. If the patient has a neurologic deficit on one side of the face and a deficit involving the extremities on the other side, this suggests a brain stem lesion. An exception is loss of vision in one eye and paralysis and/or sensory loss in the opposite extremities. This suggests a lesion of the internal carotid artery affecting its ophthalmic artery branch.

5. Patients with neurogenic claudication feel better when walking uphill (spinal flexion).

6. All voluntary movement is produced through controlled activation of motor units achieved through an interaction of descending suprasegmental inputs and segmental circuitry impinging upon motor neuron pools in the anterior horn of the spinal segment. The motor neuron and associated motor unit is the "final common pathway" for all voluntary movement.

7. After a burn injury, heterotopic ossification most commonly occurs at the elbow, followed by the shoulder (in adults) or the hip (in children).

8. One does not need to be totally blind to benefit from vision rehabilitation services. Ensure that patients are referred for early evaluation.

9. Screening for hearing loss is important in the elderly (in whom it can mimic dementia) and in infants (in whom diagnosis and treatment are critical).

10. Rehabilitative history-taking that includes review of sexuality and relationships not only identifies patient- and couple-centered goals but also recognizes patients as whole persons and facilitates positive self-perceptions and aspirations with therapeutic expectations.

11. In order to recognize the geriatric patient's wants, needs, and goals, talk directly to the individual, not only to or through the patient's caregiver. Adequate pain control is mandatory in order to maximize functional abilities.

12. Four sectors of the environment surround patients—immediate (clothes, braces, mobility equipment), intermediate (personal home, office, motor vehicle), community (neighborhood,

public spaces), and natural (minimally modified land, waterways, sky). All can be modified to enhance patient activity and participation.

13. The main cause of hypoxia in patients with restrictive lung disorder is **airway mucus plugging,** rather than **lung infection**. A cardinal rule in managing restrictive lung disorder is to always attempt to normalize the oxyhemoglobin saturation by providing adequate ventilation and assisted coughing before considering intubation.

14. A physiatric consultation recognizes patient life roles, identifies unique aspects of disablement, formulates a patient-centered goal-driven treatment plan, and orchestrates interdisciplinary interventions that can enable patient life aspirations.

15. The physiatric examination confirms the diagnosis, quantifies impairment, reveals capabilities for adaptive function, screens for complications, and provides a baseline for reassessment.

16. Human gait analysis can be practiced daily by observing people walking at different speeds, on varied surfaces, and while carrying loads in common places such as the workplace, malls, and airports.

17. Rehabilitation is the process of development of a person to his or her fullest physical, psychological, social, educational, and vocational potential by eliminating or compensating for any biochemical pathophysiology, anatomic impairment, activity limitation, or environmental barrier.

18. During electrodiagnostic studies, skin temperature should be maintained above 33°C in upper extremities and 30°C in lower extremities to avoid temperature-related artifactual changes in findings.

19. Somatosensory evoked potentials (SSEPs) and motor evoked potentials (MEPs) are viewed as sensory and motor continuity checks, respectively, of peripheral nervous system (PNS) and central nervous system (CNS) pathways. SSEPs can be viewed as a central extension of the sensory nerve conduction study, whereas MEPs can be viewed as a central extension of the motor nerve conduction study.

20. Radiculopathies can cause radiating pain, numbness, tingling, hyporeflexia, and/or weakness. The outcomes are overwhelmingly favorable for persons with cervical and lumbosacral radiculopathies. In general, rapid return to normal activities as symptoms permit is encouraged.

21. Polyneuropathies can be classified based on the primary pathologic process as axon loss, demyelinating, or combined and based on the fibers involved as motor, sensory, or combined.

22. Axonal neuropathies affect the distal territories of the longest nerves and therefore affect the feet first. Proximal nerve conduction is faster secondary to increased warmth, thicker myelination, and greater distance between the nodes of Ranvier.

23. Myasthenia gravis is postsynaptic due to antibodies against the ACh receptors and its associated functional proteins.

24. Lambert-Eaton myasthenia syndrome (LEMS) is due to presynaptic abnormality at the neuromuscular junction and is associated with bronchial carcinoma.

25. People with disabilities can return to work with vocational rehabilitation interventions focused on the person (e.g., transferable skills to a new job, retraining) and/or the environment (e.g., workplace modifications, assistive technology).

26. The Henneman size principle states that motor units are recruited from smaller motor units to progressively larger motor units, allowing for initial fine motor control and progressive gross muscle strength.

27. Malnutrition is caused by a lack of calories, protein, essential fats, or micronutrients. Surveillance for deficiencies through early dietary and nutritional consultation helps to maximize outcomes.

28. Targeting medications at risk factors for disease, pathophysiology, impairments, activity limitations, and barriers to participation will contribute to life's longevity and allow progress on person-centered goals.

29. During periods of complete inactivity, the rate of muscle strength decline is 1–3% per day, and 10–15% per week, until it plateaus at approximately 25–40% of the baseline strength.

30. Cryotherapy may produce longer-lasting effects than heat.

31. Classical massage involves stroking and gliding movements (effleurage), kneading (pétrissage), and percussion (tapotement). When prescribing traction, manipulation, and massage, clinicians must be cautiously aware of contraindications, including vertebral malignancy, active inflammatory arthropathy, ligamentous instability, tumor or metastasis, active spinal infection or osteomyelitis, acute fracture or dislocation, severe osteoporosis, acute myelopathy, and cauda equina syndrome.

32. Manual therapies include osteopathic manipulation, massage therapy, and chiropractic manipulation. Referral for manipulation is common when there is restricted quality of range of motion or limitation of motion because of pain.

33. Electrotherapy, also called electrotherapeutics, uses currents directed through the body to reduce symptoms, stimulate healing, and improve function. Muscles treated with functional electrical stimulation will increase in size, strength, and endurance, with a change of some type II glycolytic fibers to type I oxidative fibers.

34. Heel pain in the absence of tenderness of the Achilles enthesis may represent an injectable pain emanating from the retrocalcaneal bursa. The etiology of plantar foot pain may be associated with contracture of the Achilles that can be diagnosed by dorsiflexion of the ankle in a subtalar neutral position.

35. In an extraforaminal (far lateral) lumbar disc herniation, the superior spinal nerve will be affected (e.g., extraforaminal herniation of L4-L5 disc will affect the L4 spinal nerve). In a central lumbar disc herniation, the inferior spinal nerve root will be affected (e.g., central herniation of L4-L5 disc will affect the L5 spinal nerve).

36. All facet joints are innervated by two nerve branches from the posterior ramus above and at the same segmental level. The L4 medial branch and the L5 dorsal ramus innervate the L5-S1 facet joint.

37. Controlled trials have supported acupuncture to be useful in treating osteoarthritis, lower back pain, headache, extremity pain, post-operative pain, respiratory and urologic problems, and substance abuse.

38. Dysvascular diseases (peripheral vascular disease and diabetes mellitus) are the most common causes of amputation in the United States and have increased by 27% over the past 30 years, whereas other causes of amputation have decreased or remained stable.

39. Determining amputation level is best done in a multidisciplinary setting that takes into account the ability for the surgical wound to heal, functional goals, and patient preference.

40. Upper extremity orthotics can be used to reduce inflammation, promote healing, correct deformity, prevent contractures, substitute for function, and enhance exercise.

41. Early rehabilitation management after upper limb amputation improves acceptance of prosthetic use. Quality of training determines how well individuals use the prosthesis for the rest of their lives.

42. The effectiveness of lower limb orthoses is optimized under the following conditions: (1) use of stable, firm-soled footwear, (2) application of ankle joints (customized to the patient), (3) attention to knee stability, and (4) consideration of adjunctive functional electrical stimulation.

43. Patients with long unilateral or bilateral transtibial amputations caused by trauma consume less energy and walk faster than those with unilateral transfemoral amputation, regardless of etiology.

44. Even with optimal fit, the halo allows intersegmental cervical movement, particularly in the lower segments of the neck. This is the "snaking phenomenon" described in radiographs.

45. All orthoses utilize a three-point pressure system. The more contact the brace has with the wearer, the greater the pressure distribution, comfort, and compliance.

46. Although the wheelchair is arguably the most important therapeutic tool in rehabilitation, acute and chronic wheelchair-related injuries are common, and many wheelchair users do not achieve as much community mobility as they could. Proper wheelchair prescription, setup, and training have the potential to enhance wheelchair use and to prevent overuse injury.

47. Pain generators in the cervical spine include muscle, ligaments, joints, the annulus fibrosis, and nerve roots.

48. Acute low back pain (LBP) is usually a self-limited disorder treated expectantly with reassurance and minor medication. Imaging in LBP has not been shown to correlate with symptoms and can be more misleading than helpful. Chronic disabling LBP is a completely different disorder that requires consideration of and addressing of nonorganic issues.

49. LBP is a nonsurgical disorder; therefore, patients with LBP should be assessed first by musculoskeletal experts who are nonsurgeons. There is *no* definite evidence for effectiveness of surgical fusion as a treatment for LBP.

50. Posture, force, repetitions, and endurance are key components when defining restrictions for a patient.

51. Rehabilitating the shoulder cannot be performed in isolation. In terms of the musculoskeletal system, the body can be thought of as a kinetic chain of multiple joints linked together by muscles, ligaments, and bones; thus, all parts of the chain should be examined to determine faulty mechanics, away from the site of tissue injury, that are contributing to persistent pain and/or dysfunction.

52. The first step in treating shoulder pain and dysfunction is understanding the role of the scapula as the platform of support for shoulder girdle function. Thus, neuromuscular retraining and

strengthening of the scapular stabilizers (to improve scapular mechanics and positioning) are early goals in rehabilitation of shoulder injuries.

53. Forearm fractures account for 40–50% of all childhood fractures, and elbow fractures account for 10% of all fractures in children. These are the most common childhood fractures.

54. Hand numbness and/or pain that worsens at night is/are most likely carpal tunnel syndrome. A flexed finger that hesitates to open and opens eventually with a snap is most likely a trigger finger.

55. Hip fracture patients with an inability to transfer or ambulate, incontinence, dementia, fewer hours of physical therapy, and lack of family involvement may require institutionalization. Maintain total hip precautions for 10–12 weeks.

56. Hydrotherapy provides the appropriate environments for patients with osteoarthritis to exercise at intensities that improve strength and mobility.

57. Potential surgical indications for a meniscal tear include persistent locking of the knee, restricted knee motion despite physical therapy, instability, which may predispose to further intra-articular damage, persistent Baker's cyst, resulting from a meniscal tear, and persistent pain despite physical therapy.

58. Osgood-Schlatter disease is probably the most frequent cause of knee pain in children, and it is most often characterized by activity-related pain that occurs at the proximal tibial tubercle.

59. The anterior talofibular ligament is the most commonly injured ligament in an ankle sprain.

60. In the elderly, the problems of osteoporosis, falls, and fractures are found to coexist, and these factors should be considered together in the total management of the patient.

61. Strain affects the musculotendinous region, and sprain affects the ligaments.

62. To treat soft tissue injuries effectively, the clinician must do a comprehensive musculoskeletal and neurologic evaluation, looking for abnormalities of posture, flexibility, strength, endurance, and proprioception, as well as determining what perpetuating factors (e.g., overload, psychosocial) may contribute to the patient's presentation.

63. Important components that need to be incorporated in an exercise program for an ambulatory patient with Duchenne muscular dystrophy include daily stretches to the Achilles tendons, hamstrings, hip flexors, and iliotibial bands. Eccentric activities such as running downhill and excessive downstairs negotiation are to be avoided.

64. Although recovery of function from CNS injury is generally greatest in the weeks and months following the event, significant recovery is still possible in the post-acute and chronic stages, as demonstrated by constraint-induced movement therapy (CIMT) and other emerging therapies.

65. Disablement is a summary term for collective consequences of disease for a person. Consequences are considered with three interrelated domains: (1) the organ or system, (2) the whole person, and (3) society. In the International Classification of Disability Functioning and Health terminology, limitations or barriers within these domains are named **impairments** (organ domain), **activity limitations** (person domain), and **barriers to participation** (societal domain).
   - **Impairment** is any loss or abnormality of anatomic structure or physiologic or psychological function of an organ or system.

- **Activity limitation** is any deficit in a person's ability to complete a task that would otherwise be within the range considered normal for a person of a particular age.
- **Participation** refers to all the areas of life in which an individual is involved or has access to— societal opportunities in the process of meeting goals.

66. Head injury typically results in a variety of focal as well as diffuse brain damage requiring global assessment, synergistic effects of multiple therapies, and community reintegration with optimal application of the patient's capabilities. Rehabilitation focuses on assessment of baseline, behavioral management, detailed promotion of neuroplastic recovery, reestablishment of maximal independence, and return to societal roles.

67. If a patient with intracerebral hemorrhage, subarachnoid hemorrhage, or placement of a ventriculoperitoneal shunt fails to make significant gains during rehabilitation, obtain a head CT to assess for hydrocephalus.

68. The greatest sustained success in rehabilitation of the person with spinal cord injury comes through education and compliance with self-care, demonstration of ability to meet life goals, adapting skills in development of mutually positive relationships, and reestablishment of a meaningful contribution to community.

69. A guiding principle is to start L-dopa treatment in Parkinson's patients when symptoms interfere with the performance of activities of daily living (ADLs). A resting tremor alone does not usually impede function.

70. All patients with symptoms attributable to multiple sclerosis should be assessed by a multidisciplinary rehabilitation team with specific attention to problems associated with fatigue, bladder dysfunction, pain, spasticity, and cognition.

71. Classic features of motor neuron diseases most commonly include atrophy, weakness, spasticity, and fasciculations. Motor neuron diseases do not affect sensation.

72. Bone density is built throughout childhood and early adulthood and is largely dependent on sufficient calcium intake. Proper nutrition can forestall the effects of age-related bone loss and reduce the risks of fracture.

73. Functional assessment and interventions are critical to optimal treatment of osteoporosis and its comorbidities (e.g., falls, fractures). Considerations should include exercise, gait training, mobility devices, body mechanics, devices for activities of daily living, home and work modification, pharmacologic and nonpharmacologic approaches to pain, minimizing medications that cause dizziness or cloud consciousness, assessment and treatment of mood disorders, and nutrition.

74. The minimum requirement for maintaining the optimal level of functioning and fitness includes 30 minutes per day of moderate to vigorous physical activity in increments of at least 10 minutes at a time 5 or more days per week.

75. Pressure ulcers are not skin problems. They are soft-tissue problems and are usually much more than "skin-deep." If a pressure ulcer fails to show evidence of healing in a reasonable time period, the problem usually is not the dressing but rather an untreated underlying factor, such as malnutrition, infection, or poor vascular supply.

76. Categories of neurogenic bladder dysfunction are anatomically defined by nervous system lesions and include cranial (uninhibited), supraconal (hyperreflexic), conal (mixed contractile, hypocontractile), and infraconal (hypocontractile) bladder.

77. During attempted voiding, there are three distinct areas of focus: (1) detrusor activity, classified as normal, underactive, or acontractile; (2) sphincter activity, classified as normal, detrusor sphincter dyssynergia, or nonrelaxing sphincter; and (3) sensation, classified as normal, overactive/increased, underactive/reduced, absent, or nonspecific.

78. A bowel program is a treatment plan designed to minimize or eliminate the occurrence of unplanned or difficult evacuations, to evacuate stool at a regular, predictable time, and to prevent complications.

79. Bowel care is the process of assisted defecation, which includes one or more of the following components: triggering agent (digital rectal stimulation, suppository, or mini enema), positioning, assistive techniques, and adaptive equipment.

80. Following a stroke, if a patient demonstrates variable and unpredictable substitutions of sounds, blockages and repetitions similar to stuttering, and slow effortful output without evidence of weakness of oral structures, do not automatically label this as aphasia; it more likely represents apraxia of speech.

81. Cardiac rehabilitation is a three-phase process (phase I in hospital, phase II outpatient monitored, phase III independent maintenance) that is designed to assess risk, monitor for complications, treat risk factors, and gradually regain full mobility and cardiovascular fitness. The long-term goals are to maximize life span, minimize cardiac complications, and maintain maximal function.

82. The main cause of hypoxia in patients with restrictive lung disorder is "airway mucus plugging" rather than "lung infection." A cardinal rule is to always first attempt to normalize SpO_2 by providing adequate ventilation and assisted coughing before considering intubation.

83. If a patient with a history of cancer presents with neck or back pain, particularly if new or increasing severity or worsened by Valsalva or recumbency, obtain an MRI study with gadolinium enhancement to search for metastatic disease.

84. The main goal of rehabilitation for arthritis is to enhance the effects of medical treatment in reducing physical impairment and improving function. The rehabilitation evaluation should occur soon after the diagnosis of arthritis, and interventions should be started, if indicated, to help prevent the onset of disabilities.

85. If a patient with upper extremity burns has decreased range of motion of the elbow, it may be caused by contracture of the skin, but evaluate for heterotopic ossification (HO). After a burn injury, HO most commonly occurs at the elbows.

86. An important rule of pain medicine is to believe that the patient's pain is real. The goals of treating pain with medications are to decrease the subjective pain levels, improve the patient's functional status, monitor and control for potential treatment side effects, and monitor and observe for the proper use or abuse of the medications.

87. Unlike most other medications used in pain, opiates do not have a pharmacologic "ceiling effect" and should be titrated to therapeutic efficacy or side effects.

88. The segmental neuromyotherapy approach to pain management can produce immediate as well as long-term relief by reducing or eliminating central sensitization with techniques that desensitize the involved spinal segments and eradicate peripheral sensitized pain generators.

89. Central pain is defined as pain associated with lesions of the CNS. The most commonly cited central pain syndromes are central post-stroke pain and spinal cord injury pain.

90. Neuropathic pain is initiated or caused by a primary lesion (pain generator) or dysfunction in the nervous system. It can be reduced with modalities, various topical anesthetics, and oral medications from the anticonvulsant and antidepressant groups, targeted at various pain mechanisms.

91. Treatment of myofascial trigger points (MTrPs) is most effective if both the peripheral and central (segmental) sensitization are addressed.

92. If complex regional pain syndrome (CRPS) is suspected, start aggressive treatment quickly. The best treatment is a combination of pain control with medications, rehabilitation, and psychotherapy.

93. If the clinical history does not explain physical finding of trauma in a child, *always* suspect nonaccidental trauma, regardless of your personal opinion of the family.

94. Development progresses in a head-to-toe fashion and from mass activity to individual, specific actions. Hand dominance is established at about two years of age. Dominance before that age *may* suggest unilateral upper extremity deficit.

95. Cerebral palsy is a nonprogressive condition. It is critical to determine that there has been no loss of milestones when making the diagnosis.

96. Maternal ingestion of 0.4 mg/day of folic acid (standard dose in most multivitamins), beginning three months prior to conception and continuing through the end of the first trimester, reduces the risk of a neural tube defect by 70%.

97. Differential diagnoses of groin pain in dancers include torn acetabular labrum, femoral neck stress fracture, adductor sprain, and rectus femoris tendinitis and myofascial pain (especially in a poorly trained dancer who incorrectly uses this muscle to raise the leg forward).

98. Magnetic resonance imaging scans are much better than plain films for initial diagnosis of lower extremity stress fractures, as evidence of fracture may not immediately appear after the onset of symptoms.

99. Spiritual beliefs and practices can aid in healing; many patients desire the discussion of spiritual beliefs.

100. International rehabilitation involves a synergistic exchange of ideas and resources among diverse nations and cultures. Technologic innovations have made the world a smaller place and have helped to promote worldwide physiatric humanitarianism.

WHAT IS PHYSICAL MEDICINE AND REHABILITATION?

Mark A. Young, MD, MBA, Bryan O'Young, MD, and Steven A. Stiens, MD, MS

CHAPTER 1

The Art of Improving Quality of Life for People with Disabilities

A true friend knows your weaknesses but shows you your strengths; feels your fears but fortifies your faith; sees your anxieties but frees your spirit; recognizes your disabilities but emphasizes your possibilities.

–William Arthur Ward (1921–1997)

Alone we can do so little, together we can do so much.

–Helen Keller (1880–1967)

1. **What is physical medicine and rehabilitation (PM&R)?**
   PM&R, also known as physiatry, is a medical specialty that emphasizes prevention, diagnosis, and treatment of patients who experience limitations in function resulting from any disease process, injury, or symptom. Physiatrists utilize medications, injections, physical modalities, exercise, and education individualized to the patient's needs. PM&R specialists provide care for patients with neuromusculoskeletal disorders who have acute and chronic disabilities requiring rehabilitation services. The goal of physiatry is to restore optimal patient function in all spheres of life, including the medical, social, emotional, and vocational dimensions. Physiatry has been aptly branded the "quality of life medical specialty" and has grown in international recognition because of its commitment to meeting the quality-of-life and nonoperative neuromusculo-skeletal needs of an aging society.

   http://www.aapmr.org/

2. **What are the mission and motto of PM&R?**
   PM&R strives to promote a person's quality of life and functional outcomes through a dynamic team-oriented approach. Often the physiatrist plays a leadership role in this process. Valuable members of the physiatry team include the physical therapist (PT), occupational therapist (OT), speech-language pathologist, respiratory therapist, nursing staff, and others. By blending the best of the traditional medical approach ("adding years to life") with the functional model ("adding life to years"), the PM&R team accomplishes its noble mission.

   Like a true friend, a physiatrist must be an optimistic spirit, a team player, and one who gives life to the immortal words of William Arthur Ward, "a true friend knows your weakness but shows your strength; feels your fears but fortifies your faith; sees your anxieties but frees your spirit; [most importantly] recognizes your disabilities but emphasizes your possibilities."

   http://World Health.Net3. Is there a prototypic "physiatric personality"?

3. **What concepts are reflected in the name physical medicine and rehabilitation?**
   The official name of the field reflects the two essential concepts of the specialty:
   - **Physical medicine:** Diagnosis and treatment of neuromusculoskeletal disorders with the use of medications, modalities, procedures, and exercise

- **Rehabilitation:** The process of transforming a person with functional limitations to a person with "maximal ability" through the application of medical treatment, therapy, and adaptive equipment.

  http://www.acrm.org/

4. **What makes the practice of PM&R particularly satisfying and gratifying?**
   Physicians choose PM&R for many reasons:
   1. Physiatric practice is collaborative. Physiatrists seldom work alone. They practice as part of an interdisciplinary team. All team members have knowledge and skills that complement those of other team members in meeting patients' needs. The physiatrist is often the team leader, orchestrating the collaborative effort.
   2. Physiatric practice requires an intimate knowledge of the patient's resources and pitfalls as well as the patient's environment. By witnessing the "enablement" of the patient, the physiatrist becomes more "enabled" and achieves a profound sense of pride and satisfaction that is shared with patients when they achieve functional recovery. One of the deep satisfactions in physiatry arises from supporting patients as they achieve their goals and sharing successes with the entire rehabilitation treatment team.
   3. The nature of physiatric practice requires skills in interpersonal communication, multisystem diagnostics, mechanical interventions and electrodiagnostics, and therapeutics.
   4. Working individually with patients to design unique life-enhancing solutions is creative and fun for physiatrists. They often follow patients for years and help them solve a variety of problems as they age and engage in new activities.

   All of these aspects involve the continuing rediscovery of patients and team members and the existing options within their environments. Physiatrists make possible the synergistic efforts that the patient and the rehabilitation team, by working together, can use to maximize each other's potential.

   http://www.physiatry.org/field/index.html

5. **Which medical conditions are treated by physiatrists?**
   Although many physiatrists view themselves as primary care physicians for people with disabilities (and therefore offer comprehensive care for persons with diverse medical conditions), a growing number of physiatry specialists have elected to focus on specific rehabilitation areas. Common conditions treated by physiatrists include amputations, arthritis, brain injuries, burns, cancer, cardiac disorders, fibromyalgia, industrial injuries, multiple sclerosis, neuromuscular diseases, neuropathies, orthopedic injuries, pain disorders, pediatric disorders, pulmonary disorders, spinal cord injuries, stroke, and trauma. Physiatrists are uniquely suited to treat painful neuromusculoskeletal conditions through a holistic and balanced combination of exercise, medication, and procedures and moral and psychosocial support.

6. **Why should *all* physiatrists dedicate a portion of their daily work schedule to working with people with disabilities?**
   People with disabilities occupy an essential and ever-growing segment of the health care continuum. Physiatrists must always be true to the altruistic roots and traditions of the field and their education by being available to manage the unique needs of persons with disabilities. Whether the task involves readily accepting a consultation on a newly quadriplegic inpatient or rendering assistance to a community-based elderly patient who has had a stroke, the physiatrist by virtue of his/her training can truly "make a difference." As noted by one academic physiatrist in a recent issue of *JAMA*:

   > As practitioners of the healing arts, we are often swept away by the mundane minutiae of providing expert technical care to our patients. Often overlooked [however] is the "human side" of caring–that transcendent sense of seeing life through the eyes of our patients.

Physiatry admirably answers that calling, and because *all* physiatrists have been invested with that training, they must respond unabashedly. No matter which direction your subspecialty takes you, always remember that you are a physiatrist!

Young MA: Review of Still Lives: Narratives of Spinal Cord Injury by Jonathan Cole. JAMA 293(4): 497, 2005.

7. How did PM&R get started?

Around the middle of the 20th century, a major shift in thinking among health care providers began to take place. Holistic, comprehensive, team-oriented care for people with disabilities began to be recognized as an important societal obligation. This powerful philosophy sparked a burgeoning interest among health care providers to treat people with disabilities.

The year 1936 was a banner year for physiatry. Dr. Frank Krusen inaugurated the first residency training program at the Mayo Clinic. Dr. Krusen coined the term *physiatrist* and is credited as the author of the first comprehensive rehabilitation textbook. Dr. Krusen's monumental work has had a lasting imprint on the field.

Improvements in acute medical care (e.g., penicillin) during World War II saved the lives of many soldiers with disabilities who returned home in dire need of rehabilitative care.

Pioneer physicians in the field helped to plant the seeds for an exciting new specialty that cared for the whole person, not just the disease.

8. When did PM&R become recognized as a specialty?

Although the American Academy of Physical Medicine and Rehabilitation traces its origins to 1938, the American Board of PM&R (ABPM&R) was established in 1947 by members of the academy in response to the urgent need for a certifying authority. The ABPM&R was approved in 1947 by the Advisory Board of Medical Specialties as one of twenty-four "official" medical specialties.

9. How does one become a "card-carrying" physiatrist?

First, there is medical school (4 years). Then there is an internship (one year of a coordinated program of experience in fundamental clinical skills such as an accredited transitional year or six months or more in accredited training in family practice, internal medicine, obstetrics and gynecology, pediatrics, or surgery, or any combination of these patient care experiences). This 1-year internship is followed by a 3-year residency. For some, there is a fellowship (from 1 to 3 years in disciplines such as spinal cord injury, traumatic brain injury, electromyography, musculoskeletal medicine, or pain medicine). Similar to many medical specialization career paths, the road to becoming a PM&R diplomate is exciting and challenging because the field draws from so many sources of knowledge and practice. At the conclusion of PM&R residency, qualified candidates take a written certification exam (part 1) given by the ABPM&R. When they have completed residency, another exam (oral; part 2) is administered after the first year of practice. Upon successful completion of parts 1 and 2, students can proudly display a numbered board certification "sheepskin," recognizing their achievement.

10. What about recertification in physiatry?

You never stop learning. Recertification is required every 10 years.

11. What is the best way to prepare for certification?

1. Get to know your patients. Individualize their treatments. Be good to your patients.
2. Always provide high-quality and compassionate care.
3. Remember that your patients are good teachers as well.
4. Fashion your practice after caring role models, such as attending physiatrists.
5. Link your learning to your patients' problems.
6. Throughout training, read major contemporary texts (see Bibliography).
7. Complement your learning and practice knowledge by reading *PM&R Secrets, 3rd ed.*

12. **How can I learn more about PM&R in medical school?**

Some medical schools have established elective mandatory rotations in PM&R, some have a mandatory rotation, whereas others offer it as an elective. A growing number of academic departments have created educational opportunities such as lectures, courses, seminars, and symposia for interested medical students. Some have even created "shadow experiences" for undergraduates interested in an early exposure to physiatry. As part of the physical diagnosis curriculum established in many medical schools, students may spend their time in rehabilitation service where patients are medically stable and exhibit a broad array of pathologies, which lends itself to good learning.

Stiens SA, Berkin DI: A clinical rehabilitation course for college undergraduates provides an introduction to the biopsychosocial interventions that minimize disablement. Am J Phys Med Rehabil 76:462–470, 1998.

13. **Tell me about PM&R residency training programs.**

With over 75 accredited residency programs in PM&R in the United States, there are ample opportunities for postgraduate education. All accredited programs adhere to program requirements written and administered by the Residency Review Committee for PM&R. This hopefully ensures uniformity in high-quality training experience and exposure to the various programs. As an added bonus, some programs offer opportunities for advanced degrees (MBA, MD, PhD), specialized electives, and research opportunities. A select group of senior residents who become chief residents may have the opportunity to develop additional administrative and leadership skills. Some institutions offer combined programs such as PM&R/neurology, PM&R/pediatrics, and PM&R/internal medicine.

http://www.abpmr.org/certification/index.html

14. **What about subspecialty training in physiatry?**

For those who want to specialize in specific areas, subspecialty fellowships accredited by ABPM&R are currently available in Spinal Cord Injury Medicine, Pain, and Pediatrics (2002), Sports Medicine (2006), Hospice and Palliative Medicine (2006), and Neuromuscular Medicine (2006). Other nonaccredited fellowship opportunities exist in many areas.

KEY POINTS: WHAT IS PM&R?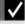

1. Like a good friend, a "good" physiatrist follows the words of William Arthur Ward: "A true friend knows your weaknesses but shows you your strengths; feels your fears but fortifies your faith; sees your anxieties but frees your spirit; recognizes your disabilities but emphasizes your possibilities."

2. PM&R, also known as physiatry, is a medical specialty emphasizing prevention, diagnosis, and treatment of patients who experience limitations in function resulting from any disease process, injury, or symptom.

3. Physiatrists are uniquely suited to treat painful neuromusculoskeletal conditions through a holistic and balanced combination of exercise, medication, procedures, and psychosocial support.

4. The most effective physiatrists get to know their patients and design care plans with them that are directed specifically to meet their goals. This is accomplished with clear awareness of each patient's strengths and weaknesses, an empathic reflection of each patient's unique capabilities, and a clear vision of each patient's realistic future possibilities.

5. Physiatrists work with patients and transdisciplinary teams to achieve patient-centered goals by using a broad synergistic variety of biomedical, modality, exercise, prosthetic, orthotic assistive technology, psychological, and educationally based treatments that require full patient participation.

15. **What about accreditation of PM&R education?**
    The Accreditation Council for Graduate Medical Education (ACGME) delegates authority to the Residency Review Committee for PM&R to confer *direct* certification of PM&R residency training programs. Accreditation is a voluntary process and confers a stamp of approval to a given program. The ACGME is an offspring of several important organizations, including the American Board of Medical Specialties (ABMS), Council on Medical Education (CME), American Medical Association (AMA), American Hospital Association (AHA), and Association of American Medical Colleges (AAMC).

16. **What is the role of a practicing physiatrist?**
    Physiatrists treat patients with acute and chronic pain and neuromusculoskeletal disorders. They often practice in major rehabilitation centers, hospitals, and private settings as either a primary caregiver or a specialist. Often, a physiatrist coordinates a team of doctors and other health care professionals. A comprehensive rehabilitation program may include physical therapists, speech therapists, occupational therapists, recreational therapists, nurses, psychologists, social workers, and specialists in allied medical specialties.

17. **What diagnostic tools are used in physiatry?**
    Diagnostic tools include those used by other physicians (medical history, physical examinations, x-rays, and laboratory tests), as well as special techniques in electrodiagnostic medicine such as electromyography (EMG), nerve conduction studies, and somatosensory and motor-evoked potentials. EMG examinations and nerve conduction studies are the most common procedures used. Musculoskeletal ultrasound is a rapidly developing technique that is also performed by many physiatrists.

18. **What treatments do a physiatrist offer?**
    Treatment options include the use of medications; modalities such as hot packs, cold packs, ultrasound, and electrotherapy; assistive devices, such as a brace or artificial limb; massage; biofeedback; traction; and therapeutic exercise. Surgery is not used. Physiatrists, with added training, also perform injections, interventional procedures, including peripheral articular injections (increasingly guided by ultrasound), spinal blocks, botulinum toxin injections, and acupuncture.

19. **Is physiatry a recognized specialty in other countries? Has it achieved international prominence?**
    Known in many countries as physical and rehabilitation medicine (P&RM), physiatry has achieved an unprecedented high level of popularity throughout the world. This field continues to be a drawing card for international doctors because of the aging population internationally and the focus on functional restoration. The International Society of Physical Medicine and Rehabilitation (ISPRM) is a unique global organization that works to assist P&RM specialists, doctors as well as other health care workers, to become more effective practitioners and to improve the quality of life of people all over the world with impairments and disabilities. Major efforts to achieve this are the convening of international congresses every two years and providing rehabilitation medicine input to international health organizations such as the World Health Organization (WHO). Many countries maintain special boards of PM&R analogous to the ABPM&R. Notable examples are the European Board of PM&R and the Australasian Faculty of P&RM. (See Chapter 83 on International PM&R.)
    www.isprm.org

20. **Are there international learning opportunities in PM&R?**
    Operation Global Goniometry (OGG) (www.isprm-edu.org), a unique international educational project sponsored by the ISPRM Faculty Student Educational Exchange Committee, serves as a central clearinghouse for novel educational, humanitarian, and learning opportunities in

PM&R across all continents. OGG is comprised of an international faculty of physiatrists and committee members representing all implied countries. The primary functions and responsibilities of the committee include:

- To serve as a central clearinghouse for international learning opportunities in rehabilitation
- To facilitate placement of medical students, residents, faculty physicians, and allied rehabilitation professionals in global voluntary didactic rotations
- To share information about global P&RM educational opportunities with the membership of the organization
- To track the outcomes, progress, and successes of the committee's educational initiatives
- To interface and network with other rehabilitation educational organizations in pursuit of international education and scholarship in the field
- To track the individual accomplishments and endeavors of the committee
- To provide academically-based, PM&R-related humanitarian assistance (recent examples: Hurricane Katrina, the Tsunami in the Indian Ocean).

A special photo album has been established at www.isprmedu.org.

21. **How can I review the fundamentals of PM&R in an entertaining and engaging way?**

Read *Physical Medicine and Rehabilitation Secrets,* share the knowledge through Socratic discussions with colleagues, and utilize *Secrets* as a bridge text to broader or more specific resources according to your learning needs. Read on and find out.

WEBSITES

1. http://www.aapmr.org

2. http://www.abpmr.org

3. http://www.isprm-edu.org

4. http://www.isprm.org

5. http://www.physiatry.org

6. http://www.acrm.org

BIBLIOGRAPHY

1. Banja JD: Ethics, values, and world cultures: The impact on rehabilitation. Disabil Rehabil 18:279–284, 1996.
2. Braddom RL (ed): Physical Medicine and Rehabilitation, 3rd ed. Philadelphia, W.B. Saunders, 2007.
3. DeLisa JA, Gans BM (eds): Rehabilitation Medicine: Principles and Practice, 4th ed. Philadelphia, Lippincott Williams & Wilkins, 2005.
4. Grabois M, Garrison SJ, Hart KA, Lehmkul LD (eds): Physical Medicine and Rehabilitation: The Complete Approach. Cambridge, MA, Blackwell Science, 2000.
5. Honet JC: PM&R education. In O'Young B, Young MA, Stiens SA (eds): PM&R Secrets, 2nd ed. Philadelphia, Hanley & Belfus, 1997, pp 15–17.
6. Stiens SA, Berkin DI: A clinical rehabilitation course for college undergraduates provides an introduction to the biopsychosocial interventions that minimize disablement. Am J Phys Med Rehabil 76:462–470, 1998.
7. Young MA, Stiens SA, Hsu P: The PM&R chief resident: A balance between administration and education. Am J Phys Med Rehabil 75:257–262, 1996.

CHAPTER 2

ANATOMY AND KINESIOLOGY OF THE MUSCULOSKELETAL SYSTEM

Carson D. Schneck, MD, PhD

Anatomy is Destiny.

–Sigmund Freud (1856–1939)

PRINCIPLES OF KINESIOLOGY

1. **What role do agonist, antagonist, and synergistic muscles play in facilitating joint motion?**
   - An **agonist,** or prime mover, is any muscle that can cause a specific joint motion. For example, the biceps brachii contracts to cause elbow flexion.
   - An **antagonist** is any muscle that can produce a motion opposite to the specific agonist motion. For example, triceps brachii is an antagonist to elbow flexion. Antagonists are normally completely relaxed during contraction of an agonist (except near the end of a rapid ballistic motion).
   - **Synergistic** muscles normally contract to remove unwanted actions of agonists or to stabilize other (usually more proximal) joints. For example, during elbow flexion by the biceps brachii, the forearm pronators contract to remove the undesirable supination that the biceps would produce.

2. **Which forces typically act to produce motion at joints?**
   Gravity and muscle contraction, with each serving as the prime mover for about 50% of all joint movements.

KEY POINTS: TYPES OF MUSCLE CONTRACTION

1. **Concentric, isotonic, or shortening contraction** occurs when the muscle's force exceeds the load. Hence, the muscle shortens to produce joint motion while maintaining constant tension.

2. **Isometric or static contraction** occurs when the muscle force equals the load. The muscle maintains the same length and the joint does not move.

3. **Eccentric or lengthening contraction** occurs when muscle force is less than the load. This normally occurs when gravity is the prime mover. To control the effect of gravity, eccentric contraction occurs in the muscle(s) that oppose(s) the direction that gravity tends to move the joint.

3. **Two muscles often perform the same function. How can the examiner eliminate one of the muscles to evaluate the other muscle in relative isolation?**
   Three muscle isolation procedures are commonly used:
   - Place a muscle at a **mechanical disadvantage** by positioning the part so that the muscle to be eliminated will have no substantial vector component in the direction of the function to be tested.
   - Place a muscle at a **physiologic or length disadvantage** by positioning the part so that the muscle is slackened or has much of its shortening capability used up by performing a function other than the one being tested.
   - If the muscle to be eliminated has several functions, **reciprocally inhibit** it from participating in the tested function by forcibly performing a function antagonistic to one of its other functions.

4. **How is muscle strength graded?**
   Manual muscle strength assessment is accomplished by proceeding cephalad downward in the order of innervation from the brachial plexus, through the lumbosacral plexus. If specific nerves are in question, examine muscles in the proximal-to-distal order in which they receive their motor branches. Resistance is best assessed using the "make and break" technique, in which the examiner overpowers a patient's fixed midmuscle length contraction. For ordinal-ranked categories used in clinical practice, see Box 2-1.

BOX 2-1. ORDINAL-RANKED CATEGORIES FOR GRADING MUSCLE STRENGTH[*]

5 = Normal power against gravity and the usual amount of resistance
4 = Muscle contraction possible against gravity and less than the normal amount of resistance
3 = Muscle contraction possible only against gravity, not with resistance
2 = Joint movement possible only with gravity eliminated
1 = Flicker of contraction with no movement
0 = No contraction detectable

[*]For greater reproducibility, a continuous measure such as hand-held dynamometry is superior.

SPINE

5. **Name the major ligaments of the spine and the spine motions they resist.**
   - Anterior longitudinal ligament: extension
   - Posterior longitudinal ligament: flexion
   - Ligamenta flava and facet joint capsule: flexion
   - Interspinous and supraspinous ligaments: flexion

6. **What are the parts of the intervertebral disc?**
   A peripheral, laminated, fibrocartilaginous anulus fibrosus and a central, gel-like nucleus pulposus. The **anulus fibrosus** contains the **nucleus pulposus** between the adjacent vertebral bodies (Fig. 2-1). The nucleus pulposus serves as a hydraulic load-dispersing mechanism, so that as the spine bends in any direction, the compressive loads borne by that side of the disc are redistributed over a larger surface area, thereby reducing the pressure.

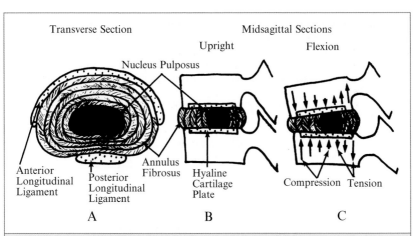

Figure 2-1. The intervertebral disk. *A,* A transverse section. *B,* A midsagittal section through the intervertebral disk with the spine in an upright neutral position to display its normal structure and relationships. *C,* A midsagittal section of the disk with the spine in flexion to demonstrate the compressile and tensile stresses in this position. (From Schneck CD: Functional and clinical anatomy of the spine. Spine State Art Rev 9:571–604, 1995.)

7. **Why do most intervertebral disc protrusions occur posterolaterally?**
    1. The disc is reinforced anterolaterally by the anterior longitudinal ligament and posteromedially by the posterior longitudinal ligament. Posterolaterally, there are no extrinsic supporting ligaments.
    2. The nucleus pulposus is eccentrically located closer to the posterior aspect of the disc, causing the posterior anulus to have the smallest radial dimension and offer the least support.
    3. The posterior anulus is thinnest in the superior–inferior dimension at cervical and lumbar levels, causing it to suffer the greatest strain.
    4. Because flexion is the most predominant spine motion, the posterior anulus receives the most repetitive tensile stresses.
    5. The posterolateral anulus is subject to the highest intralaminar shear stresses, causing intralaminar separation.

8. **Describe the course of the spinal nerves in relationship to the spine.**
    At most levels, **dorsal and ventral roots** join to form **spinal nerves** as they enter the intervertebral foramen. The **dorsal root ganglia** are located on the spinal nerve at this point. As spinal nerves exit the intervertebral foramen, they terminate by dividing into **dorsal and ventral rami**. Cervical spinal nerves exit above the vertebra of the same number. The C8 spinal nerve emerges between the C7 and T1 vertebrae, which causes all thoracic, lumbar, and sacral nerves to exit below the vertebrae of the same number. Because lower spinal nerves must descend to their intervertebral foramina from their higher point of origin from the spinal cord, they typically occupy the upper portion of their intervertebral foramen (Fig. 2-2).

9. **Why do herniated lumbar intervertebral discs commonly miss the nerve that exits at that level and instead affect the next lower spinal nerve roots?**
    Lumbar intervertebral foramina are large, and because the nerves occupy the upper part of the foramen and the disc is related to the lower part of the foramen, posterolateral disc herniations commonly miss the nerve in the foramen. Instead, they tend to affect the roots of the next lower spinal nerve, which occupy the most lateral part of the spinal canal before exiting from the next lower intervertebral foramen. For example, a herniated L4–L5 disc will typically miss the L4 nerve and affect the L5 roots.

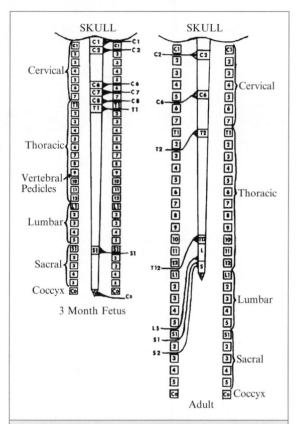

Figure 2-2. Dorsal view of spinal nerves in relation to vertebral levels and spinal cord segments in the 3-month fetus and adult. (From Schneck CD: Functional and clinical anatomy of the spine. Spine State Art Rev 9:571–604, 1995.)

10. What are the uncovertebral or Luschka's joints?

The lower five cervical vertebrae contain uncinate processes that protrude cranially from the lateral margins of the superior surface of their bodies. Luschka's joints begin to develop in the second decade of life as degenerative clefts in the lateral part of the intervertebral disc just medial to the uncinate processes. Degeneration begins at this point because it is where the cervical discs are narrowest in their superior-inferior dimension and hence subject to greatest tensile stresses during motion. Hypertrophic degenerative changes can involve Luschka's joints or the posterior portion of the cervical disc, which is the next thinnest part of the disc. Hypertrophic bars developing in the posterior disc can encroach both nerve roots and spinal cord.

Hayashi K, Yabuki T: Origin of the uncus and of Luschka's joint in the cervical spine. J Bone Surg 67A:788–791, 1985.

Schneck CD: Clinical anatomy of the cervical spine. In White AH, Schofferman JA (eds): Spine Care. St. Louis, Mosby, 1995, pp 1306–1334.

11. What are lateral recesses? What is their significance?

Lateral recesses are a normal narrowing of the anteroposterior (AP) dimension of the lateral portion of the spinal canal at the L4, L5, and S1 levels. They occur because the pedicles become

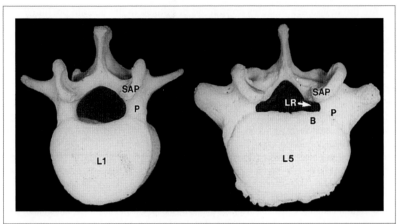

Figure 2-3. Lateral recesses are absent at L1 and present at L5. (From Schneck CD: Functional and clinical anatomy of the spine. Spine State Art Rev 9:571–604, 1995.)

shorter in their AP dimension at these levels. This brings the superior articular processes and facet joints close to the posterior aspect of the lateral part of the vertebral bodies. The pedicle forms the lateral wall of the recess (Fig. 2-3).

As the L4–S1 nerve roots descend the spinal canal, they each course through a lateral recess before exiting their intervertebral foramen. When hypertrophic degenerative changes involve the superior articular process, it can reduce the distance between this process and the vertebral body to <3 mm, producing **lateral stenosis** with the potential for nerve root encroachment. Hypertrophic changes involving the more medially situated inferior articular process will more likely produce a **central stenosis** of the spinal canal. Facet joints also form the posterior boundary of the intervertebral foramen, where hypertrophic changes can produce **foraminal stenosis**.

12. **What anatomic and mechanical features of the lumbosacral junction predispose L5 to spondylolysis and spondylolisthesis?**

The steep inclined plane of the sacral angle (commonly 50 degrees from horizontal) predisposes the L5 vertebra to slide forward on S1 under a gravitational load. This slippage is resisted by the impaction of the inferior articular processes of L5 against the superior articular processes of the sacrum. These forces and their reactions concentrate substantial shearing stresses on the **pars interarticularis** of the L5 lamina. Hence, **spondylolysis** is most commonly a stress fracture. Whether a **spondylolisthesis** develops depends on the ability of the intervertebral disc, anterior longitudinal ligament, and iliolumbar ligaments to resist anterior displacement of the L5 vertebral body (Fig. 2-4).

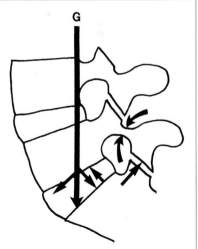

Figure 2-4. Spondylolysis at L5. (From Schneck CD: Functional and clinical anatomy of the spine. Spine State Art Rev 9:571–604, 1995.)

13. **Are the deep back muscles contracted or relaxed in the upright position?**
    In the upright position, the spine is in relatively good equilibrium, because the line of gravity falls through the points of inflection of each of the curves of the spine. As a result, activity in the major **deep back muscles** (erector spinae, semispinalis, multifidus, and rotators) is negligible, and the ligaments of the spine are the major resistors of any applied moment.

14. **Which muscles are responsible for producing the major spine motions?**
    - **Flexion:** The **anterior abdominal muscles** initiate flexion, but as soon as the spine is out of equilibrium, gravity becomes the prime mover under the control of an eccentric contraction of the **deep back muscles**. A concentric contraction of the deep back muscles returns the spine to an upright position.
    - **Extension:** Spinal extension is initiated by the **deep back muscles,** with gravity becoming the prime mover as soon as the spine is out of equilibrium. The **anterior abdominal muscles** control gravity with an eccentric contraction and return the spine to an upright position with a concentric contraction.
    - **Lateral bending:** Lateral bending is initiated by the ipsilateral **deep back, abdominal, psoas major,** and **quadratus lumborum muscles**. Once started, gravity becomes the prime mover under the control of eccentric contraction of the same muscles on the contralateral side, which also contract concentrically to return the spine to the upright position.
    - **Rotation:** Rotation of the front of the trunk to one side is produced by the ipsilateral **erector spinae** and **internal abdominal oblique muscles** and the contralateral **deeper back muscles** and **external abdominal oblique**. Rotation of the face to one side is also produced by the ipsilateral **splenius**, contralateral **sternocleidomastoid**, and other **cervical rotators**.

15. **What do dorsal rami of spinal nerves innervate?**
    Dorsal rami innervate the skin of the medial two-thirds of the back from the interauricular line to the coccyx (top of the head to the tip of the tail), deep muscles of the back, posterior ligaments of the spine, and the facet joint capsules.

UPPER LIMB

16. **What structure provides the strongest support for the acromioclavicular joint?**
    The **coracoclavicular ligament,** which descends from the distal clavicle to the coracoid process. This ligament must be torn to produce the major stepdown of the acromion below the clavicle in grade 3 acromioclavicular joint injuries.

17. **What structural features cause the shoulder (glenohumeral) joint to be a highly mobile but relatively unstable joint?**
    The relatively poor bony congruence between the glenoid and humeral head and a relatively slack capsule.

18. **What dynamic features help maintain shoulder joint contact through the full range of abduction?**
    The **rotator cuff muscles** stabilize the shoulder by varying their medially directed vector forces. In early abduction, the **deltoid** tends to sublux the humeral head superiorly. This is offset by increased tension in the superior capsule by the simultaneous contraction of the **supraspinatus** and by the slightly downward vector pull of the **subscapularis, infraspinatus,** and **teres minor** muscles. In the middle range of abduction, the **subscapularis** turns off to allow the **infraspinatus** and **teres major** to externally rotate the humerus and bring the greater tubercle posteriorly under the acromion (which is the highest part of the coracoacromial arch). This prevents its impingement against the arch.

    Inman VT, Saunders JB, Abbott LC: Observations on the function of the shoulder joint. J Bone Joint Surg 26A:1–30, 1944.

19. **How does medial and lateral winging of the scapula occur?**

    The medial border of the scapula is normally kept closely applied to the thoracic wall by the resultant vector forces of its medially and laterally tethering muscles, the **trapezius** and **serratus anterior**. If the serratus anterior is paralyzed, the medial border will wing away from the chest wall and be displaced medially by the unopposed retraction of the trapezius **(medial winging)**. If the trapezius is paralyzed, the medial border will also wing but will be displaced laterally by the unopposed protraction of the serratus anterior **(lateral winging)**.

20. **What are the two major "crutch-walking" muscles of the shoulder?**

    The upward vector force of the crutches at the shoulder is primarily offset by the downward pull of the **lower pectoralis major** and **latissimus dorsi muscles** acting on the humerus.

21. **Why is the elbow a relatively stable joint?**

    The trochlear notch of the ulna has a good grip on the humeral trochlea, and there are strong, relatively taut radial and ulnar collateral ligaments.

22. **Where is the axis for pronation and supination of the forearm located?**

    Proximally, it passes through the center of the radial head; distally, it passes through the ulnar head. Hence, during pronation and supination, the radius scribes half a cone in space about the ulna.

23. **How are major loads transferred from the radius at the wrist to the ulna at the elbow?**

    They are transferred across the **interosseous membrane,** whose fibers run primarily from the ulna upward to the radius. Hence, loads ascending the radius will tense this membrane and be transferred to the ulna.

WRIST AND HAND

24. **Which carpal bones are most frequently injured?**

    The major weight-bearing carpal bones are most frequently injured: the **scaphoid** by a neck fracture and the **lunate** with a palmar dislocation. In one-third of scaphoid fractures, there is nonunion because about one-third of scaphoids receive a blood supply only to their distal end. The lunate tends to dislocate palmarly during hyperextension injuries because it is wedge-shaped with the apex of the wedge pointing dorsally.

25. **Why doesn't carpal tunnel syndrome cause sensory abnormalities over the proximal palm?**

    The palmar cutaneous branch of the median nerve passes superficial to the flexor retinaculum.

26. **How can the flexor digitorum profundus be eliminated in order to test the flexor digitorum superficialis tendons in isolation?**

    To test the ability of the flexor digitorum superficialis to flex the proximal interphalangeal (PIP) joint of a finger, hold the rest of the fingers into forcible hyperextension by resistance over the distal phalanges. This is effective because the individual tendons of the profundus generally arise from a common tendon that attaches to its muscle mass, whereas each of the tendons of the superficialis has its own separate muscle belly. Hence, placing the other fingers into extension puts all of the profundus under stretch and eliminates it as a PIP joint flexor.

27. **How can the extensor digitorum be eliminated to isolate and test the extensor indicis as the last muscle innervated by the radial nerve?**
The extensor indicis is tested by metacarpophalangeal (MP) joint extension of the index finger with the other fingers held in tight flexion at their MP and IP joints. This is effective because the tendons of the extensor digitorum are cross-linked over the dorsum of the hand by intertendinous connections. Therefore, if the rest of the tendons are pulled distally over their MP and IP joints by forcible flexion, they tether the tendon to the index finger distally and make the extensor digitorum ineffective as an index finger MP joint extensor.

28. **Why are the motions of the thumb at right angles to the similar motions of the fingers?**
In the resting hand, the thumb is internally rotated 90° relative to the fingers. Hence, flexion and extension of the thumb occur in a plane parallel to the plane of the palm, and abduction and adduction of the thumb occur at right angles to the plane of the palm, with the thumb moving away from the palm in abduction and toward the palm in adduction. Opposition involves almost 90° of further internal rotation of the thumb at its carpometacarpal joint.

29. **What is the normal digital balance mechanism of the fingers?**
At the MP joint, there is one extensor, the extensor digitorum (although there is an additional extensor of the index and little fingers), balanced against four flexors: the interossei and lumbrical and flexor digitorum profundus and superficialis. At the PIP joint, there are three extensors (interossei and the lumbrical and extensor digitorum) balanced against two flexors (flexor digitorum profundus and superficialis). At the distal interphalangeal (DIP) joint, there are three extensors—interossei and the lumbrical and extensor digitorum—balanced against one flexor, flexor digitorum profundus. The muscles contributing to the extensor balance form an extensor hood mechanism, which splits into lateral and central bands over the PIP joint, with the central band inserting into the base of the middle phalanx and the lateral bands inserting into the base of the distal phalanx. Over the PIP joint, all three bands are connected by the **triangular membrane,** which holds the lateral bands in their normal dorsal position. An **oblique retinacular ligament of Landsmeer** splits off the lateral bands to tether them ventrally to the proximal phalanx.

LOWER LIMB

30. **What structural features make the hip a relatively stable joint?**
   1. Good congruence between the femoral head and the deeply concave acetabulum, which with its labrum forms more than half a sphere
   2. Strong capsular ligaments, two of which—the iliofemoral and ischiofemoral ligaments—are maximally taut in the extended upright position (the usual weight-bearing position)

31. **What are the unique features of the hip joint capsule and its blood supply? What is their clinical significance?**
The anterior hip joint capsule attaches to the **intertrochanteric line** of the femur, thereby completely enclosing the anterior femoral neck. The posterior capsule encloses the proximal two-thirds of the femoral neck. Therefore, the femoral head and most of the femoral neck are intracapsular. This has two clinically important effects. First, it requires that most of the blood supply to the femoral head (mostly from the **medial femoral circumflex artery**) must ascend the femoral neck. Hence, except for the small branch of the **obturator artery** that enters the head with the ligament of the femoral head (ligamentum teres), most of the blood supply to the femoral head is compromised by femoral neck fractures. Second, because the capsule attaches to the femoral neck so low, the upper femoral metaphysis is intracapsular. Because the

metaphysis is the most vascular part of a long bone, hematogenously spread infection to the upper femoral metaphysis can easily produce a septic arthritis. In most other joints, the metaphyses are extracapsular.

32. **Even though the long, obliquely situated femoral neck predisposes the hip to high shearing forces and fracture, are there any physiologic advantages to this unique design?**
The long, obliquely situated femoral neck has the salutary effect of displacing the greater trochanter farther from the abduction-adduction axis of the femoral head, thereby lengthening the moment arm of the gluteus medius and minimus muscles. In standing on one leg, the gravitational vector acting on the adduction side of the hip joint is on a moment arm approximately three times as long as the gluteus medius and minimus moment arm. Therefore, these muscles have to produce a force approximately three times as great as the gravitational vector to offset its hip adduction tendency. If the femoral neck were any shorter or more vertically oriented, as in a valgus hip, the gluteus medius and minimus moment arm would be shortened, requiring these muscles to apply more force to offset the gravitational vector. The long moment arm of the normal femoral neck thereby reduces the loads across the hip and helps protect the hip from degenerative arthritis.

Turek SL: Orthopedics: Principles and Their Application. Philadelphia, J.B. Lippincott, 1984.

33. **What is the best way to test the right gluteus medius and minimus muscles?**
Ask the patient to stand on the right leg. If these muscles are weak or paralyzed, the left side of the pelvis will sag under the influence of the gravitational adduction vector (Trendelenburg sign).

34. **At what point in the gait cycle is the gluteus maximus most active? Why?**
At heel strike of the ipsilateral limb. This offsets the effect of the ground reaction vector, which acts anterior to the hip at this point and therefore tends to cause the trunk to flex on the thigh.

35. **When is the iliopsoas most active during the gait cycle? Why?**
At toe-off, the iliopsoas acts as a hip flexor to offset the ground reaction vector, which is then acting posterior to the hip and tending to cause hip extension.

36. **Why is the knee joint most stable in extension?**
1. Because the anterior portion of the femoral condyle is less curved than the posterior portion, the congruence and area of contact between the **femoral and tibial condyles** are greatest in extension. Hence, the pressures acting across the knee are lowest in extension.
2. The **tibial and fibular collateral ligaments** are maximally taut in extension.
3. The **anterior cruciate ligament** is completely tense only in extension.

37. **Why are the gastrocnemius and soleus muscles the most active lower limb muscles in standing?**
In quiet standing, the line of gravity falls slightly behind the hip joint, slightly anterior to the knee, and 2 inches anterior to the ankle joint axis. At the hip, the tendency of the line of gravity to hyperextend the hip is resisted by the tension in the iliofemoral (and ischiofemoral) ligaments. Therefore, hip flexor muscle activity is generally unnecessary. The line of gravity tends to hyperextend the knee, and tension in the posterior capsule probably helps resist this. However, the activity in the gastrocnemius muscle, which is primarily to stabilize the ankle, also helps prevent back-knee. At the ankle, the long moment arm of the line of gravity acting anterior to the ankle makes it a strong ankle dorsiflexor. The activity in the gastrocnemius and soleus muscles resists this ankle dorsiflexion tendency.

FOOT AND ANKLE

38. **What is the most osteologically stable position of the ankle? Why?**
Dorsiflexion. Both the talar trochlea and tibiofibular mortise have wedge-shaped articular surfaces that are wide anteriorly and narrow posteriorly. In dorsiflexion, the wide anterior part of the talar trochlea is wedged back into the narrow posterior part of the tibiofibular mortise.

39. **At what joint does most of the pronation and supination of the foot occur?**
The subtalar joint permits most of the pronation (eversion) and supination (inversion) of the foot, but the transverse tarsal and tarsometatarsal joints also contribute.

40. **When are the ankle dorsiflexor muscles active during gait?**
The ankle dorsiflexors are active isometrically during swing to prevent gravity from causing foot-drop and eccentrically from heel strike to flat foot (the early loading response) to control the plantar flexion vector exerted on the calcaneus by the ground reaction.

41. **Which nerve of the foot is homologous to the median nerve in the hand?**
The medial plantar nerve. It generally supplies the plantar skin of the medial two-thirds of the foot and medial three and one-half digits, the intrinsic muscles of the great toe except for the adductor hallucis, the first lumbrical, and the flexor digitorum brevis (homologous to the flexor digitorum superficialis of the upper limb). The lateral plantar nerve is also homologous to the ulnar nerve.

WEBSITES

1. http://lt3.uwaterloo.ca/Kinesiology_liaison/online.html

2. http://www.meddean.luc.edu/lumen/MedEd/GrossAnatomy/dissector/mml/mmlregn.htm

3. http://www.uchsc.edu/sm/chs/browse/browse_m.html

4. http://faculty.washington.edu/chudler/spinal.html

BIBLIOGRAPHY

1. Bland JH, Boushey DR: Anatomy and physiology of the cervical spine. Semin Arthritis Rheum 20:1–20, 1990.
2. Cailliet R: Low Back Pain Syndrome. Philadelphia, F.A. Davis, 1995.
3. Schneck CD: Anatomy, mechanics and imaging of spinal injury. In Kirsblum S, Campagnola D, Delisa JA (eds): Spinal Cord Medicine. Philadelphia, Lippincott Williams & Wilkins, 2002, pp 27–68.
4. Schneck CD: Functional and clinical anatomy of the spine. Spine State Art Rev 9:1–37, 1995.
5. Schneck CD, Goldberg G, Munin MC, Chu A: Imaging techniques relative to rehabilitation medicine. In DeLisa JA, Gans GM, Walsh NE (eds): Rehabilitation Medicine: Principles and Practice, 4th ed. Philadelphia, Lippincott Williams & Wilkins, 2005, pp 179–228.
6. Schneck CD, Jacob HAC: Basic principles of functional biomechanics. Physical Medicine and Rehabilitation: State of the Art Reviews 11:731–751, 1997.

CHAPTER 3

NERVOUS SYSTEM ANATOMY: CENTRAL AND PERIPHERAL

Stephen Goldberg, BASc, MD

> Our nervous system isn't just a fiction, it's part of our physical body.
> —Boris Pasternak (1890–1960), *Doctor Zhivago*

CENTRAL NERVOUS SYSTEM

1. **What structures comprise the central nervous system (CNS)?**
    - Spinal cord
    - Brain stem (medulla, pons, midbrain)
    - Cerebellum
    - Cerebrum
    - Diencephalon (everything that contains the name *thalamus*—thalamus, hypothalamus, epithalamus, subthalamus)
    - Basal ganglia (caudate nucleus, globus pallidus, putamen, claustrum, amygdala)

2. **How many nerve structures make up the peripheral nervous system?**
    - 12 cranial nerves (although the optic nerve technically is an outgrowth of the CNS)
    - 31 pairs of spinal nerves

3. **What is the autonomic nervous system? What role does it play?**
    The autonomic nervous system innervates smooth muscle, cardiac muscle, and glands. It includes:
    - **Sympathetic nerves,** which originate from spinal cord segments T1–L2
    - **Parasympathetic nerves,** which originate from spinal cord segments S2–S4
    - **Four cranial nerves** (CN5): CN3 (oculomotor nerve fibers to pupil and ciliary body), CN7 (facial nerve fibers to sublingual, submaxillary, and lacrimal glands), CN9 (glossopharyngeal nerve fibers to parotid glands), and CN10 (vagus nerve fibers to heart, lungs, and gastrointestinal [GI] tract to the splenic flexure).

PERIPHERAL NERVES

4. **Are all nerves created equal?**
    No. All nerves are not created equal (see further discussion).

5. **What type of nerve fibers are found in anterior (ventral) nerve roots?**
    Mainly motor axons.

6. **What type of nerve fibers are found in posterior (dorsal) nerve roots?**
    Mainly sensory axons.

7. **What structures are located in posterior (dorsal) root ganglia?**
    Posterior root ganglia contain cell bodies of sensory axons, but no synapses. This has important implications for nerve conduction studies. If the lesion is proximal to the dorsal root ganglion, then sensory conduction will be normal in the peripheral nerve, since the cell bodies are intact.

8. **Is a peripheral nerve lesion different from a CNS lesion in terms of sensory features?**
   Peripheral nerve lesions can be distinguished from CNS lesions by the different kinds of sensory and motor deficits that arise:
   - **Peripheral nerve lesions** result in **dermatome-type** sensory deficits (i.e., there is a strip-like loss of sensation along a particular area of the body corresponding to the extension of individual peripheral nerves away from the spinal cord). L4–L5 radiculopathies are particularly common, as are C6, C7, and C8 radiculopathies.
   - The CNS, however, is not organized by dermatomes. A CNS motor lesion will more likely result in a **general sensory loss** in an extremity rather than in the strip-like dermatome deficit.

9. **Which dermatomes are innervated by which nerves?**
   - **C1:** No sensory distribution
   - **C2:** Skull cap
   - **C3:** Collar around the neck
   - **C4:** Cape around the shoulders
   - **C6:** "Thumb suckers suck C6"
   - **T5:** Nipples
   - **T10:** Belly button
   - **L1** = IL (region of inguinal ligament)
   - **L4** = Knee jerk
   - **S1** = Ankle jerk

10. **Is it possible for features to distinguish a peripheral nerve lesion from a CNS lesion?**
    Peripheral nerve lesions produce lower motor neuron deficits, whereas CNS lesions produce upper motor neuron deficits (see question 37).

11. **Which roots comprise the brachial plexus?**
    The brachial plexus contains the ventral rami of C5, C6, C7, C8, and T1.

12. **Which nerves arise from the anterior (ventral) rami of the roots prior to the formation of the brachial plexus?**
    - The **dorsal scapular nerve,** from C5 to the rhomboid and levator scapula muscles, is responsible for elevating and stabilizing the scapula.
    - The **long thoracic nerve,** from C5, C6, and C7 to the serratus anterior muscle, is responsible for abduction of the scapula.

13. **Which roots form the trunks of the brachial plexus?**
    The superior trunk arises from C5 and C6. The suprascapular nerve (C5) comes off the upper trunk and supplies the supraspinatus (abduction) and infraspinatus (external rotation) muscles of the shoulder. The middle trunk comes from C7. The lower trunk comes from C8 and T1.

14. **What is the "waiter's tip" injury?**
    A lesion to the upper trunk of the brachial plexus affects the C5–C6 nerves, and hence the infraspinatus and bicep muscles. This results in shoulder inturning, with the hand held in the pronated position, as if the waiter is "asking for a tip" behind his back.

15. **What types of injury typically may cause a "waiter's tip" deficit?**
    Stab wounds to the neck, birth injuries, and falls in which the angle between the shoulder and neck is suddenly widened.

16. **Where in the brachial plexus could an injury cause a "claw hand"?**
An injury to the lower trunk of the brachial plexus affects the C8–T1 nerves, resulting in a combined ulnar and median nerve deficit.

17. **What types of injury typically may cause a brachial plexus "claw hand"?**
   - Extra cervical rib
   - Sudden pulling of the arm (as in trying to grab onto an object to break a fall)
   - Birth injury
   - Compression from lymph node metastases

18. **Where in the brachial plexus could an injury result in a wrist drop?**
An injury to the posterior cord affects the extensors of the wrist because this cord gives rise to the radial nerve.

19. **What type of brachial nerve injury could give rise to a wrist drop?**
This is commonly the result of pressure from inappropriately applied crutches that press on the axilla.

20. **What nerve is commonly affected in shoulder dislocations or humerus fractures?**
The axillary nerve is commonly affected, resulting in weakness or abduction of the shoulder and anesthesia over the lateral proximal arm.

21. **What is the thoracic outlet syndrome?**
This syndrome, usually caused by an extra cervical rib that compresses the medial cord of the brachial plexus and the axillary artery, results in tingling and numbness in the medial aspect of the arm, along with decreased upper extremity pulses.

22. **Describe the anatomy of the peripheral nerves to the upper extremity.**
See Figure 3-1.

23. **What motor functions are impaired by peripheral nerve injuries in the upper extremity?**
   - **Radial nerve (C5–C8):** Elbow and wrist extension (patient has wrist drop); extension of fingers at metacarpophalangeal (MCP) joints; triceps reflex
   - **Median nerve (C8–T1):** Wrist, thumb, index, and middle finger flexion; thumb opposition; forearm pronation; ability of wrist to bend toward the radial (thumb) side; atrophy of thenar eminence (ball of thumb)
   - **Ulnar nerve (C8–T1):** Flexion of wrist, ring and small fingers (claw hand); opposition of little finger; ability of wrist to bend toward ulnar (small finger) side; adduction and abduction of fingers; atrophy of hypothenar eminence in palm (at base of ring and small fingers)
   - **Musculocutaneous nerve (C5–C6):** Elbow flexion (biceps); forearm supination; biceps reflex
   - **Axillary nerve (C5–C6):** Ability to move upper arm outward, forward, or backward (deltoid atrophy)
   - **Long thoracic nerve (C5–C7):** Ability to elevate arm above horizon (winging of scapula)

24. **Describe the anatomy of the lumbosacral plexus.**
The roots of L1–S4 contribute to the lumbosacral plexus, which innervates the skin and skeletal muscles of the lower extremity and perineal area (Fig. 3-2). As in the brachial plexus, its nerve fibers are extensions of anterior (ventral) rami. The inferior gluteal nerve supplies the gluteus maximus. The superior gluteal nerve supplies the gluteus medius and minimus. Injury to the superior gluteal nerve (e.g., direct trauma, polio) results in the "gluteus medius limp"—the

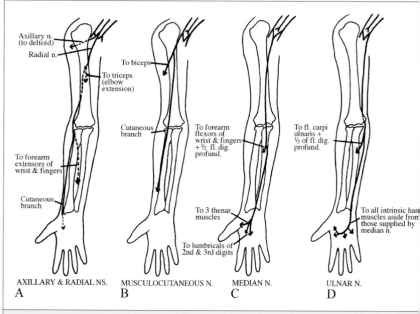

Figure 3-1. Anatomy of the nerves to the upper extremity. (From Goldberg S: Clinical Anatomy Made Ridiculously Simple, 2nd ed. Miami, MedMaster, 2001, www.medmaster.net.)

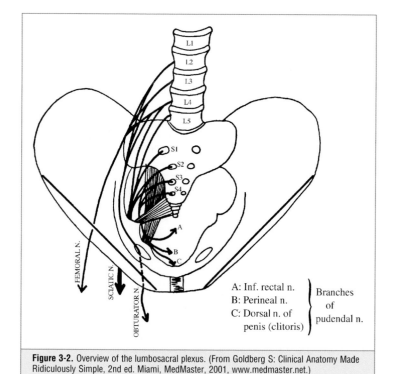

Figure 3-2. Overview of the lumbosacral plexus. (From Goldberg S: Clinical Anatomy Made Ridiculously Simple, 2nd ed. Miami, MedMaster, 2001, www.medmaster.net.)

abductor function of gluteus medius is lost, and the pelvis tilts to the unaffected side when the unaffected extremity is lifted on walking.

25. **Describe the route of the peripheral nerves to the lower extremity.**
See Figure 3-3.

26. **What motor functions are impaired by peripheral nerve injuries in the lower extremity?**
- **Femoral nerve (L2–L4):** Knee extension, hip flexion, knee jerk
- **Obturator nerve (L2–L4):** Hip adduction (patient's leg swings outward when walking)
- **Sciatic nerve (L4–S3):** Knee flexion plus other functions along its branches, the tibial, and common peroneal nerves
- **Tibial nerve (L4–S3):** Foot inversion, ankle plantar flexion, ankle jerk
- **Common peroneal nerve (L4–S2):** Foot eversion, ankle and toes dorsiflexion (patient has high-stepping gait due to foot-drop)

27. **Name the other branches of the lumbar plexus.**
- **Iliohypogastric nerve (L1):** Supplies abdominal muscles and skin over the hypogastric and gluteal areas

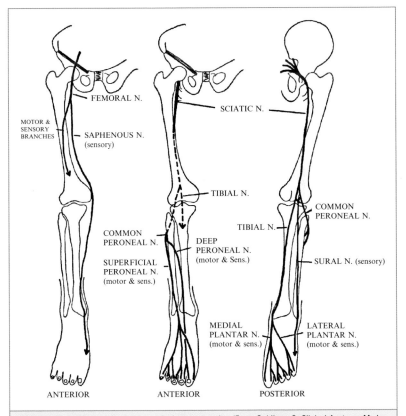

Figure 3-3. Anatomy of the nerves to the lower extremity. (From Goldberg S: Clinical Anatomy Made Ridiculously Simple, 2nd ed. Miami, MedMaster, 2001, www.medmaster.net.)

- **Ilioinguinal nerve (L1):** Innervates skin over the groin and scrotum/labia
- **Genitofemoral nerve (L1, L2):** Runs in the inguinal canal to reach the skin at the base of the penis and scrotum/clitoris and labia majora

28. **What is meralgia paresthetica?**
Commonly found in obese individuals, it is a numbness over the lateral thigh that results from compression of the lateral femoral cutaneous nerve where it runs under the inguinal ligament.

29. **Which nerve supplies the perineum?**
The pudendal nerve (S2, S3, and S4). Parasympathetic branches of S2, S3, and S4 supply the bladder and are critical in bladder emptying. Sympathetic fibers to the bladder (T11–L2) promote retention of urine, but severing of sympathetic fibers to the bladder does not significantly affect bladder function.

30. **Which nerve roots are usually affected by a herniation of the disc between vertebrae L4 and L5?**
Although the L4 nerve root exits between vertebrae L4 and L5, it is generally the L5 nerve root that is compromised by a herniation, while L4 is spared. Similarly, a herniation between vertebrae L5 and S1 typically affects S1, even though the L5 root exits between L5 and S1.

SPINAL CORD

31. **Name the five major divisions of the spinal cord.**
Cervical, thoracic, lumbar, sacral, and coccygeal.

32. **Where does the spinal cord end?**
The spinal cord ends about at the level of vertebrae L1–L2.

33. **How many nerves exit the spinal cord?**
There are 31 pairs of spinal nerves: 8 cervical, 12 thoracic, 5 lumbar, 5 sacral, and 1 coccygeal. Each spinal nerve is the fusion of a dorsal and ventral nerve root.

34. **What are the coverings (meninges) of the spinal cord?**
The meninges surround the entire CNS and consist of the **pia,** which hugs the spinal cord and brain; the **arachnoid membrane;** and the **dura,** which is closely adherent to bone.

35. **Where do you find the cauda equina?**
The cauda equina ("horse's tail") is the downward extension of spinal cord roots at the inferior end of the spinal cord.

36. **A Brown-Sequard lesion that compromises one side of the spinal cord will cause ipsilateral deficits except for one sensory modality. Which one?**
Pain-temperature sensation below the site of the lesion will be lost on the contralateral side; the pain-temperature pathway crosses over soon after it enters the spinal cord.

MOTOR AND SENSORY PATHWAYS

37. **What are the major motor pathways to the extremities?**
- **Corticospinal tract (pyramidal tract):** Extends from the motor area of the cerebral frontal cortex (Brodmann's areas 4, 6) through the internal capsule, brain stem, and spinal cord, crossing over at the junction between the brain stem and spinal cord at the level of the foramen magnum. Therefore, lesions to the corticospinal tract above the level of the

foramen magnum result in contralateral weakness, whereas lesions below the level of the foramen magnum result in ipsilateral weakness.
- **Rubrospinal tract:** This connects the red nucleus of the midbrain with the spinal cord.
- **Tectospinal tract:** This connects the tectum of the midbrain with the spinal cord.
- **Reticulospinal tract:** This connects the reticular formation of the brain stem with the spinal cord.
- **Vestibulospinal tract:** This connects the vestibular nuclei of the brain stem with the spinal cord.

38. **What distinguishes an upper motor neuron lesion from a lower motor neuron lesion?**
- An **upper motor neuron** lesion generally refers to an injury to the corticospinal tract. The corticospinal pathway synapses in the anterior horn of the spinal cord just before leaving the cord.
- A **lower motor neuron** lesion is an injury to the peripheral motor nerves or their cell bodies in the gray matter of the anterior horn on which the corticospinal tract synapses. See Table 3-1.

TABLE 3-1. UPPER VERSUS LOWER MOTOR NEURON DEFECTS

Upper MN Defect	Lower MN Defect
Spastic paralysis	Flaccid paralysis
No significant muscle atrophy	Significant atrophy
No fasciculations or fibrillations	Fasciculations and fibrillations
Hyperreflexia	Hyporeflexia
Babinski reflex may be present	Babinski reflex not present

39. **How do the effects of corticospinal tract injuries differ from those of cerebellar and basal ganglia injuries?**
All of the injuries produce motor problems:
- **Corticospinal tract** injuries cause paralysis.
- **Cerebellar** injuries are characterized by awkwardness of movement **(ataxia),** not paralysis. The awkwardness is on intention—i.e., at rest, the patient shows no problem, but ataxia becomes noticeable when the patient attempts a motor action. There may be awkwardness of posture and gait, poor coordination of movement, dysmetria, dysdiadochokinesia, scanning speech, decreased tendon reflexes on the affected side, asthenia, tremor, and nystagmus.
- **Basal ganglia** disorders, like cerebellar disorders, are characterized by awkward movements rather than paralysis. The movement disorder, however, is present at rest, including such problems as Parkinsonian tremor, chorea, athetosis, and hemiballismus.

40. **Name three major sensory pathways in the spinal cord.**
- **Pain–temperature:** Spinothalamic tract
- **Proprioception–stereognosis:** Posterior columns—(Proprioception is the ability to tell, with the eyes closed, if a joint is flexed or extended. Stereognosis is the ability to identify, with the eyes closed, an object placed in one's hand.)
- **Light–touch:** Spinothalamic tract and posterior columns

41. **Name the three parts of the brain stem.**
Midbrain (most superior), pons, and medulla (most inferior).

42. **What are the functions of the cranial nerves?**
    - **CN1 (olfactory):** Smell
    - **CN2 (optic):** Sight
    - **CN3 (oculomotor):** Constricts pupils, accommodates, moves eyes
    - **CN4 (trochlear), CN6 (abducens):** Move eyes
    - **CN5 (trigeminal):** Chews, feels front of head
    - **CN7 (facial):** Moves face, taste, salivation, crying
    - **CN8 (vestibulocochlear):** Hearing, regulates balance
    - **CN9 (glossopharyngeal):** Taste, salivation, swallowing, monitors carotid body and sinus
    - **CN10 (vagus):** Taste, swallowing, lifts palate; communication to and from thoracoabdominal viscera to the splenic flexure of the colon
    - **CN11 (accessory):** Turns head, lifts shoulders
    - **CN12 (hypoglossal):** Moves tongue

43. **What is Horner's syndrome?**
    Horner's syndrome is ptosis, miosis, and anhydrosis (lack of sweating) from a lesion of the sympathetic pathway to the face. The lesion may lie within the brain stem or the superior cervical ganglion brain stem, the superior cervical ganglion, or its sympathetic extensions to the head.

44. **Which cranial nerves exit from the three parts of the brain stem?**
    - Midbrain—CN3, CN4
    - Pons—CN5, CN6, CN7, CN8
    - Medulla—part of CN7 and CN8, CN9, CN10, CN12

    CN11 exits from the upper cervical cord, goes through the foramen magnum, touches CNs 9 and 10, and then returns to the neck via the jugular foramen. The optic nerve lies superior to the brain stem. The olfactory nerve lies in the cribriform plate of the ethmoid bone.

45. **What CNS structures connect with the brain stem?**
    The midbrain connects with the diencephalon above the brain stem. The medulla connects with the spinal cord below it. Each section of the brain stem has two major connections (right and left) with the cerebellum: two superior cerebellar peduncles connect with the midbrain, two middle cerebellar peduncles connect with the pons, and two inferior cerebellar peduncles connect with the medulla.

46. **What are the two pigmented areas of the brain stem?**
    The substantia nigra, which lies in the midbrain, and the locus coeruleus, which lies in the pons.

KEY POINTS: RAPID LOCALIZERS OF NEUROLOGIC LESIONS

1. Pain in an extremity or a sensory deficit along a dermatome suggests a lesion outside the spinal cord.

2. A facial deficit on one side and an extremity deficit on the other side suggests a brain stem lesion.

3. A visual deficit that only affects one eye suggests a lesion anterior to the optic chiasm.

4. Paralysis and loss of proprioception—stereognosis on one side of the body combined with pain-temperature loss on the other side—suggests a spinal cord lesion.

5. Paralysis along with hyperactive reflexes suggests a CNS lesion.

6. A cerebellar lesion is characterized by awkwardness of intended movements. A basal ganglia lesion is better characterized as unintended movements while at rest.

47. **What is the red nucleus?**
The red nucleus lies in the midbrain. It receives major output from the cerebellum via the superior cerebellar peduncle. It has major connections to the cerebral cortex as well as to the spinal cord via the rubrospinal tract.

48. **What is the medial longitudinal fasciculus (MLF)?**
The MLF is a pathway that runs through the brain stem and interconnects the ocular nuclei of CNs 3, 4, and 6 and the vestibular nuclei. It plays an important role in coordinating eye movements with head and truncal posture.

49. **What is the Edinger-Westphal nucleus?**
It is the parasympathetic nucleus of the third cranial nerve in the midbrain. It supplies motor fibers responsible for pupillary constriction and lens accommodation.

50. **What is an Argyll-Robertson pupil?**
One of the classic signs of tertiary syphilis. The pupil constricts on accommodating but does not constrict to light. The lesion is believed to be in the midbrain.

51. **Describe the pathway for vision.**
Optic nerve fibers extend from the retina to the optic nerve, to the optic chiasm, to the optic tract, to the lateral geniculate body, and to the visual area of the brain via optic radiation fibers. These fibers extend through the parietal lobe and end up superior to the calcarine fissure in the occipital lobe. Optic radiation fibers that extend through the temporal lobe end up inferior to the calcarine fissure in the occipital lobe.

52. **What causes a left homonymous hemianopsia? Bitemporal hemianopsia? Superior quadrantanopsia?**
   - **Left homonymous hemianopsia:** A lesion to the right optic tract, right lateral geniculate body, right optic radiation, or right occipital lobe
   - **Bitemporal hemianopsia:** A lesion to the optic chiasm, generally from a pituitary tumor
   - **Superior quadrantanopsia:** A lesion in the inferior aspect of the optic radiation

53. **What is most peculiar about the exit point of CN4 from the brain stem?**
CN4 is the only cranial nerve to exit on the posterior side of the brain stem. In addition, it crosses over the midline before continuing on its course.

54. **If a child has a head tilt, how do you know if it is due to a CN4 palsy or a stiff neck?**
Cover one eye. If the head straightens out, then the tilt is due to CN4 palsy. The child tilts the head in a CN4 palsy to avoid double vision. Covering one eye eliminates double vision, so the head straightens out.

55. **Which CNs exit at the pontomedullary junction?**
CN6 exits by the midline; CNs 7 and 8 exit laterally.

56. **Where do the motor and sensory branches of CN5 exit the brain stem?**
Both exit the brain stem at the same point, in the lateral aspect of the pons.

57. **What are the sensory branches of CN5?**
   - **V1:** Ophthalmic
   - **V2:** Maxillary
   - **V3:** Mandibular

58. **Which cranial nerve nucleus extends through all sections of the brain stem?**
The trigeminal sensory nucleus. Its mesencephalic nucleus (facial proprioception) lies in the midbrain. Its main nucleus (facial light touch) lies in the pons. Its spinal nucleus (facial pain/temperature) lies in the medulla and upper spinal cord.

59. **What is the function of CN7?**
CN7 innervates the muscles of facial expression; supplies parasympathetic fibers to the lacrimal, submandibular, and sublingual glands; receives taste information from the anterior two-thirds of the tongue; and receives a minor sensory input from the skin of the external ear.

60. **How does the facial weakness that results from a CN7 lesion differ from that caused by a lesion of the facial motor area of the cerebral cortex?**
A CN7 lesion (as in Bell's palsy of CN7, which occurs in the facial nerve canal) results in ipsilateral facial paralysis, which includes the upper and lower face. A cerebral lesion results in contralateral facial paralysis confined to the lower face.

61. **What is Möbius syndrome?**
A congenital absence of both facial nerve nuclei, resulting in bilateral facial paralysis. The abducens nuclei may also be absent.

62. **What are the nucleus ambiguus, nucleus solitarius, and salivatory nucleus?**
   - The **nucleus ambiguus,** which lies in the medulla, is a motor nucleus (CNs 9 and 10) that innervates the deep throat (i.e., the muscles of swallowing [CN 9 and 10] and speech [CN10]).
   - The **nucleus solitarius** is a visceral sensory nucleus (CNs 7, 9, 10) that lies in the medulla. It receives input from the viscera as well as taste information. It is a relay in the gag reflex.
   - The **salivatory nucleus,** which contains superior and inferior divisions, innervates the salivary glands (CNs 7 and 9) and lacrimal glands (CN7).

63. **What does CN9 do?**
CN9, the glossopharyngeal nerve, innervates the stylopharyngeus muscle of the pharynx and the parotid gland. It receives taste information from the posterior one-third of the tongue, sensory tactile input from the posterior one-third of the tongue and the skin around the external ear canal, and sensory input from the carotid body and sinus.

64. **To which side does the tongue deviate if CN12 (hypoglossal nerve) is injured?**
The tongue deviates to the side of the lesion. Imagine you are riding a bicycle and your left hand becomes paralyzed. When you push on the handle bars, the wheel will turn to the left. The genioglossus muscle, which is innervated by CN12 and pushes out the tongue, operates on a similar principle.

65. **A patient has a neural deficit involving the extremities on one side but the face on the other side. Where is the lesion?**
The combination of a facial neural deficit on one side and an extremities deficit on the other suggests a brain stem lesion. The lesion cannot be below the brain stem because a cranial nerve is involved. The lesion cannot be above the brain stem because those lesions tend to cause strictly contralateral deficits.

CEREBRUM

66. **What does the frontal lobe do?**
Motor areas of the frontal lobe control **voluntary movement** on the opposite side of the body, including eye movement. The dominant hemisphere, usually the left, contains Broca's speech

area, which when injured results in motor aphasia (**language** deficit). Areas of the frontal lobe anterior to the motor areas are involved in complex **behavioral** and **executive** activities. Lesions here result in changes in judgment, abstract thinking, tactfulness, and foresight.

67. **What does the parietal lobe do?**
It receives contralateral light touch, proprioceptive, and pain sensory input. Lesions to the dominant hemisphere result in tactile and proprioceptive agnosia (complex receptive disabilities). There may also be confusion in left-right discrimination, disturbances of body image, and apraxia (complex cerebral motor disabilities caused by cutting off impulses to and from association tracts that interconnect with nearby regions).

68. **What effects do temporal lobe lesions have? Occipital lobe lesions?**
    - **Temporal lobe** lesions in the dominant hemisphere result in auditory aphasia. The patient hears but does not understand. He speaks but makes mistakes unknowingly because of an inability to understand his own words. Lesions may result in alexia and agraphia (inability to read and write).
    - Destruction of an **occipital lobe** causes blindness in the contralateral visual field. Lesions that spare the most posterior aspect of the occipital lobe do not cause blindness but cause difficulty in recognizing and identifying objects (visual agnosia). A region of the occipital lobe also controls involuntary eye movements to the contralateral side of the body.

CEREBRAL CIRCULATION

69. **Define the terms anterior and posterior cerebral circulation.**
    - The **anterior** circulation is the distribution of the internal carotid artery to the cerebrum via the anterior and middle cerebral arteries.
    - The **posterior** circulation is the distribution of the vertebral arteries to the stem, cerebellum, and cerebrum via the basilar artery and posterior cerebral artery.

70. **Which brain region is supplied by the anterior cerebral artery?**
The midline of the cerebrum, specifically, the frontal and parietal lobes and the superior portions of the temporal and occipital lobes.

71. **Which brain region is supplied by the middle cerebral artery?**
The lateral surface of the cerebrum, specifically, the frontal and parietal lobes and the superior portions of the temporal and occipital lobes (as is the case for the anterior cerebral artery).

72. **Which region is supplied by the posterior cerebral artery?**
The medial and lateral surface of the cerebrum, specifically, the inferior portions of the temporal and occipital lobes.

73. **What is the first branch of the internal carotid artery?**
The ophthalmic artery.

74. **Where does the brain stem get its blood supply?**
From the posterior circulation—namely, branches from the vertebral arteries (to the medulla) and branches from the basilar artery (to the pons and midbrain).

75. **What blood vessels supply the cerebellum?**
The cerebellar blood supply comes from branches of the basilar artery: the superior cerebellar, the anterior inferior cerebellar, and the posterior inferior cerebellar arteries.

76. **What is the blood supply of the thalamus and internal capsules?**
    The thalamus blood supply comes from branches of the circle of Willis (Fig. 3-4), including the lenticulostriate and choroidal arteries.

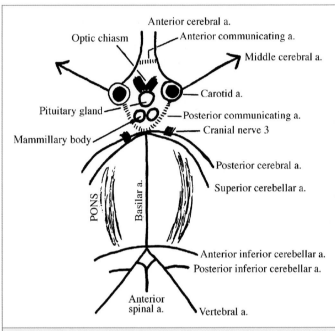

Figure 3-4. The circle of Willis. (From Goldberg S: Clinical Anatomy Made Ridiculously Simple, 2nd ed. Miami, MedMaster, 2001, www.medmaster.net.)

77. **Which vessels comprise the circle of Willis?**
    The anterior communicating artery, the two anterior cerebral arteries, the two middle cerebral arteries, the two posterior communicating arteries, and the two posterior cerebral arteries.

78. **Where does the spinal cord derive its blood supply?**
    The anterior spinal artery supplies the anterior two-thirds of the spinal cord. Two posterior spinal arteries supply the posterior third. Also, there are rich anastomoses from branches of the vertebral artery and aorta, so a stroke of the spinal cord is rare.

79. **A patient has sudden loss of vision in one eye, combined with contralateral paralysis. Where is the likely lesion?**
    The lesion most likely is in the internal carotid artery, affecting the ophthalmic artery on that side, as well as the ipsilateral brain, causing a contralateral paralysis.

CEREBROSPINAL FLUID

80. **Where is cerebrospinal fluid (CSF) produced?**
    It is produced by the choroid plexus, which may be found in the four ventricles of the brain.

81. **How much CSF is produced daily?**
    About 500 mL.

82. **How does the CSF flow through the brain?**
    The CSF flows from the two lateral ventricles (in the cerebral hemispheres), to the single midline third ventricle (between the right and left thalamus and hypothalamus), to the single midline fourth ventricle (which overlies the pons and medulla), through the foramina of Magendie and Luschka (in the fourth ventricle), to the subarachnoid space (the space between the pia and arachnoid membranes), which lies outside the brain. CSF leaves the subarachnoid space by filtering through the arachnoid granulations of the superior sagittal sinus, where the CSF joins the venous circulation.

83. **How do communicating and noncommunicating hydrocephalus differ?**
    In hydrocephalus, there is elevated CSF pressure and dilation of the ventricles secondary to obstruction to CSF flow:
    - In **communicating** hydrocephalus, the obstruction lies outside the ventricular system, beyond the foramina of Magendie and Luschka.
    - In **noncommunicating** hydrocephalus, obstruction occurs within the ventricular system before the foramina of Magendie and Luschka.

84. **Where is spinal fluid extracted during a spinal tap?**
    From the subarachnoid space between vertebrae L2 and S2. Normally, the fluid is extracted around vertebra level L4–L5.

WEBSITES

1. http://medstat.med.utah.edu/neurologicexam/html/home_exam.html

2. http://medstat.med.utah.edu/pedineurologicexam/html/home_exam.html

BIBLIOGRAPHY

1. Carpenter MB, Sutin J: Human Neuroanatomy. Baltimore, Williams & Wilkins, 1983.

2. Goldberg S: Clinical Neuroanatomy Made Ridiculously Simple, 2nd ed. Miami, MedMaster, 2001. Available at www.medmaster.net.

3. Haines DE: Neuroanatomy: An Atlas of Structures, Sections and Systems. Baltimore, Urban & Schwarzenberg, 1991.

4. Kandel ER, Schwartz JH, Jessell TM: Essentials of Neural Science and Behavior. Norwalk, CT, Appleton & Lange, 1995.

5. Martin JH: Neuroanatomy: Text and Atlas. Norwalk, CT, Appleton & Lange, 1996.

CHAPTER 4

NEUROPHYSIOLOGY AND COGNITIVE NEUROSCIENCE: FROM MEMBRANES TO FUNCTIONAL BRAIN NETWORKS

Gary Goldberg, MD, and Nachum Soroker, MD

To know the brain ... is equivalent to ascertaining the material course of thought and will, to discovering the intimate history of life in its perpetual duel with external forces.
—Santiago Ramon y Cajal (from *Recollections of My Life,* 1937)

The brain—is wider than the sky.
—Emily Dickinson (1830–1886)

1. **Explain the significance of neurophysiology and its relevance to rehabilitation.**
   Rehabilitation assesses function and treats disability. Because the lost function in many disabilities is a result of structural or physiologic impairment, all rehabilitation clinicians must have a basic understanding of normal anatomy and physiology. In Mountcastle's famous words, "Physiology is what transforms structure into action."

2. **How do neurons integrate and transmit information?**
   Via chemicals that are released at the **synapses**. These **neurotransmitters** either excite the postsynaptic neuron by depolarizing its membrane, thus creating an excitatory postsynaptic potential, or inhibit the neuron by hyperpolarizing the membrane, producing an inhibitory postsynaptic potential. The **action potential** created is conducted along the neuron's axon to other neurons via synaptic junctions.

3. **How does the voltage-dependent ion channel work to produce an action potential?**
   In neuronal and muscle specialized membrane (the neurolemma and sarcolemma, respectively), **voltage-dependent ion channels,** primarily for sodium and potassium, pop open transiently when the intracellular voltage drifts positive (i.e., the membrane depolarizes). At the threshold voltage, an explosive regenerative electrochemical process is initiated in which **voltage-dependent sodium channels** open in rapidly increasing numbers, and the transmembrane voltage rises sharply as sodium ions rush into the cell, producing a further rise in intracellular voltage and further depolarization of the cell membrane. The voltage levels off as sodium channels become less sensitive to the increased voltage and as **voltage-dependent potassium channels** open, allowing potassium to move out. The transmembrane voltage then reverses. The membrane becomes hyperpolarized for a short period called the **refractory period,** during which it is relatively resistant to excitation.

4. **What is an ectopic action potential?**
   An ectopic action potential is an *irregularly produced* action potential. Any problem with the membrane-based ion-exchange pump or the relative permeability of the membrane to any of the major ionic species can result in a major fluctuation of the resting membrane potential in nerve and muscle fibers. This fluctuation can lead to unconstrained depolarization of the membrane to the threshold level, resulting in spontaneous excitation and discharge of the membrane with the production of an aberrant, or ectopic, action potential.

5. **How do calcium ions participate in neural transmission?**
   When the action potential reaches the distal end of the axon at the presynaptic terminal, it initiates the flow of calcium ions into the presynaptic terminal through voltage-dependent calcium channels concentrated in the membrane at the presynaptic terminal. This causes a release of neurotransmitter from the presynaptic terminal, leading to excitation or inhibition of the postsynaptic cell membrane.

6. **What is a motor unit?**
   The motor unit is the *functional element of voluntary movement*. It consists of the anterior horn cell, motor axon, nerve terminals, neuromuscular junctions, and all the muscle fibers innervated by the anterior horn cell. The central nervous system activates the anterior horn cell, which in turn activates the muscle fibers in the motor unit to produce movement.

7. **How does the motor unit work?**
   The anterior horn cell typically controls several muscle fibers, ranging up to several thousand muscle fibers in a single motor unit. Each time the anterior horn cell fires, the end result is a **synchronous** twitch of all the muscle fibers in the motor unit. Tension is graded by recruiting additional motor units and by increasing the firing rate of the activated motor units in the available pool. The rate at which a motor unit starts firing when it is first recruited is called the **onset firing rate**. The rate at which a motor unit is firing when the next motor unit is recruited is called the **recruitment firing rate** or **recruitment frequency**.

KEY POINTS: MEMBRANE PUMPS

1. All membranes have a sodium-potassium ATP-dependent ion exchange pump that maintains relative electronegativity inside the cell at rest.

2. Only excitable membranes of nerve and muscle cells have voltage-dependent sodium and potassium channels to support action potential generation and conduction.

3. Muscle fibers normally contract only when "told to" by their innervating motor neuron. Spontaneous, autonomous fiber contraction is fibrillation and is abnormal.

8. **What are fibrillations and fasciculations?**
   In muscle fibers with defective membranes that "leak" sodium ions into the intracellular space, spontaneous membrane depolarization produces spontaneous generation of a muscle fiber action potential. This autonomous activation of a muscle fiber occurs when pathologic conditions either remove normal neural control over the muscle fiber or directly damage the muscle fiber membrane. This autonomous muscle fiber contraction is called a **fibrillation**.
   Electrical destabilization of the membrane of the motor neuron or motor axon leads to spontaneous generation of an ectopic nerve action potential, which is conducted to all muscle fibers innervated by the motor neuron. This results in a synchronous, isolated contraction of the fibers in the motor unit. This produces a visible twitch of the muscle called a **fasciculation**.

9. **Outline the parts and functions of the peripheral nervous system.**
   See Table 4-1.

10. **How are the sensory systems of the nervous system organized?**
    There are several major sensory systems in the brain: somatosensory, special visceral afferent (taste), vestibular, auditory, visual, and olfactory. The somatosensory system is divided into the

TABLE 4-1. COMPONENTS OF THE PERIPHERAL NERVOUS SYSTEM	
Structure	**Function**
Somatic	Controls voluntary movement
Afferent (sensory)	Transmits sensory information from periphery and surface (i.e., skin, muscles, joints) about the dynamic state of limbs, their articulation in space, and external environment
Efferent (motor)	Conducts voluntary motor control messages to skeletal muscle
Autonomic	Controls vegetative functions
Afferent	Receives sensory information about internal environment of body
Efferent	Sends control messages to smooth muscle of blood vessels, cardiac muscle, exocrine glands, and internal viscera
Parasympathetic	Maintains internal resources and internal homeostasis
Sympathetic	Involved in stress response and energy expenditure

lemniscal system, subserving epicritic sensations of light touch and vibration sense, and the spinothalamic system, subserving the protocritic sensations of pain and temperature. All systems, except for the olfactory system, transmit information to specialized regions of the thalamus.

11. **How are the extrathalamic ascending neuromodulatory systems organized?**
   In addition to the sensory system projections to the cerebral cortex, a number of widely projecting systems connect to the cerebral cortex directly from nuclei in the reticular core of the brain stem and midbrain. These extrathalamic ascending neuromodulatory systems are characterized by the major neurotransmitter that each system utilizes to modulate cortical activity. They are extremely important in controlling the overall excitability and responsiveness (or tone) of different parts of the cerebral cortex and are especially important in regulating levels of consciousness and the sleep-wake cycle. They are also involved in the regulation of mood and emotional states. Disruption of these systems is associated with the loss of consciousness that occurs with diffuse axonal injury to subcortical white matter in cranial trauma. Many neurotransmitter-based psychoactive medications function by influencing the operation of one or more of these major systems (Table 4-2).

12. **List the six major descending tracts from the brain.**
   The circuits in the spinal cord at the segmental level are controlled by the following descending tracts from the brain:
   1. Corticospinal tract (including lateral and ventral tracts), projecting from the cerebral cortex
   2. Vestibulospinal tract, projecting from the vestibular nuclei in the pons
   3. Medial reticulospinal tract, projecting from the pontine reticular formation
   4. Lateral reticulospinal tract, projecting from the medullary reticular formation
   5. Rubrospinal tract, projecting from the red nucleus in the midbrain
   6. Tectospinal tract, projecting from the superior colliculus in the tectum of the midbrain

13. **How does each of the different descending tracts affect muscle tone?**
   Each of the descending pathways has a different influence on the background tone and dynamic activation of motor neuron pools and interneuronal circuits in the spinal cord.

TABLE 4-2. MAJOR EXTRATHALAMIC NEUROTRANSMITTER SYSTEMS

Neurotransmitter	Major Source Nucleus	Typical Medication(s)
Acetylcholine	Nucleus basalis of Meynert	Benzotropine mesylate (antagonist), donepezil (agonist)
Dopamine	Substantia nigra (pars compacta), ventral tegmental area	D-Dopa, bromocriptine (agonists); droperidol (antagonists)
Norepinephrine	Locus coeruleus	Methylphenidate, nortriptyline (agonists)
Serotonin	Raphe nuclei	Fluoxetine, sertraline, escitalopram (agonists)

The **vestibulospinal** and **reticulospinal** tracts are involved in the postural biasing of muscles and anticipatory postural adjustments that precede voluntary movements. The vestibulospinal and reticulospinal output neurons are generally excitatory to extensor motor neurons, innervating extensor muscles in the arms and legs, and are under inhibitory control from the cortical level. The loss of cortical inhibitory control over these pathways tends to facilitate extensor tone in the arms and legs, resulting in **decerebrate rigidity**.

The **rubrospinal** and **corticospinal** tracts both tend to balance the extensor drive by facilitating drive to flexor muscles. The rubrospinal tract in humans extends only into the cervical cord and thus can counteract extensor drive in the arms but not the legs. The **decorticate rigidity** in humans with large cerebral hemisphere lesions is primarily one part of a net facilitation of flexors in the arms and extensors in the legs. This is because loss of descending control from the cerebral cortex releases unopposed excitatory extensor drive from the vestibular and reticular formation areas to the lower limb extensor muscles, while flexor facilitation is released from the red nucleus to upper limb flexor muscles in projections in the rubrospinal tract.

14. **What is the upper motor neuron syndrome?**
When there is dysfunction of the descending inputs to the spinal cord, there is a degrading of the dynamic control of the motor neurons, and the patterns of activation of muscles in a limb that form the basis of normal limb function become disordered. This combination of findings—changes in response to passive sustained and dynamic stretch, disinhibition of antigravity postural subroutines, and disordering of voluntary patterns of muscle activation—depends on the exact way in which the descending pathways have been affected by the damage. This combination of changes can be thought of as a type of disordered motor control or as a syndrome, the **upper motor neuron syndrome,** where the term "upper motor neuron" refers to any neuron in the central neuraxis that projects down to the spinal cord through one of the descending pathways or that influences the descending drive to the anterior horn cell.

15. **What parts of the nervous system are involved in the control of voluntary movement?**
The **motor cortex** is the cortical strip of the precentral gyrus. It is a somatotopically organized, electrically excitable region of the cerebral cortex. The motor cortex is involved in the execution of detailed aspects of voluntary fine movement, especially rapid, finely coordinated, "fractionated" movements of the fingers and toes.

Areas in the **parietal cortex** and **frontal cortex** (in the "premotor" cortex) are involved in translating the intent to act into more global aspects of the task, such as its timing, sequential linkage of different subtasks, trajectory through extrapersonal space, and coordination between postural stabilization and distal limb control in movement.

The **cerebellum** receives two inputs and has one output. One input, from the spinal cord, keeps the cerebellum informed about what is going on in the limbs. The second input outflows from the cortex, providing information about the intended action. The cerebellum generates output back to the cerebral cortex, adjusting the ongoing outflow of activity from the cortex. This circular loop involved in cerebellar circuitry is called a **re-entrant loop**, because the output re-enters the general part of the nervous system (the cerebral cortex) from which input originated.

The **basal ganglia** consist of the striatum (the caudate and putamen nuclei), the pallidal nuclei (the external and internal segments of the globus pallidus), and a set of nuclei in the midbrain, including the substantia nigra and subthalamic nucleus. The basal ganglia constitute a second, but differently connected, re-entrant loop with the cerebral cortex. Both the cerebellum and the basal ganglia reconnect to the cerebral cortex by way of distinct regions in ventral thalamus.

16. **What is the role of the cerebellum in the control of voluntary movement?**
The cerebellum is an important "meta-system" in voluntary motor control that enables *the refinement and fine-tuning of the details of motor performance* through dynamic modulation of outflows from the motor cortex. This is done by correcting "errors" detected between the sampled outflow from the motor cortex, which conveys the details of the *intended* movement, and the sensory input from the periphery, which conveys the details of the *actual* movement.

KEY POINTS: CEREBELLUM AND BASAL GANGLIA

1. Both the cerebellum and the basal ganglia operate through cortically re-entrant loops that begin and end at the cerebral cortex.

2. Outflows from cerebellum and the basal ganglia are relayed to cortex through distinct and separate regions of the ventral thalamus.

3. Cerebellar circuitry is set up to make fine-grained timing adjustments in corticospinal outflow to motor neuron pools in the spinal segments.

4. Basal ganglia is more involved in the selection and initiation of motor subroutines as well as adjustment of overall time scale of motor performance.

5. Both the basal ganglia and the cerebellum are important in different aspects of motor learning and procedural memory.

17. **What role does the basal ganglia play in voluntary movement?**
Whereas the cerebellum is involved in the control and coordination of precise timing relationships between activity in different muscles firing within a pattern, the basal ganglia seem to be involved in the *more global control of the timing of the pattern as a whole*—i.e., its relative expansion or compression in time. This may be closely related to the clocking of internal ultradian rhythms. The striatum receive widespread input from all over the cerebral cortex, and the output of the globus pallidus goes to a limited area of the thalamus connected to a very limited region of the premotor and supplementary motor areas. The striatum appears to be subdivided into segregated modules, each of which receives input from different subregions of the cerebral cortex, suggesting a highly modularized system of re-entrant loops.

18. **How does dopaminergic failure in the basal ganglia present clinically?**
Dysfunction of the dopaminergic system within the basal ganglia results in slowness of movement, impairment of initiation, and overall constriction of movement.

Dopamine acts as a promotor and energizer of movement by playing a role in the selective facilitation of specific movements. It may also serve as a controlling influence on an internal sense of time. Thus, patients with dopaminergic insufficiency associated with parkinsonism have problems with estimating time intervals and accurately reproducing time intervals presented to them.

19. **What features of the structural organization of the cerebral cortex reflect its bidirectional orientation toward the internal milieu and the external environment?**

   The structural organization of the cerebral cortex is adapted to provide responses for demands originating both in the internal milieu and in the external environment.

   - The hypothalamus plays a key role in maintaining various bodily physiologic measures within an accepted range (homeostasis). Structures within the limbic system (septum, substantia innominata, amygdala, piriform cortex, hippocampus) and paralimbic cortical areas (temporal pole, posterior orbitofrontal region, anterior insula, parahippocampal gyrus, cingulate gyrus) are closely related to this pole of cortical activity. These regions are important for evaluating the relative importance of sensory information, for the storage of information in memory, and for the regulation of emotional responses.
   - At the other end of the spectrum, highly differentiated areas of idiotypic cortex—the primary sensory areas dealing with visual, auditory, and somatosensory information (striate cortex of the calcarine sulcus, Heschl's gyri on the supratemporal plane, and the postcentral gyrus, respectively) and the primary motor area (in the precentral gyrus)—are in close connection with the external environment. These areas process afferent sensory information and act upon the environment or change the spatial position of the body within the environment.
   - Unimodal association areas of homotypical isocortex (visual, auditory, and somatosensory association areas adjacent to the respective primary sensory areas) enable complex integrated processing of information within each sensory modality and its evaluation in the light of earlier experience. Visual object recognition, face recognition, topographical orientation, recognition of auditory stimuli, and stereognosis are all functions subserved by unimodal association cortices. In addition, the lateral premotor and medial supplementary motor areas, forming the motor-association cortex, provide the neural substrate for motor programming.
   - Poorly differentiated heteromodal association areas of homotypical isocortex in the prefrontal, posterior parietal, and temporal cortical regions comprise a large part of the cortical mantle. The higher aspects of cognition and comportment are mediated by these regions of the cortex.

20. **What is the meaning of hemispheric dominance?**

   The term does not imply a state of overall dominance. Different brain functions are mediated predominantly by one hemisphere or the other.

   - For most right-handed persons, the left hemisphere (LH) plays a key (dominant) role in processing the core elements of language (phonology, lexical semantics, and syntax). Left-handed persons tend to have a more bilateral representation. In addition, the LH plays a dominant role in the organization of sequential voluntary movements.
   - The right hemisphere (RH) plays a dominant role in processing spatial relationships within and between objects, in the control of spatial attention, and in face recognition.
   - The mechanisms underlying the expression of hemispheric dominance for a given function involve inter-hemispheric inhibition. Besides this inhibitory activity, the two hemispheres interact in a cooperative and complementary manner. Within the basic spatiotemporal analysis of information characterizing all cognitive activity, the LH contributes dominantly to the temporal analysis and the RH to the spatial analysis. The global, holistic, parallel mode of RH information processing is complemented by the focal, analytic, serial processing mode on the left.

21. **What features characterize the cerebral organization of complex functions?**
Functional systems mediating complex behavior are based largely on the activity of interconnected cortical and subcortical structures forming distributed networks. These systems show substantial structural and functional interpersonal variance, and part or all of the following characteristics can be recognized in their organization:

- Bidirectional, corticostriatal connectivity, mediating the formation and activation of motor and cognitive procedures and skills.
- Bidirectional complementary modes of operation: sensory-driven (bottom-up) and data-driven (top-down). The massive cortical control of afferent transmission, which is exerted upon thalamic relay nuclei and other stations in the passage of sensory information, is one of the manifestations of top-down regulation.
- Modulation of stimulus-response relationships, enabling a flexible output of the system in the presence of a given input. The modulatory activity aims to produce an output that is adapted to the changing needs of the organism, the current general state, and the ongoing plans and goals.
- Different chemically defined systems for state-regulation (e.g., the cholinergic system of the basal forebrain, the serotoninergic system of the median raphe, the noradrenergic system of the nucleus locus coeruleus) modulate information processing in various special-purpose functional systems. The importance of this kind of modulatory activity is revealed in cases of neuro-chemical depletion, where deleterious effects are observed in various functional systems (e.g., in the case of ACh depletion in Alzheimer's disease).

22. **What are the major complex functional systems and what are their principal cortical components?**
According to Mesulam (2000), at least five large-scale networks can be identified in the human brain:

- **Spatial attention:** Epicenters in dorsal posterior parietal cortex, frontal eye fields, cingulate gyrus. RH dominance.
- **Language:** Epicenters in Wernicke's and Broca's areas. LH dominance.
- **Memory-emotion-motivation:** Epicenters in the hippocampo–entorhinal regions and the amygdaloid complex
- **Executive function-comportment:** Epicenters in lateral prefrontal cortex, orbitofrontal cortex, and posterior parietal cortex
- **Object and face identification:** Epicenters in lateral temporal and temporopolar cortices.

23. **What are the manifestations of damage in prefrontal cortex (PFC)? In what way do these manifestations reflect the functions of this cortical region?**
The PFC plays a key role in what are called "executive functions," comprising the higher aspects of behavior control. Working memory is an important element of PFC regulatory activity, helping to release the organism from "environmental dependency" (execution of primarily responsive stimulus-driven acts) and facilitating goal-directed activity.

- Damage to the dorsolateral prefrontal cortex causes executive behavior deficits: impaired data retrieval, set shifting, response inhibition, abstraction, creativity; loss of initiative, curiosity, foresight, planning; emotional blunting; slowing of thinking; apathy; loss of novelty-seeking behavior. This symptom complex is sometimes called frontal abulia.
- Damage to the orbitofrontal cortex causes primarily social behavior (conduct, comportment) deficits: disinhibited, tactless, impulsive behavior (frontal disinhibition).
- Damage to the medial prefrontal regions causes motivational behavior deficits: apathy, reduced interest and initiative, stimulus boundness (environmental dependency syndrome) with imitation and utilization behavior.

24. **What are the manifestations of left perisylvian damage, and in what ways do these manifestations reflect the functions of this cortical region?**

The cortical areas surrounding the Sylvian fissure on the left play a key role in language processing and praxis.

- Damage to the posterior-inferior frontal areas (largely Broca's area) causes speech production impairments, with phonological and syntactic processing deficits, as revealed in Broca's nonfluent aphasia and dysgrammatism.
- Damage to the posterior-superior temporal areas (largely Wernicke's area) causes speech comprehension deficits. When the processing of lexical semantics is impaired, the typical patient with Wernicke's aphasia will produce a fluent, sometimes logorrheic speech, full of verbal and phonological paraphasic errors and neologisms, which is incomprehensible to others.
- Damage to the inferior parietal regions is generally expressed in the form of acquired dyslexia, dyscalculia, ideomotor and ideational apraxia, and impaired auditory-verbal short-term memory.

25. **What are the manifestations of right perisylvian damage, and in what way do these manifestations reflect the functions of this cortical region?**

The cortical areas surrounding the Sylvian fissure on the right play a key role in spatial motor control, regulation of spatial attention, and processing of music and of prosody in speech. These areas seem to complement the activity of homologous LH regions in processing pragmatic aspects of interpersonal communication (e.g., humor, metaphors, irony, implicatures, indirect requests, speech acts).

- Damage to the posterior-inferior frontal areas may cause an expressive prosody impairment and some incompetence in pragmatics.
- Damage to the superior temporal region may cause a receptive prosody impairment and contribute to pragmatic incompetence. Patients with damage to this region may exhibit severe contralateral neglect.
- Damage to the inferior parietal region generally causes contralateral neglect. In addition to deficits in the control of spatial attention, impaired spatial motor control is revealed in the form of construction and dressing apraxia.

26. **What are the manifestations of damage to occipitotemporal and occipitoparietal regions? In what way do these manifestations reflect the functions of these cortical regions?**

The occipitoparietal and occipitotemporal regions are associated with the processing of "where" and "what" aspects of visual information. Damage to these areas impairs visual perception and visually guided behavior.

- Damage to the occipitotemporal regions causes impaired functioning of the "system of what" (ventral stream), as in the case of visual agnosia and prosopagnosia.
- Damage to the occipitoparietal regions causes impaired functioning of the "system of where" (dorsal stream), as in the case of optic ataxia and spatial neglect.

27. **What are the manifestations of damage to structures of the limbic system? In what way do these manifestations reflect the functions of the cortical regions?**

The limbic system plays a key role in the control of emotion, in the formation of long-term episodic and semantic memory, and in the control of motivational aspects of behavior and attentional selection.

- Damage to the amygdaloid complex causes impaired emotional behavior.
- Damage to the hippocampus, when bilateral and extensive, may cause severe protracted amnesia.
- Damage to the cingulate gyrus causes impaired motivational behavior and impaired attentional selection.

WEBSITES

1. www.neuroguide.com/

2. www.sfn.org/

3. www.waiting.com/brainfunction.html

BIBLIOGRAPHY

1. Deecke L, Eccles JC, Mountcastle VB (eds): From Neuron to Action: An Appraisal of Fundamental and Clinical Research. New York, Springer-Verlag, 1990.

2. Dieber MP, Passingham RE, Colebatch JG, et al: Cortical areas and the selection of movement: A study with positron emission tomography. Exp Brain Res 84:393–402, 1991.

3. Dumitru D: Electrodiagnostic Medicine, 2nd ed. Philadelphia, Hanley & Belfus, 2002.

4. Frackowiak RSJ, Weiller C, Chollet F: The functional anatomy of recovery from brain injury. In Chadwick DJ, Whelan J (eds): Exploring Brain Functional Anatomy with Positron Tomography (CIBA Foundation Symposium 163). New York, Wiley, 1991, pp 235–249.

5. Gazzaniga MS (ed): The New Cognitive Neurosciences, 2nd ed. Cambridge, MA, MIT Press, 2000.

6. Gazzaniga MS, Ivry RB, Mangum GR: Cognitive Neuroscience: The Biology of Mind, 2nd ed. New York, Norton, 2002.

7. Glenn WB, Whyte J (eds): The Practical Management of Spasticity in Adults and Children. Philadelphia, Lea & Febiger, 1990.

8. Goldberg G: From intent to action: Evolution and function of the premotor systems of the frontal lobe. In Perecman E (ed): The Frontal Lobes Revisited. New York, IRBN Press, 1987, pp 273–306.

9. Goldberg G: Neurophysiologic models of recovery in stroke. Phys Med Rehabil Clin North Am 2:599–614, 1991.

10. Goldberg G: Premotor systems, attention to action and behavioral choice. In Kien J, McCrohan CR, Winslow W (eds): Neurobiology of Motor Programme Selection. New York, Pergamon Press, 1992, pp 225–249.

11. Jenkins WM, Merzenich MM, Ochs MT, et al: Functional reorganization of primary somatosensory cortex in adult owl monkeys after behaviorally controlled tactile stimulation. J Neurophysiol 63:82–104, 1990.

12. Kandel ER, Schwartz JH, Jessel TM (eds): Principles of Neural Science, 4th ed. New York, McGraw-Hill, 2000.

13. Mesulam MM (ed): Principles of Behavioral and Cognitive Neurology, 2nd ed. Oxford, Oxford University Press, 2000.

14. Pastor MA, Atreida J, Jahanshahi M, Obeso JA: Time estimation and reproduction is abnormal Parkinson's disease. Brain 115:211–225, 1992.

15. Patton HD, Fuchs AF, Hille B, et al (eds): Textbook of Physiology: Vol. 1. Excitable Cells and Neurophysiology, 21st ed. Philadelphia, W.B. Saunders, 1989.

16. Posner MI, Raichle ME: Images of Mind. New York, Scientific American Library, 1994.

17. Raichle ME, Fiez JA, Videen TO, et al: Practice-related changes in human brain functional anatomy during non-motor learning. Cerebral Cortex 4:8–26, 1994.

II. PERSON-CENTERED CARE

COMMUNICATION STRATEGIES FOR REHABILITATION MEDICAL PROFESSIONALS: DISABILITY ETIQUETTE AND EMPOWERMENT MEDICINE

Margaret G. Stineman, MD, Ashley E. Kurz, BA, Harlan Hahn, PhD, and Steven A. Stiens, MD, MS

We reject the notion that we need "experts" to tell us how to live, especially experts from the able-bodied world. We are not diagnoses in need of a cure or cases to be closed. We are human, with human dreams and ambitions.

—JR Woodward, *A Disabled Manifesto*

1. **How is disability etiquette important in communication?**

   Etiquette refers to being polite and courteous to all people, including those with disabilities. Beyond this, disability etiquette puts the humanity of the person first and any disabilities second. Any disability etiquette principle that implies dominance and subordination is incompatible with the principle of equality and must be rejected. People with disabilities have the same needs for respect, dignity, and autonomy as anyone else.

   Cohen J: Disability Etiquette. Jackson Heights, NY, Eastern Paralyzed Veterans Association, 1998.

2. **How does communication accomplish the best outcome?**

   The establishment of an optimal patient-physician relationship requires interest and sensitivity. Effective listening and perceptive questioning lead to positive patient encounters. Each person has a unique perspective and experience of disablement, and understanding that perspective is essential for collaborative rehabilitation processes. Maximal success is accomplished by designing a rehabilitation plan that leads to functional and social recovery in a sequence that empowers the patient to be independent in accomplishing his or her broader life goals. Thus, regardless of disability, whenever possible, speak directly to the patient rather than through family or companions. It is essential to hear and formulate an understanding of the patient as a person. This evolving person-first approach must be celebrated by the entire rehabilitation team.

3. **What is empowerment medicine?**

   Empowerment medicine is the process of giving power to the patient to reestablish life, self-concept, and autonomy. The goal of empowerment medicine is to use medical knowledge to increase the freedom, awareness, and civil rights of those with disabilities. Through a reciprocal patient-physician exchange, patients explain their goals and values, while working with physicians to reduce physical, attitudinal, and societal barriers to achievement. Ultimately, this type of an approach to treatment helps the patient gain maximal control over his or her life. This process captures the patient's values, reducing physical, attitudinal, and societal barriers. As the acute phase of injury or illness subsides, a return to personal autonomy is sought for the patient through simultaneous rehabilitation and removal of environmental barriers. While emphasis on pathology and its treatment remains essential to the medical management of acute injury and illness, this approach alone is too narrow for long-term disabilities.

Hahn H: An agenda for citizens with disabilities: Pursuing identity and empowerment. J Voc Rehabil 9(1):31–37, 1997.

Nosek MA: Women with disabilities and the delivery of empowerment medicine. Arch Phys Med Rehabil 78(12 Suppl 5):S1–S2, 1997.

Stineman MG: Medical humanism and empowerment medicine. Disabil Stud Q 20(1):11–16, 2000.

4. **How does empowerment medicine relate directly to communication with patients?**

Empowerment medicine leads to a greater depth of communication, providing the patient with the optimal medical information necessary for him or her to make informed choices that will maximize quality of life. It is the opposite of patriarchal medicine and is intended to increase trust by sharing between the patient and clinician. This increased trust can positively affect how patients view themselves, their lives, and their futures, thus positively influencing patient outcomes.

5. **What stimulated the development of empowerment medicine?**

People with disabilities are viewed by some as pathetic, helpless victims who are useless to society. As a result of this stigma, people with disabilities develop attitudinal barriers, and medical goals are aimed at normalization. These attitudes create some of the most restrictive barriers that people with disabilities face. This devaluation of people with disabilities and stigmatization of pathology led to the ideas put forth by the **independent living movement** and exemplified in the *Disabled Manifesto* (excerpt at the beginning of this chapter).

The best way for clinicians to become familiar with the problems faced by people with disabilities (as well as other oppressed and disadvantaged segments of the population) is to study their history, their culture, and the discriminatory barriers they face. Effective clinicians develop the fullest understanding of patient problems by seeking knowledge about successful adaptation techniques from people with disabilities who are successful. Through disability studies, role playing, and exposure of clinical trainees to people with disabilities who live full lives, a more realistic perspective emerges.

DeJong G: Health care reform and disability: Affirming our commitment to community. Arch Phys Med Rehabil 74:1017–1024, 1993.

6. **What is the independent living movement?**

Like the civil rights and equal rights movements of the 1960s, the independent living movement in the 1970s led to major changes in the way people with disabilities are viewed. The movement was developed primarily by young people with disabilities wanting to be respected as equal members of society. The movement challenges health care providers to re-evaluate the way we relate and connect with patients. The dignity of persons with disabilities must be honored at all times, and they must be integrated into society as self-determining contributors. The passage of the Americans with Disabilities Act (ADA) gives people with disabilities rights to pursue and participate in socially meaningful activities. Ideas embodied within the movement declare that people with disabilities have the right to live in the least restrictive setting possible of their choice. The movement confirmed that life in a community is preferable to that in an institution. The ADA and federally funded independent living centers support these values. The independent living movement celebrated the dignity and individuality of each person with a disability as a self-determining contributor, integrated into society.

Batavia IA: Independent living centers, medical rehabilitation and managed care for people with disabilities. Arch Phys Med Rehabil 80:1357–1360, 1999.

Cohen J: Disability Etiquette. Jackson Heights, NY, Eastern Paralyzed Veterans Association, 1998.

U.S. House of Representatives. Americans With Disabilities Act of 1990. Public Law 101–336, July 25, 1990, 104 Stat.327.

Woodward JR: A Disabled Manifesto: http://www.empowermentzone.com/manifest.txt

7. **What are some publications outside the medical literature that are important for understanding how people with disabilities live?**

To be an effective communicator, the physiatrist needs to be familiar with a basic disability studies bibliography and to remain current with prominent disability issues as reported in magazines such as *Mouth, New Mobility,* and *Ragged Edge.* Knowledge of disability studies will enhance clinical skills, forge a deeper connection with patients, and make it possible for health professions to recommend readings to people with disabilities that can provide valuable sources of meaning and purpose in their lives.

Mouth. A bimonthly magazine usually only in print, but excerpts are available online at: http://www.mouthmag.com/

New Mobility. A magazine available in print or online at: http://www.newmobility.com/

Ragged Edge magazine online: http://www.ragged-edge-mag.com/

8. **Are there any tools for enhancing the depth and meaningfulness of communication with patients?**

Recovery preference explanation (RPE) is an emerging technology based on the Features Resource Trade-Off Game. It is intended to enhance the quality, depth, and meaningfulness of discourse among patients, family members, and clinicians. Patients or family members are first introduced to the Functional Independence Measure (FIM) or other set of functional status items to be addressed in therapy. Next, they are asked to imagine complete disability in all items and to show patterns of optimal recovery, assuming they could control all aspects of their recovery. See "Game Board" and instructions in the citations below.

Stineman MG, Maislin G, Nosek M, Fiedler R, Granger CV: Comparing consumer and clinician values for alternative functional states: Application of a new features trade-off Consensus Building Tool. Arch Phys Med Rehabil 79(12):1522–1529, 1998.

Stineman MG, Ross RN, Maislin G, et al: Recovery preference explanation. Am J Phys Med Rehabil 2007, in press.

Stineman MG, Wechsler B, Ross R, Maislin G: A method for measuring quality of life through subjective weighting of functional status. Arch Phys Med Rehabil 84(1):S15–S22, 2003.

9. **How have Health Insurance Portability and Accountability Act (HIPAA) regulations affected communication with patients?**

HIPAA prohibits the disclosure of a patient's personal health information for any purpose unless the individual has signed and authorized this disclosure. Furthermore, a patient has the right to restrict disclosure of his or her health information from individuals such as family members. These regulations can put limitations on communication between health care providers, patients, and families and can compromise care.

HIPAA: Notice of Privacy Practices: http://www.hhs.gov/ocr/hipaa/finalreg.html

10. **A barrier to open discourse: Why do some people with disabilities object to being referred to as "patients?"**

A number of individuals with disabilities do not like to be called "patients." They believe the word inherently implies too much passivity and subordination. Some health care systems have chosen the term "person served," "consumer," or "client" to reinforce their participation as the prime beneficiary of services. It is inappropriate to refer to people living with fixed impairments that are not under treatment as "patients."

11. **What is the difference between disability and illness?**

The concept of being "a patient" is seen by some people with disabilities as permanent confinement to the "sick role." The sick role, as defined by Parsons, involves people's exemption from ordinary social obligations in exchange for the promise that they will follow medical directives without questions and devote themselves exclusively to the goal of "getting well." As is the case with most disabilities (almost by definition), objectives that imply cure in the context of getting well are not always realistic. People with disabilities are not necessarily ill.

Parsons T: The sick role and the role of the physician reconsidered. Milbank Mem Fund Q Health Soc 53:257–258, 1975.

12. **What is person-first language?**

Language and the images it promotes mirror attitudes toward particular groups of people. When communicating with or about people with disabilities, most (but not all) people with disabilities argue that it is essential to use **person-first language** (Table 5-1) and to avoid focusing on the disability before recognizing the person. Saying, "person with a disability" or "person who uses a wheelchair" re-contextualizes the relationship rather than defining the person with these characteristics. Also, avoid using "normal" as the opposite of disabled. "Normal" implies that people with disabilities are not normal. Use "nondisabled" or "persons without disabilities."

Young MA, Morgan SB: Strategies for fostering communication between physician and patients with disabilities. Wis Med J 96:36–37, 1997.

Messiah College: Disability related language. Grantham, PA, Messiah College, 1999: http://www.messiah.edu/disability/terms.htm

United Nations ESCAP: Asian Pacific Decade of Disabled. Persons 1993–2002. Using the correct terminology, 1999: http://www.unescap.org/decade/terminology.htm

Woodward JR: A Disabled Manifesto: http://www.empowermentzone.com/manifest.txt

13. **What are the pitfalls to be avoided in communicating about people with disabilities?**

The Life Span Institute guidelines for "Reporting and Writing about People with Disabilities" recommends avoiding terminology that is not person-first:

- Do not focus on disability to the exclusion of the person's capabilities.

TABLE 5-1. PERSON–FIRST TERMINOLOGY

Poor Terms	Better Terms	Explanation
Cerebral-palsied	Has cerebral palsy	Use person-first, nonemotional language that describes the condition.
Cripple, invalid	Has a disability	
Paralytic	Has paralysis or is paralyzed	
Hunchback	Person with spinal curvature	
Wheelchair bound/confined	Uses a wheelchair	Wheelchairs are liberating to people with severe walking impairments.
Home bound/confined	Is limited by barriers outside the home	People are not tied to the device. Homes should be places of refuge and hopefully comfort.
Physically challenged	Has limitation in activity	
Afflicted/victim	Simply state that the person has a particular condition.	The terms *disabled* and *handicapped* are still accepted by many but are being replaced by more neutral terms.
Normal or healthy	People without disabilities or nondisabled	Avoid "tragic" but "brave" and "courageous" stereotypes.
		Emphasize abilities, but do not describe successful people with disabilities as "superhuman."
		Avoid terms that imply serious misfortune and emotional disability.

- Use of the term wheelchair-bound does not portray the mobility-enhancing effect of that adaptive tool.
- Do not portray successful people with disabilities as superheroes or necessarily extraordinary.
- Do not sensationalize disability by referring to the person as afflicted with, crippled with, victim of, or suffers with the illness or diagnosis.
- Do not use euphemisms such as physically inconvenienced or physically challenged.
- Do not use generic labels generalizing about groups such as the deaf or retarded.
- Do not imply active disease processes when not present. If persons live with fixed impairments that are not under treatment, use of the term *patient* is not appropriate.

http://www.lsi.ku.edu/lsi/internal/guidelines.html

14. **What terminology is recommended when writing about people with disabilities?**

Use **person-first language** in the descriptions. For example, use "person living with HIV," "person who is blind," or "person who uses a wheelchair." The term "nondisabled" is most appropriate for those without disabilities. Less appropriate are "normal," "able-bodied," "temporarily able-bodied," "healthy," or "whole." Portrayal of people with disabilities should emphasize their capabilities.

15. **Are there any classifications of functioning and disability that are consistent with person-first concepts?**

The World Health Organization's International Classification of Functioning, Disability and Health (ICF) is a common language for describing health and health-related states. In reflection of the need to de-emphasize pathology, the ICF focuses on how an individual's health state affects his or her ability to execute important tasks and participate in life situations.

World Health Organization: International Classification of Functioning, Disability, and Health. Geneva, Switzerland, WHO 2001.

16. **What are some possible biasing effects of medical training?**

Pathology-focused training tends to encourage physicians to see cure as success and chronic disease and progressive disability as failure. Physicians often focus on pathology to the detriment of the patient's function. A functional review of systems provides patients with excellent opportunities to openly discuss concerns about their disabilities. It should include activities of daily living (ADLs), instrumental activities of daily living (IADLs), mobility and environmental barriers, and facilitators. **RPE** (see previous discussion) provides a way to communicate the meaning of the functional limitations disclosed.

World Health Organization: International Classification of Functioning, Disability, and Health. Geneva, Switzerland, WHO, 2001.

17. **What are masked concerns in communication?**

Masked concerns occur when the patient describes one symptom, feeling, or condition that is related to but not representing the primary complaint. Sometimes patients raise issues explicitly—noting difficulty getting out of the house for social occasions or excessive fatigue. Digging deeper, the professional might find that the patient fears falling (because of weakness), is limited in ambulatory endurance by severe arthritic pain, or will not leave for fear of incontinence.

18. **How should the physiatrist balance short- and long-term goals in facilitating treatment by the interdisciplinary team?**

The realities of practice today may leave insufficient time to personally follow all problems through to their optimal resolution at each clinical encounter or admission. This makes timely and appropriate referral to other rehabilitation providers essential.

A complete and individualized problem list should be maintained and balanced with constant awareness of the patient's life passions and aspirations. Understanding of all these aspects contributes to a more holistic approach, even in a short problem-focused visit. By talking with the patient about the outcomes of referral at the next visit, the physiatrist provides continuity of care and closure. Mundane aspects of care, such as exercise or testing, need to be linked through conversation with the life goals that drive the patient's compliance.

19. **What are some special issues with regard to communicating with people with life-long disabilities?**
Recognize and respect the lessons of long-life experience. People are the experts on their own unique life methods, personal histories, and goals. Make them your teachers. Recognize and express your appreciation for and interest in the way they solve problems and how they have adapted. Ask them to teach you how they decided on various adaptive equipment and techniques. People with life-long disabilities have the opportunity to incorporate disablement experiences into their self-concept. They have the benefit of an entire lifetime to sharpen their skills. Yet they remain at a potential disadvantage in communicating with others who have had the experiences that people without disabilities share.

20. **How can patients empower the physiatrist?**
Some unique experiences of life with disability can result in creative solutions that escape the attention of people who are able-bodied. Yet many people have difficulty living independently in a society designed for those with average capacity. Nevertheless, if disability is regarded as an *experience* rather than a source of pathology, it can provide a different perspective that is enriching and can lead to innovation. When a physician acknowledges these creative responses, the therapeutic bond is strengthened, giving the physician an opportunity to learn and grow with the patient.

21. **What are some special issues in communicating with the person who becomes disabled later in life?**
People with disabilities are a minority that anyone is eligible to join at any time. Fortunately, people who become disabled later in life have the benefit of knowing how society works and have had the opportunity to develop their social skill sets as able-bodied people. Yet they carry the burden of knowing what it is like to live without disability. The process of facing and living with the real and often extreme changes in their lives can be overwhelming or depressing. The health professional, through his or her communications with the individual, has the opportunity to lead them toward autonomy and away from more self-destructive feelings. Frame these challenges positively, and facilitate successful adaptation and life role performance.

22. **How can I communicate effectively with a person who uses crutches, a wheelchair, or is in bed?**
The patient and physician should both feel comfortable and respect each other's personal space. People who use wheelchairs live below the eye level of average-sized standing adults. Even positioned in the full view of others, those with disabilities are commonly ignored. Communication is facilitated by being at the person's eye level. Sitting down goes a long way in establishing contact. People without disabilities need to be conscious of their gait speed while accompanying a person using crutches or a manual wheelchair. The best situation for communication is to be comfortably physically close to one another with respect for the other person's personal space. When walking with someone using an assistive device for gait, allow them space and let them set the pace. Use eye contact from the side and invite them to sit with you and talk. For those in a wheelchair or a bed, sit or kneel on one knee beside them. If the conversation lasts for longer than a few minutes, find some place to sit comfortably so that they know you are comfortable. Pull up a chair to be at eye level with them.

Iezzoni LI: What should I say? Communication around disability. Ann Intern Med 129:661–665, 1998.

23. **How do you communicate the need for assistive technology in a positive manner?**
    Some health professionals loathe discussing the need for a wheelchair or other type of assistive technology because of its association with infirmity and loss. Present the wheelchair or other device to the patient as an adaptive tool used to meet life goals rather than as a symbol of infirmity. The wheelchair can help return lost mobility. Appearance is key. Encourage the patient to select elegant features. The appropriate wheelchair can open life to new possibilities, give tremendous relief, and provide wonderful liberation from a restricted circumstance.

24. **If you believe a person with physical disabilities may need help getting into your office, undressing, or getting onto your examination table, how should you approach this need?**
    Ask the individual if he or she would like some help. Put the individual in charge and enable him or her. Respect the person's answers. Unless the circumstance clearly warrants quick action to avoid injury, do not provide physical assistance unexpectedly to a person who is already walking or standing. Never assume that a person needs help just because he or she has some visible physical disabilities.

    Iezzoni LI: What should I say? Communication around disability. Ann Intern Med 129:661–665, 1998.
    United Nations ESCAP. Asian Pacific Decade of Disabled Persons 1993–2002. Using the correct terminology, 1999. Available: http://www.unescap.org/decade/terminology.htm

KEY POINTS: COMMUNICATION STRATEGIES

1. The disablement experience of each person is a unique resource for that person and those caring for that person.

2. Communication is the exercise of the therapeutic encounter and results in mutually understood and attainable goals.

3. Empowerment medicine is the process of recognition of patients' personhood and full enablement of their capabilities and life roles.

4. The independent living movement defined and manifested the rights of all to live in the least restrictive setting possible.

5. Empowerment medicine utilizes the therapeutic relationship to reestablish patients' self-concept, autonomy, life roles, and their unique contribution to society.

25. **What are some common pitfalls in examining people with disabilities?**
    Doing an examination while a patient remains in a wheelchair can lead to a suboptimal pulmonary, abdominal, musculoskeletal, and neurological assessment compared to a person who is disrobed on an examining table. Determining the degree to which the person is able to stand, walk, and move around on the examination table is an essential part of the examination. Of course, if the patient has serious mobility difficulties, take appropriate safety precautions. Ask the patient whether he or she can stand and transfer onto the examination table. Ask patients to explain how they do it, how much help they need, and how difficult it is. This communication ahead of time will help plan transfers and avoid unsafe situations. It is also a good way to check the patient's insight and safety awareness.

26. **What is the "lump syndrome?"**
    In hospitals, medical equipment, food or laundry carts, and people sitting in wheelchairs or lying on litters are all hauled about and left sitting in corridors for future transport. Never begin pushing patients in wheelchairs or on litters without greeting them and saying where you are

taking them and asking if they need assistance. Never leave a person sitting somewhere without an explanation. State where they are and why you are parking them there. Introduce them to someone in that environment, a receptionist or a nurse. Thoughtful gestures take little time and go a long way. For example, "Would it be okay to leave you here in the waiting room until transportation comes for you? This is Wilma, the receptionist. She can call if they need a reminder," or "Would you like a magazine to read?" Remember, some people who use wheelchairs are stuck where you leave them. Effective and thoughtful positioning and communication prevent the lump syndrome.

27. **What is "the shock response"? How can the health professional guard against this normal response to unexpected or unusual pathology?**
   The **shock response** occurs when the professional is distracted by the most visible or unusual aspects of the patient's job, life role, history, or physical presentation. This can eclipse recognition of more important symptoms, signs, and other patient attributes in a way that may negatively influence treatment. The best ways to avoid the shock response are to listen to the patient, look at all aspects of the person, and evaluate the person's presentation. Physicians should always begin by addressing the same fundamentals as with any other patient, seeking guidance when necessary (as with any patient). If the patient brings up the characteristic in question, frankly request the patient's opinion, then address the characteristic as it relates to achievement of the patient's goals.

28. **Is it normal to have negative responses to or feel uncomfortable around people with some types of disabilities or problems?**
   Yes. Most people resist the suggestion that they might harbor negative emotions. By confronting and analyzing such feelings directly, rehabilitation professionals will be better able to prevent them from emerging inadvertently in their interactions with people. It is important for all clinicians to have close friendships with a few peers in order to discuss such responses and share their honest impressions and feelings in a confidential manner.

29. **What are invalidating responses and turn-offs?**
   The first step in an effective therapeutic interaction requires suspension of judgment in order to allow the fullest communication from the patient's perspective. Invalidating statements arise from partial truths, when the clinician judges (prejudges) the patient through the misuse or misperception of some bit of history or medical information. By responding with opinions or invalidating statements, nonspecific medical knowledge is used in ways that are insensitive or distorted or that fails to address the full circumstances of the patient's life. The "turn-off" occurs after the physician has alienated or embarrassed the patient in such a way that he or she no longer wants to communicate about an important issue or need. These interactions can have detrimental and lasting impressions on patients and hinder successful patient communication and rehabilitation.

   Iezzoni LI: What should I say? Communication around disability. Ann Intern Med 129:661–665, 1998.

30. **Give an example of an invalidating response.**
   Invalidation occurs when the physician has a faulty perception of how a disease is influencing a person's abilities or makes a broad generalization and then expresses it in a way that causes the patient to have nagging and inappropriate self-doubts. Invalidation is a conversation stopper. One example is attributing a legitimately cheerful mood to the "inappropriate euphoria of MS."

31. How can invalidating responses be avoided?

Use medical knowledge to positively support and empower the patient. This requires creativity, the ability to listen, and the ability to see beyond medical aspects to the humanity of the person. It is essential to use medical knowledge to empower and not to tear down the patient. Avoid conflicts with the patient that pit "medical knowledge" against the patient's "knowledge of him- or herself." Again, see the person as separate from the processes of his or her diseases and disabilities. Remember that disability-experienced disablement is not the same as being sick, experiencing symptoms, or living through a finite illness.

Albrecht C, Seelman K, Bury M: The Handbook of Disability Studies. Thousand Oaks, CA, Sage Publishers, 2001.

CHAPTER 6

REHABILITATION OF PATIENTS WITH SEVERE VISUAL OR HEARING IMPAIRMENTS: INNOVATIONS FOR PERSON-CENTERED FUNCTION

Stanley F. Wainapel, MD, MPH, J. Michael Anderson, MD, and Mouli Madhab Ghat

All our knowledge has its origins in our perceptions.

–Leonardo da Vinci (1452–1519)

1. What are common causes of visual impairment?
- Older adults: cataract, glaucomal, age-related macular degeneration, diabetic retinopathy
- Young/middle-aged adults: diabetic retinopathy, retinitis pigmentosa
- Children: congenital (cataract, albinism), prematurity, or neurologic disease (retinopathy of prematurity, anoxic or postinfectious cortical vision loss)

  http://www.eyesite.ca/7modules/Module7/html/Mod7Sec1.html

2. How are visual impairments classified nationally and internationally?
In the United States, legal blindness is defined as:
- Corrected visual acuity of 20/200 or less in the better eye, or
- A visual field of 20 degrees or less in the better eye.

  Low vision includes corrected acuity between 20/70 and 20/200 or visual fields exceeding 20 degrees. The World Health Organization (WHO) defines low vision as corrected acuity between 6/24 and 3/60, equivalent to 20/80 and 20/400, respectively.

3. Does visual impairment affect physical function?
Visual impairment in older people produces deficits in basic and instrumental activities of daily living (ADLs) and can be associated with increased risk of falls and resulting hip fractures.

  Branch LG, Horowitz A, Carr C: The implications for everyday life of incident self-reported visual decline among people over age 65 living in the community. Gerontologist 29:359–365, 1989.
  Carabellese C, Apollonio I, Rozzini R, et al: Sensory impairment and quality of life in a community elderly population. J Am Geriatr Soc 41:401–407, 1993.
  Felson DT, Anderson JJ, Hannah MT, et al: Impaired vision and hip fracture: The Framingham Eye Study. J Am Geriatr Soc 37:495–500, 1989.

4. How can patients gain access to vision rehabilitation services?
An ophthalmologic evaluation documenting the degree of vision loss is sent to a state agency for the blind/visually impaired, which authorizes low vision, vision rehabilitation, and vocational rehabilitation services.

5. Describe the two basic strategies of vision rehabilitation.
Vision enhancement uses devices or techniques that maximize the utility of any remaining visual function, whereas vision substitution uses technology or techniques that do not require any vision at all.

DiStefano AF, Aston SJ: Rehabilitation of the blind and visually impaired elderly. In Brody SL, Ruff DL (eds): Aging and Rehabilitation: Advances in the State of the Art. New York, Springer Publishing, 1986.

6. **What are some vision enhancement techniques?**
   They can be remembered with the mnemonic **IMAGE:**
   - **I** = **I**llumination
   - **M** = **M**agnification
   - **A** = **A**ltered contrast
   - **G** = **G**lare reduction
   - **E** = **E**xpanders of visual field

7. **Classify the common vision substitution techniques into related groups.**
   - **Mobility:** Cane, guide dog, sonic devices
   - **Tactile:** Braille books/devices, raised markings
   - **Recorded:** Talking books, radio reading services
   - **Synthetic speech:** Computers with verbal output, talking watches/calculators, Newsline for the Blind (newspapers via telephone)
   - **Computer-generated vision systems**
   - **Special ADL techniques:** Cooking, money identification

8. **Name some visual enhancement aids for the person with low vision.**
   - **Optical aids:** Magnifiers (hand-held, stand-alone, illuminated), telescopic lenses (monocular or binocular), closed-circuit television videomagnifier computer software providing magnification, reverse telescopic lenses, Fresnel prisms, or mirrors mounted on glasses for field expansion
   - **Nonoptical aids:** Appropriate lighting, visors, tinted glasses, heightened color contrast (e.g., bold print pens, paper with extra-thick lines, white-on-black, reversal images for slides)

   Faye EE: Clinical Low Vision. Boston, Little, Brown, 1984.
   Wainapel SF, Bernbaum M: Rehabilitation of the patient with visual impairment. In DeLisa JA, Gans BM (eds): Physical Medicine and Rehabilitation: Principles and Practice, 4th ed. Philadelphia, W.B. Saunders, 2005, pp 1891–1905.

9. **How can computers help visually impaired people?**
   Computers with synthetic speech output, screen reading software, optical character recognition software/scanner, Braille output, or voice-activated operation enhance informational and professional opportunities for people unable to read ordinary-sized print, allowing them to use the Internet and other computer programs. This includes access to the Internet, e-mail, and word-processing functions.

10. **What are the functional outcomes in patients with combined visual and neuromusculoskeletal disabilities?**
    They are surprisingly good, particularly when vision loss preceded the more familiar physiatric diagnosis. In a study of 12 blind amputees, 75% became functional prosthetic users, and blind stroke patients have had similar results in inpatient settings.

    Altner PE, Rusin JJ, De Boer A: Rehabilitation of blind patients with lower extremity amputations. Arch Phys Med Rehabil 61:82–85, 1980.
    Wainapel SF: Rehabilitation of the blind stroke patient. Arch Phys Med Rehabil 65:487–489, 1984.
    Wainapel SF, Kwon YS, Fazzari PJ: Severe visual impairment on a rehabilitation unit: Incidence and implications. Arch Phys Med Rehabil 70:439–441, 1989.

11. **Who pays for vision rehabilitation services?**
    Usually they are covered through a state Commission for the Blind rather than by standard third-party payers such as Medicare and Medicaid. Some occupational and/or physical therapists

have vision rehabilitation services. Under these circumstances services have been reimbursed.

12. **Where can patients get more information on vision rehabilitation resources?**
American Foundation for the Blind
11 Penn Plaza, Suite 300
New York, NY 10001
212-502-7600
800-232-5463
www.afb.org
National Federation of the Blind
1800 Johnson Street
Baltimore, MD 21230
410-659-9314
www.nfb.org
National Library Service for the Blind and Physically Handicapped
1291 Taylor Street NW
Washington, DC 20542
800-424-8567
www.loc.gov/nls
Council of Citizens with Low Vision International
5707 Brockton Drive, #302
Indianapolis, IN 46220
800-733-2258
317-254-1155
www.cclvi.org
Resources for Rehabilitation
33 Bedford Street, Suite 19A
Lexington, MA 02173
617-862-6455
Lighthouse International
111 East 59 Street
New York, NY 10021
212-821-9200
www.lighthouse.org

13. **How many people have hearing impairments?**
Hearing problems affect over 20 million people in the United States, and a minimum of 12 million have hearing loss sufficient to produce functional limitations. Over 2 million Americans are either totally deaf or lack sufficient hearing to understand speech.

14. **When is hearing loss a rehabilitation problem?**
Difficulty hearing impairs communication, education, the exchange of ideas, carrying out of orders, and the pure pleasure of listening and responding. A person begins to be socially incapacitated when hearing loss in both ears reaches 40 dB in the speech frequencies (500–3000 Hz). The term *deafness* is applied only when the hearing loss is total or near-total (>85–90 dB below normal).

15. **What clinical tests help to distinguish the common types of hearing loss?**
Both the Rinne and Weber tuning fork tests help determine types of hearing loss. Pathology in the external or middle ears results in conductive loss, whereas abnormalities of the inner ear or auditory nerve cause sensorineural loss. The Rinne and Weber tuning fork tests can help with this determination. In both tests, use a 512-Hz tuning fork (not 128-Hz or 256-Hz). With the

Weber test, conductive loss localizes sound to the impaired ear. In a sensorineural loss the sound is localized to the unaffected ear. Because sound lateralizes even in mild hearing loss, the Weber test is the more sensitive of the two. In the Rinne test, sound is louder when conducted by bone in conductive hearing loss, whereas in normal hearing or sensorineural hearing loss, the air conduction is louder.

http://www.ftc.gov/bcp/conline/pubs/health/hearing.htm (Federal Trade Commission advice on hearing aids)

16. What is the bottom line on hearing aids?
A licensed practitioner (certified audiologist) should provide hearing aids. Aids ordered via mail, phone, or over the Internet may be cheaper but are not likely to be fitted or prescribed for the individual patient's needs. The result is poor function and poor compliance. Proper hearing tests include an audiogram performed by a certified audiologist, which identifies hearing loss and its severity, determines whether the loss is conductive or sensorineural, and provides information about inner ear function and the patient's reliability in reporting hearing quality.

http://www.emedicine.com/ent/topic478.htm (overview article on hearing aids with current references)
http://www.nidcd.nih.gov/health/hearing/hearingaid.asp (National Institute on Deafness and Other Communication Disorders overview of hearing aid information for consumers and a good list of support groups for the hearing impaired)

17. Why are hearing aids underutilized?
Hearing aids can cost hundreds to thousands of dollars without coverage by most medical plans. Pride and discomfort with wear prevent use, and small dials make them difficult to tune.

Schuller DE, Schleuning II AJ: Rehabilitation of nonsurgical hearing loss and hearing loss. In DeWeese, S: Otolaryngology—Head and Neck Surgery, 8th ed. St. Louis, Mosby, 1994, pp 479–488.
Woodson GE: Ear, Nose and Throat Disorders in Primary Care. Philadelphia, W. B. Saunders, Philadelphia, 2001.
Lucente FE, Har-El G: Hearing testing. In Lucente FE (ed): Essentials of Otolaryngology, 4th ed. Philadelphia, Lippincott Williams & Wilkins, 1999.

KEY POINTS: SEVERE VISUAL OR HEARING IMPAIRMENT

1. About 65% of patients with low vision or blindness are over age 65.

2. Magnification results in a progressively narrower visual field; conversely, expansion of visual field minimizes the image.

3. Stroke and traumatic brain injury produce frequent and sometimes subtle visual impairments, which will adversely affect outcome if unrecognized and untreated.

4. One should utilize a 512-Hz tuning fork for bedside hearing assessment.

5. Aphasic/neurologically impaired patients can be assessed for hearing loss.

18. How reliable is a hearing test in an aphasic or neurologically impaired patient?
A neurologically impaired individual can often be tested reliably because the ability to detect tones does not require the higher centers of the brain. If the individual can be trained to respond to tones, a valid hearing test can be obtained. If such training cannot be completed, often speech threshold can be obtained with a little creativity. For example, ask the patient to

follow instructions such as clapping hands or finishing the words to a familiar song. In a nonresponsive patient, physiologic tests such as brain stem-evoked audiometry can be utilized.

19. **Describe the treatment options for various hearing problems.**
    Treatments for sensorineural and conductive loss include hearing aids, assistive listening devices, and aural rehabilitation. For the profoundly deaf, cochlear implants can be surgically placed to stimulate the auditory nerve and provide awareness of sound, although the sound will differ from sound as a "normal" hearing person knows it. Some conductive losses can be helped through medical intervention, depending on their cause. A hearing aid generally does not help a purely central hearing loss since the problem is not one of decreased volume. Aural rehabilitation, using speech-language pathology or audiology services, can be useful as a focusing technique. An assistive listening device can improve signal-to-noise ratio for improved focus on auditory information during therapy sessions.

20. **At what age can training begin in hearing-impaired children?**
    With the advent of infant hearing screening programs in the past several years, significant hearing loss is being identified in infancy and often is treated by 3 months of age with amplification. The important speech development period, therefore, is not lost. When amplification is not adequate, cochlear implants may be an option. In all cases, aural rehabilitation is imperative to provide proper stimulation and auditory training.

21. **How old should a child be before using a hearing aid or other device?**
    With accurate physiologic testing now available, infants can be fitted with hearing aids as soon as the hearing loss is verified. A child of 3–4 months of age can wear a hearing aid, with the hopes that speech and language development can begin. A hearing loss of a moderate to severe degree or worse warrants intervention.

SEXUAL EXPRESSION, INTIMACY, AND REPRODUCTION: METHODS FOR INTERDISCIPLINARY ROMANTIC ENABLEMENT

Steven A. Stiens, MD, MS, Rafi J. Heruti, MD, Ronit Aloni, PhD, Ruth K. Westheimer, EdD, and Mitch Tepper, PhD

I wouldn't join any club that would have me for a member.

—Groucho Marx (1890–1977)

1. **What is sexual literacy?**

   Sexual literacy is the working knowledge of anatomy, physiology, psychology, and recent research pertaining to human sexuality theory and practice. The "sexually literate" health professional must be comfortable with his or her own sexuality, able to suspend judgment, and express genuine willingness to pursue understanding and solutions with patients and partners. At the end of a consultation with a patient, the sexually literate clinician should be able to formulate a biopsychosocial problem list with goals that address patient and partner impairments.

   > http://sexualhealth.com (disability and chronic conditions channel)
   > http://sexualhealth.com/channel.php?Action=view&channel=3

2. **How does clinical knowledge in sexual literacy guide patient sex education?**

   Sex education is often suppressed, delivered in subtherapeutic doses, poorly translated, and without thoughtful design for target audiences. A clinician's knowledge of physical and social development, recovery patterns, and the relationships between various impairments and activity limitations allows for person-centered curriculum design. In interviewing patients, life circumstances, self-perceptions, and expectations are revealed. Patients' needs are met through a variety of educational media, impromptu discussions, a core series of lectures, guided self-discovery assignments, specific suggestions to enhance intimate performance, and demonstrations of equipment. During initial rehabilitation, sexuality should be on the problem list, and one team member should have primary responsibility to see that the basic education has been completed.

   > http://www.sexsupport.org/DisabilityLinks.html (excellent collection of sex- and disability-related links)

3. **What are the subcomponents of personal sexual expression?**
   - **Sexual identity:** Phenotypic sex with objective expression and function of secondary sexual characteristics, anatomy, and physiology
   - **Gender identity:** The person's subjective sense of self as man or woman
   - **Sex role:** Behavior to demonstrate that he/she is a man or woman
   - **Orientation:** The focus of desire for sexual relationship; sexual orientation is a fluid continuum ranging from exclusively heterosexual to primarily homosexual
   - **Intention:** Degree of aggression inherent in sexual fantasy and behavior
   - **Sexual desire:** Interest in a variety of activities, frequency

4. **What is sexuality?**
Sexuality is the expression of a person's femaleness or maleness through personality, body, dress, and behavior; it is the personification of biologic gender, gender identity, and sexual orientation. It develops through physiologic cues from the body, experiences of self, maturation, socialization, societal reflection of the person, and intimate relationships. Sexuality, therefore, requires an evolving self-understanding, and ongoing opportunity for communication of self-perception, and informed, proactive clinician support for the patient's goals. The clinician's positive anticipation of patients' sexuality as a facet of their roles in relationships is but one example of the power of **therapeutic expectation**.

5. **How can sexual history-taking and intervention be made less of an ENIGMA?**
The **ENIGMA model** is a series of steps that makes the process more conceivable:
- **E** = **E**ngage the patient in conversation by finding common ground validating his or her personal aspiration.
- **N** = **N**ormalize the sexual self-expression by permissively exploring interests, activities, and barriers to success.
- **I** = **I**nform and educate the patient and his or her partner.
- **G** = **G**uide them by mirroring their style of interaction, validating their success, and suggesting alternatives for next steps. Use their lingo!
- **M** = **M**aximize achievement by prescribing and providing adjuncts such as educational materials, medication, equipment, therapy, and experiences.
- **A** = **A**ssess and reassess by checking on the issue as one in the spectrum of problems addressed on regular visits.

KEY POINTS: CLINICAL INTERVENTION CYCLE FOR INTIMATE ENABLEMENT

1. With trust and listening, develop a working understanding of the patient's sexuality and aspirations.

2. Explore the ENIGMA model by Engaging, Normalizing, Informing, Guiding, Maximizing, and Assessing success in the patient's sexual expression that is goal directed.

3. Confirm and support each patient's healthy sexual identity, gender identity, sex role, orientation, intention, and desires.

4. Review success with patient and partner in recognizing, reaching for, or substituting the excitement, plateau, orgasm, and relaxation stages of the sexual response cycle as described by Masters and Johnson.

5. Utilize the PLISSIT model (Permission, Limited Information, Specific Suggestions, and Intensive therapy) as needed to set and meet patient-and couple-centered goals.

6. **How does disability affect body image, sexual self-concept, and adjustment?**
Body image is the mind's picture of our bodies, the perception we have of ourselves. It is closely associated with the awareness of our body (the afferent sensory barrage and central processing, "the experienced homunculus"). The expression and practice of sexuality are affected by self-esteem, body image, and interpersonal attachment. It is continually evaluated by the self. Despite adaptation to self, individuals are often confronted in society with a stigma and risk devaluation by others. Rehabilitation specialists must strive to help patients become fully self-aware and reconstruct a positive body image that they accept, like, and share. Acceptance of self as desirable

and as a source of pleasure emerges with sensual experience of self and perceptions of others. Educational resources, same sex support groups, and involved clinicians are particularly helpful.

Ekland M., Lawrie B: How a woman's sexual adjustment after sustaining a spinal cord injury impacts sexual health interventions. SCI Nurs 21(1):14–19, 2004.

http://groups.yahoo.com/group/disabledsex/?yguid=1373668 (group for the discussion of any sexuality issue as it pertains to people with disabilities and adaptation)

7. Is it important to have a relationship first?

Personal relationships begin with our attitudes about ourselves. Beyond self-perception are self-acceptance, self-esteem, and self-worth as a potential partner for another. The rehabilitation team must successfully reflect patients' unique personal attributes and reinforce the value of their companionship to others. People who project self-respect and satisfaction are most fully capable of attracting partners, graciously accepting others' attention, and sensitively meeting their needs. People who recognize their capabilities are most able to contribute to a mutually complementary relationship. Consequently, rehabilitation must teach patients the value of recognizing their unique assets and capabilities. With this confidence, they can take the necessary social risks to seek out partners who can be mutually complementary.

8. Would the treatment be more effective if a patient's sexual partner is involved? What communication must there be with the patient's partner?

For patients who have a sexual partner, intervention is most effective if the partner is included in any communication between the rehabilitation professional and the patient on matters of sexual functioning. The clinician has the opportunity to provide education to the partner, to receive input on the couple's needs, and to develop a plan of treatment that is mutually acceptable to the couple.

Sexual issues must be integrated into the entire rehabilitation plan; partners in life need full inclusion in the rehabilitation process. If possible, it is desirable to maintain a separation between roles of caretaker and sexual partner. This can be achieved with proactive planning for attendant care.

Lemon M: Sexual counseling and spinal cord injury. Sexual Disabil 11(1):73–79, 1993.

9. What is "fragile partner syndrome"?

Partners often do not have a full understanding of the patient's condition. Without direct, detailed, and specific demonstrations of safe and effective physical interactions with patients, partners may overestimate risk of physical and intimate contact. With patients' permission and guidance, partners should be educated in specific methods for transfers and positions for intimate contact and parameters for the intensity of activity.

10. What are the physiologic changes associated with the four stages of the human sexual response as outlined by Masters and Johnson?

Excitement stage I: Muscle tension, sympathetic activity, nipple erection
- Female: Clitoris swelling, vaginal lubrication
- Male: Penile erection, testes rise

Plateau stage II: Heightened excitement, pulse 100–160 bpm, sex flush
- Female: Clitoris withdrawals, vaginal vasocongestion
- Male: Testes enlarge, Cowper's secretion

Orgasm stage III: (seconds to minutes) Rhythmic muscle contractions
- Female: Uterus, vagina, and anus contract
- Male: Ejaculation, bladder neck closes

Relaxation stage IV: (minutes to hours) Return to baseline, refractory period

11. **Describe the physiology of the sexual response in women.**
    The uterus and ovaries receive sympathetic innervations from the hypogastric nerve (T10–L2). Sensory messages from the vagina and cervix travel via the pelvic, vagus (parasympathetic), and hypogastric and sympathetic nerves. Clitoral swelling is primarily parasympathetically mediated, and vaginal secretion is primarily sympathetic. At orgasm, the pelvic floor (pudendal nerve) contracts rhythmically. Functional MRI studies reveal increased metabolism at the nucleus accumbens.

12. **How do acute neurologic injuries affect female sexual function?**
    Menstruation may not occur for three or more months after central nervous system (CNS) trauma. After complete spinal cord injury at level T6 and above, psychogenic subjective arousal does not produce vaginal lubrication via sympathetic pathways. As long as the conus and autonomic connections remain intact, manual clitoral stimulation produces reflex lubrication and increased vaginal pulse amplitude.

    Spinal cord injury, neuromuscular disorders, and connective tissue diseases do not generally affect fertility. Pregnancy may be complicated by urinary tract infection, pressure ulcers, constipation, and mobility limitations. Labor is initiated and driven hormonally. The delivery can be vaginal, but it should be anticipated and monitored with autonomic dysreflexia prevention with anesthesia and preparedness for forceps use or cesarean section.

13. **How common is sexual dysfunction in the general population?**
    Community samples estimate 25–63% of women and 10–52% of men have sexual dysfunction. Sexual dysfunction for males is largely premature ejaculation, which is mostly associated with psychogenic causes. Another common dysfunction is erectile dysfunction, which is associated with risk factors for coronary artery disease, age, medications, and emotional factors such as anger and depression. For women, common complaints include trouble lubricating, postcoital and urinary tract infections, reduced libido, and psychosocial/relationship issues. Except for trouble with lubrication (which decreases with age), these problems are associated with urinary tract infections, past experiences, and psychosocial dimensions.

    Treatments are evaluated for **efficacy** (physiologic improvement in randomized controlled trials) and **effectiveness** (beneficial in clinical practice). No medications have been demonstrated to be effective for hypoactive sexual desire. Women who are hypogonadal with hypoactive sexual desire have demonstrated increased sexual fantasies, masturbation, and intercourse and report greater well-being while on brief oral estrogen and 300-μg testosterone patch.

    Heiman JR: Sexual dysfunction: Overview of prevalence, etiological factors, and treatments. J Sex Res 39(1):73–78, 2002.

14. **How do erections occur?**
    Male erection is initiated by arterial vasodilatation and venous outlet constriction, which result in engorgement of the cavernosal sinusoids. Psychogenic (imaginative) erections start with arousal in the mind and are mediated by the lumbar sympathetics hypogastric nerve (T12–L1). Reflexogenic (contact) erection is primarily cholinergic (parasympathetic [S2, S3, S4]) via the inferior splanchnic nerve or nervi erigentes and is augmented by mixed somatic innervation via the pudendal nerve, which contracts the pelvic floor and limits penile blood release. The ejaculation and detumescence process is primarily sympathetic, but a complex interplay of autonomic systems and other neurotransmitters continues to also play a role in the process.

15. **Describe the physiology of the sexual response in men.**
    Psychogenic stimuli activate the cortex, amygdala, and hypothalamus. Erection and emission containing spermatozoa occur with sympathetic facilitation. **Emission** starts with sympathetically (T10–L2 emission center) driven vas deferens transport of sperm to the posterior urethra to combine with seminal vesicle secretions. **Ejaculation** is the forceful delivery of the semen out of the urethra by the pudendal-innervated bulbocavernous and

ischiocavernosus muscle contractions. Ejaculation is typically ineffective after complete spinal cord injury (SCI) and may result in retrograde ejaculation (semen into the bladder). Ejaculation can be facilitated with a vibrator (Ferticare) stimulus (2.5 mm amplitude, 100 Hz frequency) under the glans at the frenulum or inhibited by the **squeeze technique** (firm grasp of glans). **Orgasm** is the cortical experience of extreme pleasure followed by a feeling of well-being and satisfaction.

Goetz L, Stiens S: Abdominal electric stimulation facilitates ejaculation evoked by penile vibratory stimulation. Arch Phys Med Rehab 86(9):1879–1883, 2005.

Sipski M, Alexander CJ, Gomez-Marin O: Effects of level and degree of spinal cord injury on male orgasm. Spinal Cord 44(12):798–804, 2006.

16. **What information should be included in a proper sexual history?**
    Patient's behaviors, needs, and expectations as well as areas that require education, counseling, reassurance, and treatment.

17. **What are the rehabilitation options for producing erections after neurologic injuries?**
    - Without erection, satisfying intromission can be accomplished with the **stuffing technique** (pushing the flaccid penis into the vagina and stimulating the woman with friction and sustained pressure at the introitus) or the use of penile splinting.
    - **Vacuum tumescence and constriction therapy** works by engorging and expanding the penis for retention. The corpora expand under negative pressure, and a custom circular rubber-tension ring is slipped around the base of the penis.
    - **Phosphodiesterase PDE-5 inhibitors** potentiate erections by preventing the degradation of cyclic guanosine monophosphate (GMP), which is a direct vasodilator. The three currently available compounds have the following onset times and durations of activation: vardenafil (Levitra), 20 min/12 hours; sildenafil (Viagra), 30 min/4 hours; and tadalafil (Cialis), 60 min/36 hours. Use of PDE-5 inhibitors is contraindicated with all nitrate-producing medications and strong vasodilators because of the risk for hypotension.
    - Intracorporal injections with **papaverine** or **prostaglandin E_1** (alprostadil) produce erections by smooth muscle relaxation. Management of side effects such as priapism is treated with observation and needle aspiration of the corpora.
    - **Penile implants** may be noninflatable (rigid or semirigid) and are seldom used because of the risk for skin breakdown with foreign body.

    Nehra A, Moreland RB: Neurologic erectile dysfunction. Urol Clin North Am 28(2):289–308, 2001.

18. **Does spinal cord injury affect male fertility?**
    Yes. Deficits in spermatogenesis documented by testicular biopsy have included tubular atrophy, spermatogenic arrest, and interstitial fibrosis. Seminal parameters show decreased sperm counts and motility as well as abnormal morphology and white blood cells. Repeated ejaculation reduces stasis and can improve sperm quality. White blood cell counts can be reduced, with short courses of antibiotics covering cultured urinary contaminants.

    DeForge D, Blackmer J, Garrity C, et al: Fertility following spinal cord injury: A systematic review. Spinal Cord 43(12):693–703, 2005.

19. **What are the fertility options for males with spinal cord injury?**
    Even though the majority of men with spinal cord injuries can achieve erections and have sexual intercourse, male infertility caused by inability to ejaculate is a common phenomenon. The high threshold for ejaculation has prompted the design of a sequential series of interventions, including penile vibratory stimulation (PVS), electroejaculation, and microsurgical aspiration of sperm from epididymis and testicular biopsy. PVS is a custom-designed mechanical vibrator

that is placed at the base of the glans penis and induces a reflex ejaculation. This technique works in patients with thoracic and cervical SCI with an intact sacral ejaculatory reflex and is the preferred choice in patients with lesions above T10. With electroejaculation, a low-current stimulation of the ejaculatory organs via a rectal probe is done. The semen typically exhibits low sperm count, low motility, and white blood cells. Assisted reproductive techniques such as sperm washing, intrauterine insemination, in vitro fertilization (IVF), and intracytoplasmic injection (ICI) of sperm into eggs can be utilized.

Heruti RJ, Katz H, Menashe Y, et al: Treatment of male infertility due to spinal cord injury using rectal probe electroejaculation: The Israeli experience. Spinal Cord 39(3):168–175, 2001.

20. **What is the PLISSIT model of sex therapy?**
- **P**= **P**ermission to be sexual
- **LI**=**L**imited **I**nformation
- **SS**=**S**pecific **S**uggestions
- **IT**=**I**ntensive **T**herapy

This model presents a spectrum of interventional areas that can be addressed, in part, by each member of the interdisciplinary team.

21. **Explain the components of the PLISSIT approach.**
- **Permission:** Sensitive questions in history-taking regarding sexual function are therapeutic affirmations of the patient's sexuality and role in the lives of others. Questions such as "Are you sexually active?" and "How has this condition affected your sexual function?" open conversation about sex. Teaching patients and partners range of motion, massage, and management techniques for angina, bronchospasm, autonomic dysreflexia, and prevention of incontinence prepares them for their own problem-solving in sexual exploration. Physicians' permission to resume intercourse can often be a prescription for success.
- **Limited information:** All rehabilitation programs should include lectures and discussion that educate the patient about the basic physiology and pathophysiology of the sexual response cycle and reproduction. One-to-one explanation of the unique effects of a patient's disease or injury should complement this review. This primary education should be the designated responsibility of one rehabilitation team member, with appropriate interdisciplinary and peer referrals.
- **Specific suggestions:** Ideally, all team members contribute to successful sexual adjustment and function. For example, the training of the patient by the primary nurse for skin examination for sores can lead to reflections on body image. A suggestion may include an assignment for the patient or couple to experiment with visual body exploration and survey patient sensation. Such a couple can later be assigned **sensate focus exercises** and then advanced to a search for new erogenous zones. Physical therapy education for a spouse on transfers and mat mobility might easily be adapted by couples for use in transferring into the Jacuzzi and sexual positioning.
- **Intensive therapy:** The presence of impairments that contribute to role performance deficits demands formal attention and the response of a rehabilitation team member. On most teams, this is the psychologist.

http://groups.yahoo.com/group/SexDisabilityResearc/?yguid=1498415 (The purpose of this list is to discuss research on issues of sexuality and disability.)

22. **Is there sex after a heart attack?**
Yes! Myocardial infarction or heart disease in general need not preclude resumption of sexual activity. The metabolic cost of sex in middle-aged married men is no more than 5 metabolic equivalents (METs) (1 MET = calories/minute at complete rest), the exertion of going up two flights of stairs. Rest before intercourse, postpone for 3 hours after meals and alcohol, take nitrates as needed before intercourse to prevent chest pain, and use familiar positions.

Remember though that nitrates are contraindicated with PDE5 inhibitors.Foreplay may be a metabolically favorable "warm-up" and training activity. Initial explorations can include masturbation to give the patient full control of the process. Thereafter, successive approximation of the previous routine can follow.

23. **What experiences do women with new neurologic impairments report as they adapt sexually?**
    The process of sexual readjustment after paralysis varies and may include three stages.
    1. **Cognitive genital dissociation:** Sexual ennui is accompanied by dysphoria and pessimism about desirability. There may be fear of rejection or abandonment. Therapeutic support includes exploration of the role sexuality played before injury, which validates the patient's current experience as common but not necessarily persistent.
    2. **Sexual disenfranchisement:** Sexuality becomes less of a priority, although activity may occur out of curiosity. Experiences may produce **sexual dissonance** and disappointment in the lack of sensation of the pleasure.
    3. **Sexual rediscovery:** Sexual readjustment continues and includes exploration and discovery of alternative approaches to arousal and orgasm.

    Tepper MS, Whipple B, Richards E, Komisaruk BR: Women with complete spinal cord injury: A phenomenological study of sexual experience. J Sex Marital Ther 27(5):615–623, 2001.

24. **Can the location of erogenous zones really change after injury to the CNS?**
    Recent primate and human data demonstrate central sensory reorganization in response to injuries to the spinal cord or peripheral nerve. People with SCI have reported areas in the zone of partial sensory preservation that are sexually exciting with stimulation. These areas can lead to orgasm with associated tachycardia and flushing above the lesion.

25. **Do experiments sometimes lead to satisfying discoveries?**
    Yes. Overcoming attitudinal and cultural taboos of interaction transcends barriers. Practices that bring together mutually sensate erogenous zones can become particularly satisfying parts of couples' repertoires. Possibilities for **kissing, cunnilingus** (oral and lingual vulva stimulation), and **fellatio** (oral and lingual penile stimulation) should be explored. Unfortunately, a major barrier to sexual fulfillment after disability is fear. Fears of poor acceptance by a partner and issues related to involuntary loss of urinary or bowel control are particularly ominous. Planning for sexual encounters reduces anxiety and makes them more conceivable.

26. **How does traumatic brain injury affect sexual function?**
    The sequelae of brain injury are diverse and may include many functional deficits, cognitive movement, communication, behavior, and emotional expression. Full participation in an intimate and sexual relationship requires the integration of all these capabilities. Sexual functioning is a comprehensive activity that involves the motivation to engage in the activity and appropriate planning, including inhibition of inappropriate behavior. Sexual dysfunction may be the consequence of the primary damage as well as other factors surrounding the survivor, such as personal relationships, responses of family to the person, and moral attitudes of the society. Therefore, the sexual dysfunction that follows traumatic brain injury (TBI) may result from the neurologic deficits, survivors' reactions to the injury, premorbid personality, or some combination of these factors. Intervention requires generating and sequentially prioritizing sexually specific goals that may relate to other problems on the problem list (e.g., varied problems with mobility, neurogenic bladder, cognition difficulties, depression) within varied disablement domains, up and down the hierarchy of biopsychosocial systems. (See Chapter 14, Person Centered Rehabilitation.)

    Aloni R, Katz S: Sexuality Difficulties after Traumatic Brain Injury and Ways to Deal with It. Springfield, IL, Charles C Thomas, 2003, pp 20–41.
    Kreutzer JS, Zasler ND Psychosexual consequences of traumatic brain injury: methodology and preliminary findings. Brain Inj 3:177–186, 1989.

27. **How does brain damage relate to sexual function?**

Although sexual function is not necessarily associated directly with higher cognitive abilities, severe concentration problems may impair the arousal phase of sexual responses in both survivors and their partners. Cognitive dysfunction can adversely affect the intimate relationship and can cause sexual difficulties due to a loss of mutual interest or as a result of role changes and/or a decline in the survivor's self-esteem. Frontal and temporal lobe damage, impaired judgment, and extreme mood swings can result in inappropriate sexual behaviors that are not tolerated by a partner or by society.

Loss of memory and difficulties in concentration may require modification of the educational methods and documentation of the intervention program. Memory loss can cause the survivor to demand sex repeatedly. Integration of events into a memory book can help. Altered verbal and nonverbal patterns of communication can impede the establishment of new relationships for single survivors or disrupt marital relationships, as they may create misunderstandings and cause frustration, anger, withdrawal, and rejection. Depression and anxiety may act as inhibitors of sexual desire and function. Emotional regression, mood swings, and irritability can alter a couple's intimate relations through role changes or an inability to predict the partner's reaction to the initiation of sexual activity.

Aloni R, Katz S: Sexuality Difficulties after Traumatic Brain Injury and Ways to Deal with It. Springfield, IL, Charles C Thomas, 2003, pp 20–41.

Kaplan SP: Five-year tracking of psychological changes in people with severe TBI. Rehabil Consel Bull 36:152–159, 1993.

Lezak MD: Brain damage is a family affair. J Clin Exp Neuropsychol 10:111–123, 1988.

28. **How can a stoma affect sexuality?**

Patients with stomas face many physical, psychological, social, and sexual difficulties. More than 40% have problems with their sex lives. Many patients find it difficult to discuss their sexual feelings, especially after a body image change, causing most of them to leave the hospital distressed and unprepared for sexual life. They lack confidence and are not aware of the anticipated problems, including irregular bowel movements and diarrhea, discharge of gas and unpleasant odor, and diminished sexual and social life. Some of the nerves important for genital sensation and sexual function (lubrication in females; erection and ejaculation in males) may be severed during the operation. Apart from the physical changes that a stoma and surgery might cause, there are psychosocial aspects concerning self-concept with the change of body image in relation to bodily functions. Patients report restrictions in their level of social functioning. A sensitive and informed approach to discuss sexuality can provide effective support. The elements of successful dialogue are presented in the PLISSIT model. Patients will more readily adapt to their new body image and way of life if they receive professional counseling concerning sexuality from the preoperative stage through rehabilitation and their return to the community.

Nugent KP, Daniels P, Stewart B, et al: Quality of life in stoma patients. Dis Colon Rectum 42(12):1569–1574, 1999.

BIBLIOGRAPHY

1. Anderson KD, Borisoff JF, Johnson RD, et al: The impact of spinal cord injury on sexual function: Concerns of the general population. Spinal Cord 44(10):1–10, 2006.

2. Annon J: The PLISSIT model: A proposed conceptual scheme for the behavioral treatment for sexual problems. J Sex Educ Ther 2:1–15, 1976.

3. Shuttleworth RP: The search for sexual intimacy for men with cerebral palsy. Sexual Disabil 18(4):263–282, 2000.

4. Silverberg C, Kaufman M, Odette F: The Ultimate Guide to Sex and Disability. San Francisco, Cleis Press, 2003.

5. Sipski ML, Alexander CJ: Sexual Function in People with Disability and Chronic Illness: A Health Professional's Guide. Gaithersburg, MD, Aspen Publication, 1997.

EVALUATION OF THE GERIATRIC PATIENT

Susan J. Garrison, MD, and Gerald Felsenthal, MD

CHAPTER 8

1. **Describe the characteristics of the geriatric population.**
   The difference in physiologic age compared to chronologic age can be amazing. Psychologically, people tend to become exaggerations of their adult selves as they age. Research shows that people who live through their middle years (ages 45–65) without major illness will live to be a part of the geriatric population. Medicare benefits begin at age 65.

2. **How do the basic principles of rehabilitative management differ for the geriatric patient?**
   The basic rehabilitation principles are the same for all adults. Those specific to the geriatric population include physiologic changes, multiple impairments, and a focus on small improvements.

3. **What neurologic changes are found in the elderly? How are these significant?**
   See Table 8-1.

4. **What changes in biologic functions occur in response to aging, as compared to inactivity and exercise?**
   See Table 8-2.

5. **How does functional impairment affect this population?**
   As one ages, comorbidities accumulate and result in functional impairment and difficulty with simple tasks. This is particularly true for women, who may live 7–12 years longer than their same-aged spouse.

6. **Which geriatric patients are candidates for rehabilitation, and where should this care be delivered?**
   Candidates should be physically well enough to participate in therapy sessions. If an acute care inpatient cannot tolerate a rigorous program of 3 hours of therapy per day, they should be considered for admission to a skilled nursing facility (SNF = slower, not faster) or long-term acute care. Other options include a subacute care facility, nursing home, home health care, and outpatient services.

   Garrison SJ, Felsenthal G: Geriatric rehabilitation. In Garrison SJ (ed): Handbook of Physical Medicine and Rehabilitation, 2nd ed. Philadelphia, Lippincott Williams & Wilkins, 2003, pp. 140–141.

7. **How should motivation be utilized in addressing this population?**
   Lack of motivation is not a reason to exclude a person from therapies. The person is motivated to do something; it may simply be to stay in bed. Many older patients are unwilling to exercise after a life of physical labor. They may also succumb to their own ageism. Make certain that the patient is not medically/surgically ill, depressed, or nutritionally impaired.

TABLE 8-1. NEUROLOGIC CHANGES AND THEIR SIGNIFICANCE IN THE ELDERLY

System	Findings	Significance
Visual	Diminished ROM on convergence and upward gaze Small, irregular pupils Diminished reaction to light and near reflex	Combination of restricted vertical gaze and cervical motion can make it difficult to see information posted on walls, such as exit signs.
Motor	Decreased muscle strength: legs > arms, proximal > distal Atrophy of interossei Short-stepped or broad-based gait with diminished associated movements	Hip extensors may no longer be strong enough to lift the body from sitting to standing; arm strength can be used to push up.
Sensory	Diminished vibratory: legs > arms	Poor sensory input from feet indicates risk for falls.
	Mildly increased threshold for pain, temperature, and light touch Possible change in proprioception	Patients are at risk for injury from topical heat modalities.
Reflexes	Absent or diminished ankle jerks Reduction in knee, biceps, and triceps reflexes Babinski's sign may not be present when it normally would occur.	Radiculopathies may be overlooked or misdiagnosed.

ROM = range of motion.
Adapted from Ham RJ: Assessment. In Ham RJ, Sloane PD (eds): Primary Care Geriatrics: A Case-Based Approach, 2nd ed. St. Louis, Mosby, 1992, p. 87.

KEY POINTS: TYPICAL CAUSES OF FALLS IN THE ELDERLY

1. Syncope

2. Visual problems

3. Peripheral vascular disease

4. Weakness, balance, or joint problem

5. Inappropriate footwear

6. Inappropriate use of gait devices

7. Use of sedative hypnotics

8. Accident or environment related

TABLE 8-2. CHANGES IN BIOLOGIC FUNCTIONS IN RESPONSE TO AGING, INACTIVITY, AND EXERCISE

Function	Aging	Inactivity	Exercise
VO_{2max}	Decreased	Decreased	Increased
Cardiac output	Decreased	Decreased	Increased, not for older adults
Systolic blood pressure	Increased	—	Decreased
Orthostatic tolerance	Decreased	Decreased	Increased
Body water	Decreased	Decreased	—
Red blood cell mass	Decreased	Decreased	—
Thrombosis	Increased	Increased	Decreased
Serum lipids	Increased	Increased	Decreased
High density lipoprotein	Increased over age 80 yr	—	Increased
Lean body mass	Decreased	Decreased	—
Muscle strength	Decreased	Decreased	Increased
Calcium	Decreased	Decreased	—
Glucose tolerance	Decreased	Decreased	Increased
EEG dominant frequency	Decreased	Decreased	Increased

EEG = electroencephalogram.
Adapted from Felsenthal G, Garrison SJ, Steinberg FU: Rehabilitation of the Aging and Elderly Patient. Baltimore, Williams & Wilkins, 1994, pp 511–522.

8. **What is the concept of functional presentation of disease?**
   While a young adult may quickly become febrile in response to an acute infection, an elderly patient may become confused or begin falling rather than demonstrating a temperature elevation. Stopping eating or drinking, urinary incontinence, acute confusion, weight loss, falling, dizziness, dementia, and failure to thrive are functional presentations of disease.

9. **Why is cognition important in this group?**
   Most rehabilitation is based on learning compensatory skills for lost functional abilities. Standard rehabilitative techniques do not benefit severely demented patients. Also, medications a patient may be taking can affect cognitive performance.

10. **Does diagnosis of vascular dementia prevent participation in rehabilitation?**
    Patients with vascular dementia are often excluded because of their inability to learn new material and retain information. Today, earlier diagnoses and more effective treatments can modify the usual progression of vascular dementia. Medications such as selective serotonin reuptake indicators (SSRIs) can improve responses and performance. A multidisciplinary approach may involve psychiatrists, risk-management personnel, adult protective services, legal counsel, and neuropsychologists. Discharge requires 24-hour supervision for safety.

    Garrison SJ, Lindeman J (eds): Vascular dementia: Implications for stroke rehabilitation. Top Stroke Rehabil 7(3):11–28, 2000.

11. **What is polypharmacy?**
Polypharmacy, the use of multiple medications, often results in compliance problems. Patients become confused about dosage and scheduling and may forget to take medications, causing potential adverse drug effects. Attempt to limit the total number of medications. Additionally, medications may represent a significant out-of-pocket expense. See Table 8-3 for tips on how to write safer prescriptions for elderly patients.

12. **Why is nutrition important?**
Nutrition is important for maintaining good health and quick healing, particularly in the elderly. The description "malnourished" can signify obesity or cachexia. Obesity causes immobility and poor endurance. The underweight are at risk for skin breakdown, poor exercise tolerance, and peripheral edema due to low serum albumin levels. There are many factors that affect the

TABLE 8-3. SEVEN STEPS FOR WRITING SAFER MEDICATION PRESCRIPTIONS FOR THE ELDERLY

Physician Behavior	Purpose
1. Start at half of the lowest recommended dose; increase slowly to obtain the desired effect: "start low and go slow."	The desired response in the elderly may occur at a lower dosage than that required in the younger population.
2. Use a simple dosing regimen, with the fewest medications possible; encourage lifestyle modifications rather than drugs.	Noncompliance and the incidence of adverse drug reactions decrease as the total number of doses and medications decline.
3. Whenever adding a new medication or changing the dosing of a current one, make certain that the instructions are understood.	Detailed information can assist in preventing problems. Write explicit instructions for the patient or significant other.
4. Be aware of medication costs.	Patients are unlikely to be compliant with numerous expensive medications. Also, they may continue to take a previously prescribed medication because they have already paid for it.
5. Periodically review patient medications, including over-the-counter drugs. Eliminate those not being used; keep the total number low.	This assists in preventing the possibility of drug-drug interactions, potentially reduces costs, and may prevent the accidental ingestion of medication.
6. Create a written prescription list for the patient to keep with him/her at all times.	This record is helpful to other physicians and pharmacists who may then review the list for possible drug problems. It is invaluable for the geriatric traveler and for ER visits.
7. Instruct home health nurses or aides to communicate directly with the physician about any medication problems.	The sooner a problem is noticed, the sooner action can be taken to correct the situation.

Adapted from Stein BE: Avoiding drug reactions: Seven steps to writing safe prescriptions. Geriatrics 49:28–36, 1994.

geriatric patient's nutrition, including socioeconomic status, food preferences, depression, dental and/or swallowing problems, in addition to underlying medical conditions that may result in malabsorption.

13. **Why is the maintenance of routine physical activity important?**
"Use it or lose it." Muscle groups must be exercised in order to stay strong.

14. **What housing options are available for the elderly who can no longer live independently?**
Living arrangements are related to the patient's financial status and functional abilities and deficits. Alternatives to living independently include nursing homes, assisted living, homecare, or living with relatives.

   Garrison SJ, Felsenthal G: Geriatric rehabilitation. In Garrison SJ (ed): Handbook of Physical Medicine and Rehabilitation, 2nd ed. Philadelphia, Lippincott Williams & Wilkins, 2003, pp 139–151.

15. **Are there specific equipment needs in the elderly?**
Many elderly patients resist using gait devices or use inappropriate ones. They may also request scooters or other electric mobility when standard wheelchairs are best. Remember that less is more. Too many adaptive devices may overwhelm people. Other concerns include environmental modifications such as entrance ramps and grab bars in bathrooms. Also, equipment is expensive, even when partially reimbursed by third-party payers, and must be maintained.

16. **Why is a hip fracture of such concern in a geriatric patient?**
Poor balance following hip fracture is significantly associated with increased hospitalizations and nursing home placement. The mortality rate in the year following hip fracture is 14–36%, and 25–75% experience prolonged functional impairment.

17. **What treatment is best for osteoarthritis? When is surgery indicated?**
The drug of choice is acetaminophen. Other options include nonsteroidal anti-inflammatory inhibitor drugs (NSAIDs), topicals (salicylate/capsaicin), or tricyclic antidepressants. Therapeutic modalities such as heat, cold, transcutaneous electrical nerve stimulation (TENS), and exercise may be helpful in pain management. Intra-articular joint injections of glucocorticoids should be limited to four. At that time, total joint replacement should be considered. Indications for total knee replacement include varus angulation of greater than 10°, ligamentous instability and valgus deformity, severe knee pain unrelieved by medications, and back pain. Total hip replacement is indicated when nonsurgical strategies have failed to provide functional improvement and pain relief.

   Garrison SJ, Felsenthal G: Geriatric rehabilitation. In Garrison SJ (ed): Handbook of Physical Medicine and Rehabilitation, 2nd ed. Philadelphia, Lippincott Williams & Wilkins, 2003, pp 139–151.

18. **What are the rehabilitative goals of total knee replacement in this population?**
To achieve ability to ambulate household distances (of approximately 100 ft) using a rolling walker and achieve active range of motion of the affected knee, approaching full extension and greater than 90° of flexion.

19. **What is significant about undergoing total hip replacement secondary to osteoarthritis?**
Postoperative rehabilitation involves teaching the patient independence in bed mobility, sitting to standing, and dressing, while following hip precautions. Joint protection and nutrition should also be stressed.

20. **What are the risk factors for stroke in this population?**
    The primary risk factor for stroke is age; the second is previous stroke. Use the Functional Independence Measure (FIM) to predict the need and projected outcome of stroke rehabilitation. Dynamic sitting balance is a good indication of the ability to participate in an intensive stroke rehabilitation program.

21. **What is the goal of stroke rehabilitation? How can patients maximize their learning efforts?**
    The goal is to teach compensatory skills to substitute for lost functional abilities. Cognitive strengths and weaknesses should be identified, and the strengths are emphasized.

22. **Can the geriatric stroke patient regain the ability to walk?**
    All unilateral-hemispheric, nonoperative stroke patients who were ambulatory prior to the stroke eventually regain some ability to ambulate if they do not sustain a second stroke or die of some other cause first.

23. **What factors may hinder lower limb prosthetic restoration in the geriatric amputee?**
    Limiting factors include inability to learn, neurologic deficits, poor endurance, hip or knee contractures of either leg, poor upper limb strength, poor skin integrity of the residual limb, and emotional effects.

24. **Describe the specific prosthetic modifications that may be helpful for the geriatric lower-limb amputee.**
    Various suspension methods, safety-type joints, and energy-storing feet may assist in providing more stability during ambulation. A cosmetic lower limb may be emotionally beneficial.

25. **What is the risk of contralateral limb loss in the geriatric amputee?**
    Approximately 15–20% of geriatric amputees experience contralateral limb loss within 2 years. After 4 years, it increases to 40%. The remaining limb should be protected with meticulous foot care, use of an appropriate shoe, and maintenance of joint active range of motion (AROM) and muscular strength.

26. **What factors increase the risk of an older driver having a motor vehicle accident?**
    Medical conditions with episodic events, such as syncope, angina, seizure, transient ischemic attacks, hypoglycemia, and sleep attacks, increase the risk of motor vehicle accidents. The use of medication and polypharmacy, in addition to functional deficits (vision, cognition, and motor function), create a combination that increases the risk. Older driver accidents typically involve inattention or slowed perception and response and include multiple vehicles in intersections, particularly during attempted left-hand turns.

    Wang CC, Carr DB: Older driver safety: A report from the older drivers project. J Am Geriatr Soc 52:143–149, 2004.

27. **What role should the physiatrist play in assessing the older driver?**
    Physical and mental changes associated with aging have been shown to result in an increased accident rate. For their safety, advise your patients to modify their driving schedules, avoiding night driving, or to alter routes using surface streets only. Identify those who should totally refrain from driving. Discuss this with the patient and caregivers, and document your recommendations.

    American Medical Association/National Highway Traffic Safety Administration/U.S. Department of Transportation: Physician's Guide to Assessing and Counseling Older Drivers: Chicago, AMA, June 2003, p 18.

WEBSITES

1. American Association of Retired Persons
   www.aarp.org/bulletin

2. American Medical Association
   www.ama-assn.org/go/olderdrivers

3. Consumer Consortium on Assisted Living
   www.ccal.org

ENVIRONMENTAL BARRIERS: SOLUTIONS FOR PARTICIPATION, COLLABORATION, AND TOGETHERNESS

Steven A. Stiens, MD, MS, Shoshana Shamberg, OTR/L, MS, Aaron Shamberg, MLA, and Alessandro Giustini, MD

Rehabilitation is often like surgery from the skin...out.

—Steven A. Stiens (1993)

1. **From a rehabilitation perspective, what aspects of the environment require evaluation and prospective treatment?**

   The environment is everything that surrounds and interacts with the patient, providing a unique habitat for each person:

   - The **physical aspects** include the object constellation and morphology as well as the energy distribution.
   - The **social aspects** are the responses of the living community surrounding the patient: family, neighbors, interdisciplinary team, and any others who may have contact with the patient.
   - The **political aspects** dictate laws and specify characteristics of the built and community environments as well as the rights of persons living with disablement.

   Various models of the environment are described in the current literature. The **World Health Organization** model divides the environment into human-made changes; support and relationships; attitudes; services; and systems and policies. Other similar models include the **Quebec Model** (1995), the **Institute of Medicine** (1997), and the recent **Craig Hospital Inventory of Environmental Factors (CHIEF),** designed as a questionnaire.

   IDEA—Center for Inclusive Design and Environmental Access: www.ap.buffalo.edu/~idea
   Whiteneck G, Harrison-Felix C, Mellick D: Quantifying environmental factors: A measure of physical, attitudinal, service, productivity, and policy barriers. Arch Phys Med Rehabil 85:1324–1335, 2004.

2. **Describe the relationship between personhood and the physical environment.**

   Human behavior is carried out through interaction with the physical environment. Normal human development requires in-depth perception and manipulation of the environment as well as self-propulsion through the environment. From these interactions, one develops a working knowledge of the environment. The capabilities acquired from these interactions define our freedom to move about and modify the environment to our personal specifications. These experiences of "mastery" are internalized as self-discovery. Mastery becomes a behavioral pattern that is successful and is acted out in relationship to the surrounding world. It is uniquely human to adapt to the environment, and to adapt the environment to our specifications.

3. How does a new injury or illness affect the person–environment relationship?
Immediately after a catastrophic illness or injury, the experience of the body is radically distorted. **Body image** may be altered because of new deficits in perception, sensation, motor performance, and loss of body parts. Environmental perception may be altered as a result of sensory deficits or neglect. This situation is compounded by the **depersonalization** of hospitalization; patients are separated from the familiar, immediate environment of their clothes and personal items and may be confined to a bed in a horizontal position. Initially, communication as a means to share personal identity and to affect the physical environment frequently dominates the interaction. During this vulnerable period, patients' requests should be encouraged and fulfilled as reassurance that patients can meet their needs in spite of new functional limitations. Effective nursing, adaptive call lights, and access to television and telephone provide critical personal environmental control.

A person in a new body interacting with their new environment is like an infant testing the environment of their crib. Testing and modifying the environment through verbal and physical interaction are crucial for beginning the problem-solving process and eliminating potential barriers to independence. Patients carry old memories, impressions, and attitudes into their current experience of disablement. Early "experiments" of environmental interaction in the new state confirm or refute their expectations and adaptive behavior. The ongoing process of adaptation is an **operant process** that is shaped in a variety of perceptual and physical interactions, including multiple spontaneous activities, repetitions, and problem solving. In this context, rehabilitation is a process of acquisition of functional skills, known as **disability-appropriate behaviors,** and extinction of maladaptive, **disability-inappropriate behaviors.** The adaptive habits need to be cued, supported, and enabled by the adapted habitat. Many of the limitations experienced by persons with physical cognitive and sensory limitations can be attributed to their environment.

Adaptive Environments Center (AEC): www.adaptenv.org

4. Can physical environment be divided into spaces that guide intervention from a person-centered perspective?
Figure 9-1 depicts the spaces of the environment from a person-centered perspective:
1. Rehabilitation treatment within the **immediate environment** (in constant direct contact with the person) includes specialized dressings, orthotics, prosthetics, adaptive clothing, communication devices, adaptive or assistive technology for toileting and feeding, and mobility devices. These aspects can be addressed in any care-giving setting.
2. The **intermediate environment** (adapted specifically for inhabitants, adapted home or office) includes designs emphasizing function, safety, and personal style.
3. The **community environment** (surrounds the homes) not only includes the physical structure, but also includes people and institutions governed by a common culture and law.
4. The **political component** specifies access and rights of persons with disabilities.
5. The **built environment component** includes public and private buildings. Many structural changes have been implemented in accordance with the Americans with Disabilities Act (ADA), the Rehabilitation Act (Section 504), and Fair Housing Act (FHA) legislation.
6. Finally, the **natural environment** (surrounds the community-modified space) presents access challenges that can be overcome with specialized skill acquisition, adaptive landscaping, and terrain-specific mobility aids.

Stiens SA: Personhood disablement and mobility technology: Personal control of development. In Gray DB, Quatrano LA, Liberman M (eds): Designing and Using Assistive Technology: The Human Perspective. Towson, MD, Paul Brookes, 1998, pp. 29–49.

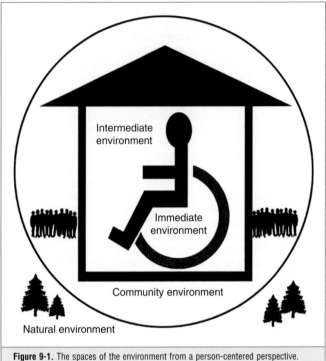

Figure 9-1. The spaces of the environment from a person-centered perspective.

5. **How can the rehabilitation team enhance patient interactions with the environment?**

   Environmental spaces are a substrate for rehabilitation intervention. The goal is for the patient to rediscover a healthy, productive interaction with the environment that allows the achievement of life goals. Clinicians and therapists should explore patient memories of particular satisfaction, prowess, and access in certain places. Through analysis of these interactions an intervention plan is formulated to make stepwise changes to the patient's environment, progressing from the immediate environment out. The interdisciplinary team also addresses the patient's person-centered goals and links them to adapted tasks.

6. **What assessment techniques can be used by the interdisciplinary team to target environmental barriers and formulate solutions to maximize functional independence?**

   Patient life behaviors can be elicited with **retrospective sociobehavioral mapping,** which is a step-by-step review of where patients have gone, who they were with, what they were doing, as well as their intentions for activities. Negative findings are often the most significant intervention foci: where patients don't go, what they are not doing. The information can be diagramed on floor plans or community maps.

   Intervention in the form of adaptive equipment often evolves as a continuum, starting with the design of the person's immediate environment (e.g., braces, wheelchair) and progressing to the intermediate environment (the patient's home). The community and natural environments are emphasized during the latter phases of the process.

Assessment of the home environment can include drawn floor plans, photographic/video depictions, or home visits. Success in the home and community is achieved with passes, predischarge home visits, and community outings. In essence, the goal is to progressively design an environment that enhances personhood (with objectives of safety and independence) and reflects the characteristics and goals of the patient in concert with others. Successive approximation of the home environment is through adaptation of the hospital room and trial living quarters as trial environments.

Giustini A: Activity and participation: New technologic possibilities to estimate and correlate them to rehabilitation treatments. Third World Congress of the International Society of Physical and Rehabilitation Medicine, Sao Paulo, Brazil, April 10–15 2005. Acta Fisiatrica 12(Suppl 1):S10, 2005.

Keysor J, Jette A, Haley S: Development of the home and community environment (HACE) instrument. J Rehabil Med 37:37–44, 2005.

7. **Describe four transitional environments in current use as part of community rehabilitation units today.**
   1. **Hospital beds and rooms on a series of units** are designed for various independence levels: intensive care, step down, telemetry, and rehabilitation unit.
   2. **Independent living trial apartments** have real-world, generic, unmodified, and modifiable characteristics to adapt for home simulation and to challenge the patients, caregivers, and family to develop adaptive solutions.
   3. **Simulated community environments** are designed for trial life scenarios without leaving the hospital.
   4. **Selected community environments** are for activity-specific trials.

KEY POINTS: ENVIRONMENTAL ADAPTATIONS

1. Environmental modifications can improve activity, participation, role function, and vocational success.

2. A functional history combined with a sketch of a home floor plan and community map is an effective method for documenting life activity.

3. Use of retrospective sociospatial mapping and family scenario mapping can suggest environmental changes and allow for virtual projection of the proposed impact as well as actual outcome assessment.

8. **In planning discharge to home, what other assessments are needed to help change the patient's immediate environment to meet personal needs?**
   Role changes may result from functional limitations that prevent the patient from performing various activities or home duties. Preparation is accomplished through **family scenario mapping** (i.e., verbal review of family activities to redefine tasks by interest and aptitude). In addition, transitions can be facilitated by practice with therapy, as needed for bathroom and kitchen activities, housekeeping, gardening, home maintenance, childcare, and marital relations.

ADA Barrier Removal Checklist: www.usdoj.gov/crt/ada/racheck.pdf

Fange A, Iwarsson S: Changes in accessibility and usability in housing: An exploration of the housing adaptation process. Occup Ther Int 12(1):44–59, 2005.

9. **What adaptive options should be focused on in a functional home assessment that will enhance a patient's activity and participation?**

An occupational therapist should accompany the patient and other occupants to follow the sequence of movements he or she would take to, and through, the home. The therapist should consider such environmental elements as:

- **Public transportation access** (stops, sidewalks, shelter safety)
- **Parking** (wide, covered, and level; motion-activated lighting)
- **Steps** (ramp, 20/1 inch length over rise; ratio, 4 degrees or 12/1 is maximum steepness)
- **Entrances and doorways** (level porch, flat or ramped threshold, light switch, security system)
- **Telephones** (cordless, multiple, headset options)
- **Exterior walkways and driveway** (level, lighted, rails)
- **Interior stairs** (gates, bilateral rails, lift options)
- **Bathroom** (door, commode height, grab bars, shower transfer, hand-held sprayer, controls, drainpipe insulation)
- **Kitchen** (reach ability, storage, food prep, cooking sequences, clean up, and reach for dish storage)
- **Security** (on-person alert system for falls, building wide with intercom, cameras, remote lock control)
- **Storage** (including closets and dressers)
- **Laundry facilities** (front loading, reacher)
- **Interior hallways** (avoid loose rugs)
- **Access to floors** (outside walks, entrances, stair lifts, elevators)
- **Living/dining room** (furniture height, serving access)
- **Breaker/fuse boxes** (location labeling)
- **Floor surfaces** (durable, nonslip)
- **Environmental control units (ECUs)** (location, power backups)
- **Interior lighting** (touch-, voice-, motion-, or ECU-activated)
- **Emergency** (lighting, escape pathways, fire extinguisher, smoke alarms)

Accessible Home Tour—Assistive Technology Partners: www.uchsc.edu/atp/adapted_home/adapthome.htm
Easter Seals home mods checklist and accessible home virtual tour: www.easterseals.com/site/
PageServer?pagename=ntlc_easyaccesshousing
Fange A, Iwarsson S: Accessibility and usability in housing: Construct validity and implications for research and practice. Disabil Rehabil 25:1316–1325, 2003.
Livable Homes Tour—Universal Design Teaching Aide: www.livablehomes.org
Ramp Building Design Guide: design.ncsu.edu/cud/pubs_p/pwoodramp.htm

10. **How is accessibility defined in the community environment?**

In the United States the **Federal Access Board** does extensive accessibility research with a variety of experts in design, architecture, medicine, and technology. Guidelines are generated for the federal level, but state and local guidelines vary. The access board in Washington, D.C., has extensive information, publications, and technical assistance services to address the government regulations for compliance with such laws as ADA, the Rehabilitation Act, Architectural Barriers Act, etc. A hard copy of accessibility guidelines can be obtained by calling 202-272-5434.

Access Board: www.access-board.gov/ada-aba/final.htm

11. **What are the rights of a tenant with disability?**

The **Fair Housing Act of 1988** mandates accessibility compliance and civil rights protection in private housing. Persons with disabilities are provided equal access. The resident cannot be denied the opportunity to modify the rented home to meet individual accessibility needs. The cost of modification is paid by the renter. In addition, the landlord may require that the work be done by an approved professional, and an escrow account may be established in which the tenant must place funds for returning the residence to its original state. Modifications that are easily used by future renters (universal design) can be left intact. A physician's prescription for modifications as "medically necessary" permits a tax deduction for expense. Section 504 of the **Rehabilitation Act of 1973** mandates that public housing and housing subsidized with federal funds be accessible and adaptable to meet the needs of tenants with disabilities.

Fair Housing Act Design Manual: www.huduser.org/publications/destech/fairhousing.html
Fair Housing Tool Kit: www.knowledgeplex.org/
Universal Design Accessibility article: www.resna.org/taproject/goals/other/univdesign/UDStrategies.htm

12. **Discuss environmental adaptations for bathrooms.**
    - Multilevel or adjustable sink heights and countertops provide accessibility from standing and seated positions.
    - Plumbing should be installed toward the back wall with hot water pipes insulated and water temperature set to prevent burns.
    - Single-levered faucet handles are universal.
    - Automatic faucets, hand dryers, wall-mounted electric toothbrushes, and soap/shampoo dispensers may be installed for a person with limited hand function and upper body strength.
    - Toilet height of 17–19 inches allows horizontal transfers from wheelchairs and eases standing and sitting. However, child access with a stool and/or exclusion with lidlock may be needed for safety.
    - An ideal grab bar system is individualized for tub and toilet access that enables greatest efficiency and safety.
    - A hand-held showerhead on an adjustable-height track can be used for bathing from a seated or standing position.
    - Padded shower chairs with back support are safe and practical.
    - Tub lifts, which lower a person into a tub, can be controlled by hydraulic, battery, or manual mechanisms.
    - A rubberized mat and tub strips provide a nonslip surface.
    - An angled mirror and a side-mounted medicine cabinet can be used from a standing or seated position.
    - Adequate lighting is nonglare, preferably with sconces and multiple bulbs or adjustable intensity.
    - A ground fault intercept (GFI) outlet prevents electrocution from the use of electrical appliances near a sink or other source of water.
    - Contrasting the color of surfaces, especially background and foreground, enables people with visual or cognitive impairments to see and define surfaces.

    Adaptable Bathrooms Manual: www.abilitycenter.org/webtools/links/adaresources/AdaptableBath.pdf
    Wheelchair Mobility Standards: www.ap.buffalo.edu/idea/Anthro/index.asp

13. **Which is the most dangerous room in the house?**
    The bathroom. Bathroom accidents are one of the leading causes of death and disability in the older population. Shower and tub falls rank as the third leading cause of accidental death in the 50-plus age group. More than half of all accidents could be prevented with some sort of environmental modification.

    Adaptable Bathrooms Manual: www.abilitycenter.org/webtools/links/adaresources/AdaptableBath.pdf

14. **List design possibilities and features for mobility-challenged adaptations for kitchens.**
    Access-friendly kitchens should have cabinets with high, deep kick plates for toe space, a U- or L-shaped floor plan for traffic flow, an appliance and storage sequence for recipe completion to service and clean up, and a stove in lowered countertop with side or front controls and angled mirror overhead. For ease of mobility, a side-swinging oven door, pullout shelves, and lazy Susans are helpful. Also, continuous countertops for sliding heavy vessels, pullout or lap cutting

boards, shallow sinks, long, retractable sprayer hoses, task lighting, reachable fire extinguishers, and strip outlets with on/off switches are popular innovations.

15. **A single woman with mild dementia had to be discharged home. Suggest possible environmental solutions for challenges she may face.**
    1. Providing environmental cues to address safety, memory, and communication deficits.
    2. Personal emergency response system with medication management and training in the use of the devices, with monitoring of her ability to learn.
    3. Automatic medication management system set up weekly by a home care nurse.
    4. Burglar alarm and posted fire escape plan that has been learned, practiced, and monitored regularly.
    5. Smoke alarms hot-wired with battery backup.
    6. Emergency lighting in case of power failure.
    7. Daily calls to monitor her ability to care for herself.
    8. Meals on Wheels and use of microwave with electric hot-water pot.
    9. Electric range or microwave oven. Avoiding use of a gas stove. Automatic turn-off controls to address memory deficits.
    10. Posted instructions on the step-by-step use of all appliances and their safety issues.
    11. Preprogramming frequently used telephone numbers for one-button speed calling.
    12. Use of a tape recorder to record daily instructions or for message taking.
    13. Providing opportunities for the patient to access as many community resources as needed to maintain her independence, health, and safety and to promote socialization (e.g., support groups, religious associations, social service agencies, and transportation).

    ADA Documents Center: www.jan.wvu.edu/links/adalinks.htm
    ADA and IT: www.adainfo.org/accessible/it/
    ADA Accessibility Guidelines on Recreational Facilities: www.access-board.gov/recreation/guides/index.htm

16. **What is visitability? Why is this movement important?**
    Visitability is a design concept for residential households that promotes the creation of communities in which people of all abilities and disabilities, especially mobility impairments, can get into the door and use at least one bathroom when visiting neighbors. This concept provides a bridge from the intermediate to the surrounding community environment and fosters social interdependence (neighbor role) and relationships that can offer natural supports for persons with disabilities.

    Center for Universal Design: www.design.ncsu.edu/cud
    Concrete Change/Visitability Resources: http://concretechange.org
    Experience Universal Design Project: www.experienceuniversaldesign.com/index.htm

17. **What interior home and community features enhance success for persons with visual impairments?**
    Interior: home
    - Increase lighting and reduce glare to increase acuity.
    - Contrast solid colors to define surfaces and edges.
    - Post large print with raised letters or use voice output on signage and controls.
    - Vary textures to define edges and boundaries.
    - Illuminate switches.
    - Install nonskid, matte-finish floor surfaces.

    Exterior: public spaces
    - Use auditory signals for crosswalks
    - Record short verbal messages about opportunities or barriers in the area.

    Iwamiya S, Yamauchi K, Takada M: Design specifications of audio-guidance systems for the blind in public spaces. J Physiol Anthropol Appl Human Sci 23: 267–271, 2004.

18. **What might aid persons with hearing impairments?**
Facing furniture arrangements with good lighting and wall-mounted mirrors to present faces for interpretation. Communication technology such as telecommunications device for the deaf (TDD) telephone, fax machine, and telephone relay system. Vibrating or light cues for clocks, telephones, doorbells, and baby monitors.

19. **What does the phrase "aging in place" mean?**
Over the past decade, older persons have overwhelmingly reported that they would prefer to remain in their homes as long as possible. Single-level homes with wide floor plans, or attached separate apartments on bus lines, near shopping, and potential attendant help are most ideal.

   AARP Home Modifications Guide: www.aarp.org/families/home_design/
   Administration on Aging—remodeling resources: www.aoa.gov/eldfam/Housing/Home_Remodeling/ Home_Remodeling.asp
   CASPAR Extended Home Living Services—home mods assessment tool: www.ecaspar.com/ec/CASPAR.pdf
   Universal Home Design Guide: www.mhfa.state.mn.us/homes/Access_Remodeling.htm

20. **Describe a series of steps that might identify safety risks, functional barriers, and an economical response to identified needs.**
   1. Client activities of daily living (ADLs)/home safety screening survey by direct mail or telephone visit
   2. Home environment: on-site home safety assessment in cases as defined by survey thresholds
   3. Functional and environmental assessment with individualized modification and patient rehabilitation on program operated by specially trained occupational and physical therapists
   4. Occupational and physical therapy with trial of interventions and specified planning for modifications and installations
   5. Product installation and home modification
   6. Client/caregiver training to help maximize the client's independence, wellness, and quality of life, as well as increasing the efficiency and safety of caregiver assistance

   National Organization on Disability (NOD)—Access to Worship Checklist: www.nod.org/index.cfm? fuseaction=page.viewPage&pageID=1430&nodeID=1&FeatureID=399&redirected=1&C FID=5162137&CFTOKEN=16611784
   Practical Guide to Universal Home Design: www.uiowa.edu/infotech/universalhomedesign.pdf
   Removing Barriers to Health Care Guide: www.fpg.unc.edu/~ncodh/RemovingBarriers/ removingbarrierspubscfm
   United Spinal Association publications: www.unitedspinal.org/pages.php?catid=7

21. **What should be considered when formulating solutions to functional and environmental barriers to maximize independence and safety?**
   - Consider the goals of the client to achieve the maximum level of independence and safety for daily activities at home to the jobsite/school environment/community.
   - Consider the caregivers and others living in the home.
   - Consider strengths and weakness in sensorimotor, cognitive, and psychosocial functions.
   - Consider the progressive nature of the client's illness/disability and future needs.
   - Target environmental barriers along a route from parking to building entrances and throughout the interior space, considering safety, maximum independence, and adaptablity of the environment.
   - Assess the need for specialized equipment and training in its use. Internet product research is now a very effective way to find products, evaluations of those products, and distributors.
   - Prioritize all suggestions (client/caregiver in consult with the team) according to the immediate requirements needed for functioning/caregiving, including getting in and out of the home, training in transfers, ADLs, mobility, compensation techniques, stress management, and safety issues according to the financial resources available to the client.

- Provide resources for the client and caregivers of specially trained professionals, support services, and funding options if needed.
- Provide ongoing consultation to designers, building contractors, and client during the design and construction phase.
- Consider financial constraints and potential resources from medical insurance, community resources, and loans/grants.

Consideration of all these factors will ensure greater levels of success in carryover of the rehabilitation process and community integration of the person once discharged from inpatient, intermediate care, and home-care therapy. In addition, **periodically monitor progress and challenges** once environmental modifications and assistive technology are in place and in use. Address issues of the person when functioning in his or her environment, as well as issues of the caregiver. Adjust elements as needed to promote success, maximum safety, function, and independence.

WEBSITES

1. Designing a More Usable World
www.trace.wisc.edu/world

2. Future Home Foundation
www.thefuturehome.net

3. Government Disability Information and Agencies
www.disabilityinfo.gov/digov-public/public/DisplayPage.do?fparentFolderId=500

4. National Resource Center on Supportive Housing and Home Modification
www.homemods.org

BIBLIOGRAPHY

1. Shamberg S: Optimizing access to home, community, and work environments. In Trombley CA, Radomski MV (eds): Occupational Therapy for Physical Dysfunction, 5th ed. Philadelphia, Lippincott, Williams & Wilkins, 2001.

2. Shamberg S: Occupational therapy practitioner: Role in the implementation of worksite modifications. IOS 24:185–197, 2001.

3. Stiens DW, Stiens SA: Environmental modifications and role functions: Redesign of a house for a family with a paraplegic father. J Am Parapleg Soc 16:278–279, 1993.

4. Wylde M, Baron-Robbins A, Clark S: Building for a Lifetime: The Design and Construction of Fully Accessible Homes. Newtown, CT, Taunton, 1994, p. 304.

RESOURCES

1. ABLEDATA (www.abledata.com): a database of information on assistive technology and rehabilitation equipment designed to serve persons with disabilities and rehabilitation professionals. Contact Kathryn Belnap: 800-227-0216.

2. Abilities OT Services and Seminars (www.aotss.com): see www.aotss.com for a complete listing of organizations and publications (3309 W. Strathmore Ave., Baltimore, MD 21215-3718; phone: 410-358-7269; fax: 410-358-6454). Technical assistance, publications, and Internet and on-site training programs for medical and design/build professionals on home modifications, job-site modifications, disability legislation compliance, and assistive technology.

3. American Occupational Therapy Association (AOTA): www.aota.org or 800-729-2682: a list of environmental access specialists in occupational therapy by region and technical assistance information on home modifications and assistive technology.

4. American Society of Interior Designers (ASID): www.asid.org or 608 Massachusetts Ave., NE, Washington, DC 20002–6006; phone: 202-546-3480; fax: 202-546-3240.

5. ADAPT (advocacy for independent living): www.adapt.org

6. Adaptive Environments Center (AEC): www.adaptenv.org

7. Andrus Center: at-home modification publications and information/directory of consultants; www.homemods.org

8. Association of Assistive Technology Act Programs: www.ataporg.org

9. Center for Universal Design: www.design.ncsu.edu/cud

10. Delaware Assistive Technology Initiative (DATI) Fair Housing and AT Resources: www.dati.org/newsletter/issues/2002n3/MultifamilyConstruction.html

11. Designing a More Usable World: www.trace.wisc.edu/world

12. Easter Seals: www.easterseals.com/site/PageServer?pagename=ntl_resource_room&s_esLocation=res, or 230 W. Monroe St., Suite 1800, Chicago, IL 60606; phone: 800-221-6827; 312-726-6200; 312-726-4258 (TTY).

CHAPTER 10

LEGISLATION, DISABILITY, AND PHYSICAL MEDICINE AND REHABILITATION: ENHANCING PARTICIPATION OF PERSONS WITH DISABILITIES

Leighton Chan, MD, MPH, Mary Richardson, PhD, MHA, and Richard Verville, JD

Life, liberty, and the pursuit of happiness.

–Thomas Jefferson, Declaration of Independence, 1776

1. **Why is legislative action important for persons with disabilities?**

   Currently, nearly 54 million people in the United States—approximately 20% of the population (according to the 2001 report of the Census Bureau Survey of Income and Program Participation)—have at least one disability. The federal government has attempted to protect the rights of these citizens and provide opportunities for them. Legislation has addressed rights to health care, education, housing, public access, income, vocational training, and employment. These laws have had a potent effect on patient outcomes by specifying many aspects of the social and physical environment in which they live.

2. **What is the Americans with Disabilities Act (ADA)?**

   The ADA was signed into law by President George Bush in 1990. Most people are aware that the ADA requires the removal of architectural barriers in some facilities; however, the ADA is much more than just a set of building codes and regulations. The ADA takes aim at discrimination and articulates goals for equal opportunity, full participation, independent living, and economic self-sufficiency. It documents that people with disabilities, as a group, maintain an inferior status in our society and are severely disadvantaged socially, vocationally, economically, and educationally. In response, the ADA calls for a "clear and comprehensive national mandate for the elimination of discrimination against individuals with disabilities" and provides enforceable standards to achieve this goal.

   Specifically, the ADA is designed to prevent discrimination against those with disabilities in several settings: employment, public services, public accommodations, telecommunications, and transportation. These rights had been partially protected by the Rehabilitation Act of 1973, which prohibited discrimination in programs receiving federal assistance. The ADA extends these rights to cover entities not receiving such funds. This means that private concerns, such as businesses and restaurants, must abide by the ADA.

   Like much federal legislation, the ADA's language is specific in some places and vague in others. Therefore, some of the operational details of the ADA have required interpretation by the judicial system through a series of ongoing legal actions, and many of the ADA's implementation issues are not yet resolved. In addition, state and local disability laws may duplicate or contradict ADA guidelines. Complete, up-to-date information about specific regulations in your area can be obtained by contacting your regional Disability and Business Technical Assistance Center (www.adata.org).

3. **How does the ADA define disability?**

The ADA defines disability as "(A) a physical or mental impairment that substantially limits one or more of the major life activities of such individual; (B) a record of such an impairment; or (C) being regarded as having such an impairment." Thus, those with physical disabilities *and/or* mental disabilities that are the result of a physiologic or mental disorder are covered under the act. The ADA protects those who are recovering alcoholics and former drug abusers, but it will not protect an alcoholic who is unable to perform his or her job because of alcoholism, nor will it protect current drug abusers.

4. **What are the employment provisions of the ADA?**

The ADA defines an *employer* as anyone engaged in an industry affecting commerce who has 15 or more employees. The ADA prohibits discrimination by the employer against any *qualified individual* with a disability in regard to hiring, promotions, discharge, compensation, training, or other privileges of employment. Qualified individuals are those who "with or without *reasonable accommodation, can perform the essential functions of the employment position that* such person holds or desires." Reasonable accommodations must be made by the employer unless they pose *undue hardship* on the operation of the business.

The ADA specifically prohibits an employer from using screening methods and selection criteria that do not pertain to the requirements of the job and/or are meant to deny opportunity to the candidate because of his or her disability. Furthermore, the employer must clearly articulate the skill demands of the position and the performance expectations. If a person can meet those required demands and expectations with reasonable accommodation by the employer, then he or she must be considered equally with other candidates, regardless of disability. The **Equal Employment Opportunity Commission** (EEOC) is in charge of issuing regulations concerning employment as well as the ADA (www.eeoc.gov/).

5. **What are the public service provisions of the ADA?**

Title II of the ADA states that "no qualified individual with a disability shall be excluded from participation in, or be denied the benefits of, the services, programs, or activities of a public entity or subjected to discrimination by such entity." Public entities are defined as state and local governments and the National Railroad Passenger Corporation.

Title II goes on to describe specific requirements for public transportation. In general, all public rail systems must have accessible cars. Retrofitting existing public buses is not required, but all new vehicles purchased or leased must be accessible, and good-faith efforts must be made to acquire accessible used vehicles.

In a far-reaching rehabilitation case of 1999 (Olmstead), the Supreme Court held that Title II required a state to deinstitutionalize persons with disabilities when treating professionals thought that a community setting was the least restrictive environment that made them most able.

6. **What are the public accommodation provisions of the ADA?**

Title III of the ADA specifies that "no individual shall be discriminated against on the basis of disability in the full and equal enjoyment of the goods, services, facilities, privileges, or accommodations of any place of public accommodation by any person who owns, leases (or leases to), or operates a place of public accommodation." The title lists places of public accommodation including hotels, restaurants, professional offices, museums, etc. Religious organizations and private clubs are exempt from this portion of the ADA.

Title III of the ADA requires that preexisting places of public accommodation remove architectural barriers only if this is readily achievable—that is, "if this is easily accomplished and able to be carried out without difficulty or expense." Among the basic changes that may be needed for compliance are:

- Making curb cuts
- Installing ramps

- Widening doorways
- Assuring an accessible path from parking lot to areas of service provision
- Removing high-pile carpeting to allow wheelchair accessibility
- Installing paper cup dispensers at water fountains
- Installing accessible toilets

7. What is the role of the physiatrist in regard to the ADA?

A good, responsible physiatrist must know the rights afforded to persons with disabilities by the ADA and make sure the patient and the rehabilitation team are well versed in them so that these goals can be achieved. In regard to the **employment provisions** of the ADA, a physiatrist may be called on by an employer to state the work limitations of a particular patient and specify any job modifications that might be necessary. Therefore, a physiatrist must be aware of what questions to ask an employer and have a good grasp of assistive technology that might help a patient perform specific job-related tasks.

In addition, a physiatrist, like other physicians in practice, is obligated to have accessible facilities for disabled patients and provide reasonable communication accommodations for those with sensory impairments such as deafness. The accommodation may include communication by computer, by written notes, or through use of an interpreter. However, no accommodation is required if it would impose an unreasonable financial hardship.

KEY POINTS: AMERICANS WITH DISABILITIES ACT (ADA)

1. The ADA defines disability as a mental impairment or physical impairment that is a result of a disorder.

2. Ongoing alcohol or drug abuse is not covered.

3. The ADA requires that local, state, and federal governments, as well as companies with 15 or more employees, not discriminate against an *individual* with a disability, provide reasonable physical and other accommodations, and remove architectural barriers.

8. How do individuals with disabilities acquire medical insurance?

For those who do not have private insurance, the most common way is through Medicare and Medicaid. Persons who are injured while working may have their medical bills covered through Workers' Compensation.

9. What is Medicare?

Medicare is a federal program that provides health care coverage to those who have paid a Medicare payroll tax during their working years. In addition, family members of those who qualify may also be covered. In 2007, Medicare provided health care coverage for 43.7 million people. In general, Medicare benefits begin at age 65. An individual can apply for benefits earlier in life if he or she is disabled or on renal dialysis (www.medicare.gov).

Centers for Medicare and Medicaid Services: 2006 Data Compendium: www.cms.hhs.gov/DataCompendium

10. How is Medicare organized?

Medicare coverage is divided into several parts. **Part A** covers the cost of inpatient hospitalization and home health services, as well as stays in skilled nursing facilities and hospices. **Part B** is a voluntary program that requires additional payments by the beneficiary and covers the services of physicians, outpatient clinic visits, and many ancillary services, such as x-rays, lab tests, and durable medical equipment. Many private insurance companies offer Medicare supplemental coverage for those items not covered in Part A or B. On January 1, 2006, **Part D** came into effect. This benefit provides coverage of medically necessary prescription drugs, but it is voluntary and requires a premium payment.

11. **How does Medicare pay for inpatient rehabilitation?**
    To classify as an inpatient rehabilitation facility, a hospital or unit must satisfy the "75% rule"; that is, 75% of patients must fall into one of several diagnostic categories: stroke, spinal cord injury, congenital deformity, amputation, major multiple trauma, fracture of femur (hip fracture), traumatic brain injury, neurologic disorders, burns, active polyarticular rheumatoid or psoriatic arthritis, seronegative arthropathies, systemic vasculitides with joint inflammation, severe/advanced osteoarthritis involving two or more major weight-bearing joints, and selected joint replacements.

    Medicare pays rehabilitation hospitals through a **prospective payment system**. Patients in rehabilitation facilities are assessed using the Inpatient Rehabilitation Facility-Patient Assessment Instrument (IRF-PAI) and are then placed in certain groups based on characteristics such as age, diagnosis, and functional status (Functional Independence Measure [FIM] scores). Rehabilitation facilities are given a fixed amount of money for each patient based on the category they fall into, no matter how long the patient stays. Additional payments may also be given to facilities based on their location, whether they train residents, the income status of their patients, and for "outliers" (patients whose extended stay might be particularly expensive) (www.cms.hhs.gov/InpatientRehabFacPPS/downloads/irfpai-manual040104.pdf).

KEY POINTS: MEDICARE

1. Medicare insurance covers people over age 65, people with a disability, and people on dialysis.

2. It pays inpatient, outpatient, and some drug costs.

3. It reimburses inpatient rehabilitation facilities through a prospective payment system.

12. **What is Medicaid?**
    Medicaid provides health insurance to low-income patients who receive public assistance, including families with children, the aged, individuals with disabilities, as well as medically needy individuals. The Medicaid program is funded jointly by federal and state dollars. The federal government issues broad guidelines to the states, who then administer the programs. Regulations concerning eligibility, coverage, and reimbursement vary from state to state. In 2006, Medicaid enrollment was approximately 63.2 million people.

    Centers for Medicare and Medicaid Services: 2003 Data Compendium. www.cms.hhs.gov/DataCompendium

13. **How does a person qualify for Medicaid?**
    In general, Medicaid is a means-tested program. That is, if an individual's income and resources are below a certain level, he or she is eligible for coverage. However, not all indigent individuals qualify. For instance, healthy adults without children cannot be covered by Medicaid, regardless of their income and resources. Individuals who might qualify include pregnant women, families

with children, and people who are elderly, blind, medically needy, institutionalized, or disabled. Often, these individuals have to "spend down" their resources until they qualify.

To qualify for Medicaid on the basis of disability, an individual needs to be receiving federal Supplemental Security Income (SSI) payments for that disability. The SSI program requires that an individual must be "unable to engage in any substantial gainful activity by reason of a medically determined physical or mental impairment expected to result in death or that has lasted or can be expected to last for a continuous period of at least 12 months." In addition, recipients may also have to pass a means test.

14. What is covered under Medicaid?
Medical coverage varies widely from state to state. In general, Medicaid requires that states cover the cost of hospital stays, physician care, and nursing homes. Several states, such as Oregon, have Medicaid waivers to design their own package of benefits.

Coverage of many items such as prescription drugs and dental care is optional, and states are not required to include them in their Medicaid package. Some states have waivers enabling them to provide community-based living for persons with disabilities in lieu of nursing home care.

KEY POINTS: MEDICAID

1. Medical insurance covers disabled persons, children, and pregnant women.

2. Patients often have to exhaust their own resources before they qualify for Medicaid benefits.

3. State and federal governments split the cost.

4. Each state defines the benefits.

5. Benefits are usually less than those for Medicare patients.

15. How can individuals with disabilities receive income assistance?
Poverty is commonly associated with disability. With costly medical bills and poor earning potential, many people with disabilities are economically disadvantaged and may come to rely on public assistance. There are two major federal programs to provide income assistance to individuals with disabilities: SSI and Social Security Disability Insurance (SSDI) (www.ssa.gov/disability).

SSI is linked to the Medicaid system and provides financial assistance to low-income individuals who are elderly, blind, or disabled. To qualify on the basis of disability, a person must be "unable to engage in any substantial gainful activity by reason of a medically determined physical or mental impairment expected to result in death or that has lasted or can be expected to last for a continuous period of at least 12 months." (Note: SSI determination for children is different and based on a categorical definition of disability.)

SSDI is similar to SSI, but the benefits are more generous. In addition, it is linked to the Medicare system. To get SSDI benefits, one must have worked and paid into the Social Security system. Applicants for SSDI must meet a definition of disability similar to that for SSI. Physicians assess when a person cannot work or is ready to return to work and eligibility is reevaluated approximately every 3 years.

16. What has the federal government done to educate children with disabilities?
Federally mandated education for children with disabilities began in the mid-1970s, when several studies revealed that only a few states attempted to educate more than half their disabled children. In 1975, Congress passed the Education for All Handicapped Children Act. This act was later incorporated into Individuals with Disabilities Education Act (IDEA), and together they have

served to define state obligations in regard to education of the children with disabilities (www.ed.gov/policy/speced/guid/idea/index.html).

17. **Who is covered under IDEA?**

By law, any state that accepts federal funds under IDEA must have a "zero reject" policy and provide assistance to all who qualify. In general, all children aged 3–21 years are eligible for educational assistance under IDEA if they meet specific eligibility criteria. A child must have 1 of 13 specific conditions listed in the Act, or they must fall under the category of "other health impairment." In addition, this health condition must "adversely affect educational performance" and require special education.

18. **What type of education is the state required to provide?**

Under IDEA, all qualified children must be provided with a free appropriate public education, which includes special education and related services in the least restrictive setting. The Act further mandates that "to the maximum extent appropriate, children with disabilities. . .are educated with children who are not disabled." States are obligated to provide the necessary assistive technology and other personnel necessary to achieve these goals.

The intent of IDEA is to promote the "mainstreaming" of children with disabilities into regular classrooms with the rest of their peers, which improves the education of both disabled *and* nondisabled students. Clearly, however, "mainstreaming" is not appropriate for all children with disabilities, and for some individuals a more controlled setting may represent the "least restrictive environment." The educational goals for children with disabilities, including the educational setting, are set out in an Individual Education Plan (IEP) produced by the school district for each student. Educational goals vary depending on the student's capabilities. Some goals may be similar to those of students without disabilities or they may be focused on achieving "self-help skills."

19. **What is the physiatrist's role in the education of children with disabilities?**

The physiatrist can be helpful in educating pediatricians about screening for disabilities and defining specific impairments and activity limitations. Specific explanation of the deficits can be provided to schools with advice for treatment and adaptive devices. This information can be included in the IEP.

Although the physiatrist is not directly involved in creating the IEP, he or she can be very helpful in (1) identifying children who might be candidates for educational assistance; (2) providing written guidance to the school concerning the educational impact of the disability; and (3) outlining a child's health maintenance activities, such as medication prescriptions, urinary catheterization, and g-tube feedings, as well as writing therapy orders.

20. **What has the federal government done to promote assistive technology?**

The Technology-Related Assistance for Individuals with Disabilities Act of 1988 (The Tech Act) was signed into law in response to the growing awareness of the role of technology in the field of rehabilitation. The Act defines assistive technology as a combination of both devices and services. The term *assistive technology device* is defined as "any item, piece of equipment, or product system whether acquired commercially off the shelf, modified, or customized that is used to increase, maintain, or improve the functional capabilities of individuals with disabilities." Assistive technology services means "any service that directly assists an individual with a disability in the selection, acquisition, or use of an assistive technology device." These definitions were later amended into IDEA in 1990. The Tech Act also provides funding to each of the states for research efforts, demonstration projects, and educational programs, as well as direct provision of assistive technology to patients (www.ataporg.org/index.asp).

WEBSITES

1. Disability Business Technical Assistance Center (DBTAC): 800-949-4232 V/TTY
   www.dbtac.vcu.edu

2. Rehabilitation Engineering & Assistive Technology Society of North America
   www.resna.org

ACKNOWLEDGMENT

This research was supported in part by the Intramural Research Program of the NIH.

BIBLIOGRAPHY

1. Balanced Budget Act of 1997: Public Law 105–33. Subtitle E, Chapter 2, sections 4401–4421.

2. Carter GM, Relles DA, Wynn BA, et al: In Interim Report in an Inpatient Rehabilitation Facility Prospective Payment System. No. DRU-2309-HCFA. Santa Monica, CA, Rand Corp, 2000, pp 1–235.

3. Centers for Medicare and Medicaid Services: 2003 Data Compendium. www.cms.hhs.gov/researchers/pubs/datacompendium/current

4. Fast Facts and Figures about Social Security. Social Security Administration, Office of Research, Evaluation and Statistics, Aug 2000.

5. Julnes R, Brown S: Assistive technology and special education programs: Legal mandates and practice implications. Law Educ Desk Notes 3(4):54, 1993.

6. Melvin D: The desegregation of children with disabilities. DePaul Law Rev 44:603, 1995.

7. Perlman L, Kirk F: Key disability and rehabilitation legislation. J App Rehabil Counsel 22(3):25, 1991.

8. Price R: Medicaid: Eligibility for the Aged, Disabled, and Blind. CRS Report for Congress, 94–297 EPW, April 4:39, 1994.

9. Public Law. Americans with Disabilities Act of 1990, pp 101–336.

10. Richardson M: The impact of the Americans with Disabilities Act on employment opportunity for people with disabilities. Annu Rev Public Health 15:91–105, 1994.

11. Rothstein L: In Disabilities and the Law. New York, McGraw-Hill, 1992.

THE PHYSIATRIC CONSULTATION: ACUTE TREATMENT, IMMEDIATE REHABILITATION, AND FUTURE ENABLEMENT

Steven A. Stiens, MD, MS, Rina Reyes, MD, and Jelena N. Svircev, MD

Electric communication will never be a substitute for the face of someone who with their soul encourages another person to be brave and true.

–Charles Dickens (1812–1870)

1. **What is a physiatric consultation?**
   In the past, a consultation consisted of two physicians evaluating the patient together. Today, this process is asynchronous and requires collaborative coordination. **Consultation** provides expert medical advice to the patient's attending physician and treatment team. Consultations are unique because physicians and their views of patients and interventions are formulations as unique as physiatric assessments of patients and anticipated outcomes. The essential tasks include identification of the foci for intervention, tailoring the treatment options for the setting, and communication and agreement on outcome and orchestration of the team to meet the identified goals.

2. **Why are physical medicine and rehabilitation (PM&R) consultations requested?**
   Typically, various patients do not have sufficient capabilities for transition in care settings or life roles. Patient needs include inpatient rehabilitation, pain management, disability determination, musculoskeletal treatment, electrodiagnosis, and assumptions of primary care. Ideally, physiatrists are consulted to keep patients maximally capable in order to enable them to meet life demands and aspirations. Early involvement of physiatrists minimizes impairments, speeds recovery, and prepares patients for change in the environmental settings. Typically, there are activity limitations that prevent patient progress or sufficient independence for discharge home. Most consults, however, are requested too late in the course. Consultations are an opportunity to provide education to the treating team, patient, and family.

   Musick DW, Nickerson RB, McDowell SM, Gaters DR: An exploratory examination of an academic PM&R inpatient consultation service. Disabil Rehabil 25(7):354–359, 2003.

3. **How can physiatric consultation fit into the medical continuum?**
   The medical continuum includes **prevention, acute treatment,** and **rehabilitation.** Although Howard Rusk referred to rehabilitation as the "third phase of medical care," the interdisciplinary team can intervene throughout the medical continuum. Physiatric consultations can address risk for disability, proactive life management in anticipation of deterioration, disease-appropriate self-care, and function preservation during acute care as well as rehabilitation thereafter.

4. **Should rehabilitation be limited to this late stage of medical care?**
   The interdisciplinary rehabilitation team can intervene throughout the medical continuum. Early intervention with rehabilitation during or before acute treatment can shorten the overall time

required for rehabilitation and prevent morbidity and mortality, especially in stroke, cardiac, spinal cord, and amputation rehabilitation.

For example, contemporary rehabilitative intervention for a patient who requires a limb prosthesis includes a collaborative effort among vascular surgery, orthopedic surgery, and the interdisciplinary rehabilitation team to prompt appropriate medical attention as soon as infection, ischemia, or other processes threaten a limb. In this consultative model, the physiatrist contributes throughout the medical continuum. If a wound is discovered, the rehabilitation team can advise on dressings, protective footwear, bracing, assistive devices for ambulation, and foot care for the opposite limb. Should preventive efforts fail, the physiatrist and prosthetist can contribute during the acute phase of the medical continuum by planning for level of amputation and applying rigid dressings with pylons immediately after surgery, as indicated for early weight-bearing and ambulation. Thereafter the rehabilitation team will define and fit the definitive prosthesis and continue both prevention with systemic interventions to interrupt pathophysiology and treatment for risk factors and risk behaviors. Preventive measures to protect the opposite limb include diabetes management, prevention of platelet adhesion, foot-care training, and foot protection with custom footwear with Plastizote inserts and a large toe box. Inclusion of the physiatrist in this early intervention produces the best results for the patient.

5. **What skills and knowledge are necessary for the savvy consulting physiatrist?**
First and foremost, physiatrists are patient-centered function doctors. Therefore the physiatrist should be knowledgeable about the daily routine and life goals of patients with new impairments and activity limitations. The primary theme of the physiatric visit is that rehabilitation can help the patient maximize his or her abilities for the most promising future. The physiatrist must know people, personalities, and coping styles and be able to estimate patient's tolerances for treatment and equipment **(gadget tolerance).** The consultant should know the hospital or practice setting very well, including diets, supplies stocked, therapies, other ancillary support, and pass policies. Finally, it is good to know the "territory" of the community from which patients come and return. Knowledge of the surrounding community, landscape, housing designs, transportation, and access to places of business helps the physiatrist prepare the patient for the fullest community participation upon discharge.

6. **What are the objectives of a comprehensive physiatric consultation?**
   1. **Confirm the diagnosis,** pathology, and active pathophysiology.
   2. **Quantify functional levels** and provide a functional prognosis.
   3. **Design a rehabilitation problem list** (*see* Chapter 14).
   4. **Answer the question** of the initial consultation and then educate the team about the rehabilitation interventions.
   5. **Formulate** short-term, intermediate, and long-term rehabilitation **goals.**
   6. **Translate the plans** and interventions for the originators of the consult and for the patient and family, and arrive at agreement on treatment plans.
   7. **Orchestrate the secondary consultations** and direct interventions through the interdisciplinary process to immediately begin to achieve goals on schedule and advance function.
   8. Should a **transfer to inpatient rehabilitation** be planned, confirm with the treating team if acute medical interventions have been completed and/or which treatments need to be continued.

7. **When you go into the room to take the patient's history, how many experts will be present?**
At least two: the **patient** and (hopefully) the **physiatrist.** Every experience of an injury or disease is unique because the course of injury and recovery always varies and the person impacted by the bodily changes has a unique development, life experiences, and goals. The patient is an expert on his or her **illness experience** (a subjective sense of not being well) and the impact of

disablement (sum total of impairments, activity limitations, and barriers to participation). Other "experts" in the room may include family, close friends, attendants, and roommates. Each has a perspective of the challenges that the patient faces and may have a vision of what recovery is and their role in it. These expectations need to be elicited and addressed in the design of a cohesive rehabilitation plan that the patient and the interdisciplinary team can adopt. In acute inpatient cases, it is often necessary to conduct ward-based patient, family, and **team goal-setting meetings** to explain the rehabilitation process and decide on the facility for future postacute rehabilitation.

8. **How do you elicit information on the actual and specific help the patient gets at home from family, friends, and attendants?**
   The establishment of an **atmosphere of acceptance** permits patients' and families' honest expression of functional solutions and requests for improvement in the system that is in place. Keep the patient in charge of his or her life activity. Ask: "Whom do you direct in assisting you with transfers such as dressing, bathing, and meal preparation?" The role of the clinician is to frame the interaction as a learning activity. Each patient then becomes an anthropologist reporting on his or her experience in a unique environmental matrix. It is the work of the physiatrist to recognize, define, and negotiate goals in the context of the patient's life and to commit to achieving solutions. Indeed, each situation is a perception, activity, psychosocial, and economic equation in itself. The challenge is to understand the patient's specific self-care methods and refine these processes with new techniques and equipment.

9. **What options are there for sequencing the history taking from the patient?**
   First, an introduction of the clinician and his or her role is presented; then an understanding of the patient as a whole person is derived. Next, the menu of rehabilitation services is presented as a directory related to patient-centered needs. A medical and functional history is elicited from the patient's detailing of the impact of the illness on life activity. One sequence is to record the history chronologically, starting by asking the patient "how you noticed your injury, pain, or diagnosis, and what worried you most about how it would affect your life?" If the patient is newly injured, exploration for immediate goals may be a next step. If the patient is being seen in an outpatient setting or has a chronic disability, proceed from the history into a description of the disablement, as experienced by the patient. Another approach would be to focus on the patient's function before the injury or illness, and then review the changes afterward in a format guided by a problem list or by organ systems. Be sure to elicit comments about function as well as symptoms. Identify immediate barriers and focus the rehabilitation process on barriers to transfer to rehabilitation and then on return home.

10. **How can the examination be an education for the patient and provide therapy that could contribute to recovery?**
    Many patients with pain, paralysis, and on anesthesia are not fully aware of their capabilities and learn much from a guided examination. In addition, spouses, attendants, and nurses caring for the patient may have questions about methods for improving the patient's care. Sensory testing allows discussion of the receptive fields of various peripheral nerves and dermatomes. In the patient with myelopathy, sacral sparing can be explained and used as an incentive to be attentive to and attempt to regain control of bowel, bladder, and sexual function. Range-of-motion (ROM) testing allows for instruction in self-stretching and ROM with assistance. Strength testing permits instruction in proprioceptive neuromuscular facilitation techniques. Functional motor and coordination testing can lead to demonstration of exercises prescribed for the patient. At the conclusion of a visit, the patient can be set up with a written set of exercises and schedule for practice that can be posted at bedside or used in the home before therapy visits start.

11. **What essential components should be included in the consultation report?**
    Remember, the consultation report may be used not only by the referring provider but also by the patient, rehabilitation therapists, lawyers, and insurance providers (Box 11-1). Indicate

---

BOX 11-1. CONTENTS OF A CONSULTATION

Problem list—Include primary diagnoses, secondary diagnoses, impairments, activity limitations, and barriers to participation. Follow each of the problems with a brief assessment description.

Introduction—Record referring physician and reason for referral.

Current treatment

    a. Patient identity, life roles in past and present

    b. History of injury or disease process, life impact

    c. Interventions, medications, treatments

Past history

    a. Past medical history—diagnoses and impact

    b. Family history—risk for conditions

    c. Social history—past and current life roles, potential support options

Current function

    a. Mobility—assistive devices, transfers, ambulation, setting required

    b. ADLs—eating, hygiene, bowel/bladder management, bathing, dressing

    c. Vocational function—include volunteering, parenting, work from home

    d. Leisure activities—enjoyment, engagement with others, channels for satisfaction

    e. Equipment and home architecture, vehicles

Examination—Focus on diagnosis confirmation, impairment and activity limitation quantification, and areas of rehabilitation. Record functional neuromuscular examination, including mental status, cognition, mobility, and ADLs.

Assessment—Develop a summary statement of diagnosis, medical stability (improving, plateau, declining), preparedness for rehabilitation, and setting for further interventions.

Recommendations—List in the same order as the problem list. Record recommendations for further testing, treatment options, patient's daily schedule, and prognosis. Include short- and long-term goals and prognosis. Describe an immediate plan (i.e., acute rehabilitation), an intermediate plan (i.e., transfer to subacute rehabilitation), and a long-term plan (i.e., discharge to home).

ADLs = activities of daily living.

---

who will order necessary studies and medications and provide ongoing care for the patient. A copy of the consultation should be sent to the referring physician, as well as to the primary medical care provider and patient and family.

Keely E, Dojeiji S, Myers K: Writing effective consultation letters: 12 tips for teachers. Med Teacher 24(6):585–589, 2002.

12. **How is the problem list organized in consultation report notes?**
   As the chart is reviewed, a problem list is derived that includes **diagnoses, impairments, activity limitations,** and **barriers to participation,** arranged in that order. This process might

occur at bedside, on the phone with family, or in earshot of the patient's nurse. Specifics of the hospital course need not be recorded. The diagnoses themselves, duration of time under treatment, and recent severity measures are most useful in each problem. Each problem should be a short phrase that describes the unique situation of that patient. **Potential problem domains** are primary injury or diagnosis, other diagnoses, spine stability, neurogenic bowel, neurogenic bladder, neurogenic skin, pressure ulcers, mobility, activities of daily living (ADLs), communication, psychological adaptation, sexuality, social role function, architectural accessibility, community reintegration, and discharge management. Patient-centered domains should be included as well.

13. **Whose consult is it, anyway?**
Whose life is it, anyway? The patient's, of course. In practicing patient-centered medicine we must receive confirmation of and engage the patient's interest and willingness to participate in the evaluation process and treatment. Sensitivity and perceptiveness are required as the patient's needs are elicited and the plan of care is designed. First, the physiatric assessments and treatment recommendations should be discussed and communicated to the attending physician or the directly responsible resident for discussion and concurrence. Immediately thereafter, a report should be made to the patient for his or her concurrence with the plan. This allows the patient to know the plan before it is disseminated to other providers, minimizes misunderstanding, promotes consistency in information transmitted to the patient, and maximizes cooperation.

14. **What is a physiatric prescription?**
A prescription is a written formula for the preparation and administration of a therapeutic remedy. The physiatrist leads the interdisciplinary rehabilitation team by prescribing specific interventions to meet short- and long-term goals of various patient problem domains. Prescriptions for treatment come in the form of orders for nursing care and consultative referrals to allied health professionals and other members of the rehabilitation team. The physician as team leader must balance specific requests for interventions with the objectives or outcomes that may be achieved through a variety of means. Therefore, therapeutic prescriptions are often an amalgamation of objectives, specific requests for treatment, and requests for evaluation and problem solving to achieve various outcomes.

15. **How do you write a prescription for treatment that integrates other members of the interdisciplinary team into the rehabilitation process?**
The **basic components of the physiatric prescription** are:
- Identification of **discipline consulted** (e.g., physical, recreational, occupational therapy)
- Major and significant secondary **diagnoses**
- Pertinent **impairments, activity limitations, and barriers to participation** that may be a focus of therapy
- **Precautions:** cardiac, weight-bearing, pulmonary (O_2 sat monitoring)
- **Short- and long-term goals** and objectives of therapy, including a copy of physiatric consult as needed
- **Specific therapeutic prescription** that includes areas to be treated, modality, intensity, duration, and frequency, as needed
- **Frequency of visits** and over what period
- **Date of reevaluation**, request for a summary report detailing response to therapy

16. **How would you carry out a consultation on a 55-year-old married white man with a new left-middle cerebral artery stroke?**
On approach to the ward, identify the patient's nurse for a review of current condition and particular needs. Abstract from the chart a list of problems such as cerebrovascular accident (CVA), risk factors, and complications. Use a phrase with each problem to specify severity. For example, identify location, size, and etiology of stroke. List the risk factors for CVA as separate problems as well. For example, a description of diabetes mellitus might read, "IDDM for 10

years with HgbA1C of 8." Follow with a list of various complications, such as deep venous thrombosis, edema, and skin breakdown. Then list the impairments (perception/neglect) and activity limitations (mobility, ADLs, communication ability, cognition, leisure activities). Specific functional limitations in self-care can be included in or under the ADL limitation problems. Thereafter, problems at the barrier to participation level can be listed: psychological adaptation (depression), social role function (e.g., husband, neighbor), and architectural access (ramp to door, bathroom access). Recommendations and prioritization of short-term goals should be listed, making sure to include the family in training. Immediate progress might be achieved with medication adjustments or by posting a schedule for goal-based activity throughout the day: ROM, sitting time, Foley drainage to leg bag, dressing, supervised meals, prescribed family activities, identifying one primary nurse. After stabilization, the patient should be transferred to the least restrictive setting for continued rehabilitation.

17. **What is a clinical pathway or care map?**
A **clinical pathway,** or **clinical care map,** is a uniform procedure for coordination of interventions by a variety of medical disciplines in patients within a given diagnostic group. The development of a clinical pathway requires a sufficient number of cases seen per year to justify pathway design. Management of past cases is reviewed by all disciplines that care for patients with the diagnosis. The sequence schedule and details of interventions are designed and agreed on. Then, a form for the chart is drawn up that lists the interventions and disciplines. The pathway is typically triggered by one order made by the attending physician. Other referrals and orders are made automatically through the clinical pathway to save time and improve the quality of care. As a result, time is saved and the quality of care is enhanced.

18. **How can the PM&R consultation be used as a mechanism for teaching?**
A PM&R consultation can fulfill many teaching missions. Bringing rehabilitation to other floors of the hospital, to clinics, or to patients' homes showcases rehabilitation in process and demonstrates functional outcomes in patients with many diagnoses. Bringing medical students and premedical students on PM&R consultation rounds introduces them to patients with a wide spectrum of disablement experiences who are treated in various settings. The consult service offers an opportunity to provide a broad overview of a number of various medical problems and rehabilitation solutions.

Stiens SA, Berkin DI: A clinical rehabilitation course for college undergraduates provides an introduction to biopsychosocial interventions that minimize disablement. Am J Phys Med Rehabil 76:462–470, 1998.

KEY POINTS: ESSENTIAL COMPONENTS OF THE PHYSIATRIC CONSULTATION

1. Discover the patients' life roles and future aspirations.

2. Confirm current diagnoses and risk factors.

3. Quantify impairments, disabilities, and barriers to participation.

4. Develop a problem list.

5. Formulate a goal-driven treatment plan.

6. Orchestrate interdisciplinary team interventions.

7. Reevaluate progress toward goals.

ACKNOWLEDGMENT

The authors thank Walter Stolov, MD, for his PM&R consult format, used for decades at the University of Washington.

BIBLIOGRAPHY

1. Fredrickson M, Cannon NL: The role of the rehabilitation physician in the postacute continuum. Arch Phys Med Rehabil 76:SC5–SC9, 1995.
2. Marin EL, Colandner AS: Therapeutic prescription. In O'Young B, Young MA, Stiens SA (eds): PM&R Secrets. Philadelphia, Hanley & Belfus, 1997, pp 509–512.
3. Zimmermann KZ, Brown RD: Rehabilitation technology prescription: Determinations of failure and elements of success in advances in rehabilitation technology. Phys Med Rehabil State Art Rev 11:1–12, 1997.

CHAPTER 12

NEUROLOGIC EVALUATION OF THE REHABILITATION PATIENT: LOCALIZING LESIONS, ACCESSING CAPABILITY, AND PLANNING THERAPY

Rajiv R. Ratan, MD, PhD, Tom Jackson, MD, Ian B. Maitin, MD, and Albert C. Recio, MD, PT

Nearly all men can stand adversity, but if you want to test a man's character, give him power.
—Abraham Lincoln (1809–1865)

1. **What are the major parts of the neurologic examination?**
   The neurologic evaluation of the rehabilitation patient includes:
   - Mental status
   - Cranial nerves
   - Motor function (tone, reflexes, strength, adventitial movements)
   - Sensory function (touch, pain, temperature, proprioception, vibration, stereognosis, two-point discrimination)
   - Cerebellar function
   - Functional motor activity (screening for apraxia, dressing, and gait)

   Caplan L, Hollander J: The Effective Clinical Neurologist, 2nd ed. Oxford, Butterworth-Heinemann, 2001.
   Internet Handbook of Neurology: www.neuropat.dote.hu/neurology.htm
   Neuroexam.com: www.neuroexam.com

2. **What should bedside cognitive or mental status testing include?**
   Standard mental status testing is extensive, making it difficult for physicians to remember. To encourage use of the examination, the mnemonic **COMO ESTAS,** the Spanish phrase for "how are you?", can be used to denote the components of the examination:
   - **C** = **C**ognitive functions (i.e., calculation, concentration, insight, judgment)
   - **O** = **O**verview (i.e., appearance, attitude, level of consciousness, movements)
   - **M** = **M**emory (i.e., recent and remote)
   - **O** = **O**rientation (i.e., to person, place, and time)
   - **E** = **E**motion (i.e., affect and mood)
   - **S** = **S**peech (i.e., fluency, form, comprehension)
   - **T** = **T**hought (i.e., process, content, perceptual disturbances)
   - **A** = **A**ttention (i.e., abstract thinking, recall, intelligence)
   - **S** = **S**omething else that the practitioner has forgotten that might be important for the patient

   The level of wakefulness and attention should be evaluated and used as a guideline to interpret performance on other tasks. If arousal is significantly compromised, testing of memory, language, and other cognitive functions may not be valid.

   Astrachan JM: Como estas, a mnemonic for the mental status examination [letter]. N Engl J Med 324:636, 1991.

3. **Define *dementia*. What are the differences between delirium and dementia?**
   Dementia is a clinical state characterized by a significant loss of function in multiple cognitive domains, to the point of interfering with activities of daily living (ADLs). Dementia does not necessarily indicate any specific etiology. Thus, its diagnosis is not synonymous with a progressive course, and it does not imply irreversibility. The differences between delirium and dementia are summarized in Table 12-1.

   eMedicine site: www.emedicine.com/neuro/index.shtml

TABLE 12-1. COMPARISON BETWEEN DELIRIUM AND DEMENTIA		
	Delirium	**Dementia**
Onset	Acute	Insidious
Course	Fluctuating	Chronically progressive
Duration	Days to weeks	Months to years
Orientation	Impaired initially	Intact initially
Sleep	Disrupted cycle	Less disruption
Hallucination	Visual common	Less common, except sundowning
Memory	Recent markedly impaired	Recent > remote impaired

4. **Define *unilateral neglect*.**
   Unilateral neglect is a lack of orienting responses to stimuli presented unilaterally. Neglect cannot be diagnosed unless the primary sensory or motor modalities required to sense or orient the particular stimulus are intact. Neglect can be unimodal (i.e., visual neglect) or multimodal (i.e., performing complex tasks, such as dressing, in which the patient fails to cover the neglected side). Hemineglect is most commonly associated with right hemisphere strokes but can be seen with strokes or with tumors affecting either hemisphere. Neglect is prognostic of poor functional recovery.

   Jehkonen M, Ahonen JP, Dastidar P, et al: Visual neglect as a predictor of functional outcome one year after stroke. Acta Neurol Scand 101:195–201, 2000.

KEY POINTS: OBJECTIVES OF THE NEUROLOGIC EXAMINATION IN PM&R

1. Confirm the diagnosis.

2. Quantify impairment.

3. Identify adaptive capabilities.

4. Screen for complications, deterioration, and additional neurologic disorders.

5. Record a baseline for future comparison.

5. **After excluding visual field defects and disorders of eye movements, how does one evaluate neglect at the bedside?**
   ■ **Line bisection:** Have the patient mark the center of five horizontal lines, each presented separately on a sheet of paper.

- **Line cancellation:** Present the patient with a single sheet of paper on which 20 lines in varying orientations are drawn on each half of the page.
- **Letter cancellation:** Instruct the patient to mark all the A's on a sheet of paper. There should be 8 A's on the sheet, 4 on each side, with 70 distractor letters (e.g., D, L, F, R).
- **Clock construction:** Have the patient place numbers as they would appear on a clock face, with a circle outline on a piece of paper.

With the aforementioned tests, performance on the left side can be compared with performance on the right side.

Butter C, Kirsch N: Combined and separate effects of eye patching and visual stimulation on unilateral neglect following stroke. Arch Phys Med Rehabil 73:1133–1139, 1992.

CRANIAL NERVE EVALUATION

6. **How should one evaluate the integrity of the patient's visual fields?**
Stand approximately 3 feet in front of the patient, and ask him or her to focus on your nose. Hold your hands to either side of your face, midway between your eyes and the patient's. Briefly present one or two fingers from each hand, and ask the patient to indicate the number of fingers on each hand. Give the patient one or two trials to make sure that the nature of the trial is understood. The hands should be moved so that all four quadrants of the visual field are tested. These tests will enable detection of a field defect or neglect.

During testing, encourage the patient to maintain fixation on your nose. If the patient is uncooperative, bedside confrontation of the visual fields can provide diagnostic information. In the patient who is uncooperative, dysphasic, or lethargic, visual threat may cause an asymmetric blink response if there is field deficit or neglect.

7. **What do defects in the separate visual fields indicate?**
See Table 12-2 and Figure 12-1.

TABLE 12-2. LOCATION OF LESIONS IN VISUAL FIELD DEFECTS

Visual Field Defect	Location of Lesion
Right anopsia (monocular blindness)	Right optic nerve
Bitemporal hemianopsia	Optic chiasm (classically caused by pituitary tumor)
Left homonymous hemianopsia	Right optic tract
Left upper quadrant anopsia	Right optic radiations in the right temporal lobe
Left lower quadrant anopsia	Right optic radiations in the right parietal lobe
Left homonymous hemianopsia with macular sparing	Right occipital lobe (from posterior cerebral artery occlusion)

8. **How do you distinguish a field defect caused by malingering or hysteria from an organic field defect?**
In nonorganic field loss the most frequently encountered defect remains the same size, regardless of distance from the eye, and is often described as tunnel vision. In organic field loss the size of the intact field increases with the distance from the eye.

9. **What is the first question to ask a patient who complains of diplopia (double vision)?**
"Does the diplopia go away when you cover one eye?" **Monocular diplopia** (double vision that persists with only one eye viewing) is usually caused by a problem with the lens or cornea.

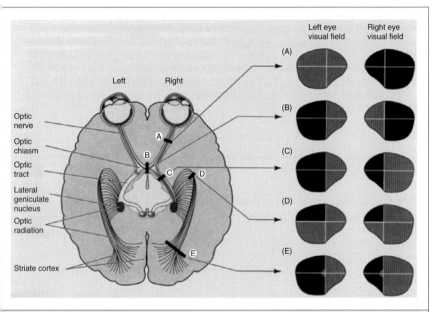

Figure 12-1. Neurologic location of visual fields.

Binocular diplopia (double vision that disappears with only one eye viewing) is usually a result of paralysis of extraocular muscles.

10. **How does one evaluate the seventh cranial nerve?**
    Paying particular attention to the nasolabial folds and palpebral fissures, look for facial asymmetry at rest and during spontaneous facial movements. Then systematically test the frontalis muscle ("raise your eyebrows"), orbicularis oculi ("close your eyelids and don't let me open them"), buccinator ("blow out your cheeks"), elevators of the lips ("show me your teeth; smile"), orbicularis oris ("purse your lips and don't let me open them").
    Upper motor lesions generally cause lower facial weakness, with slight asymmetry of the palpebral fissures and little or no weakness of the orbicularis oculi or frontalis muscles. Lower motor neuron lesions result in weakness of the upper and lower parts of the face and can involve taste (chorda tympani) and tearing (greater superior petrosal nerve).

MOTOR FUNCTION

11. **Define spasticity and rigidity.**
    - **Spasticity** is the increased resistance appreciated by the examiner when he or she moves a joint briskly. The hypertonicity is sometimes called *clasp-knife spasticity* because, like a pocketknife blade, the initial resistance fades away as the joint is flexed. Spasticity usually involves some specific groups of muscles more than others. For instance, after a brain lesion, a patient may become hemiplegic and have a greater increase in flexor muscles in the upper extremity and extensor muscles of the lower extremity.
    - **Rigidity** is defined as increased resistance appreciated by the examiner throughout the range of joint movement. It is like bending a lead pipe and thus is referred to as *lead pipe rigidity*.

The *cogwheel sign* corresponds to an intermittent but regular resistance to passive motion. The resistance affects flexor and extensor muscles in the involved limb equally.

eMedicine site: www.emedicine.com/neuro

12. **What diseases are commonly associated with rigidity?**
Diseases that involve damage or dysfunction of the extrapyramidal system (basal ganglia) such as idiopathic Parkinson's disease or drug-induced parkinsonism (e.g., metoclopramide, haloperidol, reserpine).

13. **What historical features suggest proximal muscle weakness?**
Legs
- Inability to get up from a chair or toilet without using one's hands
- Inability to get out of a car

Arms
- Inability to comb one's hair or brush one's teeth
- Inability to carry grocery bags or young children

14. **What are the clinical features of myopathy?**
Nearly asymmetric proximal muscle weakness without muscle wasting, with normal sensory examination, and with intact or slightly decreased reflexes.

15. **List some of the common causes of myopathy in the rehabilitation setting.**
- Steroids
- Alcohol
- Zidovudine (AZT)
- Hypothyroidism
- Duchenne's muscular dystrophy
- Polymyositis
- AIDS
- Mitochondrial diseases

16. **What is the critical clinical difference between myopathies and disorders of the neuromuscular junction (e.g., myasthenia gravis)?**
Although the distribution of weakness is similar in these disorders, neuromuscular diseases are characterized by **fatigability**. They worsen with use and recover with rest.

17. **What historical features suggest distal weakness?**
- **Arms:** Inability to fasten buttons, open jars, or hold onto things
- **Legs:** Frequent tripping or unusual wear on the toes of the shoes

18. **What are the clinical features of peripheral neuropathies?**
Distal weakness, which may be asymmetric or symmetric, with atrophy, possible fasciculations, sensory loss, and absent reflexes.

19. **How can peripheral neuropathies be distinguished from spinal cord lesions?**
Spinal cord lesions usually cause weakness that is distal more than proximal. They are characterized by a sensory level below which there is a decrease in sensation, distal symmetric weakness, hyperreflexia, and bowel and bladder problems. Peripheral neuropathies may have a glove-and-stocking, dermatomal, or single nerve distribution type of sensory loss. They are characterized by loss of reflexes rather than hyperreflexia. Some types of neuropathies involve the bladder or bowel. However, peripheral neuropathies cause bladder disorders of emptying, whereas spinal cord lesions usually cause bladder disorders of storage.

20. **What pattern of weakness is commonly seen after hemispheric stroke?**
Hemispheric stroke involving the internal capsule (subcortical) or cortical motor strip results in hemiparesis of the contralateral limb. The pattern of weakness is typically extensors greater than flexors in both the upper and lower extremities. In subcortical strokes the face, arm, and leg are usually affected equally, whereas in cortical strokes the face, arm, and leg are usually affected unequally.

21. **Describe one grading system for reflexes.**
- Grade 0 = absent reflex
- Grade 1 = hypoactive reflex, or normal reflex that can only be elicited with reinforcement
- Grade 2 = normal reflex
- Grade 3 = hyperactive reflex (A clear indicator is elicitation of other reflex responses when testing one reflex; for example, if testing the biceps, the brachioradialis and finger flexor reflexes are also elicited, suggesting hyperreflexia.)
- Grade 4 = clonus

22. **What can you do if you get no response when eliciting a reflex? What is Jendrassik's maneuver?**
Make sure to strike the blow crisply on the muscle, vary compression of the tendon with your finger, or try reinforcement. Reinforcement can be done by having the patient perform a strong voluntary contraction of a muscle you are not testing. Jendrassik's maneuver is a reinforcement for the patellar reflex. The patient hooks hands together by the flexed fingers and pulls apart as hard as possible.

   Gregory JE, Wood SA, Proske U: An investigation into mechanisms of reflex reinforcement by the Jendrassik's manoeuvre. Exp Brain Res 1383: 366–374, 2001.

23. **How is clonus at the ankle elicited?**
Quick dorsiflexion of the foot followed by continuous light pressure against the ball of the foot. The continuous light pressure opposes the reflex plantar flexion elicited by quick dorsiflexion.

24. **What does the presence of clonus indicate?**
Hyperreflexia caused by a lesion. Nonsustained clonus can also be elicited in patients who are anxious.

25. **What happens to the abdominal and cremasteric reflexes in a cervical spinal cord lesion?**
They are usually absent. When testing this reflex, remember that the abdomen should be relaxed. The abdominal reflex response is difficult to obtain if the muscles are too tense. **Cremasteric reflex** is elicited by stroking the superior and medial part of the thigh in downward direction. Normal response in males is a contraction of cremasteric muscle that pulls up the scrotum and testis on that side.

26. **What is the Babinski sign?**
The Babinski sign is dorsiflexion of the great toe in response to a plantar stimulus. It indicates an interruption of upper motor neuron tracts to the lumbosacral reflex centers, as seen in spinal cord injury, stroke, and multiple sclerosis.

27. **What are the four Babinski-like signs?**
- Chaddock's sign (obtained by stroking the lateral malleolus)
- Gordon's sign (squeezing the patient's calf)
- Oppenheim's sign (running the metal handle end of the reflex hammer along the crest of tibia and the tibialis anterior muscle)
- Gonda's sign (pressing one of the patient's toes downward and releasing it with a snap)

RANGE OF MOTION

28. **Define active range of motion (AROM) and passive range of motion (PROM).**
    AROM is the ROM through which the patient can move the joint. PROM is the ROM through which the examiner can move the joint.

29. **When is PROM less than AROM?**
    Never. PROM must be greater than or equal to AROM.

30. **Can fluid in the knee limit ROM?**
    Yes. Small amounts of fluid in the knee (bulge sign) probably limit flexion and extension of the joint.

31. **What joints do the ROM of shoulder abduction measure?**
    Glenohumeral and scapulothoracic.

32. **In shoulder abduction ROM, how does the glenohumeral joint move as the scapulothoracic joint moves?**
    There is approximately 2 degrees of glenohumeral joint motion for every degree of scapulothoracic joint motion.

33. **What is the instantaneous axis of rotation (IAR) of a joint?**
    The IAR of the joint is the center about which both members of the joint move. IAR varies throughout the ROM of a joint. Thus, it is difficult to maintain the axis of the goniometer always on the axis of the joint.

34. **Does the straight-leg-raising test measure full ROM of hip flexion?**
    No. The knee must be flexed to measure the full extent of hip flexion.

35. **Approximately how much variation occurs with repeated ROM examinations of the same joint by the same examiner?**
    10%.

36. **Early inflammatory arthritis of the hip usual limits what ROM?**
    Internal rotation.

37. **What does the Schober test measure?**
    Loss of mobility of the spine. The posterior spinous processes do not spread apart, and flexion occurs because of hip motion.

38. **What does the Spurling test detect?**
    Cervical spine radiculopathy demonstrated by simultaneous cervical lateral flexion and cervical spine extension.

39. **What does the Thomas test evaluate?**
    The presence of a hip flexion contracture. It is measured when the patient is lying flat on a firm surface, and the hip opposite the side measured is flexed to the chest as much as possible.

40. **Are there other forms of ROM besides PROM and AROM?**
    - **Active-assisted ROM:** Patient assisted by the therapist
    - **Self ROM:** Hemiparetic patient uses one arm to assist the other

MANUAL MUSCLE TESTING

41. **Why perform manual muscle testing (MMT)?**
Results help define impairment and develop a program to improve function.

42. **In MMT, how are muscles graded?**
   - 0/5 = No motion at all
   - 1/5 = Trace motion observed
   - 2/5 = Poor strength; full range of motion (FROM) when not against gravity only
   - 3/5 = Fair strength; FROM against gravity, but not against additional resistance
   - 4/5 = Good strength; FROM against gravity and moderate resistance
   - 5/5 = Normal strength; FROM against gravity and normal resistance

   Hislop HJ, Montgomery J: Daniels and Worthington's Muscle Testing: Techniques of Manual Examination, 7th ed. Philadelphia, W.B. Saunders, 2002.

43. **What does MMT provide result for?**
The one-repetition maximal contraction of the muscle.

44. **How is muscle endurance tested?**
Muscle endurance is tested by counting the seconds the muscle contraction is maintained or by counting repetitions against a given weight.

45. **What factors may limit the results of MMT?**
   - **Lack of full effort:** The patient should try his or her hardest. The examiner can determine this by observing or feeling other muscle groups contracting. A person cannot maximally move one muscle without contracting many others.
   - **Inappropriate positioning:** The patient must be stable while being tested. If the patient feels off balance, he or she will not be able to perform maximal contraction.
   - **Abnormal muscle tone:** Spasticity, for example, may give a false result.

46. **Does deconditioning cause focal muscle weakness?**
No. Deconditioning leads to decreased endurance in all muscles.

47. **What can cause focal muscle weakness?**
Focal neuropathies, nerve entrapment, mononeuritis, injuries, trauma, or myopathies.

48. **Does MMT include mostly concentric or eccentric muscle contractions?**
Mostly concentric.

49. **What does a hand-held dynamometer measure?**
It measures force in pounds or kilograms of the contracting muscle.

   Andrews AW, Thomas MW, Bohannon RW: Normative values for isometric muscle force measurements obtained with hand-held dynamometers. Phys Ther 76:248–259, 1996.

SENSORY EXAMINATION

50. **Define the primary and secondary sensory modalities.**
Primary sensory modalities include pain, temperature, light touch, proprioceptive, and vibratory sensation. Primary sensory loss can be caused by a lesion in the periphery, spinal cord, brain stem, or thalamus. Stereognosia (form sense, as in identifying a nickel or penny placed in the hand) and topognosia (ability to localize skin stimuli) are **secondary sensory** or cortical sensory modalities.

51. **What is the proper way to test pain sensation?**
   With a clean safety pin. The advantage of a safety pin is that it has a blunt end and a sharp end, thus allowing the reliability of the patient to be tested. The pin should be disposed of after the examination.

52. **What is the proper way to test position sense?**
   Position sense should be tested in the hands or feet. The distal end of the third or fourth digit or toe should be used, because these have the least cortical innervation and are thus the most sensitive to a loss in position sense. The digit should be grasped laterally and moved up or down or maintained in the neutral position. It is helpful to perform the test a few times with the patient's eyes open to be sure communication is established. With the eyes closed, the patient should make no mistakes on five trials. If abnormalities are found in one digit or two, other digits or toes should be tested.

53. **What frequency tuning fork should be used for vibration testing?**
   256 Hz.

54. **How is the Romberg test performed? What does a positive Romberg sign signify?**
   The Romberg test examines the integrity of the dorsal columns. It is not a test of cerebellar function. The patient is asked to stand with his or her heels together. With the patient's eyes open, note whether he or she sways. Instruct the patient to close his or her eyes. The visual information for balance is being removed, thus placing the responsibility for balance solely on the proprioceptive system. If the swaying is dramatically worse and the patient almost falls, it is considered "positive." Patients normally sway slightly with the eyes closed, but never fall. Patients with cerebellar disease usually sway more with the eyes open as well as closed.

55. **Name the anatomic landmarks that mark different dermatomes.**
   - C2—angle of the jaw
   - C6—thumb
   - C7—middle finger (third digit)
   - C8—little finger (fifth digit)
   - T4—nipple
   - T10—umbilicus
   - L4—knee cap
   - L5—big toe
   - S1—lateral foot
   - S4, S5—perianal area

CEREBELLAR TESTING

56. **What are the clinical features of cerebellar disease?**
   The main features of cerebellar dysfunction can be remembered by the mnemonic
   HANDS Tremor:
   - **H** = **H**ypotonia
   - **A** = **A**synergy (lack of coordination)
   - **N** = **N**ystagmus (ocular oscillation)
   - **D** = **D**ysarthria (speech abnormalities)
   - **S** = **S**tation and gait (ataxia)
   - **Tremor** = Coarse intention tremor

57. **How can cerebellar ataxia be distinguished from a sensory ataxia?**
    - Cerebellar ataxia
    - Nystagmus
    - Hypotonia
    - Coarse intention tremor
    - Dysarthria
    - Sensory ataxia
    - Loss of vibration and position sense
    - Loss of reflexes
    - Ataxia worse with eyes closed (positive Romberg sign)

58. **What is the best way to describe someone with cerebellar dysfunction?**
    They look drunk.

59. **What is the typical stance of someone with cerebellar dysfunction?**
    A broad-based gait.

60. **How can gait coordination be tested?**
    Have the patient tandem walk or step along a straight line, placing the heel of one foot directly in front of the toe of the other foot.

61. **How can coordination of the arms be tested?**
    Have the patient perform a finger-to-chin test. Instruct the patient to touch the examiner's finger, then touch his or her own chin. Repeat this sequence several times while altering the position of your finger with each trial. The chin is used instead of the nose because many patients with cerebellar dysfunction have such poor coordination that they are in danger of poking their own eye. If the patient undershoots or overshoots the examiner's fingers, the test is considered indicative of cerebellar dysfunction.

    Detailed neurologic exam of the adult: www.uptodate.com

62. **What is the heel-to-shin test?**
    This is another test of leg ataxia. While lying down or sitting, the patient is instructed to place the heel of one leg on the opposing knee and to run the heel down to the shin.

63. **Name some common causes of cerebellar dysfunction seen in the rehabilitation setting.**
    Strokes, multiple sclerosis, and anticonvulsants (phenytoin, phenobarbital, carbamazepine).

64. **What is apraxia?**
    Apraxia is a neurologic disorder characterized by loss of ability to execute or carry out learned (familiar) movements, despite having the desire and physical ability to perform the movements. There are several types: ideomotor (inability to carry out a motor command), ideational (inability to create a plan for or idea of a specific movement), constructional (inability to draw or construct simple configurations), verbal (difficulty coordinating mouth and speech movements), limb-kinetic (inability to make fine, precise movements with a limb), and oculomotor (difficulty moving the eyes).

    Strub R, Black WF: The Mental Status Examination in Neurology, 4th ed. Philadelphia, F.A. Davis, 2000.

BIBLIOGRAPHY

1. Bickley LS: Bates' Guide to Physical Examination and History Taking, 7th ed. Philadelphia, Lippincott Williams & Wilkins, 1999.
2. DeMeyer W: Technique of the Neurologic Examination: A Programmed Text, 3rd ed. New York, McGraw-Hill, 1980.
3. Hoppenfeld S: Physical Examination of the Spine and Extremities. New York, Prentice-Hall, 1976.
4. Kendall FP, McCreary EK, Provance PG: Muscles Testing and Function, 4th ed. Baltimore, Williams & Wilkins, 1993.
5. O'Dell MW, Lin CD, Paganos A, et al: The physiatric history and physical examination. In Braddom RL (ed): Physical Medicine and Rehabilitation, 3rd ed. Philadelphia, W.B. Saunders, 2007, pp 1–35.

CHAPTER 13

GAIT: BIOMECHANICAL AND CLINICAL ANALYSIS

D. Casey Kerrigan, MD, MS, and Fred Newton, MD, MS

All truly great thoughts are conceived by walking.

—Fredrich Nietzsche (1844–1900)

1. **Define gait cycle and other terms commonly used in discussing gait.**
   - **Gait cycle** = basic unit of gait, defined from one foot strike to repeat of same foot strike
   - **Stride length** = distance between sequential corresponding points of contact by the same foot
   - **Step length** = distance between sequential corresponding points of contact by opposite feet (normally approximately 38 cm)
   - **Cadence** = number of steps per unit time (steps/min)
   - **Speed** = cadence × step length

2. **Describe the terminology of gait analysis.**
   The classic terminology of gait, such as heel strike, heel-off, and toe-off, is dated, because these terms are often not applicable in certain disabilities. Figure 13-1 illustrates gait divided into three functional tasks: weight acceptance, single limb support, and limb advancement. The first two terms comprise the stance period, whereas the latter comprises the swing period. Stance can be further subdivided into the following phases: initial contact, loading response, midstance, terminal stance, and pre-swing. Swing consists of three phases: initial swing, midswing, and terminal swing.

Gait Cycle							
Stance ~60%				Swing ~40%			
Weight Acceptance		Single Limb Support		Limb Advancement			
Initial Contact	Loading Response	Midstance	Terminal Stance	Preswing	Initial Swing	Midswing	Terminal Swing
Preswing Opposite leg	☐ = Double limb support ~ 25%						

Figure 13-1. Periods, tasks, and phases of the gait cycle.

3. **How much of a typical walking cycle is spent in the stance phase? How much in the swing phase?**
   At normal walking speed, approximately 60% of a gait cycle is spent in stance and 40% in swing. The relative amount of time in stance decreases as the speed of walking increases.

4. **What is the difference between walking and running?**
Double limb support usually comprises 20–25% of a normal walking gait cycle. As walking speed increases, the time spent in double support decreases, and walking becomes running when there is no longer a period of double support.

5. **What are the determinants of gait?**
The determinants of gait were originally described by Saunders, Inman, and Eberhart as natural mechanisms in human gait utilized to minimize the movement and smooth the path of the center of mass. Recently, it has been shown that three of the determinants originally described (pelvic rotation, pelvic tilt, and knee flexion), in fact, do not significantly minimize the vertical displacement of the center of mass. Instead, heel rise of the trailing limb in double-limb support has been shown to be the major contributor in minimizing the vertical displacement of the center of mass.

6. **Where is the normal center of mass (COM)? How much does it move during ambulation?**
The normal COM is approximately 5 cm anterior to the second sacral vertebra. The average total displacement of the COM is approximately 5 cm in the vertical axis and 5 cm in the horizontal axis for an average adult male step. The actual displacement of the COM varies depending on individual height and step length, but it is always approximately half of what it would be if it were not for the determinants of gait.

KEY POINTS: THE DETERMINANTS OF GAIT AND HOW THEY WORK

1. **Heel rise:** Reduces center of mass's (COM) overall displacement by approximately 6–8 mm; has been shown to be the major contributor to reducing COM displacement

2. **Pelvic rotation:** Effectively raises the COM's predicted lowest point by approximately 2.0–2.5 mm

3. **Pelvic tilt (also called list or obliquity):** Occurs at midstance, increases the effective leg length, and lowers the COM's predicted highest point by approximately 2–3 mm

4. **Knee flexion:** Occurs at midstance and lowers the COM's predicted highest point by 2 mm

5. **Foot and knee motion:** Ankle pivots on the posterior heel at initial contact; pivot point progresses to the forefoot by terminal stance; knee and foot motions act to smooth the motion into a sinusoidal curve

6. **Lateral displacement of the pelvis:** Valgus alignment at the knees combined with hip adduction places the feet closer together, which allows less excursion of the center of gravity in the horizontal plane

7. **When is the center of gravity at its highest and lowest points in walking? In running?**
In walking, it is highest in midstance during single-limb support and lowest at initial contact during the double support. Interestingly, in running, it is at its highest point in the "flight" phase and at its lowest point in midstance of single-limb support.

8. **Why is walking more costly in energy terms than wheelchair ambulation?**
The body's center of mass must rise and fall with each step during gait, whereas in wheelchair ambulation the center of mass remains horizontal. The work done in walking a certain distance

can be estimated by multiplying the vertical displacement of the center of mass by the body weight and then by the number of steps.

9. **What is considered a comfortable walking speed?**
A comfortable walking speed (CWS) is one in which the energy cost per unit distance is at a minimum (i.e., comfort equates with efficiency). In a normal adult, this is approximately 80 m/min or 3 mph, with an energy cost of 0.15 mL O_2 per kg per meter. Abnormal biomechanics result in an increased energy cost, which is usually compensated for by a slower walking speed.

10. **How do gait deviations and assistive devices affect energy expenditure?**
The degree of energy expenditure is highly dependent on the type of gait abnormality and the assistive device used. See Table 13-1.

TABLE 13-1. TYPES OF GAIT	
Gait Type	**% Increase in Energy Cost**[*]
Normal	—
Ankle fusion	13
Knee immobilized	33
Hip fusion	47
Knee flexed 15 degrees	13
Knee flexed 30 degrees	27
Traumatic TT	7
Traumatic TF	33
Vascular TT	13
Vascular TF	87
Bilateral TT/TT	33
Bilateral TF/TF	120
Hemiplegic	80
Crutches PWB	18–36
Crutches NWB	41–78

TT = transtibial amputation, TF = transfemoral amputation, PWB = partial weight-bearing, NWB = non–weight-bearing.
[*]Energy expenditure typically measured at comfortable walking speed, with prosthesis in place and without upper extremity assistive device, except for crutches.

11. **Does a plastic or metal ankle-foot orthosis (AFO) reduce the energy cost of hemiparetic ambulation?**
An AFO reduces energy cost by simulating pushoff and raising the center of gravity in terminal stance (most important). Walking speed is increased and foot-drop is prevented in the swing phase. In hemiplegic subjects, energy expenditure per unit distance is 74% above normal using an AFO but 88% without one. There is no significant difference in energy expenditure between the types of AFOs.

12. **What is the difference between kinematics and kinetics?**
Kinematics is the study of the motions of joint and limb segments. Kinetics is the study of forces or torques that cause joint and limb motion. Modern gait laboratories use a multicamera system for collecting kinematics and a computer to combine ground reaction forces from forceplates to obtain joint forces and torques.

13. **When is a gait laboratory analysis indicated?**
It is particularly useful in cases of upper motor neuron pathology, in which the static evaluation of strength and tone may be deceptive. For instance, spasticity evident on static examination may not be apparent during ambulation. Gait analysis provides a respectable quantifiable measure of the requirement and result of a therapeutic intervention. It can be useful to assist in selecting the correct orthosis, therapy program, or surgical procedure. It may suggest a different treatment plan for a patient whose performance has plateaued.

14. **In quiet standing, which muscles maintain the body in erect position?**
The ground reaction force in this case acts along the line of gravity through the center of mass and passes in front of the ankle and knee and behind the hip. This allows the hip to be supported by the iliofemoral ligament and the knee to be supported by the posterior popliteal capsule with no muscular effort. Ankle stability is maintained by continuous contraction of the gastrocsoleus to produce a stabilizing ankle joint moment (torque).

15. **What is antalgic gait?**
In an ambulator with lower extremity pain, gait is modified to reduce weight-bearing on the involved side. The uninvolved limb is rapidly advanced to shorten stance on the affected side. Gait is often slow and steps are short to limit the weight-bearing period.

16. **What is steppage gait?**
It is a compensatory gait using excessive hip and knee flexion to assist a "functionally long" lower leg and foot to clear the ground. It may be seen with equinus (excessive plantar flexion) during swing caused by heel cord contracture, gastrocsoleus spasticity, or weak dorsiflexors.

17. **Which gait can be detected before the patient enters the room?**
The foot-slap of a patient with a partial foot-drop can be heard as the foot rapidly moves from initial contact to loading response. Moderately weak (grade 3 or 4) dorsiflexors are the cause. During the period from initial contact to loading response, they must eccentrically contract to slow the forward fall of the body. If dorsiflexors are very weak (grade 2 or worse), a steppage gait is used because there is not enough strength to lift the forefoot off the ground; this gait is silent.

18. **What are possible causes of genu recurvatum during the stance period of gait?**
   - Plantarflexion contracture (causing a knee extension moment through the closed kinetic chain)
   - Quadriceps weakness
   - Plantarflexor spasticity
   - Quadriceps spasticity

19. **What is Trendelenburg or gluteus medius gait? What is the cause?**
A Trendelenburg gait is caused by either weak hip adductors (gluteus medius) or hip pain from osteoarthritis and is first seen with increased pelvic tilt opposite the affected side. To compensate, the trunk will bend toward the affected side to keep the center of gravity directly above the hip during the stance phase. This maneuver decreases the large adductor moment,

eliminates the need for hip abductors, and decreases the forces across the hip joint. A useful intervention is the introduction of a cane to be used contralaterally during the stance period of the affected side. With increasing speed and less time in stance, this gait deviation is less visually evident.

20. **What is the gait pattern in a person with weak hip extensors?**
The person walks with an extensor lurch. The trunk is hyperextended at the hip to prevent rapid forward fall at initial contact (jackknifing).

21. **When does an infant acquire the ability to walk supported? To walk unsupported? To run?**
   - Walks with support by 1 year
   - Walks unsupported by 15 months
   - Runs by approximately 18 months
   - A mature gait pattern is established by 3 years old

22. **How does a toddler's gait differ from that of an adult?**
   - Wider base of support
   - Reduced stride length with a higher cadence
   - No heel strike
   - Little knee flexion during standing
   - Absence of reciprocal arm swing
   - External rotation of the entire leg during the swing phase

23. **What are the only two consistent kinematic/kinetic differences between elderly people and young adults that both (1) persist when elderly people are asked to walk faster and (2) are exaggerated in elderly people who recurrently fall?**
There are many differences in lower extremity joint parameters in the elderly when compared to young adults. However, the only difference that persists when elderly subjects walk at an increased speed consistent with younger subjects is decreased peak hip extension. Peak hip extension has also been found to be further reduced in elderly patients with a history of falls when compared to elderly patients who have no history of falls.

24. **At how many degrees does a knee flexion contracture significantly interfere with gait?**
At 30 degrees, all phases of the gait cycle will be abnormal. Contractures of this severity or greater essentially produce a leg-length discrepancy.

25. **Does varus or valgus knee alignment affect progression of knee osteoarthritis with ambulation?**
Yes. It has been shown that ambulating with greater than 5 degrees of varus alignment increases the risk for progression of medial compartment knee osteoarthritis with similar results for valgus alignment and lateral compartment knee osteoarthritis. Increased varus knee torques have been correlated with the progression of medial compartment knee osteoarthritis.

26. **Can a shoe insole modify joint biomechanics in patients with knee osteoarthritis?**
In fact, a 5-degree lateral-wedge insole has been shown by quantitative gait analysis to significantly reduce peak knee varus torques by 6%. Although a 10-degree lateral-wedge insole reduces the same torques by 8%, it was less well tolerated by study subjects.

27. Do high-heeled shoes increase the risk for osteoarthritis of the knees?
Performing gait analysis of women wearing high-heeled shoes (2.5 in.) has demonstrated increased force across the patellofemoral joint and a 23% greater compressive force on the medial compartment of the knee (23% greater) during walking in high heels versus walking barefoot. With osteoarthritis of the knee being twice as common in women as it is in men and usually occurring bilaterally, it appears likely that high heels can predispose to osteoarthritis of the knees.

28. What about the effects of moderately high–heeled shoes?
Even moderately high–heeled shoes (1.5 in.) have been shown by gait analysis to significantly increase the varus torque (14%) and knee flexor torque (19%) thought to be relevant in the development and progression of knee osteoarthritis.

WEBSITES

1. American Society of Biomechanics
www.asb-biomech.org

2. Clinical Gait Analysis
http://guardian.curtin. edu.au:16080/cga/

3. Gait and Clinical Movement Analysis Society
www.gcmas.net/index.html

4. International Society of Biomechanics
www.isbweb.org

5. University of Virginia Physical Medicine and Rehabilitation Gait Lab
www.healthsystem.virginia.edu/ internet/pmr/Biomechanics.cfm

BIBLIOGRAPHY

1. Fisher S, Gullickson G Jr: Energy cost of ambulation in health and disability. Arch Phys Med Rehabil 59:124–133, 1978.
2. Gard SA, Childress DS: The effect of pelvic list on the vertical displacement of the trunk during normal walking. Gait Posture 5:233–238, 1997.
3. Gard SA, Childress DS: The influence of stance-phase knee flexion on the vertical displacement of the trunk during normal walking. Arch Phys Med Rehabil 80:26–32, 1999.
4. Gonzalez E, Corcoran PJ: Energy expenditure during ambulation. In Downey JA (ed): Physiological Basis of Rehabilitation Medicine, 2nd ed. Boston, Butterworth-Heinemann, 1994, pp 413–446.
5. Harris GF, Wertsch JJ: Procedures for gait analysis. Arch Phys Med Rehabil 75:216–225, 1994.
6. Kerrigan DC, Della Croce U, Marciello M, Riley PO: A refined view of the determinants of gait: Significance of heel rise. Arch Phys Med Rehabil 81:1077–1080, 2000.
7. Kerrigan DC, Johansson JL, Bryant MG, et al: Moderate-heeled shoes and knee joint torques relevant to the development and progression of knee osteoarthritis. Arch Phys Med Rehabil 86:871–875, 2005.
8. Kerrigan DC, Lee LW, Collins JJ, et al: Reduced hip extension during walking in healthy elderly and fallers versus young adults. Arch Phys Med Rehabil 82:26–30, 2001.
9. Kerrigan DC, Lelas JL, Goggins J, et al: Effectiveness of a lateral-wedge insole on knee varus torque in patients with knee osteoarthritis. Arch Phys Med Rehabil 83:889–893, 2002.
10. Kerrigan DC, Riley PO, Lelas JL, Della Croce U: Quantification of pelvic rotation as a determinant of gait. Arch Phys Med Rehabil 82:217–220, 2001.

11. Pease WS, Bowyer BL, Kadyan V: Human walking. In Delisa JA, Gans BM (eds): Physical Medicine and Rehabilitation Medicine Principles and Practice, 4th ed. Philadelphia, Lippincott Williams and Wilkins, 2005, pp 155–167.

12. Saunders JB, Inman VT, Eberhart HD: The major determinants in normal and pathological gait. J Bone Joint Surg Am 35-A:543–558, 1953.

13. Sharma L, Song J, Felson DT, et al: The role of knee alignment in disease progression and functional decline in knee osteoarthritis. JAMA 286:188–195, 2001.

14. Waters RL, Mulroy S: The energy expenditure of normal and pathologic gait. Gait Posture 9:207–231, 1999.

CHAPTER 14

PERSON-CENTERED REHABILITATION: INTERDISCIPLINARY INTERVENTION TO ENHANCE PATIENT ENABLEMENT

Steven A. Stiens, MD, MS, Bryan J. O'Young, MD, and Mark A. Young, MD, M

The mainspring of creativity appears to be the same tendency we discover so deeply as the curative force in psychotherapy, man's tendency to actualize himself, to become his potentialities. By this I mean the organic and human life, the urge to expand, extend, develop, mature—the tendency to express and activate all the capacities of the organism, or the self.

—Carl Rogers (1902–2002)

1. How are the person and personhood relevant to rehabilitation?

The **person** is a living human being with characteristic unique genetic, physical, mental, social, and spiritual dimensions. He or she is guided by past experiences and developmental changes and has the free will to make his or her own life decisions. The person, therefore, is the "real self," the subject of rehabilitation intervention. As such, **personhood** is the dynamic process of being and becoming the self. Awareness of the patient's self-understanding is critical to the rehabilitation success. The person has the right of choice in solving his or her own problems and plays an essential role in health goal-setting. As Carl Rogers explains: "The hypothesis is that the patient has within him or herself the capacity latent, if not evident, to understand those aspects of life and the capacity to reorganize a relationship to life in a direction of self actualization and maturity with resulting inner comfort."

Kirschenbaum H: Carl Rogers's life and work: An assessment on the 100th anniversary of his birth. J Counsel Devel 82:116–124, 2004.

2. Define health, illness, and disease.

- **Health** is the optimum condition of a person's physical, mental, and social well-being. Health is not merely the absence of disease or infirmity.
- An **illness** is the patient's unique subjective experience of "unwellness," distress, or failed function. Illness is not only a biologic state but can also be an existential transformation that affects trust in the body and reliance on the future. The illness experience contributes to the psychological state, which influences the perception of the body's ability to function in the present and future.
- A **disease** is a medical construct that diagnoses a disorder as characterized by a set of symptoms, signs, and pathology and is attributable to infection, diet, heredity, or environment.

3. Define patient, case, client, and customer.

- A **patient** is a person who is affected by injury, illness, or disease and is under active medical treatment to return to better health. Working with a person as a patient implies an active medical relationship with expectations beyond that of a case, client, or customer.
- A **case** is an instance of disease or injury with its attendant contributing circumstances as abstracted from the person for scientific study or education.
- A **client** is one for whom services are rendered, a patron, and does not require the person's participation in the relationship. Services are performed for clients.
- A **customer** merely buys goods or services.

4. **What are the five responsibilities of the physician in the physician–patient relationship?**
   1. **Suspension of judgment** means respect for the patient's personal and cultural values and priorities without imposing your own. Through empathy, the physician seeks the patient's perspective.
   2. **Evaluation** requires acquiring knowledge of the patient as a person, the illness experience, symptoms, and signs. Functional evaluation requires assessment of impairments, activity and participation, and the patient's unique disablement experience.
   3. **Diagnosis** requires an integration of many symptoms, signs, findings, and test results to deduce a pathophysiologic process or syndrome.
   4. In **reporting**, the physician interprets the diagnosis and prognosis that is appropriate as expected for the patient's unique life circumstances and provides the education required for informed choices.
   5. **Treatment** requires a formulation, prescription, or plan, which is then offered to the patient for informed consent.

5. **What are the three responsibilities of the patient in the physician–patient relationship?**
   - **Presentation:** Patients make known aspects of their experience through medical history and by revealing their bodies, equipment, and home for examination. They contribute to the evaluation process by demonstrating their functional capability. Patients get the very most from rehabilitation when they reflect on their unique aspirations.
   - **Understanding:** Patients with evaluations from their care team gain the capability to consider the risks, investments, and benefits of treatment options. They consider the impact on their goal attainment and the lifestyle they aspire.
   - **Compliance:** The concept of compliance requires that patients understand and accept the plan and work toward its goals.

   Emanuel EJ, Emanuel LL: Four models of the physician–patient relationship. JAMA 267:2221–2226, 1992.

6. **How does understanding suffering contribute to patient care?**
   Suffering must be differentiated from pain: **pain** is the psychophysiologic process of perception in response to nociceptive stimuli, whereas **suffering** is the perception of a threat to personhood (i.e., the person's satisfaction with the present and anticipation of the future, as related to family and society). Suffering may include but is not limited to physical pain. Suffering can be relieved when the perception of threat is reinterpreted into a positive meaning.
   An understanding approach to suffering includes an open exploration of the patient's concerns about the impact of the illness on their lifestyle, family, occupation, and future plans. The patient's experience of illness may be reframed as new possibilities are generated as goals.

   Cassell EJ: The nature of suffering and the goals of medicine. N Engl J Med 306:639–645, 1982.

7. **How can the effects of the disease on a person be practically classified?**
   The World Health Organization originally published the *International Classification of Impairments, Disabilities, and Handicaps* (ICIDH) in 1980, then published a revised version in 2001, *International Classification of Disability Functioning and Health* (ICF). *Disablement* is a summary term for collective consequences of disease for the person. Consequences are considered with three interrelated domains: (1) the **organ** or system, (2) the whole **person**, and (3) **society**. In the ICF ICIDH-2 (revised 2000) terminology, limitations or barriers within these domains are named **impairments** (organ domain), **activity limitations** (person domain), and **barriers to participation** (societal domain).

World Health Organization: www3.who.int/icf

Gray DB, Hendershot GE: The ICIDH-2: Development for a new era of outcomes research. Arch Phys Med Rehabil 81(suppl 2):S10–S14, 2000.

8. **Define impairment.**

Impairment is any loss or abnormality of anatomic structure, physiologic, or psychological function of an organ or system. Examples include loss of limb, weakness, sensory deficit, and facial disfigurement.

9. **Define disability and activity.**

These terms refer to capabilities in the person domain. A **task** is a purposeful activity that requires engagement of the whole person. **Disability** is the ICIDH-1 term for the inability of a person to complete a task that would otherwise be considered normal for a human of a particular age. Examples are an inability to perform activities of daily living, such as dressing, driving, shopping, or cooking. Disabilities reflect the consequences of impairment on activities of the whole person. **Activities** (ICF) (ICIDH-2) are the performance of personal-level tasks or human endeavors.

10. **How is handicap defined in the relationship of the person to society?**

Handicap is a historic term that evokes a variety of experiences, images, fears, and situations for many. The term comes from the phrase "cap in hand," referring to holding a hat out for a contribution that in some way may economically equalize the disadvantage. Operationally, handicap results from the interaction of the person (including impairments and disabilities) with the environment. The **environment** is everything that surrounds the patient and therefore has a profound impact on his or her self-perception and function. Specifically, the characteristics of the environment that need to be considered are physical, psychological, social, and political.

- The **physical environment** provides the conduit for travel through obstructive barriers that may limit access. Adaptations are modifications for task and participation enablement.
- The **psychological environment** is all the stimuli uniquely experienced by the person living with disablement, including communicated attitudes and expectations of the person.
- The **social environment** includes the predominant cultural role with expectations for acceptance in family, work, and leisure activities.
- The **political environment** includes the laws and guaranteed rights of each person, regardless of handicap.

The resultant **handicap** is the disadvantage for a given individual, stemming from impairments or disabilities, in performing a role otherwise normal (age or sex appropriate) for an individual. **Disadvantage** is defined as socially perceived failure to conform to expected role behaviors, either by deficit or excess behavior. Full subclassification of (handicap) **barriers to participation** circumstances is unique to the person and dynamic. Environmental factors have been written into ICF ICIDH-2 by considering the range of handicap circumstances that can affect participation in the environment immediate to the person and beyond.

Iwarsson S, Stahl A: Accessibility, usability and universal design of concepts describing person-environment relationships. Disabil Rehabil 25:57–66, 2003.

11. **What is the relationship between handicap and participation?**

The relationship is reciprocal. **Participation** is defined as the person's involvement in life situations. **Involvement** means inclusion and contributions to life activities in the context of the person's own community. As participation increases, handicap decreases. The restriction of participation or involvement in life activities by external factors (social roles) is termed **participation limitation/restriction.**

KEY POINTS: IMPORTANT DEFINITIONS

1. The **rehabilitation problem list** is a sequence of diagnoses, impairments, activity limitations, and participation barriers that guide goal setting. It is organized as a spectrum starting from active injuries and diagnoses through the domains of disablement.

2. **Impairment** is any loss or abnormality of anatomic structure, physiologic, or psychological function of an organ or system.

3. **Activity limitation** is any deficit in a person's ability to complete a task that would otherwise be within the range considered normal for a person of a particular age.

4. **Participation** includes all the areas of life in which an individual is involved, or has access to, societal opportunities in the process of meeting goals.

12. **What are contextual factors?**

Contextual factors are the situations within and around the person. ICF ICIDH-2 describes environmental and personal contextual factors as follows:

- **Environmental factors** include many categories, such as natural environments; man-made changes to the environment; products and technology; support and relationships; attitudes, values, and beliefs; services; and systems and policies.
- **Personal factors** refer to patient characteristics that may contribute to or limit adaptation. They include gender, age, diagnoses, fitness, lifestyle, upbringing, coping styles, social background, education, profession, past experiences, character style, and physical and psychological assets.

13. **Has functional loss been addressed on a more universal or spiritual level? If so, how does this apply in the rehabilitation setting?**

We propose that the term *suffering* be used to describe loss of function on a spiritual level. The term is useful because it addresses a spiritual dimension that is not specifically included in the three domains of disablement. It is essential that rehabilitation specialists identify and address a person's needs on different levels in order to maximize a person's potential. For many, the highest form of need to be addressed is the spiritual need. Instilling meaning into a patient's illness can empower a person to maximize his or her health to live with meaning. This serves as a seed that can be tended by a health care professional into a fruitful discussion with patient and others in the field of rehabilitation and beyond.

14. **What is rehabilitation?**

Rehabilitation is the process of development of a person to his or her fullest physical, psychological, social, educational, and vocational potential, by eliminating or compensating for any biochemical pathophysiology, anatomic impairment, activity limitation, or environmental barrier. In contrast to classic medical therapeutics, which emphasize diagnosis and focused treatment directed against the pathologic process, rehabilitation directs treatment against the pathologic process but also applies multiple simultaneous interventions addressing both the cause and secondary effects of injury and illness **(biopsychosocial model).** Traditionally, medical science has directed treatment at the cause of disease **(biomedical model),** neglecting the secondary effects of illness. The very nature of rehabilitation includes assessment of the individual's personal capacities, role performance, and life aspirations.

Comprehensive rehabilitation can be further considered to require five necessary and sufficient subcomponents:

1. A unique, patient-centered plan formulated by the patient and rehabilitation team
2. Goals derived and prioritized through an interdisciplinary process

3. Patient participation required to achieve the goals
4. Results in improvement in the patient's personal potential and spontaneous activity
5. Outcomes demonstrate **enablement** (i.e., improved organ system function, activity, and participation)

Imrie R: Rethinking the relationships between disability, rehabilitation, and society. Disabil Rehabil 19:263–271, 1997.

Wade DJ, deJong B: Recent advances in rehabilitation. BMJ 390:1385–1388, 2000.

15. **What is patient-centered rehabilitation medicine?**
It is a process of interaction and intervention that requires collaboration with the patient as a whole person, derivation of goals specifically to meet the patient's life plan, and interventions that maximize all of the patient's capabilities and potential. The process has the following seven interactive components:
1. **Understanding of the whole person:** Identity, occupation, lifestyles, ideology, and aspirations
2. **Exploration of the illness experience:** Pathologic process, disablement, and capabilities for compensation
3. **Formulation of a comprehensive problem list** with patient contributions
4. **Derivation of short- and long-term goals:** Prioritizing goal attainment and environmental interventions to allow for rapid transition to least restrictive settings
5. **Incorporating prevention, health promotion, and patient education**
6. **Enhancing the treatment relationships** among the interdisciplinary team and the patient, family, friends, and volunteers
7. Establishing **home- and community-based habits, a routine of self-care,** and scheduled follow ups with new goals upon discharge

Cott CA: Client-centered rehabilitation: Client perspectives. Disabil Rehabil 26:1411–1422, 2004.

Martin D: Martin's Map: A conceptual framework for teaching and learning the medical interview using a patient-centered approach. Med Educ 37:1145–1153, 2003.

Ozer MN, Payton OD, Nelson CE: Treatment Planning for Rehabilitation: A Patient-Centered Approach. New York, McGraw-Hill, 2000.

16. **What is the multidisciplinary practice of patient care? How does it differ from interdisciplinary practice?**
Multidisciplinary teams consist of various professionals treating the patient separately, with discipline-specific goals. Patient's progress with each discipline is communicated through documentation and/or or at meetings for information exchange.

In the **interdisciplinary** collaborative practice model, each distinct profession evaluates the patient separately and then interacts together at team meetings, where they share options for short- and long-term goals. The team collectively develops a vision for patient outcomes, as informed by their assessments and patient aspirations. The goals of each discipline are combined into a unified, coordinated plan through the synergistic interaction of the team. Photographs of successful events in the past can be meaningfully applied in setting the goals for a disabled patient.

In addition, the team collaboratively participates in problem solving and decision making as the plan is executed. Evidence for decision making includes measurements of various disablement domains and task performances. Patients with intellectual disabilities can contribute to the process with photographs of successful life activities that can be prioritized by the team for goal setting. The **whole outcome,** therefore, is more than the sum of the component parts.

17. **What nine conditions maximize the success of interdisciplinary rehabilitation teams?**
1. Allegiance to a mission statement (i.e., person-centered rehab in the least restrictive setting)
2. Specifically delineated roles for each discipline
3. Balance of participation by each professional

4. Agreement on, and implementation of, ground rules for interaction
5. Clear and effective communication and documentation
6. Scientific approach to patient problems
7. Clearly defined, measurable goals
8. Working knowledge of group process
9. Expedient procedures for coming to consensus and decision-making

18. How does a transdisciplinary team interact?

Transdisciplinary teams are designed through cross-training of members and procedure development to allow **overlap of responsibilities** between disciplines (Fig. 14-1). This overlap allows flexibility in problem solving and produces greater interdependence of team members. Leadership may differ for each patient served by the team. Disciplines with extensive involvement with the patient may become **case managers** and coordinate team efforts. Establishment and achievement of goals starts with unconditional positive regard but may require a more directive approach, such as **motivational interviewing,** in patient interactions at times during rehabilitation. The four basic principles are as follows:

1. Share understanding and express empathy.
2. Relax and supportively discuss client resistance and argument.
3. Gently explore discrepancies between the patient's current behavior and desired future.
4. Support self-efficacy and help the patient gain confidence in self-commitment.

Britt E, Blampied NM, Hudson SM: Motivational interviewing: A review. Australian Psychol 38:193–201, 2003.

Wagner CC, McMahon BT: Motivational interviewing and rehabilitation counseling practice. Rehabil Counsel Bull 47:152–161.

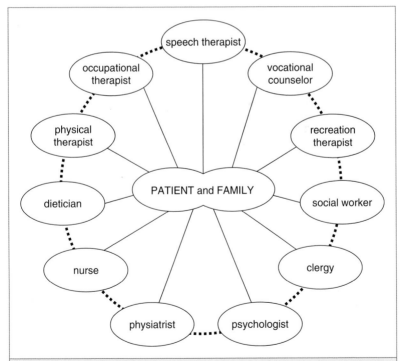

Figure 14-1. Interdisciplinary team interaction. (From Mumma CM, Nelson A: Models for theory-based practice of rehabilitation nursing. In Hoeman SD [ed]: Rehabilitation Nursing: Process and Application. St. Louis, Mosby, 1995, 32–53.)

19. **Describe the phases in the rehabilitation process.**

Rehabilitation intervention is best orchestrated to achieve outcomes in a sequence that advances the patient efficiently to the fullest function in the least restrictive setting. These phases are guidelines for intervention, with an emphasis on efficiently achieving life-enhancing outcomes, results using a comprehensive problem list, a baseline, continuous index measures of pathophysiology, and key functional capabilities in the three domains of disablement: impairment, activity, and participation.

- **Phase I (evaluation).** Rehabilitation intervention is best orchestrated with the patient's personal history and disablement experience to achieve outcomes in a sequence that advances the patient to the fullest function in the least restrictive setting.
- **Phase II (initial treatment)** emphasizes treatment to arrest the pathophysiologic processes causing tissue injury, prevent complications, and establish psychological support and planning.
- **Phase III (therapeutic exercise)** focuses on enhancement of organ performance, remobilization, and healing.
- **Phase IV (task reacquisition)** emphasizes the total person's knowledge, adaptive techniques, and spontaneous disability-appropriate behavior.
- **Phase V (patient-family adaptation and environmental modification)** directs efforts toward environmental enhancement (physical, psychological, social, and political) to maximize participation.

These phases approximate the emphasis of the team's interventions during a continuum that guides the patient out of acute treatment and into reintegration with the community. The **rehabilitation problem list** (Box 14-1) is a sequence of diagnoses, impairments, activity limitations, and participation barriers that guide goal setting. Members of the rehabilitation team

---

BOX 14-1. REHABILITATION PROBLEM LIST

Primary rehabilitation diagnosis or anatomic injury

Other associated diagnoses with severity measures

Impairments (e.g., neurogenic, bladder, bowel, sexual function)

Activity limitations (e.g., mobility, ADLs, communication)

Education

Participation barriers

Psychological adaptation

Social role function

Architectural accessibility

Community reintegration

Vocational adaptation

Spiritual practice

ADLs = activities of daily living.
*The rehabilitation problem list is organized as a spectrum of areas for intervention starting from active injuries and diagnoses through the dimensions of disablement. It is individualized for each patient and organizes short- and long-term goals.

derive goals from their encounters with the patient as a whole person. The patient drives the process by demonstrating his or her particular predicament with disablement. Adaptation is achieved by enhancing the patient's personal characteristics that mediate or limit the disablement. The overall goal is the fullest personal enablement and action toward fulfillment of life roles that are actively played out.

de Kleijn-de Vrankrijker M, Seidel C, Tscherner U: The International Classification of Impairments, Disabilities, and Handicaps (ICIDH): Its use in rehabilitation. World Health Statist Q 42:151–156, 1999.

WEBSITE

World Health Organization
www.who.org

BIBLIOGRAPHY

1. Granger CV, Gresham GE: International Classification of Impairments, Disabilities, and Handicaps (ICIDH) as a conceptual basis for stroke outcome research. Stroke 21(Suppl II):1166–1167, 1990.
2. Stiens SA, Haselkorn JK, Peters DJ, Goldstein B: Rehabilitation intervention for patients with upper extremity dysfunction: Challenges of outcome evaluation. Am J Ind Med 29:590–601, 1996.
3. World Health Organization: In International Classification of Functioning and Disability: ICF Pocket Size Book, Beta-2 draft, short version (ICIDH-2). Geneva, WH, 2001, p 228.
4. Young MA, Baar K: Women in Pain. New York, Hyperion Publishers, 2002.

IV. ELECTRODIAGNOSTIC FUNDAMENTALS

BASIC ELECTRODIAGNOSIS: INTERPRETATION OF ELECTRICAL MANIFESTATIONS OF NEUROMUSCULAR DISORDERS

Janet C. Limke, MD, James M. Plunkett, MD, Elliot B. Bodofsky, MD, and Lawrence R. Robinson, MD

CHAPTER 15

Genius hath electric power which earth can never tame.

–Lydia M. Child (1802–1880)

1. **What is the role of electrodiagnosis in the evaluation of a patient?**
   Electrodiagnosis is a direct extension of the history evaluation and physical examination. It can help localize and quantify pathophysiologic causes of pain, numbness, tingling, weakness, fatigue, and muscle cramping. Electrodiagnostic studies include electromyography (EMG), nerve conduction studies, somatosensory evoked potentials, and motor evoked potentials. A properly trained physician can assist the referring physician by establishing or narrowing diagnoses, determining prognosis, and providing advice on management of neuromuscular disorders.

2. **What are the limitations of the nerve conduction and electromyographic studies?**
   1. The nerve conduction studies (NCSs) selectively examine only the large myelinated fibers and do not reveal diseases of the smaller nerve fibers. Nerve conduction velocities do not correlate with functional deficit, although motor amplitudes may correlate with strength and prognosis. Neither motor nor sensory nerve conduction studies correlate with pain.
   2. Motor conduction studies are currently not reliable for many proximal nerve segments.
   3. Sensory nerve conduction studies (SNCs) only evaluate lesions distal to the dorsal root ganglion (DRG) and not the lesions proximal to the DRG. SNCs are not useful for evaluating conduction block because of the great degree of temporal dispersion and excessive cancellation.
   4. Needle EMG evaluates the early recruitment of mainly the small type 1 motor units. It cannot be used to differentiate the large motor units that are recruited later. The needle electrode only detects signals close to the tip of the needle. Needle EMG provides only pathophysiologic information and does not translate directly to an etiology.
   5. Needle EMG and NCSs can be greatly affected by technical artifacts (e.g., cold temperature, improper filter or gain settings, electronic noise) and operator-dependent factors (e.g., nerve or muscle selection, localization, measurement error, stimulation intensity). These factors need to be standardized and optimized for valid results.

3. **How are the electrodiagnostic parameters affected by the frequency of the filters?**
   Compound motor action potential (CMAP) is more profoundly affected by raising the low-frequency filter than sensory nerve action potential (SNAP) because the CMAP contains mostly low frequencies. On the other hand, CMAP is not significantly affected by slightly lowering the

high-frequency filter. Fibrillation and initial sharp components of positive sharp waves can be affected by lowering the high-frequency filter because these are potentials with predominantly high frequencies (*see* Table 15-1).

TABLE 15-1. EFFECT OF FILTER FREQUENCY ON SNAP PARAMETERS

Parameters of SNAP	Elevated Low-Frequency Filter	Lowered High-Frequency Filter
Onset latency	No change	Increased
Peak latency	Decreased	Increased
Amplitude	Decreased	Decreased

SNAP = sensory nerve action potential.

4. **What is spontaneous activity?**
   After insertion of an EMG needle into normal muscle at rest, no electrical activity is usually seen after the initial burst of insertional activity unless the needle is near an end-plate zone. **Spontaneous activity** refers to involuntary electrical potentials recorded in resting muscle after movement of the recording electrode has ceased.

5. **Name the commonly observed spontaneous activities and describe their characteristic sounds.**
   - Fibrillation potentials: regular clicking noises, such as raindrops on the roof or static (very common)
   - Positive sharp waves: pop, pop, pop, regular 2–20 Hz (very common)
   - End-plate spikes: irregular clicks, such as fat in a frying pan
   - Fasciculation potentials: spontaneous isolated loud snaps or pops
   - Complex repetitive discharges: motorboat or machine-like drone that starts and stops abruptly
   - Myokymic discharges: marching soldiers
   - Myotonic discharges: dive-bomber or revving motorcycle
   - Neuromyotonic discharges: high-pitch whining sound of a racecar
   Historic point: The first EMG machines had no screens, only a speaker.

   www.aanem.org/publications/cdrom_page1.cfm (to order CD-ROMs for auditory recognition of waveforms)

6. **What are the EMG characteristics of a fibrillation potential?**
   Fibrillation potential is defined as a spontaneous action potential recorded from a single muscle fiber by a needle electrode located outside the end-plate zone. The precise mechanism for generation of fibrillation potentials is not known, although the prevalent hypothesis is "**acetylcholine hypersensitivity.**" When a muscle fiber loses innervation either through nerve injury or segmental necrosis, there is increased production of acetylcholine receptors and other membrane proteins, which are widely distributed on the muscle cell membrane. This reduces the threshold for depolarization. Fibrillations are also found in inflammatory myopathies, neuromuscular transmission disorders, and in some upper motor neuron disorders.

Fibrillation potentials are usually regularly firing and have amplitudes from 20 to 1000 μv. The amplitude of the fibrillation is often more than 200 μv early on, but falls over time and is typically less than 100 μv after 1 year of denervation. Firing rates range from 0.5 Hz to 30 Hz.

7. **What are positive sharp waves (PSWs) and their EMG characteristics?**
PSWs are often seen along with fibrillations (Fig. 15-1). A PSW is a spontaneous depolarization of a single muscle fiber recorded close to the tip of the needle electrode with biphasic morphology consisting of a sharp initial positive (downward) deflection followed by a return to baseline. Amplitudes range from 10 μv to 3 mv and have firing rates between 0.5 Hz and 30 Hz.
Positive sharp waves appear earlier than fibrillation potentials after a nerve injury and have similar clinical significance. PSWs can be seen in the nonpathologic foot intrinsics and paraspinal muscles of some normal individuals. When the recording electrode is near the tendon area, upcoming propagation of motor unit action potentials may look like PSWs.

Gatens PF, Saeed MA: Electromyographic findings in the intrinsic muscles of normal feet. Arch Phys Med Rehabil 63:317–318, 1982.

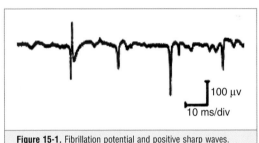

100 μv
10 ms/div

Figure 15-1. Fibrillation potential and positive sharp waves.

8. **Describe the EMG characteristics of end-plate spikes (EPSs) and miniature end-plate potentials (MEPPs).**
End-plate spikes are single muscle fiber action potentials originating from the end-plate zone, triggered by the needle electrode. They usually have an initial negative muscle fiber action potential, although they can be initially positive if recorded just outside the end-plate zone. EPSs are irregular in rhythm and, unlike fibrillations, are only recorded at the end-plate zone. MEPPs are also known as **end-plate noise** and sound like the noise heard when holding a seashell to one's ear. MEPPs are nonpropagating potentials recorded from the end-plate zone and result from spontaneous release of acetylcholine vesicles during the resting state.

9. **What are complex repetitive discharges (CRDs)?**
CRDs are continuous trains of complex action potentials that may begin spontaneously or after needle movement (Fig. 15-2). They have a constant frequency, polyphasic shape, and amplitude, with abrupt onset or change in configuration. Firing rates are typically 20–150 Hz. They probably originate from **ephaptic activation** (i.e., direct activation by local electrical currents) of groups of adjacent muscle fibers and are seen in both neuropathic and myopathic disorders.

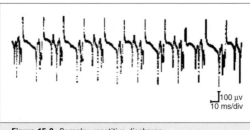

Figure 15-2. Complex repetitive discharge.

10. **What are fasciculation potentials?**

    Fasciculation potentials result from the spontaneous discharge of either the entire group of muscle fibers belonging to a **motor unit** or a portion of its fibers. Fasciculations are often visible in the superficial muscles but may not be visible in the deep muscles. The source is usually either the motor neuron cell body or its axon.

    Fasciculations can be seen in normal individuals. Benign and pathologic forms of fasciculations can look similar and are best distinguished by looking for associated abnormalities such as fibrillation potentials or abnormal motor unit morphology. Morphology and amplitudes are similar to voluntary motor unit action potentials, but firing rates are random and irregular.

KEY POINTS: FASCICULATION POTENTIALS ✓

1. A fasciculation potential is an involuntary discharge of a motor unit or part of a motor unit.

2. Fasciculation potentials are often seen in normal individuals.

3. They are characterized by an irregular or isolated loud snap or pop.

4. They may be pathologic if present with other abnormalities.

11. **What are the EMG characteristics of myokymic discharges? Neuromyotonic discharges?**

    - **Myokymic discharges** are rhythmic, spontaneous bursts of a group of motor unit potentials (i.e., grouped fasciculations) probably resulting from ephaptic transmission between the motor axons. There are variable numbers of potentials in each group or burst. Interburst frequency is 0.1–10 Hz, whereas the intraburst potentials fire at 20–150 Hz.
    - **Neuromyotonic discharges** are bursts of motor unit action potentials that originate in motor axons, fire at high rates (150–300 Hz) for a few seconds, and often start and stop abruptly. These discharges can be seen in many conditions, including neuropathies, tetany, spinal muscular atrophy, and Isaac syndrome.

    Gutmann L: Diseases with abnormal muscle activity. In Tan FC (ed): EMG Secrets. Philadelphia, Hanley & Belfus, 2004, pp 217–219.

12. **Define a motor unit.**

    The **motor unit** consists of the motor neuron, the axon and its branches, and all the muscle fibers (10–1500 fibers) innervated by that motor neuron. A motor unit territory is 5–10 mm in diameter. Normally, each muscle fiber produces an action potential duration of approximately

1–3 ms. It is often difficult to differentiate the small motor unit with short duration (i.e., facial muscles) from "myopathic motor unit potentials" or fibrillation potentials.

13. **Describe the EMG characteristics of a motor unit action potential (MUAP).**
The most important parameters of a MUAP are duration, firing rate, variability, phases, and amplitude, in decreasing order.
   - The **duration** is the most reliable and informative parameter (normal MUAP durations vary according to muscle but are typically 6–15 ms). The duration of a MUAP becomes longer with monopolar needle recording, lower temperature, larger motor unit size, advanced age, and neuropathy.
   - **Firing rate** and **variability** can provide additional clues for differentiating neuropathy, neuromuscular transmission disorders, and myopathy.
   - The **phases** are determined by counting the deflections of the waveform away from and back to the baseline.
   - The **amplitude** is determined by fiber density (the number of muscle fibers in the same motor unit in close proximity to the recording electrode) and not by the total number of muscle fibers in that motor unit (size), because only several fibers close to the needle determine the amplitude.

14. **What are "myopathic" MUAPs?**
MUAPs with short duration and small amplitude are often somewhat erroneously called **myopathic MUAPs**. These MUAPs can be seen in conditions involving decreased number of contributing muscle fiber action potentials (i.e., neuromuscular transmission diseases, early regeneration of nerve fibers after injury, neuropathies affecting the terminal branches of the nerve fiber and myopathies). Instead of using the term "myopathic MUAP," it is recommended that the parameters of the observed MUAP be described (e.g., small amplitude, short duration MUAP).

15. **Explain the size principle in motor unit (MU) recruitment. What is the recruitment rate and ratio?**
The primary mechanism for increasing muscle force is the additional activation of more MUs (**spatial recruitment**) rather than an increased firing rate of MUs (**temporal recruitment**). MUs are recruited in size order from small to large, because larger units require greater facilitation for depolarization than smaller MUs (Henneman **size principle**). The recruitment is a function of the central nervous system, not a function of the peripheral nervous system.
   - **Recruitment rate** is defined as the firing rate of the first MU when the second is recruited (usually 10–12 Hz, <15 Hz in normal individual). A single MU firing rate can be as rapid as 50 Hz in pathologic conditions.
   - **Recruitment ratio** is calculated by the highest firing rate of MU among all on the screen, divided by the number of MUs recruited. Recruitment ratio is normally <5.

   Henneman E, Somjen G, Carpenter DO: Functional significance of cell size in spinal motor neurons. J Neurophysiol 28:560–589, 1965.

16. **Describe the significance of both decreased and increased MUAP recruitment rates.**
In the early phase of proximal nerve or root lesions (i.e., early radiculopathy), the only electrodiagnostic clue is **decreased recruitment** with high firing rate of MUs. Early or **increased recruitment** signifies that too many MUAPs are recruited in proportion to the level of muscle force upon initiating contraction. This can be observed in myopathies, neuromuscular transmission disorders, or even end-stage neuropathy in which the force contributed by each MU is decreased because of the loss of the muscle fibers.

17. **What information can be obtained with a nerve conduction study (NCS)?**

An NCS induces and detects the waves of depolarization along the nerve axons and muscle depolarization. The types of nerves tested are sensory, motor, or mixed. Nerve conduction velocity (NCV) represents the velocity of the fastest fibers depending on axon diameter, quality/thickness of the myelin sheath, internodal distance, and temperature. NCV is decreased in demyelinating disease with relatively preserved amplitude unless significant conduction block coexists. NCV may remain normal with reduced amplitude in diseases with axonal degeneration. Some slowing of the NCV occurs with loss of fast, large-diameter fibers during progression of an axonal neuropathy.

18. **What is the mixed nerve study (MNS)? When is it useful?**

MNS is technically the same as sensory NCS, using an **orthodromic sensory** and **antidromic motor** to avoid volume conduction from compound muscle action potentials. Median and ulnar MNS across the wrist is useful for diagnosis of carpal tunnel syndrome. Medial and lateral plantar MNS across the ankle is useful for diagnosing tarsal tunnel syndrome, because a SNAP is technically difficult to obtain from toe stimulation.

The electrodiagnostic instrument should be set for the sensory conduction study mode because it is only recording compound nerve action potentials. The initial deflection of the compound mixed nerve potential probably represents the larger myelinated sensory fibers.

19. **How does temperature affect electrodiagnostic measurements?**

- **Nerve conduction velocities:** Cooling results in a longer time for the action potential to propagate and a net slowing of conduction. For each 1°C drop in temperature, there is an approximately 5% decrease in nerve conduction velocity.
- **SNAP and CMAP amplitude:** When cool, the duration of an action potential gets longer and the amplitude gets larger. Because of prolonged opening times of the sodium channels, larger action potentials are seen from individual axons and the nerve as a whole.
- **Conduction block:** With low temperature, slow opening and even slower closing of ion channels lead to prolonged ion channel opening time and increased influx of Na^+, resulting in prolonged action potential duration. This extra duration may be just long enough to excite or skip a short demyelinated segment. Therefore, conduction block can be overcome by cooling.
- **Spontaneous and voluntary EMG potentials:** Cooling leads to desynchronization, which results in an increase in the duration of the MUAP and increased polyphasicity. The amplitude of the MUAP may or may not increase depending on the pattern of cooling. Fibrillations and positive waves decrease in frequency with cooling, whereas fasciculations may increase.

Rutkov SB: AAEM minimonograph #14: The effects of temperature in neuromuscular electrophysiology. Muscle Nerve 24:867–882, 2001.

20. **How does the F-wave differ from the H-reflex?**

- **The F-wave** is a late motor potential recorded with supramaximal stimulation as a result of backfiring of 3–5% of the motor neuron pool. The F-wave latency is approximately 30 msec in the upper limb (side-to-side difference <2 msec) and 50–60 msec in the lower limb (side-to-side difference of <4 msec).
- **Hoffman (H) reflexes** are the electrical equivalent of the muscle stretch reflex and are usually only recorded in the soleus and flexor carpi radialis at rest in healthy adults. H-reflexes may be recorded in a variety of muscles in infants, in some types of central neuropathology, and in healthy adults during an isometric contraction.

F-wave and H-reflex are most useful for suspected proximal-segment pathologies when the other electrodiagnostic parameters are normal, especially in the early stage of disease (*see* Table 15-2).

Bodofsky EB: Contraction-induced upper extremity H reflexes: Normative values. Arch Phys Med Rehabil 80(5):562–565, 1999.

TABLE 15-2. F-WAVE VERSUS H-REFLEX

	F-wave (not a reflex)	H-reflex
Afferent arc	Alpha motor neuron	I-A fiber
Efferent arc	Alpha motor neuron	Alpha motor neuron
Stimulation intensity	Supramaximal	Submaximal
Stimulation duration	Same as motor conduction study	Long duration (>500 msec for I-A fibers)
Muscles recorded	All distal muscles	Soleus, flexor carpi radialis
Consistency	Variable latency and configuration	Consistent latency and configuration
Amplitude	3–5% of M-response	Can be higher than M-response
Side-to-side difference	<2 msec in upper extremity <4 msec in lower extremity	<2 msec in soleus

21. **Describe the types of nerve injury according to the Seddon classification system.**
    - **Neurapraxia:** Failure of impulse conduction across the affected nerve segment combined with normal conduction above and below the affected segment; carries a good prognosis for recovery; no Wallerian degeneration involved
    - **Axonotmesis:** Disruption of axonal continuity with Wallerian degeneration
    - **Neurotmesis:** Severance of entire nerve; carries a poor prognosis, and surgical repair is needed for functional recovery

22. **What is the purpose of electrodiagnosis soon after nerve injury (10 days after injury)?**
    The goal of EMG early after injury is to distinguish neurapraxia from axonotmesis or neurotmesis. Axonotmesis and neurotmesis are not easily distinguished from each other because the difference is primarily integrity of supporting structures, which have no electrophysiologic function.
    The best way to distinguish neurapraxia from axonotmesis or neurotmesis is by examining the amplitude of the distal CMAP. In neurapraxia the distal CMAP (stimulating and recording distal to the lesion) is maintained, whereas in axonotmesis or neurotmesis the distal CMAP disappears after 10 days as a result of Wallerian degeneration. The larger the distal CMAP, the better the prognosis.
    Robinson LR: AAEM minimonograph #28: Traumatic injury to peripheral nerves. Muscle Nerve 23(6):863–873, 2000.

23. **What is the meaning of a lesion proximal to the dorsal root ganglion (DRG)?**
    In most, but not all, cases of radiculopathy the pathology is proximal to the DRG. Despite sensory loss, routine sensory conduction studies in the limb show no abnormalities. This is because the distal sensory fibers continue to be supplied by axoplasmic flow from the DRG. An abnormal SNAP occurs infrequently in discogenic radiculopathy such as when a far lateral disc causes damage to the DRG. The DRG can also be damaged in diseases such as diabetes mellitus and herpes zoster (ganglionopathy).

KEY POINTS: REPORTING ELECTRODIAGNOSTIC FINDINGS

1. Present the most likely diagnoses first.

2. Explain limitations of the study.

3. Use caution when commenting on severity of a process.

4. Use neuromuscular localization, not musculoskeletal landmarks.

24. **List common reasons for an unstable baseline during electrodiagnostic studies.**
    - Poor contact between ground electrode and patient
    - Broken recording electrode wire (G1 or G2)
    - Cathode/anode reversal and anodal block: placing stimulating cathode near the recording electrode and stimulating anode away from the nerve trunk minimizes anodal block
    - Excessive stimulus duration and intensity
    - Crossing of stimulation wire leads with the other leads and cables
    - Recording electrodes contacting parts of body other than recording site

    Stolov WC: Instrumentation and measurement in electrodiagnosis: AAEM minimonograph #16. Muscle Nerve 18:799–811, 1995.

25. **List five common pitfalls in reporting electrodiagnostic results.**
    1. The use of vague terminology and the inclusion of too many findings and differential diagnoses can confuse the referring physicians.
    2. Diagnoses should not be outlined in a random order without explanation. Organize diagnoses from the most likely to least likely.
    3. Absence of explanation of the limitations of electrodiagnosis to the referring physician.
    4. Qualitative grading of the lesion by "mild to severe" (radiculopathy, carpal tunnel syndrome) or "one plus to four plus" (fibrillation, positive sharp waves) should be done cautiously because the grading is rather subjective.
    5. The lesion should be described in terms of neuromuscular localization rather than musculoskeletal localization. For example, a radial nerve lesion should be described as "distal to innervation of the triceps, proximal to innervation of brachioradialis" instead of "lesion in spiral groove," because the specific fascicular lesion at proximal site can mimic the lesion at a distal location.

    Johnson EW: Why and how to request an electrodiagnostic examination and what to expect in return. Phys Med Rehabil Clin North Am 1:149–158, 1990.

ACKNOWLEDGMENT

The authors of this chapter and the editors would like express appreciation for the fine scholarship that went into the General Principles of Electrodiagnosis chapter in the second edition of *PM&R Secrets*, which provided an example for the development of this chapter.

WEBSITES

1. www.aanem.org/education/education.cfm

   Test questions, go to each issue of *Positives Waves,* a publication of the AANEM
   www.aanem.org/publications/positive_waves/positive_waves.cfm

   Ordering CD-ROMs for auditory recognition of waveforms
   www.aanem.org/publications/cdrom-page1cfm

   Patient resource information
   www.aanem.org/education/PatientInfo/patientinfo.cfm

2. Online NCS/EMG guides, anatomy tools, and doctor's discussion forum
   www.teleemg.com/index.htm

BIBLIOGRAPHY

1. Bodofsky EB: Contraction-induced upper extremity H reflexes: Normative values. Arch Phys Med Rehabil 80(5):562–565, 1999.

2. Dumitru D: Electrodiagnostic Medicine, 2nd ed. Philadelphia, Hanley & Belfus, 2002.

3. Gatens PF, Saeed MA: Electromyographic findings in the intrinsic muscles of normal feet. Arch Phys Med Rehabil 63:317–318, 1982.

4. Gutmann L: Diseases with abnormal muscle activity. In Tan FC (ed): EMG Secrets. Philadelphia, Hanley & Belfus, 2004, pp 217–219.

5. Henneman E, Somjen G, Carpenter DO: Functional significance of cell size in spinal motor neurons. J Neurophysiol 28:560–589, 1965.

6. Johnson EW: Why and how to request an electrodiagnostic examination and what to expect in return. Phys Med Rehabil Clin North Am 1:149–158, 1990.

7. Katirji B, Kaminski HJ, Preston DC, et al: Neuromuscular Disorders in Clinical Practice. Boston, Butterworth-Heinemann, 2002.

8. Preston DC, Shapiro BE: Electromyography and Neuromuscular Disorders. Boston, Butterworth-Heinemann, 1998.

9. Robinson LR: AAEM minimonograph #28: Traumatic injury to peripheral nerves. Muscle Nerve 23(6):863–873, 2000.

10. Rutkov SB: AAEM minimonograph #14: The effects of temperature in neuromuscular electrophysiology. Muscle Nerve 24:867–882, 2001.

11. Stolov WC: Instrumentation and measurement in electrodiagnosis: AAEM minimonograph #16. Muscle Nerve 18:799–811, 1995.

CHAPTER 16

SENSORY- AND MOTOR-EVOKED POTENTIALS

Gary Goldberg, MD, Jeffrey L. Cole, MD, and Mark A. Lissens, MD, PhD

It is not enough to assess a person based on the question "How do you feel?" The key questions are "How do you perceive and comprehend the world? How do you attend to it and become conscious of it?"

–John J. Ratey, MD, *A User's Guide to the Brain* (2002)

1. **What is the difference between a sensory and a motor evoked potential study?**
   - **Sensory evoked potential** (SEP) is an averaged electrical signal recorded on the body surface following stimulus delivery via a sensory pathway (somatosensory, visual, or auditory). SEPs are generally recorded as voltage changes at a fixed point on the scalp, plotted against time in milliseconds following the stimulus, and reflect bioelectric activation in the central nervous system (CNS) (Fig. 16-1).
   - **Motor evoked potential** (MEP) is a compound muscle action potential produced by transcranial stimulation of the motor cortex or stimulation of the motor roots of the spinal cord (Fig. 16-2).

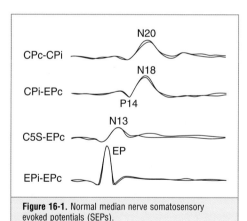

Figure 16-1. Normal median nerve somatosensory evoked potentials (SEPs).

2. **What is a somatosensory evoked potential (SSEP) study?**
   SSEP is the electrophysiologic examination of central somatosensory transmission using a peripheral afferent pathway. Often involving the body's longest axons stretching from the feet up to the base of the medulla, SSEP can be viewed as the CNS extension of the peripheral sensory nerve action potential (SNAP) study. The SSEP technique traces the afferent impulses through the plexus, root, spinal cord, brain stem, and cerebrum, and finally, the

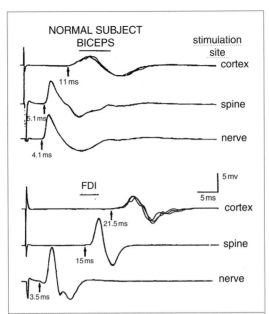

Figure 16-2. Typical motor evoked potentials. Six traces of three superimposed motor evoked potentials after magnetic transcranial motor cortex, spinal, and peripheral nerve stimulation of the biceps brachii muscle (upper three traces: biceps) and the first dorsal interosseus muscle (lower three traces: FDI) in a healthy, normal subject. Central motor conduction times (cortical–spinal latency time) are 5.9 ms and 6.5 ms, respectively. (From Lissens M [ed]: Clinical Applications of Magnetic Transcranial Stimulation. Peeters Press, Leuven, Belgium, 1992. Courtesy of Mark A. Lissens.)

primary somatosensory cortex. It is a "continuity check" of the peripheral nervous system–CNS pathway.

3. **Are only electrical stimuli used for eliciting SSEP studies?**
   Mechanical skin tapping or muscle stretch can also be used, as the first peak contains skin mechanoperceptive afferents. Electrical stimulation produces synchronous activation of the majority of low-threshold, large-diameter peripheral nerve fibers, leading to peripheral nerve activation. When a mixed nerve is stimulated, this compound sensory action potential is conducted along the large-diameter, rapidly conducting epicritic sensory system fibers (discriminative tactile and kinesthetic information), which travel along the ipsilateral spinal cord dorsal columns to synapse at the cervicomedullary junction in the dorsal column nuclei (cuneatus and gracilis).

4. **How are SSEP peaks usually labeled?**
   The most common labels for the upper-extremity SSEP studies use the **polarity** (P1 or N1, for positive or negative) and expected median **latency** (in milliseconds), such as P_{14} or N_{20}.

5. **What normal physiologic factors can affect the latency of an SSEP component?**
   Pathway length (determined by body size) and age. In developing children, while central pathways are not yet fully myelinated, the latencies are relatively prolonged because of slower conduction that is partially offset by shorter pathways.

6. **Can the scalp SSEP be conclusively interpreted without evaluating peripheral conduction?**
   No. To ascribe any SSEP latency anomaly exclusively to a central lesion, there must be no peripheral nerve conduction slowing or blockage.

7. **What is the central somatosensory conduction time (CSCT)?**
   In the SSEP recorded after stimulation of the median nerve at the wrist, the CSCT is the time interval between the major negative peak (i.e., N_{13}) identified in the cervical spine response and the initial major negative peak identified in the cortical response (i.e., N_{19}). It is typically between 5 and 6 ms. The CSCT can be helpful in detecting slowed transmission through the central neuraxis between the cervicomedullary junction and the cortex. It is especially helpful for side-to-side comparisons, where the difference in CSCT between sides should not exceed 1.1 ms.

8. **How can the abnormalities of the SSEP be classified?**
   Abnormalities of the SSEP can be divided into changes in component onset or peak latencies, changes in component amplitude or structure, or loss of specific waveform components. CNS demyelination tends to produce CSCT delays and prolongation of interpeak latencies in segments of the pathway spanning the CNS. Components may be attenuated or absent at proximal recording sites, depending on the severity of the demyelination. When there is unilateral or asymmetric extent of pathology, side-to-side comparisons of interpeak latencies or component amplitudes can be helpful.

9. **What is the main diagnostic limitation of the SSEP?**
   Abnormalities of the SSEP are etiologically nonspecific.

10. **When can the SSEP be helpful in the intensive care unit?**
    When the cortical responses of the median nerve SSEP are bilaterally absent, a patient in coma is extremely unlikely to recover from his or her condition. This is especially true for nontraumatic (e.g., anoxic) coma in adult patients.

11. **What is a visual evoked potential (VEP) study?**
    A VEP is the occipital cortex potential generated after a discrete visual stimulus. The stimulus can be a bright flash of light or a sudden change in light pattern (as with a reversing black-and-white checkerboard pattern) with constant luminance ($40-100$ cd/m^2). The latter is referred to as a pattern-shift VEP (PSVEP) and is more stable and reproducible than the flash-evoked VEP. The primary visual cortex response is best recorded from electrodes placed over the occipital scalp referenced either to the vertex or to a midfrontal electrode. The PSVEP should be recorded with corrective eyeglass lenses in place.

12. **Which PSVEP component is used primarily for clinical interpretation?**
    With pattern-shift visual stimulation the wave usually has a triphasic structure, with three peaks that are labeled by their polarity and position (N_1, P_1, N_2), or by latency (N_{75}, P_{100}, N_{140}). The most important PSVEP parameter is the P_{100} latency because of its stability, ease of recording and identification, and its clinical correlation with lesions affecting the anterior optic pathway.

13. **What type of problem is best detected with a VEP study?**
    The greatest utility of VEP is detection of retrobulbar optic nerve demyelination. This condition is associated with significant prolongation of the P_{100} latency or complete loss of this component.

Each eye is tested separately. An abnormality can be detected as an increase in the P_{100} latency of an affected eye beyond the normal range, or by an abnormal increase in the interocular latency difference between the recorded P_{100} latencies for the two eyes. With advanced demyelination, the P_{100} component from the affected eye may be absent.

14. **What are the indications for doing a brain stem auditory evoked potential/ auditory brain stem response (BAEP/ABR) in an adult?**
In adults the BAEP has found use in a variety of **audiologic problems,** including unexplained "central" losses on behavioral audiometry and in the differential diagnosis of a sudden-onset unilateral deafness or severe hearing loss. The test has superb sensitivity in diagnosing **multiple sclerosis** and other demyelinating conditions, in early diagnosis of **acoustic neuromas,** for **intraoperative monitoring of brain stem function,** for evaluating brain stem function during a **barbiturate coma,** and in intensive care unit (ICU) assessment of patients who appear to be "**brain dead.**"

15. **When is a BAEP/ABR study indicated in a child or infant?**
"Objective" audiometry using the ABR can be used in preverbal children, infants, and neonates to detect the presence of hearing impairment. These studies should be considered in:
- Infants and children suspected of hearing loss or hearing problems
- Families with a history of metabolic or genetic diseases known to cause an early or congenital hearing impairment
- Orofacial dysmorphic syndromes associated with auditory impairment
- All premature infants who have been treated in a neonatal ICU and have failed an auditory screening examination
- Term infants who had hypoxic episodes that resulted in changes in consciousness lasting >24 hr, or unexplained impaired consciousness
- Congenital infections or neonatal bacterial meningitis
- After exposure to ototoxic drugs

16. **What clinical examination should be done before performing a BAEP/ABR?**
Gross behavioral assessment of hearing before establishing threshold values. Otoscopic examination of the external auditory canal with tympanic membrane visualization to ensure that the canal is not obstructed; if the auditory canal shows significant blockage, this should be removed before the studies are performed.

17. **Which BAEP/ABR peaks are used for clinical interpretation?**
The **I–III interpeak latencies** have shown correlation with lesions in the peripheral auditory mechanism, auditory nerve, and lower pons. The **I–V interpeak latencies** have more widespread use in brain stem, thalamic, and cortical injuries when the I–III interpeak latencies are normal. There can be diffuse involvement in both the I–III and III–V interpeak latencies with multiple sclerosis and other demyelinating processes.

18. **What is a magnetically (or electrically) stimulated transcranial motor evoked potential?**
MEPs evaluate transmission along a pathway that includes the efferent corticospinal motor conduction pathway. This complements the afferent dorsal column and spinocerebellar tract information derived from SSEP studies. The transcranial MEP involves initiation of an efferent motor volley through synchronous activation of cortical motor neurons in primary motor cortex. Responses are recorded from surface electrodes placed over a targeted peripheral muscle.

19. **Where are transcranial and spinal MEPs helpful diagnostically?**
Maximization of the magnetic MEPs is best obtained on awake, cooperative patients who can voluntarily contract the "target" muscle, producing a prestimulation baseline level of low-level

voluntary activation. MEP studies can be used to examine impairment of conduction through central motor pathways traversing the brain and spinal cord. MEPs have proven useful in the study of patients with stroke, multiple sclerosis, motor neuron disease, and myelopathy. They can be used to assess and localize damage to CNS pathways that result in motor impairment.

KEY POINTS: SENSORY AND MOTOR EVOKED POTENTIALS

1. Somatosensory evoked potentials (SSEPs) and motor evoked potentials (MEPs) are viewed as sensory and motor continuity checks, respectively, of peripheral nervous system (PNS) and central nervous system (CNS) pathways.

2. SSEPs can be viewed as a central extension of the sensory nerve conduction study, whereas MEPs can be viewed as a central extension of the motor nerve conduction study.

3. Patients with anoxic encephalopathy are highly unlikely to emerge from coma if cortical SSEPs are bilaterally absent.

4. SSEPs with stimulation of lower limb nerves can be used to assess spinal cord conduction and evaluate for myelopathy.

5. Interpeak latencies and side-to-side latency differences are more sensitive measures of abnormality than absolute latencies.

6. Objective audiometry can detect hearing loss and permit institution of early aural rehabilitation efforts in young children and infants.

20. **How should EPs be reported?**
The important elements of the report are the history and physical examination and the clinical reason for the referral. Signal EP data should be attached. The traces used for analysis and interpretation must show at least two clearly superimposed runs to confirm the recording reliability. The stimulus site (type, intensity), active recording electrode site, reference location, equipment (settings), and recording parameters used for the test should be included with the data, as well as a basic summary of the technique used. Interpretation of latency, amplitude, and waveform morphology should always be based on side-to-side comparisons and statistical analysis (mean $\pm$ 2.5 SD) for all the data criteria used to differentiate abnormality from normality.

WEBSITES

1. www.emedicine.com/neuro/topic640.htm

2. www.emedicine.com/neuro/topic69.htm

3. http://en.wikipedia.org/wiki/Sensory__evoked_potentials

4. www.healthatoz.com/healthatoz/Atoz/ency/evoked_potential_studies.jsp

5. www.neurophys.com

BIBLIOGRAPHY

1. Binnie CD, Cooper R, Fowler CJ, et al (eds): Clinical Neurophysiology: EMG, Nerve Conduction and Evoked Potentials. Oxford, England, Butterworth-Heinemann, 1995.

2. Chiappa KH (ed): Evoked Potentials in Clinical Medicine, 3rd ed. Philadelphia, Lippincott-Raven, 1997.

3. Cole JL: Central nervous system electrodiagnostics. In DeLisa J (ed): Rehabilitation Medicine: Principles and Practice, 3rd ed. Philadelphia, J.B. Lippincott, 1998, pp 373–406.

4. Goldberg G: Clinical neurophysiology of the central nervous system. Evoked potentials and other neurophysiologic techniques. In Grabois M, Garrison SJ, Hart KA, Lehmkuhl LD (eds): Physical Medicine and Rehabilitation: The Complete Approach. Malden, MA, Blackwell Science, 2000, pp 196–224.

5. Mauguière F: Clinical utility of somatosensory evoked potentials (SEPs): Present debates and future trends. Electroencephalogr Clin Neurophysiol Suppl 46:27–33, 1996.

6. Misulis K, Fakhoury T: Spehlmann's Evoked Potential Primer, 3rd ed. Oxford, England, Butterworth-Heinemann, 2001.

CHAPTER 17

RADICULOPATHIES: SYMPTOMS, DIFFERENTIAL DIAGNOSIS, AND TREATMENT

Timothy R. Dillingham, MD, and Diane W. Braza, MD

Pain makes man think. Thought makes man wise. Wisdom makes life endurable.
—John Patrick, 1851

1. **What are radiculopathies?**
   Radiculopathies are conditions resulting from pathologic processes affecting the spinal nerve root. Common pathologies may include herniated nucleus pulposus, spinal stenosis, degenerative spondylosis, spondylolisthesis, and inflammatory radiculitis.

   www.spineuniverse.com/displayarticle.php/article1431.html

KEY POINTS: COMMON CAUSES OF RADICULOPATHY

1. Herniated nucleus pulposus

2. Spinal stenosis

3. Degenerative spondylosis

4. Spondylolisthesis

5. Inflammatory radiculitis

2. **What are the nondiscogenic/nonspondylitic causes of radiculopathies?**
   - Tumors
     - Primary: meningiomas, neurofibromas, lipomas (cauda equina and conus medullaris)
     - Secondary: breast, prostate, lung, colorectal, thyroid, etc.
   - Leptomeningeal metastasis (leukemias, lymphoproliferative diseases)
   - Abscess, hemorrhage, cysts
   - Infection: herpes zoster, tuberculosis, Lyme disease, syphilis, HIV infection
   - Arachnoiditis: myelogram, surgery, anesthetics, steroid injections
   - Sarcoidosis, Guillain-Barré syndrome, diabetes

3. **Describe the relationship of the exiting spinal nerve to the numbered vertebral segment.**
   In the cervical region, there are eight cervical nerve roots and only seven vertebrae. The first seven cervical roots (C1–C7) exit above the same numbered vertebrae. C8 exits above T1.

In the thoracolumbar spine the nerve roots exit the spinal canal by passing below the pedicle of their named vertebrae.

American Association of Orthopaedic Surgeons: www.aaos.org
www.spineuniverse.com/displayarticle.php/article265.html

4. **What symptoms are associated with radiculopathies?**
   - Radiating limb pain greater than axial pain; aggravated by sneezing, coughing, or Valsalva maneuver
   - Numbness or tingling
   - Weakness
   - Rarely, bowel and/or bladder retention or incontinence

KEY POINTS: AGGRAVATING AND ALLEVIATING FACTORS

1. Classic disc-related lumbosacral radicular pain is often aggravated by sitting and forward-bending and is alleviated by walking, standing, or lying supine.

2. Lumbar stenosis–related radicular pain is often relieved by sitting or flexion and aggravated by standing and walking.

3. Cervical radicular pain may be aggravated by neck extension, which causes narrowing of the intervertebral foramen.

5. **Discuss the most important elements of the examination in patients with potential radiculopathies.**
   A focused neuromuscular examination to determine the presence or absence of neurologic deficit is mandatory. For each nerve root, assessment of strength, sensation, and, when appropriate, reflex testing should be completed. Patients with radiculopathy may demonstrate subtle weakness, a reduced reflex, or sensory loss. A positive straight-leg raising test (pain radiating below the knee) can be seen despite normal strength, sensation, and reflex findings. Central nerve system (CNS) disorders (e.g., stroke or spinal myelopathy) may result in sensory loss and weakness similar to that found in radiculopathy; however, reflexes are usually increased in these CNS conditions.

   SpineUniverse: www.spineuniverse.com

6. **Describe the classic patterns of pain radiation and the corresponding physical exam findings seen in common cervical and lumber radiculopathies.**
   See Table 17–1.

KEY POINTS: PHYSICAL EXAM PEARLS

1. Upon hearing a heavy foot slap as your patient enters the room, think L5 radiculopathy (ankle dorsiflexor weakness).

2. If your patient cannot walk on his or her toes, think S1 radiculopathy.

3. If your patient cannot extend the elbow, think C7 radiculopathy.

TABLE 17-1. CLASSIC PATTERNS OF PAIN RADIATION AND PHYSICAL EXAM FINDINGS IN COMMON CERVICAL AND LUMBAR RADICULOPATHIES

Root	Pain Radiation	Reflex	Sensation	Motor Weakness
C5	Shoulder blade and lateral arm	Biceps	Lateral arm	Shoulder flexion and abduction, elbow flexion
C6	Shoulder blade, radial arm, and forearm	Brachioradialis and biceps	Radial distal arm and forearm, thumb	Elbow flexion, forearm pronation, wrist extension
C7	Posterior arm and forearm	Triceps	Posterior arm and dorsal forearm, middle finger	Elbow extension, wrist flexion
C8	Medial arm and forearm	Triceps	Medial forearm, fourth and fifth fingers	Finger flexion and abduction
L4	Anterior thigh and knee, medial calf	Patellar	Anterior thigh, medial calf/foot	Knee extension, ankle dorsiflexion
L5	Buttocks, lateral thigh and calf, dorsal foot and great toe	Medial hamstring	Lateral leg and dorsum of foot	Ankle dorsiflexion, great toe extension
S1	Posterior thigh and calf, lateral/plantar foot	Achilles	Posterior calf, lateral foot	Ankle plantar flexion

7. **What conditions can mimic cervical radiculopathy?**
   For a list of musculoskeletal conditions that commonly mimic cervical radiculopathy, see Table 17-2. Common entrapment neuropathies, plexopathies, and idiopathic brachial neuritis can present similarly. Brachial neuritis usually begins with severe proximal shoulder girdle pain and then weakness develops. The weakness is characteristically in a focal nerve distribution such as the long thoracic nerve.

8. **What conditions may mimic lumbosacral radiculopathy?**
   For a list of musculoskeletal conditions that commonly mimic lumbosacral radiculopathy, see Table 17-3. Neuralgic amyotrophy (caused by nerve ischemia) from diabetes often presents with thigh pain. On electromyography (EMG), it appears more like proximal lumbosacral plexopathy with frequent involvement of the femoral nerve. Distal mononeuropathies such as peroneal and tibial can develop similarly.

9. **Which diagnostic tools are useful for further evaluating patients with suspected cervical or lumbosacral radiculopathy?**
   In the absence of red flags (fever, trauma, weight loss, incontinences, night pain, or history of malignancy), diagnostic studies are rarely needed initially unless they will alter the treatment plan, or if progressive neurologic deficits occur.
   - **Plain radiographs** reveal bony alignment, disc space narrowing, and bony trauma but are insensitive for radiculopathy.
   - **Dynamic flexion/extension views** can reveal instability.
   - **Magnetic resonance imaging (MRI)** provides the best resolution of water, colloidal tissue, and spinal structures. Gadolinium enhancement must be used if tumor is suspected. Because of its sensitivity, clinical correlation with imaging findings is essential for optimal patient care.

TABLE 17-2. MUSCULOSKELETAL CONDITIONS THAT COMMONLY MIMIC CERVICAL RADICULOPATHY

Condition	Clinical Symptoms/Signs
Fibromyalgia syndrome	Pain all over, female predominance, sleep problems, tender to palpation in multiple areas
Regional myofascial pain	Trigger point reproducing localized or radiating pain syndrome
Polymyalgia rheumatica	Age >50 yr; pain and stiffness in neck, shoulders, and hips; high ESR
Sternoclavicular joint arthropathy	Pain in anterior chest, pain with shoulder movement, pain on direct palpation
Acromioclavicular joint arthropathy	Pain in anterior chest, pain with shoulder movement, pain on direct palpation, pain with crossed adduction of shoulder
Shoulder bursitis, impingement syndrome, bicipital tendonitis	Pain with palpation, positive impingement signs, pain in C5 distribution
Lateral epicondylitis, "tennis elbow"	Pain in lateral forearm, pain with palpation and resisted wrist extension
de Quervain's tenosynovitis	Lateral wrist and forearm pain, tender at abductor pollicis longus or extensor pollicis brevis tendons; positive Finkelstein test
Trigger finger, stenosing, tenosynovitis of finger flexor tendons	Intermittent pain and locking of digit in flexion

ESR = erythrocyte sedimentation rate.

- **Computed tomography (CT)** is especially valuable in assessing bony encroachment. Use of intrathecal contrast can enhance visualization of soft tissues and neural structures.
- **Electrodiagnostic testing** consists primarily of EMG and nerve conduction studies (NCSs). EMG/NCS studies provide an assessment as to whether motor axonal damage is occurring, help localize the lesion to a specific root level, and complement spinal imaging, particularly when the imaging findings are subtle or can be attributed to age-related changes. EMG/NCS studies are useful to assess a coexistent peripheral polyneuropathy, focal entrapment neuropathy, or myopathy, especially when presenting symptoms and signs are vague, diffuse, or nonlocalizing.
- **Laboratory testing:** Complete blood count (CBC), erythrocyte sedimentation rate (ESR), serum electrophoresis (SPEP) may be indicated if infection, tumor, or metabolic disease is suspected.

American Association of Neuromuscular and Electrodiagnostic Medicine: www.aanew.org

Mobic MT, Obuchowski NA, Ross JS, et al: Acute low back pain and radiculopathy: MR imaging findings and their prognostic role and effect on outcome. Radiology 237:597–604, 2005.

10. **How common are false-positive MRI findings?**
The false-positive rates for MRI of the lumbar spine are high; 27% of normals show a disc protrusion. For the cervical spine the false-positive rate is much lower, with 19% of subjects demonstrating an abnormality but only 10% showing a herniated or bulging disc.

TABLE 17-3. COMMON MUSCULOSKELETAL DISORDERS MIMICKING LUMBOSACRAL RADICULOPATHY

Condition	Clinical Symptoms/Signs
Fibromyalgia, myofascial pain syndrome, polymyalgia rheumatica	*See* Table 17-2
Hip arthritis	Pain in groin and anterior thigh, pain with weight-bearing, positive Patrick's test
Trochanteric bursitis	Lateral hip pain, pain with palpation over lateral and posterior hip
Iliotibial band syndrome	Pain along outer thigh, pain with palpation, tight iliotibial band (positive Ober test)
Knee arthritis	Pain with weight-bearing
Patellofemoral pain	Anterior knee pain, worse with prolonged sitting, positive patellar compression test
Pes anserinus bursitis	Medial proximal tibia pain, tender to palpation
Hamstring tendinitis, chronic strain	Posterior knee and thigh pain, can mimic positive straight-leg raise, common in runners
Baker's cyst	Posterior knee pain and swelling
Plantar fasciitis	Pain in sole of foot, worse with weight-bearing activities, tender to palpation
Gastrocnemius-soleus tendonitis, chronic strain	Calf pain, worse with sports activities, usually limited range of motion compared to asymptomatic limb

Radiculopathies can occur without structural findings on MRI and, likewise, without EMG findings. The sensitivity of MRI for identifying pathologic conditions of the spine is very high, but the trade-off is the correspondingly high rate of false-positive findings. EMG and MRI findings agree in a majority (60%) of patients with a clinical history compatible with cervical or lumbosacral radiculopathy. The correlation is greater in patients with objective neurologic findings, consistent with a radiculopathy.

Boden SD, McCowin PR, Davis DO, et al: Abnormal magnetic resonance scans of the cervical spine in asymptomatic subjects. J Bone Joint Surg 72A:1178–1184, 1990.

Boden SD, Weisel SM: Errors in decision making following radiographic investigations of the spine. Seminars in Spine Surgery 5:90–100, 1993.

Nardin RA, Patel MR, Gudas TF, et al: Electromyography and magnetic resonance imaging in the evaluation of radiculopathy. Muscle Nerve 22:151–155, 1999.

www.emedicine.com/SPORTS/topic66.htm

11. **What is the most important and useful electrodiagnostic test for radiculopathy?**
    Monopolar needle electromyography of the deep paraspinal musculature (multifidus and others) at the bony level of the clinically suspected radiculopathy will likely reveal membrane instability.

12. **Can a radiculopathy at a specific root level be diagnosed simply on the basis of positive paraspinal EMG findings?**
    No. The diagnosis of radiculopathy can be made, but the root level cannot be specified unless EMG abnormalities are found in two or more muscles innervated by a single root and by different peripheral nerves, yet muscles innervated by adjacent nerve roots are normal.

The paraspinal muscles are innervated by multiple nerve roots—not by one nerve root alone—and demonstrate considerable overlap.

13. **Are NCSs helpful in assessing for radiculopathy?**
The motor and sensory nerve conduction studies are usually normal with single-level radiculopathies. The sensory nerve action potential (SNAP) should be unaffected with a typical compressive radiculopathy given that the lesion is proximal to the dorsal root ganglion or its peripheral fibers. Traditional motor latencies and conduction velocities are normal in radiculopathy and further rule out neuropathy. With axonal degeneration, the compound muscle action potential (CMAP) may be reduced. CMAP amplitude comparison, side to side and at different times, may provide assessment of the severity of denervation and eventual recovery through reinnervation.

Late responses (H-waves and F-waves), as a measure of proximal motor conduction, are not useful at all levels. H-wave latency, compared side to side, is useful in the evaluation of S1 radiculopathy. A side-to-side latency difference of 1.8 msec or more suggests proximal slowing resulting from a radiculopathy.

www.teleemg.com/new/hrefqs.htm

14. **How sensitive is EMG for diagnosing radiculopathy?**
It is rather unimpressive. Various studies place the sensitivity of needle EMG for lumbosacral radiculopathies somewhere between 50% and 80%, depending on the diagnostic gold standard used—clinical standards, imaging standards, or intraoperative confirmation. For cervical radiculopathies, the sensitivity is roughly 60–70%.

15. **Why is the EMG normal for many people with radiculopathies?**
The needle EMG assesses only the motor axons. A radiculopathy that involves only the sensory nerve roots and causes radicular pain and numbness will demonstrate a normal EMG. Radiculopathies that cause motor neurapraxia at the nerve root level will not show spontaneous activity (fibrillations and positive sharp waves) on EMG. Radiculopathies that result in chronic, slow axonal loss that is balanced with reinnervation may not show spontaneous activity, but rather may show more subtle findings, such as polyphasic motor units or large motor units firing in a reduced recruitment pattern. Fibrillation potentials in a group of muscles innervated by a single root level with normal myotomes above and below provides compelling evidence of a radiculopathy with motor axonal loss.

16. **How many muscles must be studied to confidently identify a radiculopathy by EMG?**
Delineating an optimal EMG screening exam that allows the examiner to identify a radiculopathy (when one can be electrodiagnostically confirmed), yet minimizes the number of muscles studied, is of great clinical interest.
For optimal identification while minimizing harm, study six muscles in the leg and six in the arm.

Six lower limb muscles, including paraspinal muscles, consistently identify more than 98% of electrodiagnostically confirmable lumbosacral radiculopathies. Studying additional muscles leads to marginal increases in identification. A suggested lower-limb EMG screen with optimal identification includes the vastus medialis, anterior tibialis, posterior tibialis, short head of biceps femoris, medial gastrocnemius, and lumbar paraspinal muscles.

Six upper limb muscles, including paraspinal muscles, also consistently identify more than 98% of electrodiagnostically confirmable cervical radiculopathies. For upper-limb EMG evaluation, a suggested screen includes deltoid, triceps, pronator teres, abductor pollicis brevis, extensor digitorum communis, and cervical paraspinal muscles. For both lumbosacral and cervical symptoms, when paraspinal muscles are not reliable to study, **eight** distal muscles are necessary to achieve optimal identification.

Dillingham TR, Lauder TD, Andary M, et al: Identifying lumbosacral radiculopathies: An optimal electromyographic screen. Am J Phys Med Rehabil 79:496–503, 2000.

Dillingham TR, Lauder TD, Andary M, et al: Identification of cervical radiculopathies: Optimizing the electromyographic screen. Am J Phys Med Rehabil 80(2):84–91, 2001.

KEY POINTS: NONOPERATIVE TREATMENT FOR RADICULOPATHIES

1. Control pain with over-the-counter analgesics or prescription nonsteroidal anti-inflammatory medications.

2. Encourage positional pain relief techniques, avoiding prolonged bed rest.

3. Incorporate cervical or lumbar stabilization exercises.

4. Consider epidural steroid injections for intractable radicular pain, unresponsive to above measures.

17. **Outline the initial treatment plan for a patient with an active radiculopathy.**
The initial goals of treatment are to control pain and reduce inflammation. Treatment strategies include over-the-counter analgesics or nonsteroidal anti-inflammatory medications, prescription analgesic medications for acute intractable pain, intermittent localized icing, and positional pain relief techniques. Prolonged bed rest is not recommended. Activity modification is recommended; avoiding bending, lifting, and twisting, which tend to increase intradiscal pressure.

   Malanga GA: The diagnosis and treatment of cervical radiculopathy. Med Sci Sports Exec 29(7)Suppl: S236–S245, 1997.

18. **Describe a rehabilitation plan of care for a patient with an acute lumbosacral radiculopathy.**
Goals of physical therapy include centralization of peripheral radicular pain, improvement in basic and advanced activities of daily living, and restoration of function. Treatment includes education in proper back protection techniques, initiation and progression of core strengthening through lumbosacral stabilization exercises, and correction of lower extremity musculoligamentous imbalances. Aerobic exercise such as a walking program should be encouraged if possible. Lumbar traction has not been proven to be beneficial.

   Clarke JA, van Tulder MW, Blomberg SE, et al: Cochrane Back Group. Traction for low back pain with or without sciatica. Cochrane Database Syst Rev 4, 2005.

   Harte AA, Baxter GD, Gracey JH: The efficacy of traction for back pain: A systematic review of randomized controlled trials. Arch Phys Med Rehabil 84:1542–1553, 2003.

19. **What are the long-term outcomes for persons with a herniated cervical disc managed nonoperatively?**
Saal, Saal, and Yurth demonstrated that persons with cervical disc herniations have a favorable clinical course. Their cohort of patients were managed with pain management strategies that incorporated medications, rehabilitation with cervical traction and exercises, and epidural or selective nerve root injections if medications failed to control pain. In this series the majority (24 of 26) of patients with herniated cervical discs achieved successful outcomes without surgery. Overall, 83% of the nonoperative group had a good or excellent outcome. A total of 89% of patients with disc extrusions treated nonoperatively achieved a good or excellent outcome,

compared to 80% of patients with contained disc herniations. No patients had progressive neurologic loss or new-onset myelopathy.

Saal JS, Saal JA, Yurth EF: Nonoperative management of herniated cervical intervertebral disc with radiculopathy. Spine 21:1877–1883, 1996.

20. **What are the long-term outcomes for persons with a herniated lumbar disc managed nonoperatively?**
They are quite good. A classic investigation by Henrik Weber, a randomized, prospective study of surgery versus conservative care for herniated nucleus pulposus, demonstrated that surgery was somewhat more effective at pain control during the first year. Beyond 1 year, however, conservative treatment had equal results compared to the surgically managed group. Even for persons with motor weakness, a good outcome with conservative treatment was the norm, and surgery did not improve motor return. Other investigators in cohort outcomes studies have demonstrated that the majority of persons suffering lumbosacral radiculopathy can resolve their symptoms. In fact, on follow-up MRI studies, lumbosacral disc herniations and disc fragments resolve in 76% of patients.

Atlas S, Keller RB, Wu YA, et al: Long-term outcomes of surgical and nonsurgical management of sciatica secondary to a lumbar disc herniation: 10-year results from the Maine Lumbar Spine Study. Spine 30 (8):927–935, 2005.

Lipetz JS, Misra N, Silber JS: Resolution of pronounced painless weakness arising from radiculopathy and disk extrusion. Am J Phys Med Rehabil 84:528–537, 2005.

Weber H: Lumbar disc herniation: A controlled, prospective study with ten years of observation. Spine 8:131–140, 1983.

KEY POINTS: INDICATIONS FOR SURGICAL REFERRAL

1. Progressive neuromotor deficits

2. Cauda equina syndrome

3. Cervical myelopathy

4. Intractable pain, unresponsive to nonoperative treatment

21. **What are the indications for referral of a patient with radiculopathy to a spine surgeon?**
The indications for urgent referral to a spine surgeon include cauda equina syndrome with bowel or bladder dysfunction, saddle paresthesias, and/or bilateral lower extremity weakness, and progressive cervical or thoracic myelopathy with gait disturbance, upper/lower extremity weakness, and bowel and bladder dysfunction.

Surgical referral may be considered for
- Intractable pain despite aggressive nonoperative care
- Severe or progressive motor weakness

BIBLIOGRAPHY

1. Bush K, Cowan N, Katz DE, Gishen P: The natural history of sciatica associated with disc pathology: A prospective study with clinical and independent radiological follow-up. Spine 1:1205–1212, 1992.

2. Dumitru D (ed): Electrodiagnostic Medicine, 2nd ed. Philadelphia, Hanley & Belfus, 2002.

3. Honet JC, Puri K: Cervical radiculitis: Treatment and results in 82 patients. Arch Phys Med Rehabil 57:12–16, 1976.
4. Jensen MC, Brant-Zawadzki MN, Obuchowski N, et al: Magnetic resonance imaging of the lumbar spine in people without back pain. N Engl J Med 331:69–73, 1994.
5. Knutsson B: Comparative value of electromyographic, myelographic and clinical-neurological examinations in diagnosis of lumbar root compression syndrome. Acta Orthop Scand Suppl 49:7–135, 1961.
6. Kuruoglu R, Oh SJ, Thompson B: Clinical and electromyographic correlations of lumbosacral radiculopathy. Muscle Nerve 17:250–251, 1994.

CHAPTER 18

NEUROPATHY: HEREDITY, TOXICITY, AND ENTRAPMENT

Peter Daniel Donofrio, MD, Elliot B. Bodofsky, MD, and Steven A. Stiens, MD, MS

Strain every nerve to gain your point.

–Cicero (106–43 BC)

PERIPHERAL POLYNEUROPATHY: TOXIC, ENTRAPMENT, AND HEREDITARY

1. **Which drugs cause peripheral neuropathy?**
   Peripheral sensory and motor fibers react to toxins (in this case, medications) in a limited manner. Schaumburg and Spencer theorized that toxins cause disease at one of four regions of the peripheral nerve:
   - Distal sensory and motor axon (axonopathy)
   - Schwann cell
   - Dorsal root ganglion (ganglionopathy or neuronopathy)
   - Anterior horn cell or motor neuron
     Box 18-1 lists medications and chemotherapeutic agents based on their primary pathologic site of injury.

   Schaumburg HH, Spencer PS: Toxic neuropathies. Neurology 29:429–431, 1979.

2. **What tests are helpful to identify the cause of a diffuse polyneuropathy?**
   In longstanding diabetics, laboratory evaluation may not be necessary unless the history and physical examination suggest another etiology for the neuropathy. Commonly needed tests for the evaluation of an idiopathic distal symmetric polyneuropathy include complete blood count, fasting blood sugar, serum B_{12} level, serum protein electrophoresis, urinalysis, metabolic panel, erythrocyte sedimentation rate, and thyroid function studies. If unremarkable, additional evaluation may include HIV testing, rheumatologic studies, spinal fluid analysis, vitamin E or B_6 levels, and 24-hour urine for heavy metals.

3. **What is the role of nerve conduction studies and electromyography in the assessment of a polyneuropathy?**
   Nerve conduction studies and electromyography are useful to determine whether the primary pathologic process is demyelinating or axon loss, to identify the predominant fibers affected (motor or sensory), and to provide clues into the duration and severity of the neuropathy. They can also decipher if another neuromuscular condition is present, such as a plexopathy, polyradiculopathy, anterior horn cell disorder, or mononeuritis multiplex.

4. **What industrial and environmental toxins cause neuropathies?**
   Similar to drug-induced neuropathies, industrial and environmental agents can cause a neuropathy at one of several levels of the peripheral nerve. Box 18-2 lists these agents.

5. **How are inherited neuropathies classified?**
   Box 18-3 lists a recently published classification of inherited neuropathies. Hereditary motor and sensory and hereditary and sensory autonomic neuropathies are the most common. Other conditions, such as Tangier disease, have multisystem features in addition to polyneuropathy.

BOX 18-1. DRUG-INDUCED NEUROPATHIES

Axonopathy
Amiodarone
Amitriptyline
Chloramphenicol
Chloroquine
Cis-platinum
Clioquinol
Colchicine
Cyanate
Disopyramide
Disulfiram
Enalapril
Ethambutol
Ethionamide
Glutethimide
Gold
Hydralazine
Isoniazid
Lithium
Mercury
Methaqualone
Metronidazole
Misonidazole
Nitrofurantoin
Nitrous oxide

Phenytoin
Sulfapyridine
Sulfasalazine
Statins
Thalidomide
Vancomycin
Vinblastine
Vincristine

Anterior horn cell
Dapsone

Dorsal root ganglion
Paclitaxel (Taxol)
Pyridoxine

Schwann cell
Allopurinol
Amiodarone
Indomethacin
Perhexiline
Suramin
Zimeldine
L-tryptophan contaminant

Adapted from Donofrio PD: Electrophysiologic evaluations. Neurol Clin Neurobehav Toxicol 18:601–613, 2000.

6. **What are the genetic defects in Charcot-Marie-Tooth disease?**
   The majority of patients with Charcot-Marie-Tooth disease have mutations in one of three genes:
   - PMP 22 (peripheral myelin protein 22)
   - MPZ (myelin protein zero)
   - GJB1 (gap junction), also called connexin 32

   Greenberg SA, Welsh RJ: Molecular diagnosis of inheritable neuromuscular disorders. II. Application of genetic testing in neuromuscular disease. Muscle Nerve 31:431–451, 2005.

7. **How are diffuse polyneuropathies categorized by their underlying pathologic mechanisms?**
   The majority of polyneuropathies can be subdivided into those that are motor, sensory, or both, and into those that are axon loss, demyelinating, or combined. The demyelinating neuropathies

BOX 18-2.   ENVIRONMENTAL AND INDUSTRIAL NEUROPATHIES

Arsenic

Mercury

n-Hexane

Hexacarbons

Trichloroethylene

Organophosphorus compounds

Thallium

Lead

Acrylamide

Ethylene oxide

Carbon disulfate

Adapted from Albers JW, Wald JJ: Industrial and environmental toxic neuropathies. In Brocon WF, Bolton CF, Aminoff M (eds): Neuromuscular Function and Disease, Basic, Clinical and Electrodiagnostic Aspects, Vol 2. Philadelphia, W.B. Saunders, 2002, pp 1143–1168.

BOX 18-3.   INHERITED NEUROPATHIES

Hereditary motor and sensory neuropathy (HMSN)

Hereditary sensory and autonomic neuropathy (HSAN)

Hereditary focal neuropathy

Hereditary neuralgic amyotrophy

Hereditary neuropathy with liability to pressure palsies (HNPP)

Tangier disease

Familial amyloidotic polyneuropathy

Giant axonal neuropathy

Adapted from Greenberg SA, Welsh RJ: Molecular diagnosis of inheritable neuromuscular disorders. II. Application of genetic testing in neuromuscular disease. Muscle Nerve 31:431–451, 2005.

can be further grouped as multifocal acquired or uniformly demyelinating. Guillain-Barré syndrome is a good example of a motor greater than sensory-acquired polyneuropathy, whereas most toxic neuropathies, such as alcohol- or medication-induced neuropathies, affect primarily the axon and sensory fibers more than motor fibers. Inherited neuropathies often cause uniform demyelination of a nerve. Charcot-Marie Tooth disease is a good example of a uniformly demyelinating neuropathy.

Donofrio PD, Albers JW: AAEM minimonograph #34: Polyneuropathy: Classification by nerve conduction studies and electromyography. Muscle Nerve 13:889–903, 1990.

KEY POINTS: POLYNEUROPATHIES

1. Polyneuropathies can be classified based on the primary pathologic process as axon loss, demyelinating, or combined and based on the fibers involved as motor, sensory, or combined.

2. Axonal neuropathies affect the distal territories of the longest nerves and therefore affect the feet first.

3. Proximal nerve conduction is faster secondary to increased warmth, thicker myelination, and greater distance between the nodes of Ranvier.

MONONEUROPATHY: ENTRAPMENT

8. **How does carpal tunnel syndrome (CTS) present?**
   CTS is the most common focal nerve entrapment syndrome. The presentation includes specific symptoms of pain and paresthesias (tingling, burning, and numbness) in the median nerve distribution, often worst at night. In advanced cases, weakness of the median-innervated hand muscles is present. Minor, nonspecific symptoms include clumsiness, tightness, and complaints of dropping objects. Symptoms are often induced by overuse of the hand, especially forceful gripping or repetitive hand/wrist motion.

   Katz RT: Carpal tunnel syndrome: A practical review. Am Fam Physician 49:1371–1378, 1994.

9. **How is the diagnosis of CTS made?**
   Median nerve impingement at the wrist (CTS) can be identified using nerve conduction studies (NCSs), nerve ultrasound, magnetic resonance imaging (MRI), or open surgical exploration. Some clinicians make the diagnosis solely on clinical history and physical exam and recommend surgery after conservative measures have failed. However, many conditions can be confused with CTS. In studies in which patients were surgically treated for clinical CTS without NCS, a significant number did not improve and were eventually found to have other conditions.

   Jarvik JG, Kliot M, Maravilla KR: MR nerve imaging of the hand and wrist. Hand Clin 16:13–24, 2000.
   Keles I, Karagulle Kendi AT, Aydin G, et al: Diagnostic precision of ultrasonography in patients with carpal tunnel syndrome. Am J Phys Med Rehabil 84(6):443–450, 2005.

10. **List the differential diagnosis of CTS.**
    See Box 18-4.

11. **Explain the important components of the electrodiagnostic consultation in suspected CTS.**
    The electrodiagnostic consultation evaluates nerve and muscle function as an extension of the clinical neuromuscular examination. At the least, the consultative report should describe the patient's history, symptoms (weakness duration and distribution, exacerbating/relieving facts), physical findings (atrophy, reflexes, strength, sensation, evocative maneuvers), electrodiagnostic data, and an interpretation of findings.

12. **How is the Phalen wrist flexion test carried out?**
    The patient places his or her flexed elbows on a table and allows the wrists to fall freely into maximum flexion (no forced flexion by patient or examiner). This positioning should elicit numbness and tingling in a median distribution in 75% of patients with CTS symptoms after 2 minutes.

BOX 18-4. DIFFERENTIAL DIAGNOSIS OF CTS

Neurologic disorders

- Cervical radiculopathy (C6, C7, C8)
- Brachial plexus lesions, including thoracic outlet syndrome
- Ulnar, radial, or proximal median nerve lesions
- Syringomyelia
- Cervical cord lesions

Musculoskeletal disorders

- Tenosynovitis, including de Quervain's (inflammation of synovial tendon sheaths)
- Osteoarthritis of the metacarpal-trapezial joint (thumb carpometacarpal arthritis)
- Kienböck's disease (avascular lunate necrosis)
- Scaphoidal-trapezial arthritis
- Digital neuritis

Vascular disorders

- Raynaud's phenomenon
- Radial artery thrombosis

---

13. How is the Tinel's test performed at the wrist?

Percussion over the median nerve at the wrist with a reflex hammer produces a tingling sensation in the distribution of the regenerating injured median nerve fibers. False-positives range from 6% to 45%. Tinel's sign is not specific to the median nerve and can be elicited at other sites where nerves are superficial.

14. If median neuropathy of the wrist is suspected, what is the current standard electrodiagnostic approach?

1. Sensory NCS of the median nerve across the wrist, and if the latency is abnormal, comparison to another sensory study in the symptomatic limb.
2. If the initial median sensory NCS across the wrist has a conduction distance >8 cm and the results are normal, additional studies should be pursued: (a) median sensory NCS across the wrist over a short (7–8 cm) conduction distance or (b) comparison of median sensory NCS across the wrist to the radial or ulnar sensory conduction across the wrist in the same limb. The American Association of Neuromuscular and Electrodiagnostic Medicine (AANEM) practice parameter recommends motor NCS of the median nerve with comparison to one other motor nerve in the symptomatic limb. Electromyographic (EMG) study of the limb is considered optional.

American Association of Electrodiagnostic Medicine, American Academy of Neurology, and American Academy of Physical Medicine and Rehabilitation: Practice parameter for electrodiagnostic studies in carpal tunnel syndrome: Summary statement. Muscle Nerve 16:1390–1391, 1993.

15. What factors are associated with false-positive results in CTS?

Cold temperature, increasing age and height, and finger circumference.

16. Which technical problems can result in inaccurate results?

A cold hand will give inaccurate results (increased latencies, slowed conduction velocities, and increased amplitudes). Submaximal stimulus intensity may elicit an erroneously small amplitude response and a longer latency because the fastest fibers may not be depolarized. Sensory studies performed with less than a 4-cm electrode separation between active and reference electrodes may result in a smaller amplitude and shorter peak latency. For motor studies, the recording electrode must be centered over the motor point of the muscle.

17. **Describe anomalous innervation affecting interpretation of NCSs in CTS.**

The **Martin-Gruber anastomosis,** a median-to-ulnar connection in the forearm of motor fibers from the median or anterior interosseous nerve, occurs in 15% of individuals and affects both median and ulnar recordings. In an individual without median neuropathy at the wrist, this anomaly will result in a larger compound muscle action potential (CMAP) amplitude when stimulating the median nerve at the elbow than at the wrist. In a median neuropathy, the anastomosis causes an initial positive deflection when stimulating at the elbow, despite proper centering of the recording electrode over the belly of the thenar muscles. The same deflection is not noted on distal wrist stimulation.

18. **What does the needle EMG exam contribute to the diagnosis of CTS?**

Results of the needle exam show evidence of acute and chronic axon injury to the thenar muscles. It confirms axon loss in severe CTS and may help to determine chronicity. It is useful to assess separate or concomitant pathology, such as proximal median neuropathy, cervical or thoracic radiculopathy, plexopathy, or polyneuropathy.

Werner RA, Albers JW: Relation between needle electromyography and nerve conduction studies in patients with carpal tunnel syndrome. Arch Phys Med Rehabil 76:246–249, 1995.

19. **What other common sites of median nerve compression should be considered in the differential diagnosis of CTS?**
   - At the supracondylar **ligament of Struthers** (an anomalous ligament) or **lacertus fibrosus** (bicipital aponeurosis)
   - Between the two heads of the **pronator teres** or under the edge of the **flexor sublimis** (sublimis arch)
   - At the **anterior interosseous branch,** a pure motor branch of the median nerve in the forearm

20. **What are the nonoperative therapies for CTS?**

Nonoperative therapy includes hand splinting in a neutral wrist position, passive stretching of the transverse carpal ligament, range-of-motion (ROM) exercises, diuretics and nonsteroidal anti-inflammatory drugs (NSAIDs), ergonomic modifications, and steroid injections into the wrist. Modest doses of pyridoxine (vitamin B_6) have been advocated, although no well-designed study has demonstrated its efficacy.

Kaplan SJ, Gickel SZ, Eaton RG: Predictive factors in the non-surgical treatment of carpal tunnel syndrome. J Hand Surg 15:106–108, 1990.

21. **What are the ergonomic risk factors for CTS?**

High force, high repetition, vibration, awkward posture, and temperature extremes have been implicated as ergonomic risk factors for occupational hand and wrist disorders, including CTS. Obesity is also an independent risk factor.

22. **What surgical treatments can be performed for CTS?**

The most traditional technique for CTS release is an open decompression using a curved, longitudinal incision that provides good exposure of the transverse carpal ligament. Endoscopic techniques have recently been developed. A recent analysis of published series describes comparable rates of complications between open and closed techniques. Some case reports have described a heightened risk of complications from endoscopic release, such as transection of the median nerve. Conversely, endoscopic release is associated with higher levels of physical functioning and fewer days of convalescence compared to open release. Overall, the success rate for surgical treatment of CTS approaches 90%.

Boeckstyns ME, Sorensen AI: Does endoscopic have a higher rate of complication than open carpal tunnel release? An analysis of published series. J Hand Surg [Br] 24:9–15, 1999.

KEY POINTS: ENTRAPMENT NEUROPATHIES

1. Median nerve compression can be formed at the wrist, anterior interosseous branch, between the two heads of the pronator teres, and at the supracondylar ligament of Struthers (anomalous).

2. Entrapment neuropathies are more common at distal locations and are exacerbated by proximal entrapments.

23. **List the common sites of nerve entrapment in the upper and lower limbs.**
See Table 18-1.

TABLE 18-1. COMMON SITES OF NERVE ENTRAPMENT

Nerve	Site of Entrapment	Example
Median nerve	Wrist	Carpal tunnel syndrome
	Forearm	Anterior interosseous syndrome
Ulnar nerve	Elbow	Cubital tunnel syndrome
	Wrist	Guyon's canal syndrome
Peroneal nerve	Knee or fibular head	Cross leg syndrome
Lateral femoral cutaneous nerve of thigh	Medial to anterior superior iliac spine (ASIS)	Meralgia paresthetica
Tibial nerve	Under laciniate ligament	Tarsal tunnel syndrome

24. **What is Saturday night palsy? Honeymoon palsy?**
Saturday night palsy is one of the "sleep palsies" that results from compression of the radial nerve at the brachium as it pierces the lateral intermuscular septum in the upper part of the arm. Compression often occurs in patients who fall asleep with the arm resting against the firm edge of a chair or couch. Honeymoon palsy results from compression of the radial nerve more distally in the arm when the bed partner's head injures the nerve resting in the crook of the patient's arm.

25. **Describe the three distinct compressive ulnar neuropathies at the wrist.**
   - Compression of the superficial and deep branches within Guyon's canal
   - Compression of the ulnar nerve after it exits Guyon's canal
   - Compression of the superficial branch of the ulnar nerve in Guyon's canal

26. **What is "double-crush syndrome"?**
The double-crush nerve entrapment syndrome was described in 1973 by Upton and McComas. In this syndrome the sensory or motor fibers emanating from a particular root, if compressed

proximally, are more susceptible to compression distally. A good example is a patient with a C6 or C7 radiculopathy and entrapment of the median nerve at the wrist.

Upton ARM, McComas AJ: The double crush in nerve-entrapment syndromes. Lancet 2:359, 1973.

27. **What are the clinical and electrodiagnostic features of anterior interosseous nerve entrapment?**
Typically, the patient complains of vague aching pain in the forearm and weakness in the muscles supplied by the anterior interosseous nerve (i.e., flexor pollicis longus, flexor digitorum profundus [lateral head], and pronator quadratus). These muscles work together to make the "okay" sign with the hand. There is no sensory deficit. The anterior interosseous nerve is often entrapped in the forearm by a fibrous band.

28. **Describe the clinical features of meralgia paresthetica. How is it treated?**
Meralgia paresthetica results from compression of the lateral femoral cutaneous nerve of the thigh (a pure sensory nerve), as it passes beneath or through the inguinal ligament, medial to the anterior superior iliac spine (ASIS). This condition is often associated with pregnancy, obesity, and the use of tight belts, corsets, and underwear. The patient usually complains of paresthesias and pain over the anterolateral aspect of the thigh. There may be point tenderness, a positive Tinel's sign, or a positive compression test, medial to the ASIS. Treatment includes eliminating the causative factor, a temporary block with a local anesthetic and steroid, and surgical release of the nerve.

29. **What are the common sites of entrapment in the sciatic nerve?**
The sciatic nerve can be injured as a result of neoplasia, pelvic fractures, pelvic infection, penetrating injuries, surgical trauma, aneurysm, intramuscular injection, or entrapment by the piriformis muscle.

30. **Where does entrapment of the tibial nerve commonly occur?**
The tibial nerve is commonly entrapped under the foot flexor retinaculum or just posterior to the medial malleolus. This is popularly known as tarsal tunnel syndrome and can occur as a result of tenosynovitis, venous stasis, edema, trauma, pronated foot (pes planovalgus), arthritis of the subtalar joint, or a ganglia arising in the area of the medial aspect of the ankle. Lesions distal to the flexor retinaculum can compress the medial or lateral plantar branches of the tibial nerve. An uncommon entrapment is in the popliteal fossa by a Baker's cyst.

31. **Describe the clinical presentation of tarsal tunnel syndrome.**
   - Painful dysesthesias of the soles and toes, associated with a sensory deficit on the plantar aspect of the foot and toes and weakness in the intrinsic muscles of the feet
   - Pain occurs at rest, while the patient is sitting or in bed
   - Positive Tinel's sign (paresthesias in the nerve distribution) after percussion over the nerve at the entrapment site posterior to the medial malleolus

32. **What is Morton's neuroma?**
Entrapment of the interdigital nerve between the second and third or the third and fourth metatarsal heads. The symptoms include shooting pain and burning of the second, third, or fourth toes. Examination reveals tenderness of the sole and affected web spaces. Conservative treatment of Morton's neuroma includes positioning of a pad just proximal to the metatarsal heads and/or an injection of bupivacaine and corticosteroid.

33. **Outline the approach to prevention and treatment of entrapment neuropathies.**
See Box 18-5.

BOX 18-5.   PREVENTION AND TREATMENT OF ENTRAPMENT NEUROPATHIES

Prevention

- Avoid sustained pressure or tethering at the entrapment sites.

- Optimize control of diabetes. (Diabetics are more vulnerable to developing not only a polyneuropathy but also entrapment neuropathies.)

Treatment

Nonoperative

- Splint the limb in a neutral position; this maximizes space for the entrapped nerve.

- Modify activity and avoid positions that can be a source of nerve trauma.

- Consider the use of ice, NSAIDs, and corticosteroid injections in structures surrounding the nerves.

Operative

- Use surgical decompression.

CHAPTER 19

NEUROMUSCULAR JUNCTION DISORDERS: PHYSIOLOGY, CLINICAL PRESENTATION, AND ELECTRODIAGNOSIS

Michelle Stern, MD, Thomas McGunigal, MD, and Olajide Williams, MD

In theory, there is no difference between theory and practice. But, in practice, there is.
—Jan L.A. van de Snepscheut (1953–1994)

1. **What is the neuromuscular junction (NMJ)?**
   It is the specialized synapse between a motor nerve and a muscle fiber, consisting of a presynaptic nerve terminal, synaptic cleft, and postsynaptic end plate of the muscle fiber.

2. **What is the neurotransmitter of the NMJ? What three physiologic events occur?**
   Acetylcholine is the neurotransmitter at the NMJ. The three physiologic events that occur are (1) presynaptic storage, synthesis, and release; (2) synaptic transmission and degradation; and (3) postsynaptic coupling with receptors.

3. **Describe the presynaptic storage and release of acetylcholine.**
   Acetylcholine (Ach) storage occurs in three interrelated compartments. In the largest compartment, the main store, Ach is not immediately available for release across the synaptic cleft. It supplies a smaller compartment, the mobilization store, which in turn supplies the smallest compartment, where Ach is available for immediate release into the synapse. Here, Ach is packaged in vesicles approximately 300–500 A in diameter, each vesicle containing 5000–10,000 Ach molecules (a quantum). The main store contains approximately 300,000 quanta, the mobilization store holds 10,000 quanta, and the immediate-release store holds 1000 quanta. When an action potential reaches the presynaptic nerve terminal, it causes a voltage-sensitive influx of calcium ions, which signals the vesicles to release Ach into the synaptic cleft.

4. **Identify the common disorders of NM transmission.**
   The disorders can be classified into three categories: immune-mediated disorders, toxic/metabolic disorders, and congenital myasthenic syndrome (Table 19-1).

5. **How does NM transmission disease typically present in a patient?**
   There is progressive weakness and fatigue, especially with repetitive activities. Strength is often restored with rest.

6. **Which NM disorders are postsynaptic, and which are presynaptic?**
   The most common disorder is myasthenia gravis (MG), which is caused by a postsynaptic abnormality. Myasthenic syndrome, sometimes associated with bronchial carcinoma and botulism poisoning, is associated with a presynaptic abnormality of the NMJ.

7. **Describe the clinical presentation of myasthenia gravis.**
   Drooping of the eyelids and intermittent diplopia result from levator palpebrae (extraocular muscles) involvement, which is seen in 90% of MG cases. The muscles of facial expression,

TABLE 19-1. COMMON DISORDERS OF NM TRANSMISSION

Immune-Mediated Disorders	Toxic/Metabolic Disorders	Congenital Myasthenic Syndrome
LEMS Myasthenia gravis	Arthropod venom poisoning (e.g., black widow spider) Botulism Hypermagnesemia Medication side effects (e.g., aminoglycosides, procainamide, penicillamine) Organophosphate insecticide poisoning (e.g., malathion parathion) Snake venom poisoning Tick poisoning	Defective synthesis or packaging of (acetylchlorine) Ach Deficiency of acetylcholinesterase Deficiency of Ach receptors

LEMS = Lambert-Eaton myasthenic syndrome.

mastication, swallowing, and speech are involved in 80% of cases, leading to altered facial appearance and difficulty eating. Muscles of the neck, shoulder girdle, trunk, and hips may also be involved. Muscle weakness typically worsens as the day progresses.

8. **What are some genetic facts on MG?**
   MG occurs predominantly in people ages 20–40. Its incidence peaks in the third decade in females and in the fifth and sixth decades in males. MG occurs more commonly in females, with a female-to-male ratio of 1.5:1.

9. **Describe the clinical presentation of Lambert-Eaton myasthenic syndrome (LEMS).**
   The muscles of the trunk, shoulder girdle, and lower extremities are more likely to be initially affected. Unlike MG, LEMS patients may experience an increase in muscle power during the first few contractions.

10. **What causes LEMS?**
    The pathophysiology stems from a presynaptic abnormality of Ach release at the NMJ secondary to an autoimmune attack against the voltage-gated calcium channel on the presynaptic motor nerve terminal. Autonomic symptoms that are common in LEMS (especially involving salivation and erectile dysfunction) are absent in patients with MG.

11. **Describe the clinical presentation of botulism.**
    Symptoms of botulism usually appear within 12–36 hours of ingestion of tainted food. The typical neural symptoms of blurred vision and diplopia may be accompanied by anorexia, nausea, and vomiting. Unlike myasthenia gravis, pupils are often unreactive in botulism. Other bulbar symptoms, such as nasal or hoarse vocal quality, dysarthria, and dysphagia, follow rapidly and are soon joined by respiratory insufficiency and weakness of the neck, trunk, and limbs and respiratory insufficiency. This takes place over 2–4 days.

12. **What is the "safety factor"?**

After depolarization of the terminal axon in normal persons, there is an overabundance of Ach released, more than enough to bind receptors. This redundancy is called the "safety factor." In disease states such as MG, the NM transmission is much more tenuous. With fewer receptors available, a slight drop in acetylcholine concentration may block transmission.

13. **What is the Tensilon test?**

The Tensilon test is a diagnostic test for MG. The test consists of administering edrophonium (Tensilon) intravenously and observing for improvement in muscle strength. The most common protocol used is to give a test dose of up to 2 mg, followed by subsequent doses of 3–8 mg until there is a positive response or a total of 10 mg is given. The patient is observed for 60 seconds between doses and for 3–5 minutes after the full 10-mg dose has been administered. Improvement of strength is seen as a positive end point. Edrophonium has a rapid onset (30 seconds) and short duration of effect (5–10 minutes). Side effects from edrophonium include increased salivation and sweating, nausea, stomach cramping, and muscle fasciculations. Hypotension and bradycardia are uncommon side effects, but atropine should be available if bradycardia is severe.

14. **What is repetitive nerve stimulation (RNS)?**

RNS occurs when a motor nerve is stimulated repetitively while recording compound muscle action potentials (CMAPs) from an appropriate muscle. RNS serves to "stress" diseased NMJs by depleting the store of readily releasable acetylcholine, which causes failure of neuromuscular transmission in a portion of motor end plates, resulting in fewer muscle fibers contributing to the CMAP. Trains of supramaximal stimuli are delivered to a peripheral nerve at rates of 2–5 Hz. The decremental response is defined as the percentage of change between the amplitude or area of the fourth, fifth, or lowest potential compared with the first potential of each train. A decrement >10% is usually considered abnormal. Some laboratories require a decrement of ≥20% in proximal muscles in order to be considered abnormal, because of baseline variability.

15. **What rate is best for stimulating a motor nerve repetitively?**

The most useful information is usually obtained with a relatively low stimulation frequency (<2–3 Hz). Stimulation at faster frequencies (>5 Hz) may not detect faulty transmission because faulty transmitter release will be enhanced because of residual calcium in the presynaptic terminal. Frequencies slower than this mask a transmission disorder because very low frequencies permit mobilization of Ach into the immediately available store with enhancement of transmission.

16. **How can you increase the diagnostic yield in RNS?**

Activating the muscle by performing a maximum isometric exercise of the tested muscle for a prescribed period or by rapid-rate nerve stimulation (20–50 Hz) can increase the sensitivity of the test. The physiologic effect of such activation results from accumulation of calcium in the nerve terminal, which enhances the release of Ach.

17. **How can this strategy be used to distinguish a presynaptic from a postsynaptic disorder?**

If the initial CMAP is small, as in a presynaptic disorder, activation can produce a marked increase in the CMAP amplitude. This phenomenon is termed *postactivation facilitation*. More sustained activation, with maximum exercise for 30–60 seconds or longer, depletes the readily releasable stores of acetylcholine, which overrides the effects of calcium accumulation in the nerve terminal and also depresses end plate excitability. This effect is most marked 2–4 minutes after activation and is referred to as postactivation exhaustion. The electrodiagnostic manifestation of this phenomenon is an exaggeration of the decremental response compared with the pre-exercise values.

18. **Are abnormal RNS studies diagnostic for primary disorders of the NMJ?**
Abnormal RNS studies are not diagnostic of specific disorders but relay information about the integrity of the entire neuromuscular junction. These abnormalities may be found in several diseases, which include motor neuron disease, neuropathy, primary muscle membrane diseases, MG, congenital myasthenia, drug-induced and other acquired myasthenic syndromes, and radiculopathy.

19. **What is the most sensitive test for MG?**
Single-fiber electromyography (SFEMG) is more sensitive than RNS. Only 40% of MG patients will show decremental responses on repetitive nerve stimulation on distal muscles and 90% on proximal muscles.

20. **What is single-fiber EMG?**
SFEMG uses a specialized needle electrode that allows recording of two single fibers within a motor unit. SFEMG shows increased jitter and blocking (failure of the action potential to be propagated to one of the two fibers) in diseases of NM transmission (although it is not specific for NMJ disorders).

21. **What is jitter?**
During sustained activation of the motor nerve, the latency from nerve activation to muscle action potential varies from discharge to discharge. This variation is the neuromuscular jitter and is produced by fluctuations in the time it takes for the end plate potential at the NMJ to reach the threshold for muscle action potential generation. These fluctuations are in turn a result of the normally varying amount of Ach released from the nerve terminal after a nerve impulse. A small amount of jitter is seen in normal muscles because of this phenomenon. An increase in the jitter is the most sensitive electrophysiologic evidence of a defect in neuromuscular transmission. When the defect is more severe, some nerve impulses fail to elicit action potentials, and SFEMG recordings demonstrate an intermittent absence of one or more single muscle-fiber action potentials on consecutive firings. This is called impulse blocking and represents neuromuscular transmission failure at the involved end plate.

22. **What are the nerve conduction study (NCS) finding in patients with NMJ transmission defects?**
See Table 19-2.

23. **How do LEMS and MG differ electrophysiologically?**
Myasthenia gravis defect occurs when antibodies bind to the postsynaptic Ach receptor, resulting in destruction and reduction of surface area of the postsynaptic membrane and fewer Ach receptors. Electrophysiologically, the CMAP amplitudes are usually normal. With 2–5 Hz of repetitive stimulation, there is >10% decrement in CMAP amplitude. Decrement is typically greatest between the first and second responses, with the maximum occurring between the first and fourth to fifth responses. With continued stimulation, response amplitudes generally return to normal. A 10-sec maximum isometric contraction will usually result in an increased response amplitude, but not >50% above baseline.

LEMS occurs more often in men than women, usually presenting in the fifth decade. There is a high coexistence of malignancy, most commonly oat-cell carcinoma of the lung. LEMS appears to be caused by antibodies directed at the voltage-gated calcium channels of the motor nerve terminal, which interfere with release of Ach. Electrophysiologically, the initial CMAP is usually low in amplitude. With 2–5 Hz of stimulation, there may be a decremental response. With >10 Hz stimulation or a 10-second maximum isometric contraction (which approximates a 50-Hz

TABLE 19-2. NERVE CONDUCTION STUDY FINDINGS IN NMJ TRANSMISSION DEFECTS

NMJ Defect	Stimulation Frequency	Finding in NCS	With Exercise	Findings of NCS
Postsynaptic	2–5 Hz	>10% decrement Normal CMAP amplitude	10 sec	Repair of decrement postexercise
			30–60 sec	Postactivation exhaustion 2–4 min
Presynaptic	2–5 Hz	>10% decrement, low CMAP amplitude	10 sec	Postactivation facilitation postexercise
	20–50 HZ	>100% increase CMAP amplitude		

CMAP = compound muscle action potential, NCS = nerve conduction study, NMJ = neuromuscular junction.

stimulation), there is an increase in the CMAP amplitude that is usually much greater than 50%, often 200–400% above the single-stimulation CMAP.

24. **How is the course of events at the NMJ related to findings on repetitive stimulation?**
Motor axonal discharge frequency affects NM transmission by modulating Ach availability and calcium concentrations at the synaptic cleft. Depolarization of the nerve terminus causes the immediate release store to dump quanta of Ach into the synaptic cleft. Five to 10 sec are required for the mobilization store to replenish the lost Ach. Therefore, volleys arriving faster than every 5 sec progressively deplete the immediate-release store. On the other hand, the calcium that is released with each depolarization requires 100–200 msec to diffuse away from the nerve terminal. Therefore, stimulation that arrives at rates greater than 5–10/sec (5–10 Hz) causes calcium to accumulate.

Thus, in myasthenia gravis, repetitive stimulation at rates between 3 and 5 Hz shows a decremental response as smaller amounts of Ach are released into the NM junction, preventing some fibers from reaching critical threshold. In LEMS, the CMAP may show a decremental response similar to MG at low stimulation frequencies. At frequencies of 20–50 Hz, however, facilitation is observed. Successive CMAPs show increasing amplitude, often exceeding single-stimulation CMAPs by 200% of baseline, because rapid rates of stimulation result in accumulation of calcium at the presynaptic cleft of the NM junction, progressively allowing the release of more Ach.

25. **What is pseudofacilitation?**
Stimulation rates >10 Hz may produce a phenomenon known as pseudofacilitation: an increase in the amplitude of the M-wave accompanied by a decrease in the duration, without any change in the total area under the curve. It results from synchronization of the action potentials in muscle fibers, not an increase in the number of muscle fibers activated. It can produce an increase in M-wave amplitude of 50%, which should not be mistaken for abnormal pathologic facilitation.

KEY POINTS: NEUROMUSCULAR JUNCTION DISORDERS

1. Myasthenia gravis is postsynaptic because of antibodies against the Ach receptors and its associated functional proteins.

2. LEMS is caused by presynaptic abnormality at the NMJ and is associated with bronchial carcinoma.

3. Botulism is also associated with a presynaptic NMJ disorder.

4. SFEMG is the most sensitive test for assessing the NMJ.

5. Postsynaptic disorders show normal CMAP amplitude but have a progressive decrement on slow frequency RNS, which is exacerbated during postexercise exhaustion.

6. Presynaptic disorders show small CMAP amplitude with improvement using high-frequency stimulation and exercise.

26. Are MG and LEMS caused by antibodies?
Yes. In MG, antibodies to the Ach receptor attack and destroy the postsynaptic membrane. In LEMS, autoantibodies against the calcium channels attack the Ach-release sites at the active zone on the presynaptic membrane, resulting in failure of Ach release.

27. How does repetitive nerve stimulation compare with other laboratory tests for MG?
Fluctuating muscle weakness that is made worse by repeated use and relieved at least partially by rest is the clinical hallmark of MG. Under these conditions the diagnosis of MG is easy to make, although in certain patients with mild or restricted symptoms, such as in ocular MG, the diagnosis may be more elusive. Unfortunately, the sensitivity of RNS in MG is moderate, with false-negative results occurring not infrequently.

Abnormal decrement in a distal or proximal muscle occurs in approximately 75% of patients with generalized MG and in less than 50% of patients with ocular MG. Various methods to decrease the number of these RNS false negatives have been described, but because they are based on increased blocking rather than increased jitter, none has been able to rival the sensitivity of SFEMG. SFEMG is the most sensitive test for assessing the NMJ and is abnormal in more than 90% of patients with MG. Ach-receptor antibodies are found in 70–90% of patients with acquired MG. The advantage of these antibodies is that they confirm a diagnosis of MG, whereas SFEMG, though more sensitive, is a nonspecific test for general neuromuscular dysfunction.

28. What is neonatal MG?
Fifteen percent of infants born to myasthenic mothers have neonatal MG. It is caused by the transplacental passage of Ach-receptor antibodies. This condition resolves completely in weeks to months.

29. Describe some rehabilitation issues for patients with MG.
Weakness in MG will increase with fatigue and heat. Energy conservation techniques will be useful in this patient population, with afternoon rest periods recommended. Strength training has not been extensively studied; therefore, maximal stress exercise cannot be recommended for these patients. One small study showed that moderate-intensity isometric strengthening in the lower limbs might be allowed in patients with mild disease.

30. **Which NM disorder presents with a true reduction in reflexes?**
LEMS presents with reduced reflexes. MG, botulism, and congenital myasthenia present with normal reflexes, although they may be reduced in proportion to the degree of muscular weakness.

WEBSITES

1. Myasthenia Gravis Foundation of America
www.myasthenia.org

2. Myasthenia Gravis and Neuromuscular Junction Disorders
www.neuro.wustl.edu/neuromuscular/synmg.html

BIBLIOGRAPHY

1. Campbell W: Essentials of Electrodiagnostic Medicine. Baltimore, Williams & Wilkins, 1999.
2. Dumitru D: Electrodiagnostic Medicine. Philadelphia, Hanley & Belfus, 1995.
3. Grabois M: Physical Medicine and Rehabilitation: The Complete Approach. Boston, Blackwell Science, 2000.
4. Keesey JC: Clinical evaluation and management of myasthenia gravis. Muscle Nerve 29(4):484–505, 2004.
5. Kimura J: Electrodiagnosis in Disease of the Nerve and Muscle: Principles and Practice, 2nd ed. Philadelphia, F.A. Davis, 1989.
6. Meriggioli MN, Sanders DB: Advances in the diagnosis of neuromuscular junction disorders. Am J Phys Med Rehabil 84(8):627–638, 2005.
7. Preston D, Shapiro B: Electromyography and NM Disorders. Boston, Butterworth-Heinemann, 1998.

IMPAIRMENT AND DISABILITY RATING: ESTIMATION OF WORK CAPACITY

Richard T. Katz, MD, and Robert D. Rondinelli, MD, PhD

CHAPTER 20

Disability is a matter of perception.
If you can do just one thing well, you're needed by someone.

–Martina Navratilova (1956–)

1. **What are the differences among impairment, disablement, and being disabled for an occupation?**
   - **Disablement** is the summation of impairment, disability, and handicap as defined by the World Health Organization (1980).
   - **Impairment** is an abnormality of structure, appearance, and/or function at the end-organ level. For example, a herniated disc or ligament inflammation or a weak muscle with a trigger point is an impairment.
   - **Disability** is the inability of a person to perform an activity. For example, inability to carry a bag of groceries or walk upstairs is a disability.
   - **Handicap** is an environmentally defined abnormality reflecting societal bias experienced by the individual trying to fulfill a role.

2. **What constitutes disability in the workplace?**
   Disability as understood in relation to employment means inability to carry out the activities of an occupation. When the worker can no longer throw 400 sacks weighing 100 pounds each day, the patient is *disabled* for performing that particular job. When a nurse can no longer bend over and stoop on a frequent basis—which most job analyses require for a ward nurse—he or she can no longer work *full duty* and must be placed temporarily or permanently on *light duty*.

3. **How is disability officially defined?**
   In 2001 the World Health Organization revised terminology for impairment, handicap, and disability and promoted a new model. The new model describes body "functions and structures." Impairment is the loss of organs or deviations in organ function. Disability is renamed as activity limitation, and barriers to life opportunities are termed *barriers to participation*. The new model provides a theoretical framework for the impact of an injury on a person. Current definitions of disability vary between various institutions that provide compensation.

   Unfortunately, there is confusion because government and insurance companies have their own definitions for disability. Insurance companies typically use *disabled* to imply that the person can no longer perform the *substantial and material duties of an occupation*. To be disabled in the context of the Social Security Administration means that a person must be disabled for "all substantial gainful activity" in order to receive benefits.

4. **How are levels of disability determined?**
   When a patient with low back pain (LBP) has an acute musculoskeletal back injury, we may place the patient on *temporary disability,* but it is unlikely there will be any *permanent*

disability. When treatment for LBP has continued without improvement for more than 12 months, many would consider that the patient's *temporary disability* has become a *permanent disability*. A disability rating is then required by many Workers' Compensation jurisdictions and will determine whether the patient's disability is *total* (100% of the whole person), or some fraction thereof *(partial disability)*.

The terms *impairment* and *disability* are used somewhat interchangeably and incorrectly. For example, physicians may be asked in certain jurisdictions to use the *American Medical Association Guides to the Evaluation of Permanent Impairment* to provide a disability rating, although the title and introduction to the book clearly state it was intended to rate *impairment* and not disability. The reason is simple—different jurisdictions rate and provide compensation for physical impairments differently. There is no way the *Guides* can satisfy the rules of disability ratings in all of these different settings.

5. **How prevalent is occupational disability in Western countries?**
The prevalence of disability varies widely in different Western countries. For example, the United States, Canada, and Great Britain have a prevalence of approximately 2–3%; West Germany and the Netherlands, 4%. In Sweden the prevalence has climbed to an astonishing 8% of the population. In Great Britain, the disability rates for chronic LBP are increasing exponentially. About one in six Americans (48 million) receives a Social Security benefit today.

   www.ssa.gov/pressoffice/factsheets/young.htm

6. **What are the costs of occupational disability?**
Costs include medical expenditures, lost wages and production, consumer cost increases, employee retraining, and litigation. In 2002, the costs of Workers' Compensation claims varied from approximately $3000 in Indiana, to almost $12,000 in Louisiana.

   www.ppinys.org/reports/jtf2004/workerscomp.htm
   www.ssa.gov/policy/docs/statcomps/di_asr/2001/exp_toc.html

7. **What is Workers' Compensation?**
The critical language of Workers' Compensation statutes is that employees must suffer "accidental ... personal injury ... out of and in the scope of employment." Using LBP as an example, this language is troublesome for the clinician. LBP is an essentially ubiquitous condition, and yet statutes indicate that LBP must arise clearly through the course of employment. A key concept in the Workers' Compensation statues is that of no-fault or tort immunity. In exchange for the employer caring for the injured worker, the worker offers the employer tort immunity from legal suit in response to being injured. Workers' Compensation usually offers the worker between 50% and 70% of preinjury wages as an incentive to return to work.

Compensation varies greatly among states. Some states provide scheduled awards based on the physician-determined disability rating or the permanent partial loss of function of the body part or person as a whole. Others compensate in a nonscheduled fashion, as a function of the loss of the ability to be gainfully employed in a part of the workplace.

8. **How does the Social Security Administration define disability?**
Social Security is the second major system for providing a social safety net for persons with disability. For a worker to become eligible for Social Security disability benefits, the patient must have a disability defined as "the inability to engage in any substantial gainful activity by reason of any medically determinable physical or mental impairment(s) which can be expected to result in death or which has lasted or can be expected to last for a continuous period of not less than 12 months."

9. **What other groups of American workers have coverage for disability?**
Although most physicians are aware of the Workers' Compensation statutes and Social Security disability programs, they may not be aware that there are special programs for other specific populations. Various workers may be protected under the Federal Employees' Compensation Act, Longshore and Harbor Workers' Compensation Act, Veterans Administration, and Federal Employers' Liability Act.

10. **How does the physician determine if and when a patient is ready to return to work?**
The physician can decide based on clinical judgment, or he or she may rely on a **functional capacity evaluation** (FCE). An FCE is simply a quantified physical ability test in which various parameters are measured over time—how long and how much a given patient can perform in a given day in regard to strength, flexibility, endurance, lifting, carrying, pushing, pulling, bending, crawling, sitting, standing, walking, and ascending steps/ladders. These parameters are quantified in terms of weight and frequency. Terms used to modify frequency include *occasional,* which generally refers to ≤33% of the time; *frequent,* which is 34–66% of the day; and *constant or frequent,* which is 67% or more of the day. Although there is an intuitive attractiveness to FCE, there is debate over whether these tests are reproducible and the degree to which they are limited by patient motivation. An FCE in a highly cooperative patient may be of value. In a patient with poor motivation, it is expensive and often invalid. Utilizing FCEs, the physician may designate permanent restrictions for an employee and may indicate they can return to work within certain strength requirements from sedentary work through very heavy work. These classifications are discussed in detail at www.occupationalinfo.org/appendxc_1.html.

11. **How does the Americans with Disabilities Act define disability?**
The Americans with Disabilities Act (ADA) defines disability as a "physical or mental impairment that substantially limits one or more of the major life activities of the individual, or a record of such an impairment, or being regarded as having such an impairment." The ADA is intended to protect persons who can perform the *essential functions* of a job with *reasonable accommodation*. The employer may not inquire about a potential employee's impairment or medical history when the potential employee applies for a job. Upon offering the potential employee a job, a medical examination may be performed. The position may be withdrawn if the medical officer, based on receiving more information about the worker's abilities, impairments, or past medical history, feels that the particular position offered would be a *direct threat* to the health of the worker or those around him or her. If the worker cannot perform every single aspect of a job, the employer is obligated to make a *reasonable accommodation* by modifying the job description, providing adaptive equipment or physical assistance.

12. **If an employee is injured on the job, how are coverage and disability determined?**
If the patient is injured in a Workers' Compensation setting, the first thing to do is find out the laws of the state. These can be obtained on a search of the state's website, by contacting a human resources department, or by speaking to an attorney who handles Workers' Compensation claims. There are certain periods in which the worker must notify the employer of the injury (waiting period), and a certain period after which compensation begins (waiting period). State law varies as to whether the employer or employee selects the clinician who delivers care to be covered under the Workers' Compensation program. Certain states, such as Florida, Minnesota, and California, have their own schedules for rating disability, and the physician should consult those statues before proceeding. Veterans are rated according to their own schedule, which can be found at:

www.vetshome.com/schedule%20for%20rating%20disabilities.html

13. **Is there a standard method for evaluation and documentation of physical disability?**

In many jurisdictions, the physician will be asked to provide a disability rating, and the best available document to do so (and one that will often be mandated by that state's Workers' Compensation statute) is the *AMA Guides to the Evaluation of Permanent Impairment.*

14. **What are the *AMA Guides?***

The *Guides* began to take form in the 1950s and have evolved into a widely recognized impairment-rating document, used in 40 of 53 jurisdictions, according to a 1991 AMA survey. The proportion is approximately the same today. The fifth edition was published in 2001, and the sixth edition is well underway.

The *AMA Guides* is not a scientific document based on demographic or epidemiologic data. It was developed with a "delphi" panel to produce a consensus among informed experts. Although some complain of its inadequacies, it can be argued that no superior document is available. The *Guides* rates *impairments* (not disabilities, not schedule for compensation, not employability) for each organ system in the body.

15. **According to the *Guides,* what constitutes permanent disability?**

A suitable period must elapse before an impairment is considered to be permanent, generally 12 months, according to the present *Guides*. Raters need to determine within their jurisdiction how long a patient needs to remain at his or her "therapeutic plateau" before being considered at *maximal medical improvement*, also called *permanent and stationary.*

16. **What are long-term disability insurance and Social Security?**

It is estimated that 40 million Americans are protected by long-term disability, largely through their workplace. An important feature of long-term disability policies is whether there is *"own occupation* versus *any occupation* coverage."

- **Own occupation coverage** provides the insured with disability benefits (typically in the range of 60% of normal salary reimbursement to provide incentive to return to work) if they are not able to provide the essential elements of their particular job.
- **Any occupation coverage** means, within limits, the employee would be reimbursed only if he or she could no longer perform meaningful work in any related occupation.

Less expensive *group* long-term disability plans tend to have own occupation coverage for approximately 2 years; then the worker must be disabled from any occupation to receive further benefits. More expensive *individual* long-term disability plans tend to have more restrictive own occupation provisions.

Social Security is the second major system for providing a social safety net for persons with a disability. In order for a worker to become eligible for social security disability benefits, the patient's disability must be defined as "the inability to engage in substantial gainful activity by reason of any medically determinable physical or mental inpairment(s) that can be expected to result in death or that has lasted or can be expected to last for a continuous period of not less than 12 months."

www.ssa.gov/pressoffice/basicfact.htm

17. **What are the challenges of maintaining objectivity that the independent medical examiner faces?**

The independent medical examiner must be objective, and the challenge is significant. If the person to be evaluated is a patient, the physician must honestly offer a disability rating in an objective fashion without being biased in the patient's interest. If a physician sees a patient at the behest of a Workers' Compensation carrier, insurer, or attorney who regularly refers business to the practice, the examiner must be mindful of this potential bias.

18. **When a physician is performing an independent medical exam (IME), who assumes patient care?**

When performing an IME, the physician does not assume care of the patient. Make it clear that the evaluation is for IME purposes and that there is to be no ongoing physician–patient relationship. Have the patient sign a disclosure indicating that he or she understands that the evaluation is only for the purpose of an IME and you will not be assuming care.

KEY POINTS: IMPAIRMENT AND DISABILITY RATING

1. The occupational definition of disability varies among institutions.

2. The Social Security Administration defines disability as "inability to engage in any substantial gainful activity by reason of any medically determinable physical or mental impairment(s)."

3. The operational definition of disability in the workplace is *inability to carry out the activities of the occupation*.

4. Definitions of *disabled* by insurance companies typically imply that a person can no longer perform the substantial and material duties of an occupation.

19. **What is the legal definition of medical probability?**

The IME physician is asked to comment on causality. For example, "within a reasonable degree of medical certainty, doctor, can you state that A caused B?" The real question that the attorney is asking is "whether it *is more likely than not (greater than 50% probability)* that A caused B." If the answer is yes, you are satisfying the legal requirement that it is "probably true." This is the level of certainty that the attorney is requesting. It is not the standard of "beyond a reasonable doubt" that holds in criminal cases. If the answer is that A *possibly* caused B, the real meaning of the statement is that it is less than likely (<50% probability) that A caused B. This statement suggests evidence *against* causality.

20. **How are benefits apportioned?**

While impairment rating certainly presents an ethical dilemma, the concept of apportionment is additionally precarious. IME physicians may be asked, "Doctor, you felt the patient's back condition is worthy of a 20% whole person impairment. But the patient had back injuries in 1986, 1992, 1994, and 1996! How much of that 20% do you apportion to each injury?" It is safe to say that there is no scientific way to answer this question.

MEDICOLEGAL INTERFACE

21. **What are the two basic types of depositions?**

Finally, IME physicians may be asked, in their role as expert evaluators, to participate in depositions and trial appearances. Depositions come in two varieties—discovery and evidentiary.

- **Discovery depositions** offer the plaintiff and defense attorneys a chance to hear what the other's experts have to say and hopefully to lay out the weight of truth for each side. The rules of evidence do not apply in discovery deposition, and the physician's testimony can be introduced into the courtroom only if it conflicts with testimony that the physician offers at the time of trial.

- In distinction, **evidentiary depositions** represent legal testimony according to the formal rules of evidence and may be videotaped in lieu of the physician appearing at trial. The physician's testimony may be read verbatim at the trial (or the videotape played) as part of the trial record.

BIBLIOGRAPHY

1. American Medical Association: Guides to the Evaluation of Permanent Impairment, 5th ed. Chicago, American Medical Association, 2001.
2. Demeter SL, Andersson GBJ (eds): Disability Evaluation. St. Louis, Mosby, 2003.
3. Rondinelli R, Katz RT (eds): Impairment Rating and Disability Evaluation. Philadelphia, W.B. Saunders, 1999.
4. Social Security Administration Office of Disability Programs: Disability Evaluation Under Social Security. SSA Publication Number 64–039, ICN 468600, January, 2005.

VOCATIONAL REHABILITATION COUNSELING: ASSESSMENT, CASE MANAGEMENT, ACCOMMODATION, AND PLACEMENT

Ruth Torkelson Lynch, PhD, Rochelle V. Habeck, PhD, Steven A. Stiens, MD, MS, Mark A. Young, MD, MBA, and Rhodora C. Tumanon, MD

To find out what one is fitted to do, and to secure an opportunity to do it, is the key to happiness.

– John Dewey (1859–1952)

1. **What is the role of work and career in the lives of people with disabilities?**
   Work is a central force in defining one's life. It provides self-identity, daily structure, economic support, and social networks. When disability interferes with one's vocational role, then social status, identity, and a source of life satisfaction are also disrupted.

2. **What is vocational rehabilitation (VR)?**
   VR is a coordinated and systematic process of professional services that enables people with disabilities to obtain, retain, and sustain employment, economic self-sufficiency, self-dignity, and independence. The most efficient way to have vocational success with patients is to recognize current or potential problems with employment and refer early.

3. **Who might benefit from VR services?**
   VR can help people with disabilities to keep or maintain current employment through changes in work schedules, accommodations, and accessible/assistive technology. Those who have lost employment or who need to change careers may also benefit from transferable skills analysis, career development, or retraining. Persons who have not been employed or who have not developed career skills because of childhood disability or extended chronic illness are also recipients of VR services (e.g., career exploration through job shadowing, work skill development).

4. **How do people with disabilities access VR services?**
   VR services can be most effective if they start during inpatient rehabilitation with an onsite VR counselor (if available) and continue with a referral to a VR counselor in the patient's local community (e.g., to the local Division of Vocational Rehabilitation [DVR], a state/federal program). There are DVR offices in every state, funded by the Rehabilitation Services Administration (RSA) in partnership with state governments. To be eligible for VR services from the state DVR agency, a person must have a physical or mental impairment that is a substantial impediment to employment; be able to benefit from VR services in terms of employment; and require VR services to prepare for, enter, engage in, or retain employment. More information about RSA is available at http://www.ed.gov/about/offices/list/osers/rsa/index.html. Patients can identify offices in their local areas by searching by state at www.jan.wvu.edu/SBSES/VOCREHAB.HTM.

   Individuals may also be able to access other VR counseling services (depending on eligibility requirements) through a Workers' Compensation or personal injury insurance carrier, through transition-to-work programs in high schools, through disabled student services centers at postsecondary institutions, or through other community rehabilitation agencies (e.g., county social services, veterans' agencies, community mental health centers).

5. **Who pays for VR services?**

A DVR or a Department of Rehabilitation Services office (states use slightly different names for their RSA-funded program) serves each county within its state. These offices fund services for eligible persons through a partnership of state and federal (RSA) funds. Other VR services are sometimes provided through funding from Workers' Compensation; Social Security Disability; private health, motor vehicle, or disability insurance; county or local social services; legal settlements; or nonprofit agencies serving persons with disabilities through donations and grant funding (e.g., Easter Seals, Goodwill Industries). VR services may also be provided by large employers (e.g., disability management, employee assistance programs) or by schools, colleges, and universities (e.g., high school work transition services, university offices for students with disabilities).

6. **Who provides VR services?**

Comprehensive vocational rehabilitation to achieve work and independent living goals is a team effort that involves health care, psychosocial, educational, occupational, technological, and engineering service providers. The professionals with the most active involvement in VR services are rehabilitation counselors. Additional VR services may be provided by vocational evaluators, work adjustment specialists, job developers and job-placement specialists, job coaches, disability management case managers, low-vision specialists, rehabilitation teachers for vision impairment, and sign-language interpreters.

7. **What are the qualifications of VR professionals?**

Most of the psychosocial, occupational, and job development providers are certified rehabilitation counselors (a national credential) and/or licensed professional counselors (a state level credential). Both of these credentials require a master's degree with relevant supervised experience.

8. **What do rehabilitation counselors do?**

Rehabilitation counselors help determine rehabilitation needs, identify resources and programs, and provide counseling and skill development for independent living and vocational functioning. Specifically, they:

- Collect educational, vocational, medical, and psychological information to better understand the person's current situation, and their interests and capabilities.
- Provide and coordinate appropriate analyses (e.g., physical demands, reasonable accommodations) so the person can make an informed choice about his or her career options.
- Help design a plan for independent living and career pursuits.
- Identify skills, knowledge, and further training necessary to pursue a career consistent with the person's interests and abilities.
- Develop an individualized plan for achieving employment that lists the steps needed to reach the person's job goal.
- Provide labor market information and other resources to obtain job leads.
- Follow the person's progress at work to help in maintaining the job.

9. **What is involved in case management with a VR focus?**

VR counselors function as case managers who facilitate reintegration into work, school, recreation, and independent living. They interact with third-party payers, employers, schools, community agencies, and local health care providers to get patients involved with work and/or school as soon as possible, to minimize costs, and to obtain the resources and benefits that will facilitate outpatient rehabilitation success.

Chan F, Leahy M, Saunders JL (eds): Case Management for Rehabilitation Health Professionals, 2nd ed. Osage Beach, MO, Aspen Professional Services, 2005.

10. **How do environmental influences impact VR planning and service delivery?**
    An individual's characteristics and functional capacities are certainly not the only determinants of independent living and employment outcomes. Discriminatory policies and practices, as well as environmental barriers (e.g., poor access to transportation, limited entrance into or movement within buildings, lack of modified tools and equipment), are also major handicapping factors. VR services must address modifications in both the physical and interpersonal aspects of the worksite:
    Physical structures (e.g., equipment or architecture)
    - Modify the physical environment of the workplace.
    - Restructure job duties or processes so that essential functions can be performed.
    - Provide augmentative or assistive technology equipment, qualified readers, or interpreters.
    - Coordinate accessible transportation.
    Interpersonal elements (e.g., coworkers and supervisors)
    - Teach direct supervisors how to facilitate accommodation needs with production and performance requirements.
    - Solicit supportive coworkers (natural supports) to provide accommodations or assistance.
    - Develop endorsement by management of the accommodation plan.
    Interventions will be most effective when the client, VR counselor, and individuals from the targeted environment are in close collaboration.

11. **What are alternatives for persons who have work tolerance restrictions?**
    - Work-hardening programs (e.g., conditioning programs that focus on work-specific physical activities such as sitting, standing, lifting tolerances).
    - Modified return-to-work plans (e.g., reduced work hours, gradually increasing work tasks and hours).

12. **What are alternatives for persons when work capacities are very limited?**
    - Supported employment (e.g., provide a job coach in a competitive work environment, place and train the individual directly in the workplace, build work supports and accommodations with the employer and coworkers, and gradually modify the job coach intensity).
    - Day programs (e.g., day centers with flexible hours).
    - Home-based employment.
    - Sheltered work or enclave work (e.g., a group of workers with disabilities with their own supervisor in competitive settings).

13. **What is involved in a "determination of severity" of disability for VR services? What does "order of selection" according to disability refer to?**
    Determination of severity is terminology used by the state/federal DVR system to clarify the level of physical and mental limitations and functional capacities that may influence employment outcomes (e.g., mobility, communication, self-care, self-direction, interpersonal skills, work tolerance, work behavior skills). **Order of selection** refers to the system that state/federal agencies use to prioritize individuals eligible for service. When funding is limited, waitlists may be created, with individuals with the most severe disabilities being served first based on the order of selection system.

14. **Define these work disability terms: SSDI, SSI, SGA, PASS, trial work period, ticket to work, BPAO, IPE, and informed choice.**
    - **SSDI (Social Security Disability Insurance)** provides benefits to individuals who are "insured" by workers' contributions to the Social Security trust fund through prior social security tax paid on their earnings or those of their spouses or parents.

- **SSI (Supplemental Security Income)** makes cash assistance payments to elderly, blind, and disabled people (including children under age 18) who have limited income and resources. The federal government funds SSI from general tax revenues.

- **SGA (Substantial Gainful Activity)** refers to the earnings guidelines used by the Social Security Administration (SSA) to evaluate the extent of one's work activity for SSI or SSDI. To be eligible for disability benefits, a person must be unable to engage in SGA. A person who is earning more than a certain monthly amount (for nonblind individuals in 2007, the monthly SGA amount was $900 net after impairment-related work expenses) is ordinarily considered to be engaging in SGA and is not eligible for SSI or SSDI benefits.

- **PASS:** Under the **Plan for Achieving Self-Support**, recipients of SSI disability benefits may set aside income and/or resources over a reasonable time to enable them to reach a work goal and become financially self-supporting (e.g., use income set aside for occupational training, purchase of occupational equipment, establish a business). The set-aside income and resources in the PASS plan are not counted when determining SSI eligibility or payment amounts.

- **Trial work period:** During a trial work period, a beneficiary receiving Social Security Disability benefits may test his or her ability to work and still be considered "disabled" and receive benefits. Work activities during the trial work period are not considered as documentation that the disability has ended until substantial work activities have been performed in at least 9 months (not necessarily consecutive) in a rolling 60-month period. In 2007, any month in which earnings exceeded $640 was considered one month of work activity against the individual's 9 months of trial work. During the trial work period, there are no limits in earnings in order to retain benefits.

- **Ticket to Work program:** The intent of this program is to create a competitive market for VR services and provide choice to consumers of VR services through the provision of a "ticket" for VR services, which they may deposit with any qualified employment network (EN). Another portion of this bill is aimed at removing barriers that have essentially required people with disabilities to choose between working or retaining access to health care services through Medicare and Medicaid. Among other incentives, the program provides for several years of continued eligibility for coverage under Medicare and gives states the option of providing a buy-in provision for continued Medicaid coverage to more people ages 16–64 with disabilities who work.

- **Work Incentives Planning and Assistance (WIPA) Program of the Social Security Administration (SSA):** The aim of the WIPA program is to enable SSA's beneficiaries with disabilities to utilize work incentives and return-to-work supports (e.g., PASS, trial work period, Ticket to Work program). SSA has cooperative agreements with community agencies throughout the country to administer the WIPA Program. Each of the WIPA projects has Community Work Incentive coordinators (CWICs) who work with individual SSA beneficiaries, their families, and vocational rehabilitation agencies to maximize return-to-work and job opportunities for persons with disabilities. CWIC coordinators are often rehabilitation counselors by education with specialized knowledge and experience about work incentive programs.

- **IPE (Individualized Plan for Employment):** The IPE is used in the state/federal DVR system and is developed jointly by the person with a disability and the VR counselor. The IPE lists the steps and services necessary to achieve the employment outcome and identifies how each step will be evaluated.

- **Informed choice** refers to the decision-making process in state/federal DVR in which the individual with a disability analyzes relevant information and selects a vocational goal with the assistance of the rehabilitation counselor or coordinator. The emphasis is on primary decision-making by the person with a disability.

KEY POINTS: ACHIEVING VOCATIONAL REHABILITATION OUTCOMES

1. Set the expectation, even from the initial rehabilitation stages, that resuming or pursuing careers is a viable and desirable rehabilitation goal.

2. Optimize physical, emotional, and cognitive functioning.

3. Utilize professional VR services and return-to-work incentive programs.

4. Facilitate work adaptation through retraining, assistive technology, and work accommodations, support, and communication.

---

15. **How are disability benefits affected by return to work?**

    Disability beneficiaries receiving SSDI or SSI can still receive benefits while they test their ability to work. Employment supports are provided through the Ticket to Work program and trial work periods. The employment supports include consideration for the cost of impairment-related work expenses (e.g., attendant care services, transportation costs, work-related equipment). The SSA employment supports also offer opportunities to maintain health coverage while trying to return to work. As authorized by the Ticket to Work and the Work Incentives Improvement Act of 1999, the Social Security Administration established a grant program called Benefits Planning, Assistance and Outreach. Under this program, cooperative agreements (monetary awards) are granted to community-based organizations, called BPAO Projects, to provide all SSA beneficiaries with disabilities access to work incentives planning and assistance services.

    Rehabilitation counselors and related professionals (e.g., social workers) have required additional training or specialization in benefits counseling to master the complexities of benefit systems.

    Details of SSA's work incentive programs:http://www.ssa.gov/work
    Details regarding BPAO:www.ssa.gov/work/ServiceProviders/BPAODirectory.html

16. **Describe a possible VR plan for an individual with chronic low back pain who is returning to a preinjury job.**

    Vocational intervention at the **personal level:**
    - Effective pain management, regular physician follow-up, and use of support groups.
    - Analysis of the person's functional capacities in relation to the demands of preinjury work.
    - Counseling regarding the impact of the injury on the individual's career.
    - Coordination of rehabilitation efforts to maximize that individual's confidence, strength, endurance, and flexibility to perform the demands of the job.

    Vocational intervention at the **environment level:**
    - Detailed analysis of the work environment and job demands.
    - Modifications to accommodate current functioning and reduce chances of further aggravation of the condition; ergonomic modifications.

    Vocational plan: Developing and negotiating gradual return to work or temporary modified duty; all parties assisting the individual in an early transition back to work.

17. **Describe a plan for an individual with traumatic brain injury who was unemployed at the time of injury.**
    - Vocational intervention at the **person level**—Assess residual skills and learning style; determine interests and aptitudes; develop a career plan.

- Vocational intervention at the **environment level**—Consider requirements of suitable occupations, work environments, and potential accommodation strategies (i.e., maximize residual functioning, reduce or modify tasks to require fewer of the individual's skill or knowledge deficits).
- **Vocational plan**—Provide social skills training for use at the work environment; provide occupational retraining through continuing education or on-the-job training; use volunteer placement to develop general work behaviors or supported employment with a job coach to teach work skills at the job site; provide placement assistance or continue supported employment services depending on severity and capacities; provide adaptive technology for augmentation of work performance.

18. **An individual with a spinal cord injury wishes to return to a former job but has substantial limitations in performing essential duties of the job, even with accommodations. What are the options?**
There are other VR options besides returning to the same job with the same employer. Employment options may exist with the same employer by using existing transferable skills in a different position. In other circumstances, there may be more accommodation and flexibility options to return to a similar job but with a new employer. Volunteering, self-employment, telecommuting, and/or retraining for new job skills may be other options to lead to a paid position.

19. **Describe how physiatry and other medical specialties can facilitate VR of persons with disabilities.**
Physicians can facilitate the VR process by approaching each patient with expectations for each individual to reach his or her highest potential and by communicating an expectation of return to work with patients and their families. Other steps that can facilitate the VR process are as follows:
- To promote and build endurance for daily schedules that would accommodate work.
- To communicate with VR counselors and employers to help determine appropriate job duties and work modifications for safe and timely return to work.
- To assist in developing trial work situations or volunteer positions at medical facilities or in the community for patients who require job tryouts.
- To include return to work as a goal at medical follow-up visits.

BIBLIOGRAPHY

1. Chan F, Leahy M, Saunders JL (eds): Case Management for Rehabilitation Health Professionals, 2nd ed. Osage Beach, MO, Aspen Professional Services, 2005.
2. Clifton DW: Physical Rehabilitation's Role in Disability Management: Unique Perspectives for Success. Philadelphia, Elsevier Saunders, 2005.
3. Parker R, Szymanski E, Patterson J (eds): Rehabilitation Counseling: Basics and Beyond, 4th ed. Austin, TX, Pro-Ed, 2005.
4. Riggar T, Maki DR (eds): Handbook of Rehabilitation Counseling. New York, Springer, 2004.
5. Szymanski E, Parker R (eds): Work and Disability: Issues and Strategies in Career Development and Job Placement, 2nd ed. Austin, TX, Pro-Ed, 2003.

VI. GENERAL THERAPEUTICS

THERAPEUTIC EXERCISE: ESSENTIALS

Shashank J. Dave, DO, Ralph M. Buschbacher, MD, Gregory Strock, MD, and Mark Randall, PsyD, DrPH, MA

Lack of activity destroys the good condition of every human being, while movement and methodical physical exercise save it and preserve it.

—Plato (427–347 BC)

1. **What are the three types of muscle fibers?**
   See Table 22-1.

TABLE 22-1. MUSCLE FIBER TYPES AND THEIR CHARACTERISTICS			
Characteristic	**Type I: Slow Oxidative**	**Type IIa: Fast Oxidative Glycolytic**	**Type IIb: Fast Glycolytic**
Histology and biochemistry	Numerous mitochondria	Increased electrochemical transmission of action potentials; increased calcium release and uptake by sarcoplasmic reticulum and cross-bridge turnover	
Activity level of myosin ATPase	Low	High	High
Speed of contraction	Slow	Fast	Fast
Glycolytic/anaerobic potential	Low	Moderate	High
Oxidative potential	High	Moderate	Low
Resistance to fatigue	High	Moderate	Low
Uses	Posture/endurance muscles	Quick force contractions	

2. **What determines the fiber type of a given muscle cell?**
   The fiber type is determined by the nerve fiber that innervates it. All fibers innervated by a given motor neuron have the same physiologic and histochemical properties. The type of motor neuron and pattern of nerve impulses transmitted play the main roles in determining the mechanical and histochemical properties of the muscle fibers. After denervation, if nerve regrowth and sprouting occur, the muscle fiber will take on the characteristics determined by the new nerve fiber.

   Bacou F, Rouanet P, Barjot CP, et al: Expression of myosin isoforms in denervated, cross-reinnervated and electrically stimulated rabbit muscles. Eur J Biochem 236:539–547, 1996.

3. **What is the Henneman size principle?**
   Motor units are recruited in order of increasing size, increasing contraction strength, and diminishing fatigue resistance. Therefore, the smaller, less powerful, fatigue-resistant fibers are recruited before the larger, more powerful, fatigable fibers, regardless of speed of contraction. This makes sense because these fibers are weaker. When initially moving a muscle, not much strength is needed, and activating the weaker fibers (motor units) gives finer motor control. When more strength is needed, increasingly larger fibers are recruited to generate more gross muscle strength.

   http://jn.physiology.org/cgi/content/full/93/6/3024
   Thomas GT, Munson CK, Stein RB: The resilience of the size principle in the organization of motor unit properties in normal and reinnervated adult skeletal muscles. Can J Physiol Pharmaco 82(8–9):645–661, 2004.

4. **What are the determinants of muscle strength?**
   See Figure 22-1.

   Edstrom L, Grimby L: Effect of exercise on the motor unit. Muscle Nerve 9:104–126, 1986.

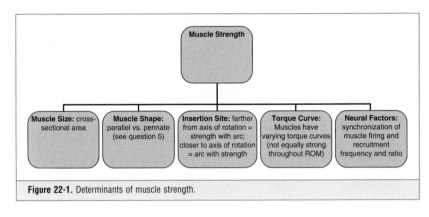

Figure 22-1. Determinants of muscle strength.

5. **Describe two different types of muscle shapes.**
   - **Parallel** muscle fibers travel the entire length of the muscle. A muscle fiber ordinarily contracts by approximately 50% of its resting length (length if removed from the body). Thus, parallel muscle fibers can generate a large amount of shortening but have lesser strength (*see* Fig. 22-2).
   - **Pennate** muscles have fibers that insert onto the muscle tendon at an angle, which allows a greater number of muscle fibers. Although the total size of the muscle may be the same as in a parallel arrangement, the total effective cross-sectional area is greater and thus provides greater strength. Because the muscle fibers shorten by approximately 50% of their resting length and the fibers attach at an angle onto the tendon, the total movement is less than in parallel muscle fibers.

   Kenny W, Humphrey R, Bryant C: ACSM's Guidelines for Exercise Testing and Prescription, 5th ed. Philadelphia, Lippincott Williams & Wilkins, 1995.

6. **What did Moritani and deVries show in regard to the relationship between strength and hypertrophy?**
   Moritani and deVries showed that in the first few weeks of a training program, there is an increase in strength not related to hypertrophy. An increase in integrated electromyographic (EMG) activity during this time period implies that there are neural factors leading to increased

strength. This may be caused by increased synchronization and coordination of muscle firing. Only later does hypertrophy take effect. They also showed that neural training effects are transferred to some extent to the opposite (untrained) limb. Moritani and deVries also found that elderly subjects had a strength increase with weight training primarily resulting from neural learning, not hypertrophy.

Moritani T, deVries HA: Neural factors versus hypertrophy in the time course of muscle strength gain. Am J Phys Med 58:115–130, 1979.
Moritani T, deVries HA: Potential for gross muscle hypertrophy in older men. J Gerontol 35:672–682, 1980.

7. **Can a muscle fiber's type be changed by exercise?**
Although a muscle fiber's type cannot be changed by exercise, Gollnick and colleagues showed that the cross-sectional area of type I muscle fibers could be increased with aerobic training. Similarly, strength training results in hypertrophy of both type I and type II muscles; however, the type II fibers respond to a greater extent than the type I fibers. There is felt to be minimal, if any, hyperplasia of either type I or type II fibers in human beings, only an increase in size of existing fibers.

Gollnick PD, Armstrong RB, Saltin B, et al: Effect of training on enzyme activity and fiber composition of human skeletal muscle. J Appl Physiol 34:107–111, 1973.

8. **Describe three types of muscle movement.**
See Table 22-2.

www.emedicine.com/pmr/topic199.htm

TABLE 22-2. TYPES OF MUSCLE MOVEMENT			
	Isometric	Isotonic	Isokinetic
Definition	Equal distance	Equal tone	Equal speed
Joint movement	No	Yes	Yes
Example	Pushing on a wall	Weight lifting	Cybex machine
Important principles	Muscle has some internal shortening, but no gross movement of the joint	Constant resistance throughout joint motion. See question 14.	Speed of movement remains constant no matter how hard the subject pushes against the machine

9. **What is the difference between concentric and eccentric muscle contraction?**
See Table 22-3.

TABLE 22-3. CONCENTRIC VERSUS ECCENTRIC CONTRACTION		
	Concentric	Eccentric
Definition	Shortening (e.g., lifting a weight)	Lengthening (e.g., lowering a weight, or a decelerating tibialis anterior contraction from heel strike to foot flat)
Characteristics	Less muscle tension	Greater muscle tension; hence more potential for tissue injury, but also more potential for hypertrophy

10. **How do open and closed kinetic chain exercises differ?**
    See Table 22-4.

TABLE 22-4. OPEN VERSUS CLOSED KINETIC CHAIN EXERCISES		
	Open Kinetic Chain	Closed Kinetic Chain
Definition	Distal end not fixed	Distal end fixed
Example	Extending leg with free weight	Squatting
Comments	More shear stress	Less shear stress

11. **What is the DeLorme technique?**
    The DeLorme technique, used to strengthen muscles, is also called **progressive resistance exercise**. Classically, the subject is tested to determine the maximum weight that he or she can lift 10 times using good form and technique—this is called the "10 repetition max," or 10 RM. DeLorme would have the person lift at various percentages of the 10 RM, starting at 10%, 20%, 30%, etc., up to 100%. The weights would progressively increase from week to week as the subject got stronger.

    deLateur BJ, Lehmann JF, Fordyce WE: A test of the DeLorme axiom. Arch Phys Med Rehabil 49:245–248, 1968.

12. **What is the DeLorme axiom?**
    The **DeLorme axiom** states that "high-intensity, low-repetition exercise builds strength, and low-intensity, high-repetition exercise builds endurance, and that each of these two types of exercise is incapable of producing the results obtained by the other type." It is now felt that the axiom is too extreme and that there is some crossover effect from one exercise type to the other.

    deLateur BJ, Lehmann JF, Fordyce WE: A test of the DeLorme axiom. Arch Phys Med Rehabil 49:245–248, 1968.

13. **What is the Oxford technique?**
    The Oxford technique basically turned the DeLorme method on its head by doing the exercises at 100% 10 RM, then 75% 10 RM, then 50% 10 RM.

    Zinovieff AN: Heavy resistance exercises: The "Oxford" technique. Br J Phys Med 14:129–132, 1957.

14. **How do the effects of free weights, pulleys, and cam-varied resistance differ during range of motion (ROM)?**
    - **Free-weight** lifting is usually considered a type of isotonic exercise. However, the actual muscle tension is *not equal* throughout the ROM because of gravity and joint position, which is a limitation of using free weights. You can only lift as much as the weakest part of the motion.
    - **Pulleys** *even out* the tension and create the same amount of resistance throughout the entire ROM of the muscle. Nevertheless, this still does not match the natural torque curve of the muscle, because the muscle is not equally strong in all parts of its ROM.
    - **Cam-varied resistance** *varies* the torque throughout the ROM of the muscle and therefore strengthens the muscle at *all* parts of its ROM because it attempts to match the torque curve of the muscle. An example is Nautilus-brand equipment.

15. **What is plyometric exercise?**
    Plyometric exercises are functional types of exercise, which apply the principle of a brief stretch followed by contraction. A brief stretch (such as during a muscle stretch reflex) will elicit a

contraction, and by briefly preloading (stretching) the muscle, this is felt to facilitate the subsequent contraction. Exercises using this principle include jumping up and down or jumping over boxes. Plyometric exercise is useful because many sports involve plyometric-type maneuvers. However, it is also more likely to cause injury.

Chu D: Jumping into Plyometrics. Champaign, IL, Human Kinetics, 1998.

16. Ouch! Why do muscles become sore after a workout?

Lengthening (eccentric) contractions are probably responsible for delayed-onset muscle soreness and are probably better at generating muscle hypertrophy than concentric contractions. This soreness usually starts a day or two after exercise and lasts a few days.

Armstrong RB: Initial events in exercise-induced muscle injury. Med Sci Sports Exerc 22:4 429–435, 1990. www.emedicine.com/pmr/topic117.htm

17. What is endurance exercise? Endurance fitness?

Endurance exercise is the prolonged reciprocal use of large muscle groups. It is differentiated from **muscle endurance**, which refers to the length of time that a muscle can contract at a given tension.

The terms *stamina, endurance fitness, cardiovascular fitness,* and *aerobic fitness* refer to the body's ability to generate adenosine triphosphate (ATP) aerobically. Aerobic energy, or the long-term energy system, is primarily measured by an individual's VO_{2max}. VO_{2max} is considered the fundamental measurement of aerobic capability in exercise physiology.

18. Define VO_2 and VO_{2max}.

The V in VO_{2max} refers to the **rate**, and the O_2 refers to the **oxygen** being consumed. Put together, this is the **rate of oxygen consumption**. VO_{2max} is the **maximum rate of oxygen consumption** and is a measure of the maximum intensity of exercise that can be sustained. VO_{2max} is limited by the oxygen-carrying and utilization capacity of the body. Exceeding the VO_{2max} for brief periods can be accomplished by reverting to glycolytic energy production; however, this creates a buildup of lactic acid and cannot be sustained.

Guyton A, Hall J: Sports physiology. In Guyton A, Hall J (eds): Textbook of Medical Physiology, 11th ed. Philadelphia, Elsevier, 2006, pp 1061–1062.

19. What are the different types of flexibility exercises?

- **Static stretching:** Static stretches involve stretching the muscle and staying in that position for some time period. Generally, at least 15–20 sec is required to provide any benefit. Static stretching is relatively safe.
- **Ballistic stretching:** Ballistic stretching involves bouncing-type maneuvers. This exercise was popular several decades ago, but it is now out of favor because the muscle stretch reflex is activated in a manner similar to plyometric exercise and will actually hinder the stretching.
- **Proprioceptive neuromuscular facilitation:** This is similar to osteopathic muscle energy techniques. For this type of stretching, the muscle is stretched to its fullest extent, and then the person contracts that muscle against the direction of the stretch. Although joint position does not change, this is felt to cause internal shortening of the connective tissues of the muscle, and after a few seconds of contraction, the muscle is relaxed and again stretched a bit more. This is generally done three times in any given position and can sometimes be done with a partner.
- **Passive stretching:** Also known as relaxed stretching or static-passive stretching, in this form of stretching exercise the person stretching assumes a position and holds it with another part of the body or with assistance from a partner or some apparatus such as a machine. For example, when standing with the ball of the foot on a step and the heels hanging down, body weight will stretch the gastrocsoleus complex.

- **Dynamic stretching:** Dynamic stretching is different from ballistic stretching in that ballistic stretching forces a limb or part of the body beyond its usual ROM. Dynamic stretching involves moving parts of the body in a controlled manner (e.g., dance or martial arts) and gradually increasing the reach and speed of movement.

Alter MJ: Science of Stretching. Champaign, IL, Human Kinetics, 1988.
Anderson R, Anderson J: Stretching: 20th Anniversary. Bolinas, CA, Shelter Publications, 1980.
www.emedicine.com/pmr/topic199.htm

KEY POINTS: TYPES OF FLEXIBILITY EXERCISES

1. Static stretching: a gradual stretch over 15 seconds

2. Ballistic stretching: repeated rapid stretching such as bouncing

3. Proprioceptive neuromuscular facilitation: stretching followed by muscle contraction, then further stretching

4. Passive stretching: a partner applying a stretch to a relaxed muscle

5. Dynamic stretching: controlled movement of body parts such as martial arts

20. **How do I measure flexibility?**
    Although there are various methods to measure flexibility, the **goniometer** is the most commonly used tool to determine joint range of motion. Measuring 0–180 degrees, values are then compared to standardized values of normal joint ROM. When measuring spine ROM, a goniometer is less reliable. An **inclinometer** is a device placed on the spine used to assess gross ROM, where sagittal plane (*not* coronal or transverse) measurements are taken. However, it has been shown that, at least in the lumbar spine, flexion measurement is more reliable than extension measurement.

    Saur PM, Ensink FB, Frese K, et al: Lumbar range of motion: Reliability and validity of the inclinometer technique in the clinical measurement of trunk flexibility. Spine 21(11):1332–1338, 1996.

21. **Do I have to warm up?**
    Warming up is generally accepted as a valid procedure before vigorous exercise. It is felt that the performer is better prepared both physiologically and psychologically for an activity and that the warm-up may reduce the chance of injury. Animal studies have shown that greater forces and increases in muscle length were required to injure a "warm" muscle than a "cold" muscle. It is suggested that warming up stretches the muscle tendon unit and allows for greater length and less tension at any given load on the unit.

    Williford HN, East JB, Smith FH, et al: Evaluation of warm-up for improvement in flexibility. Am J Sports Med 14(4):316–319, 1986.

22. **What is the difference between upper-extremity and lower-extremity exercise?**
    Blood pressure (both systolic and diastolic) is considerably higher for a given level of upper-body exercise versus lower-body exercise. This is most likely a result of the smaller muscle mass and vasculature of the upper extremities, which offer greater resistance to blood flow than the larger muscle mass and vasculature of the lower body and legs.

    Astrand P-O, Elblom B, Messin R, et al: Intra-arterial blood pressure during exercise with different muscle groups. J Appl Physiol 20(2):253–256, 1965.

23. **How does aging affect muscle strength?**
Aging reduces isometric and concentric muscle strength because of atrophy, deterioration of mechanical properties, and motor unit breakdown. Additional factors can include nutritional inadequacies, effects of disease, and sedentary lifestyle. If strength decline is primarily caused by a sedentary lifestyle or disuse of the muscles, then strength training would seem reasonable. It has been shown that conventional resistance training is possible, even for very old adults, and can reverse some of the effects of aging on muscular strength.

Fiatarone MA, Marks EC, Ryan ND, et al: High-intensity strength training in nonagenarians. Effects of skeletal muscle. JAMA 263:3029–3034, 1990.

24. **How does sex affect muscle strength and the response to exercise? Ah, I mean gender.**
Because they have lower levels of testosterone, women experience less hypertrophy of the muscles and have less of an increase in VO_{2max} with exercise. In addition, because women on average have a greater amount of body fat (and therefore less lean muscle mass as a percentage of total body mass), they are less efficient in endurance exercise.

Shepard RJ: Exercise and training in women. I. Influence of gender on exercise and training responses. Can J Appl Physiol 25(1):19–34, 2000.

25. **How does the cardiovascular system adapt (or not) to aerobic, endurance-type exercise?**
See Figure 22-2.

Rupp JC: Exercise physiology. In Roitman JL, Bibi KW, Thompson WR (eds): ACSM Health Fitness Certification Review. Philadelphia, Lippincott Williams & Wilkins, 2001, pp 26–27.

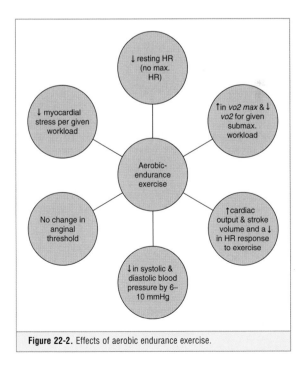

Figure 22-2. Effects of aerobic endurance exercise.

26. **How does regular aerobic exercise affect diabetes?**

For **non–insulin-dependent** diabetic persons, there is an increase in end-organ cell receptor sensitivity to insulin. Exercise will also decrease obesity, which will help in blood sugar control. Be careful to watch for the Somogyi effect when exercising, especially if exercise is performed late during the day. In addition, medication doses may need to be adjusted. Because diabetics may have silent cardiac ischemia, they should be monitored for this condition.

In **insulin-dependent** diabetic persons, exercise does not change the nature of the disease but certainly will change insulin requirements.

Kriska AM, Blair SN, Pereira MA: The potential role of physical activity in the prevention of non-insulin-dependent diabetes mellitus: The epidemiological evidence. Exerc Sport Sci Rev 22:121–143, 1994.

27. **How do I write an exercise prescription?**

A handy mnemonic is **TOIL:**
- **T** = **T**ype: remember to include components of question 8 as well as exercises the patient will most likely stick with.
- **O** = How **O**ften: per day/week/month, etc.
- **I** = **I**ntensity
- **L** = **L**ength of time

WEBSITES

1. American Alliance of Health, Physical Education, Recreation, and Dance
   www.aahperd.org/

2. American College of Sports Medicine
   www.acsm.org/

3. American Council on Exercise
   www.acefitness.org

4. American Heart Association
   www.americanheart.org/

5. National Institute for Fitness and Sport
   www.nifs.org/

6. Physiatric Association of Spine, Sports, and Occupational Rehabilitation (PASSOR)
   www.aapmr.org/passor.htm

7. President's Council on Physical Fitness and Sports
   www.fitness.gov/

CHAPTER 23

NUTRITION AND DIET IN REHABILITATION: OPTIMIZING OUTCOMES

Marlene M. Young, MA, Mark A. Young, MD, MBA, and Steven A. Stiens, MD, MS

Don't give the same food to the sick and the healthy.

–Croatian proverb

1. **Do rehabilitation professionals really need to know about nutrition?**
   Of course. A basic understanding of important key nutritional principles is critical to all rehabilitation practitioners. Physical medicine and rehabilitation (PM&R) interventions (including modalities for healing and exercise) require proper nutrition to maximize results at all biopsychosocial levels, thereby reducing impairment and optimizing outcomes. Specific nutritional substrates are essential for cellular, tissue, and organ-based function. Good nutrition is intrinsically linked to functional outcomes in all aspects of rehabilitation. People with disabilities, including those with pain, neurologic, musculoskeletal, and orthopedic diagnoses, are positively impacted by dietary optimization.

2. **What is the definition of malnutrition?**
   Malnutrition is a medical condition resulting from an imbalanced diet with either too *little* or too *much* food or a dietary intake lacking in one or more essential nutrients. People who are malnourished are frequently lacking in one or more of the following important nutritional components: **calories, vitamins,** or **trace minerals.**

   Nursal TZ, Noyan T, Atalay BG, et al: Simple two part tool for screening for malnutrition. Nutrition 21:659–665, 2005.

3. **Is there more than one form of malnutrition?**
   Yes. Common forms of malnutrition include:
   - **Protein-energy malnutrition (PEM),** which is inadequate availability or absorption of energy substrate and proteins in the body.
   - **Micronutrient malnutrition,** which is inadequate availability of essential nutrients such as vitamins and trace elements required by the body in small quantities (e.g., vitamin A, iron, iodine) for critical enzyme function and as cofactors in cellular reactions. This can lead to various clinical manifestations, including stunted growth, reduced intelligence, and decreased cognitive ability.

4. **Is malnutrition a common disorder?**
   Yes. Although malnourishment can occur in otherwise healthy, unsuspecting patients, it has a high incidence in rehabilitation patients. The incidence of malnutrition in hospitalized medical patients in the United States is between 30% and 50%. Because rehabilitation patients often have chronic long-standing illnesses that require prolonged hospitalizations, malnutrition is often an inevitable consequence. Optimal nutritional support can reduce body protein loss during critical illness by as much as half.

   Ishibashi N, Plank L, Sandok N, et al: Optimal protein requirements during the first two weeks after onset of critical illness. Crit Care Med 26(19):1429–1535, 1998.

5. **What are the common risk factors for malnutrition in older adults?**
   Sudden weight gain or weight loss, inadequate diet, underlying disease, multiple medications, economic hardship, oral pain, and tooth loss.

KEY POINTS: HALLMARKS OF MALNUTRITION IN THE ELDERLY

1. Insufficient diet

2. Oral or dental pathology

3. Recent weight change

4. Multiple medications

6. **How can the physiatrist perform a simple bedside nutritional assessment?**
   1. **Review the medical record.**
      a. Previous history of dietary or nutritional deficiency or systemic diseases (intestinal disease)
      b. Documented weights from previous clinical visits
   2. **Get a thorough nutritional history.**
      a. Changes in body weight, food diaries, gastrointestinal (GI) symptoms, ability to obtain food, general mental status, and swallowing ability
   3. **Perform a focused clinical evaluation.**
      a. Anthropometric measurements—that is, height and weight
      b. Physical examination—muscle strength, skin evaluation, neurologic exam

7. **What are the common serum markers that are diminished in malnourished patients?**
   - Total protein
   - Albumin
   - Pre-albumin
   - Cholesterol
   - Triglycerides
   - Creatinine
   - Blood urea nitrogen
   - Total lymphocyte count
   - Beta carotene

8. **Name two common methods of assessing energy requirements of a rehabilitation patient by determining the basal metabolic rate (BMR).**
   1. **Harris-Benedict equation**
      a. Male kcal: $66 + (13.7 \times \text{weight in kg}) + (5 \times \text{height in cm}) - (6.8 \times \text{age})$
      b. Female kcal: $655 + (9.6 \times \text{weight in kg}) + (1.8 \times \text{height in cm}) - (4.7 \times \text{age})$
   2. **Simple estimation**
      a. 30 kcal/kg $- 25\%$

9. **What is ideal body weight (IBW)? How is it calculated?**
   Body mass index (BMI) provides a useful measure of body fat based on height and weight. It eliminates dependence on frame size to assess differences in body composition. The formula is as follows: Weight (in kg) divided by height (in m^2)

The BMIs for men and women vary. BMI helps to categorize a person:

- Underweight = <18.5
- Normal weight = 18.5–24.9
- Overweight = 25–29.9
- Obesity = BMI ≥ 30

As BMI increases above 20 kg/m^2, there is an incremental risk of morbidity from conditions such as hypertension, type 2 diabetes, heart disease, cancer, stroke, osteoarthritis, sleep apnea, and respiratory disease. When BMI is >25, risk of morbidity and mortality from these conditions increases dramatically (National Health and Nutrition Examination Survey 3).

The weight that is considered "normal" for a particular age, sex, and body frame is IBW. It is estimated from comparison tables, the most common of these being the Metropolitan Life Insurance Tables.

www.nhlbisupport.com/bmi/bmicalc.htm

10. **How does distribution of body fat differ between men and women? What clinical implication does this have for drug bioavailability?**
Although the percentage of fat in the body is greater in women than in men in all age groups, the distribution of excess body fat is generally higher in men (abdominal) than women (thighs and buttocks). The old adage for describing the body shape is apples (men) and pears (women). The difference in percentage of body fat has significant implications for drug metabolism and bioavailability and may explain why men and women show different responses to certain medications (e.g., analgesics and other pain medications).

11. **What should rehabilitation professionals know about nutritional support?**
Nutritional support is the provision of necessary nutrients (calories, protein, water, vitamins, and minerals) to patients who are unable to ingest these nutrients on their own by oral means. The two primary ways of bypassing the oral route are the enteral route (i.e., nasogastric tube or endoscopically or surgically placed gastrostomy or jejunostomy) and the parenteral route (i.e., intravenous feeding).

12. **What are the most frequent indications for total parenteral nutrition (TPN) in hospitalized patients unable to achieve adequate nutrition?**
- Protracted nutrient losses with severe malnutrition.
- Presurgery and postsurgery with expected prolonged course before return to normal bowel function.
- Preoperative patients who are malnourished.
- Inability to eat.
- Adjunctive therapy in patients with GI disease or dysfunction (e.g., inflammatory bowel disease).
- Nonfunctioning or poorly functioning GI tract.
- Hypermetabolic conditions with decreased ability to take in nutrients (i.e., polytrauma, infection).

13. **Is it important to treat B$_{12}$ deficiencies?**
B$_{12}$ deficiencies are much more prevalent and clinically significant than previously thought, especially in the spinal cord injury population and the elderly (up to 14.5%). Deficiencies can result in peripheral neuropathy, deficits in memory and cognitive skills, poor wound healing (B$_{12}$ is a protein synthesis cofactor), and pernicious anemia. It also may be associated with high homocysteine levels, contributing to coronary artery disease. Monthly intramuscular injections are known to be effective; however, oral therapy can be used in lieu of injections, with effective dosing of 1000 µg/day.

Petchkrua W, Burns S, Stiens S, et al: Prevalence of vitamin B$_{12}$ deficiency in patients with spinal cord injury or disease: Arch Phys Med Rehabil 84:1675–1679, 2003.
www.vitamins-nutrition.org

14. **Can good nutrition play a role in pain management?**

    Poor nutrition and suboptimal appetite are common concomitants of chronic pain syndrome. Bolstering nutrition and proper hydration can significantly improve outcomes in pain patients. Scientific evidence supports the role of targeted food selection in pain reduction and rehabilitation. For example, bromelain, an extract from pineapple plant, has been shown to have anti-inflammatory and analgesic properties, possibly providing nutritionally astute treatment alternatives for pain syndromes.

WEBSITES

1. www.eatright.org/cps/rde/xchg/ada/hs.xsl/index.html

2. www.nutrition.gov/

3. www.nutrition.org/

BIBLIOGRAPHY

1. Bendich A: Vitamin Intake and Health: A Scientific Review. New York, Marcel Dekker, 1999.

2. Brien S, Lewith G, Walker AF, et al: Bromelain as a treatment for osteoarthritis: A review of clinical studies. Evidence Based Complement Alternat Med 1(3):251–257, 2004.

3. Finestone HM, Greene-Finestone LS: Rehabilitation medicine. II. Diagnosis of dysphagia and its nutritional management for stroke patients. Can Med Assoc J 169:1041–1044, 2003.

4. Heymsfield SB: Enteral solutions: Is there a solution?. Nutr Clin Pract 10:4–7, 1995.

5. Pain: Clinical Updates. New York, IASP, 2004.

6. Whitney EN, Cataldo CB, Rolfes SR: Understanding Normal and Clinical Nutrition. Belmont, CA, Wadsworth Publishers, 1998.

7. Young MA, Barr K: Nutrition and pain. In Women and Pain: Why It Hurts and What You Can Do. New York, Hyperion-AOL Time Warner, 2002, pp 18–25.

CHAPTER 24

MEDICATIONS: TOOLS FOR WELLNESS AND ENABLEMENT IN REHABILITATION

Jennifer J. James, MD, Jelena N. Svircev, MD, David J. Kennedy, MD, Karen Y. Lew, PharmD, and Steven A. Stiens, MD, MS

One of the first duties of the physician is to educate the masses not to take medicine.
—Sir William Osler

1. **Why is a chapter on medications important to me as a physiatrist?**
   Medications are tools for wellness and enablement. Because of the risks of side effects and interactions, unique approaches to medication usage are often utilized. A complete review of pharmacology is beyond the scope of this chapter. Rather, this chapter addresses medications that are used to treat common conditions that affect individuals with rehabilitation needs. Some medications commonly used to treat patients in rehabilitation are covered in other sections of this book.

2. **How does pharmacologic management fit into the process of rehabilitation and primary care?**
   Interdisciplinary rehabilitation is the process that makes the patient maximally able. The ever-expanding options in medications allow the physiatrist to target drug therapy for disease prevention, block pathophysiology, reduce symptoms, minimize organ dysfunction, enhance functional activity, and promote full social participation. Pharmacologic treatment is applied at the molecular systems level in the biopsychosocial model, but outcomes are realized at many other system levels. Drug therapy should therefore be carefully targeted in concert with other treatment modalities directed at all system levels.

3. **What principles guide the drug therapy for patients with chronic, often permanent disabilities?**
   Use medications only when necessary, and remember to dose sparingly and monitor for outcomes. Provide accessible and practical schedules and methods of administration. Recognize that the body is dynamic and may not need all medications on a continual basis for success. Reevaluate medications by reducing doses to eliminate medications no longer required. Use minimal potency and dosage of medications that will achieve the desired outcomes.

4. **What are the major classes of antidepressants, their place in therapy, and their side effects?**
   See Table 24-1.

5. **Explain the risks and benefits of neuroleptics to calm an agitated patient recovering from a traumatic brain injury (TBI).**
   If behavioral or environmental management is not effective, the recommended first-line pharmacologic treatment for agitation and delirium in a TBI patient is the **short-acting benzodiazepine** class with no active metabolite (such as **lorazepam**). The use of **neuroleptics,** such as **haloperidol,** in minimal dose is second-line therapy. This class is postulated to disrupt neural recovery, cause extrapyramidal movement disorders, lower the seizure threshold, and place the patient at risk for neuroleptic malignant syndrome.

TABLE 24-1. MAJOR CLASSES OF ANTIDEPRESSANTS

Class	Place in Therapy	Side Effects
Tricyclic antidepressants (TCAs)		
Amitriptyline	Limited use because of side effects	Anticholinergic
Imipramine		Arrhythmias
Desipramine		Antihistaminic
Nortriptyline		Weight gain
		Orthostasis
		Sedation
Selective serotonin reuptake inhibitors (SSRIs)		
Fluoxetine	Generally first line	Fatigue
Sertraline		Insomnia
Paroxetine		Sexual dysfunction
Citalopram		
Dual-action reuptake inhibitors		
Bupropion	Alternative or adjunct	Activating, decrease in seizure threshold
Venlafaxine		Increase in blood pressure
Duloxetine		
Mixed action		
Mirtazapine	Alternative or adjunct	Sedation
		Weight gain

Adapted from Mann JJ: The medical management of depression. N Engl J Med 353:1819–1934, 2005; and Gelenberg AJ, Hopkins HS: Assessing and treating depression in primary care medicine. Am J Med 120(2):105–108, 2007.

6. **What are the advantages and disadvantages of soporific agents (sleepers) prescribed by physicians?**

   Commonly used agents

   - Gamma amino-butyric acid (GABA) receptor agonists **zolpidem** (Ambien), **zaleplon** (Sonata), and **eszopiclone** (Lunesta) may be less disruptive of normal sleep architecture (stages 3 and 4 "restorative" sleep) than benzodiazepines. They are administered right before sleep because of their rapid onset and short duration.
   - **Triazolopyridines,** such as trazodone (not a tricyclic antidepressant), has a positive effect on sleep architecture, but side effects include vivid dreams and enhanced appetite. Its longer duration is helpful for sleep maintenance, but administer at least one hour before bedtime.

   Other options

   - **Hypnotics,** such as **chloral hydrate,** are effective for some patients but can cause confusion, dizziness, and physical dependence.
   - **Benzodiazepines,** such as **temazepam** (Restoril), have anxiolytic effects but can alter electroencephalographic sleep patterns and lead to dependence.

- **Antidepressants** can be given for their sedative side effects (*see* antidepressant question for further details).
- **Diphenhydramine (Benadryl)** is frequently prescribed but has significant anticholinergic side effects and is therefore not recommended.

7. **What are current recommendations for seizure prophylaxis after TBI?**
Anticonvulsant prophylaxis with **carbamazepine** or **phenytoin** has been recommended for the prevention of early post-traumatic seizures (seizure within the first week following TBI) in individuals with penetrating or nonpenetrating TBI. The prophylactic use of antiepileptic drugs is not recommended for preventing late post-traumatic seizures (seizures that occur after 1 week of injury) in individuals with nonpenetrating or penetrating TBI who have not yet had a seizure.

Brain Injury Special Interest Group of the American Academy of Physical Medicine and Rehabilitation: Practice parameters: Antiepileptic drug treatment of posttraumatic seizures. Arch Phys Med Rehabil 79:594–597, 1998.

8. **What medications are used as neurostimulants?**
A number of medications have been investigated as neurostimulants for individuals with traumatic and nontraumatic brain injury, stroke, multiple sclerosis (MS), and dementia. Goals have been increased alertness, initiation, endurance, and engagement in the therapy process. There is not enough data to support the routine use of these medications during the acute phase of rehabilitation, and there are no long-term studies that review the outcomes with these medications. Occasionally used medications include:
- Methylphenidate (Ritalin, Methylin, Concerta) and D-amphetamine (Dexedrine, Dextrostat): used for mood, attention, and to speed thought process.
- Amantadine (Symmetrel), bromocriptine (Parlodel), and carbidopa/levodopa (Atamet, Sinemet): used to improve apathy, fatigue, and cognitive impairment.
- Modafinil (Provigil): used for fatigue and excessive daytime sleepiness in patients with MS and TBI.
- Memantine (Namenda): used to improve mood, attention, fatigue, and cognitive impairment.

Fann JR, Kennedy R, Bonbardier CH: Physical medicine and rehabilitation. In Levenson J (ed): Psychosomatic Medicine. Washington, DC, American Psychiatric Publishing, 2004, pp 787–825.

9. **Are there any special considerations when using antihypertensives in those with spinal cord injuries (SCIs)?**
First, discriminate essential hypertension from autonomic dysreflexia (AD) and other secondary forms of hypertension.
- For essential hypertension, the dihydropyridine class of calcium channel blockers, which includes **felodipine** and **amlodipine** is a good choice because of the absence of negative inotropic effects but may cause reflexive tachycardia initially. **ACE inhibitors** in low doses have been successfully used and enhance renal function as well.
- **Diuretics, nitrates, ACE inhibitors,** and **clonidine** may increase orthostatic hypotension in a population that is already prone to this effect.
- Nonselective beta blockers **(propranolol, nadolol, labetalol)** may increase bronchospasm. Cardioselective beta blockers **(atenolol, metoprolol, betaxolol)** generally cause less bronchospasm but lose their cardioselectivity at higher doses. Additionally, beta blockers decrease high-density lipoprotein (HDL) and exacerbate insulin resistance.

Chobanian AV, Bakris GI, Black HR, et al: The Seventh Report of the Joint National Committee on Prevention, Detection, Evaluation, and Treatment of High Blood Pressure. JAMA 289:2560–2572, 2003.

10. **How is hypertension resulting from AD managed?**
Hypertension caused by autonomic dysreflexia is treated by eliminating the noxious stimuli that trigger the event. If pharmacologic intervention is necessary, **transdermal nitrates**

(nitropaste), **hydralazine,** or **clonidine** may be used. The use of short-acting nifedipine for the treatment of AD is strongly discouraged because of risks for sudden, profound hypotension and death (reported in patients without SCI).

A word of caution: Because of the risk of profound hypotension, the use of nitrates is contraindicated in patients who use sildenafil for erectile dysfunction. Nitrates dilate smooth muscle vasculature by increasing cyclic guanosine monophosphate (cGMP) synthesis. Sildenafil preferentially inhibits the enzyme that degrades cGMP within the vasculature of the penis, but it also has systemic effects. The use of both may have an additive effect leading to severe hypotension, which could progress to cardiac or cerebral ischemia. Sildenafil should be used with caution in individuals with chronic hypotension. Nitrate-containing medications (nitropaste) should not be used to treat autonomic dysreflexia that develops as a result of sexual activity if sildenafil has been used. Hydralazine may be considered as an alternative.

Clinical Practice Guideline. Acute Management of Autonomic Dysreflexia. Consortium for Spinal Cord Medicine, 1997; http://www.pva.org/site/PageServer?pagename=research_consort.

11. **Which medications can be used to attenuate orthostatic hypotension in the SCI population?**
One of the most effective "medications" for the treatment of orthostatic hypotension is **water!** Individuals with neurotrauma lose the ability to peripherally constrict vasculature. Encouraging adequate fluid intake and using abdominal binders and lower extremity compression wraps may adequately treat symptomatic hypotension. Should pharmacologic intervention be necessary, **midodrine,** a sympathomimetic with predominant alpha-receptor binding, dosed 30 minutes before the patient gets out of bed may be helpful. To avoid hypertension, it is recommended that patients wait 4 hours before lying back down. **Fludrocortisone,** a mineralocorticosteroid, may be effective but increases fluid retention. Salt tablets are effective but also cause fluid retention and are not very palatable.

12. **What are anticoagulant guidelines in rehabilitation patients?**
See Table 24-2.

TABLE 24-2. ANTICOAGULANT GUIDELINES IN REHABILITATION PATIENTS		
Guidelines for Deep Venous Thrombosis (DVT) Prophylaxis		
	Enoxaparin	**Heparin**
Acute SCI (complete)	30 mg SC q12h × 12 wk	5000 U SC tid × 12 wk
Acute SCI (incomplete)	30 mg SC q12h × 8–12 wk	5000 U SC tid × 8–12 wk
Chronic SCI (lower extremity fracture)	30 mg SC q12h	5000 U SC tid
Chronic SCI (febrile illness, bedrest >2 wk,other DVT risk)		5000 U SC tid
Guidelines for DVT therapy		
	Duration	**Goal INR**
DVT: first time and reversible risk factors	6 months	2.5 (2–3)
DVT: recurrent or first time with idiopathic risk factors	6–12 months	2.5 (2–3)

TABLE 24-2.   ANTICOAGULANT GUIDELINES IN REHABILITATION PATIENTS—CONT'D

Guidelines for ischemic stroke prophylaxis and prevention

	Primary Prevention	Secondary Prevention*
Ischemic stroke	Aspirin 325 mg qd	Aspirin 325 mg qd Clopidogrel 75 mg qd, Aspirin/ dipyridamole SA cap 1 bid, or ticlopidine 250 mg bid
Cardioembolic stroke		Warfarin, goal INR 2–3
Type II diabetes mellitus with or without hyperlipidemia	Simvastatin 40 mg qhs Atorvastatin 10 mg qd	
High-risk nondiabetic with or without hyperlipidemia	Simvastatin 40 mg qhs Atorvastatin 10 mg qd	

Guidelines for therapy after major orthopedic surgery

Enoxaparin, 30 mg SC q12h, or heparin, 5000 U SC tid, may be used until at least 14 days postoperatively when the patient is ambulating >250 feet per day

SCI, Spinal cord injury; *INR*, international normalized ratio.
*If the patient is not on any previous antiplatelet medications, start with daily aspirin therapy. Do not combine aspirin and another antiplatelet medication, because this may increase a patient's risk of bleeding.
Data from Heart Protection Study Collaborative Group. Lancet 360:7–22, 2002; Sever PS, Dahlof B, Poulter NR, et al. Lancet 361:1149, 2003; and Koennecke HC. CNS Drugs 2004 18:4, 2004; Proceedings of the Seventh ACCP Conference on Antithrombotic and Thrombolytic Therapy: Evidence-based guidelines. Chest 126(3 Suppl):367s–368s, 2004; www.apha.org, www.americanheart.org, and www.familydoctor.org

13. **Which medications can be used to reverse pulmonary and ventilatory impairments in individuals with tetraplegia or higher level paraplegia?**
Weakness in inspiratory and expiratory muscles impairs ventilation. Increased parasympathetic activity unbalanced by sympathetic activity promotes bronchospasm and increases secretion production. This problem is exacerbated if secretions are made more tenacious by anticholinergic agents. Mucolytic agents, such as **guaifenesin** and **acetylcysteine,** can facilitate secretion clearance when combined with adequate hydration and appropriate assisted cough techniques (mechanical insufflator/exsufflator, mechanical vests, cough assist/quad cough). **Acetylcysteine** is administered by inhalation along with albuterol to reduce the risk of bronchospasm. Purulent secretions may respond to inhaled **recombinant human DNase**, which breaks down DNA released by lysed leukocytes.

Patients with tetraplegia frequently show airway hyperresponsiveness to methacholine during pulmonary function testing, even without prior history of reactive airway disease. **Inhaled beta agonists** such as **albuterol** prevent bronchoconstriction.

14. **Can any agent be administered to safely attenuate the diarrhea associated with *Clostridium difficile* colitis?**

    Colestipol and **cholestyramine** are nonabsorbable, anion-exchange, binding resins that bind *C. difficile* toxin. They can be safely prescribed while awaiting results of a stool toxin test and culture or antibiotic therapy. Be aware that they may bind to medications in addition to the *C. difficile* toxin. Therefore, other medications should be dosed 1 hour before or 4 hours after colestipol or cholestyramine.

    Probiotics are micro-organisms with beneficial properties to the host. **Lactobacillus** is found in cultured milk products (some yogurts) and creates an environment unfavorable to some bacteria through production of lactic acid and reestablishes normal bowel flora. ***Saccharomyces boulardii*** is a nonpathogenic yeast used to prevent antibiotic-associated diarrhea by reconstituting normal colonic flora, but it is not regulated by the Food and Drug Administration (FDA). *C. difficile* can be avoided by using H_2 blockers and proton pump inhibitors (PPIs) sparingly, and using targeted antibiotic therapy in the least potent dose and duration for infections.

15. **What are some guidelines for prophylaxis against urinary tract infections (UTIs)?**

    Any residual urine in a neurogenic bladder is a culture medium for bacteria to proliferate. Most individuals who have neurogenic bladders either perform intermittent catheterization (IC) or have an indwelling Foley catheter. Invariably, the neurogenic bladder demonstrates asymptomatic pyuria or is colonized with bacteria, but this does not usually indicate a UTI. Chronic low-dose antibiotic chemoprophylaxis is not recommended because of proliferation of resistant bacteria.

    Methods of prophylaxis

    - Keep the bladder drained of urine and avoid allowing the bladder to fill beyond a volume of 400 mL. This should be accomplished by timed voiding, IC, indwelling Foley, or a combination.
    - Keep well hydrated, so that the urine is not concentrated.
    - There is some evidence to indicate that the **organic proanthocyanidins** (OPCs) in cranberries and blueberries cause the bladder wall to become more slippery, thus deterring the adherence of uropathogen bacterial fimbria. This property is not dependent on urine pH. Pure cranberry extract is not very palatable; thus it is often diluted with water and sugar is added. Rather than ingesting large quantities of cranberry cocktail, it is advised to take concentrated cranberry capsules instead. The use of this supplement, however, has not been proven effective in patients with neurogenic bladder.
    - **Methenamine** is a medication that is hydrolyzed in acidic urine to form formaldehyde, which inhibits most bacteria; exceptions include urea-splitting bacteria such as *Proteus* and *Pseudomonas*. However, it works only in the presence of a urine pH less than 6.5.
    - Up to 1000 mg of **ascorbic acid** (vitamin C) per day may assist in acidification of the urine, and doses above that should be avoided because of risk of developing nephrolithiasis.
    - Consider daily irrigation of the bladder with normal saline or **Renacidin**. If this is not sufficient, irrigation with an antibiotic such as **gentamicin** may be indicated.

16. **Why do individuals with SCI or TBI seem to produce greater volumes of urine at night versus during the day?**

    Although the precise mechanism is not known, there can often be a loss of nocturnal component of the diurnal surge of antidiuretic hormone (ADH) after neurotrauma. With the use of a nasal spray of **desmopressin** before bedtime, more than 90% of individuals with loss of nocturnal ADH surge can be successfully treated. Within a couple of days, the treatment can cause greater production of urine during the day instead of at night. This is especially beneficial in individuals performing IC for neurogenic bladder management. Additionally, after a person has been upright during the day, there is remobilization of fluid in the evening, leading to the production of greater volumes of urine at night.

17. **Nonsteroidal anti-inflammatory drugs (NSAIDs) continue to be the most widely used drugs in musculoskeletal medicine. Describe the mechanism of action and precautions when prescribing NSAIDS.**

NSAIDs inhibit prostaglandin synthesis by blocking the **cyclo-oxygenase** enzyme and therefore decrease pain, inflammation, and fever. The inhibition of gastroprotective prostaglandins is associated with gastric ulcers. NSAIDs have a **ceiling effect** for pain relief. For example, the maximum analgesic effect may occur with 600 mg q6h (pain relief may not be improved with increased dosing and side effects may increase), whereas the maximum anti-inflammatory effects may occur at 800 mg every 8 hours. Individuals may respond better to one NSAID over another.

NSAIDs are **contraindicated** in patients with active peptic ulcer, women who are pregnant or breastfeeding, and persons taking anticoagulants or having an inherent defect in coagulation (due to their platelet effects). Aspirin is contraindicated in children under 16 years of age (Reye's syndrome) and patients with aspirin allergy. **Relative contraindications** include asthma and renal, hepatic, or cardiac impairments.

COX II inhibitors: Cyclo-oxygenase II is an inducible isoform of the enzyme present at inflammatory sites. Selective inhibition of inflammatory prostaglandins provides anti-inflammatory effects with less interference on the prostaglandins that protect the stomach. Studies demonstrate less stomach ulceration than nonselective agents. No studies have demonstrated improved analgesia/anti-inflammatory properties when compared to nonselective agents. Most have been removed from the market secondary to safety concerns and side effects including increased risk of stroke and myocardial infarction. **Nabumetone** (Relafen) and **diclofenac** (Voltaren) are relatively more COX-II selective than other NSAIDs.

Ketorolac (Toradol) is used primarily as a postoperative analgesic in lieu of narcotics in patients where morphine and its derivatives are relatively contraindicated. Given the high risk of side effects, use for a limited time of 5 days or less.

18. **What are some important metabolic considerations in patients prone to repetitive or poorly healing pressure ulcers?**

- **Nutrition**. Adequate protein intake is imperative for high-density collagen matrix protein synthesis required for wound healing. Because the very presence of an open wound causes a catabolic state, most sources recommend 1.5–2 mg/kg/day of protein.
- **Appetite. Megestrol acetate** (Megace) is FDA approved for appetite stimulation. It is a progesterone and glucocorticoid analog and can therefore cause lean tissue catabolism, hyperglycemia, and adipose weight gain. It can also deplete testosterone levels, thus resulting in decreased endogenous anabolic stimulus for protein synthesis, poor skin turgor, and further risk of skin breakdown, osteoporosis, muscle wasting, and depression.
- **Anabolic hormone analog agent. Oxandrolone** is FDA approved as an adjunct medication for weight loss from a variety of etiologies and has been shown to increase lean body mass from enhanced protein synthesis. It also stimulates fibroblasts to produce the collagen that heals wounds. Low albumin is a marker for malnutrition, and low levels correlate with the presence, severity, and lack of healing of pressure ulcers. Oxandrolone is a testosterone analog with anabolic but few androgenic properties. Oxandrolone's anabolic to androgenic ratio is 16:1. It should not be given with an elevated prostate-specific antigen (PSA). It also will potentiate warfarin.
- **Testosterone**. Low levels can result from a multitude of etiologies such as SCI, advanced age, malnutrition, opioid use, or catabolic stress from pressure ulcers or multitrauma. PSA must be checked before the decision to prescribe at physiologic levels.

19. **Describe some of the anticholinergic medications and medications with anticholinergic side effects.**

Use the following medications with caution in the rehabilitation patient:

- **Oxybutynin, propantheline,** and **tolterodine** are anticholinergic agents used for bladder spasms and urinary incontinence because they decrease urge incontinence. Tolterodine is more selective for receptors in the bladder and may cause less dry mouth, constipation, and orthostatic hypotension.
- **Benztropine,** an anticholinergic agent, is used for extrapyramidal side effects associated with neuroleptic agents such as quetiapine, risperidone, or olanzapine.
- TCAs **amitriptyline, imipramine, nortriptyline,** and **desipramine** have been used for sleep, migraine headaches, and neuropathic pain. **Amitriptyline** produces significant anticholinergic side effects, dry mouth, blurred vision, constipation, and urinary retention, as well as orthostatic hypotension, whereas **imipramine, nortriptyline,** and **desipramine** have moderate to low side effects.
- **Diphenhydramine** and **chlorpheniramine** are used for allergy symptoms and are associated with significant anticholinergic side effects. **Hydroxyzine,** used for allergy symptoms and anxiety, as well as **cyproheptadine,** used for appetite stimulation, have moderate anticholinergic side effects.

20. **Is there a difference between muscle antispasmodics and antispasticity medications? What are the options and best choices for my patients?**
    Medications such as **cyclobenzaprine** (Flexeril), **carisoprodol** (Soma), and **methocarbamol** (Robaxin) are spasmolytic agents intended for transient muscle relaxation. These agents are not intended or effective for spasticity. Oral antispasticity medications include the following:

- **Baclofen** is a short-acting GABA analog that is dosed up to four times a day and is usually the first choice for both spinal and brain-mediated spasticity. Recommended maximum dosing is 80 mg/day, although some clinicians prescribe more. Higher doses may exacerbate sleep apnea and respiratory depression. Side effects also include fatigue and clouded mental status, although these usually resolve with time. Seizures may occur with abrupt discontinuation.
- **Diazepam** (Valium) is a benzodiazepine effective for attenuating spasticity.
- **Tizanidine** (Zanaflex) is an α_2-agonist similar to clonidine, although its effect on blood pressure is mild. It has a short half-life and therefore is dosed three to four times daily. Side effects include sedation and headache. Start at night with 4 mg and titrate up to maximum doses of 8–12 mg; do not exceed 32 mg/day.
- **Clonidine** is also an α_2-agonist, but its side effects of hypotension and rebound hypertension make it less popular than tizanidine as a spasticity medication.
- **Gabapentin,** a GABA analog, is FDA approved as an adjunct for partial seizures, but it is also used for neuropathic pain and spasticity. Efficacy above 600 mg four times daily has not been shown for neuropathic pain. It has a saturable absorption process per dose. It is excreted by the kidneys; therefore, the dose needs to be adjusted for renal dysfunction.
- **Lamotrigine** (Lamictal) is an antiepileptic drug of the phenyltriazine class that can be effective as an adjuvant for spasticity, but rash is a major side effect that can lead to Stevens-Johnson syndrome. This can be minimized by slowly titrating up the dose.
- **Dantrolene** is the only peripherally acting antispasticity medication, which works by decreasing the amount of calcium release at the sarcoplasmic reticulum. Known to weaken the diaphragm, this medicine should be used cautiously with SCI. Liver function tests must be monitored regularly.
- **Botulinum toxin A/B** irreversibly blocks neuromuscular junction transmission by inhibiting presynaptic acetylcholine release. Each injection lasts approximately 3–6 months, with no known long-term effects.
- **Alcohol/phenol nerve blocks** permanently denature protein in nerve fibers, thereby decreasing muscle contraction.
- **An intrathecal baclofen pump** can be considered when a patient is at the maximum dosing of oral baclofen, is requiring multiple antispasticity medications, or is having significant systemic side effects from the antispasticity medications.

KEY POINTS: MEDICATIONS IN REHABILITATION

1. Review problem list not only for diagnoses but also impairments, activity limitations, and barriers to participation that may respond to medications.

2. Add medications one at a time guided by pertinent indications and expected effectiveness.

3. Monitor for therapeutic results using sensitive measures and multiple baseline assessments and individualized single-subject designs.

4. Reduce and remove medications that are causing side effects or are no longer needed or ineffective.

5. Reinforce compliance with simplified regimens, education or mechanisms, and data documenting effectiveness.

21. **Describe some considerations used when determining if a patient is a candidate for an intrathecal baclofen pump.**

    An intrathecal baclofen pump can be considered when a patient is at the maximum dosing of oral baclofen, is requiring multiple antispasticity medications, or is having significant systemic side effects from the antispasticity medications. The patient must weigh more than 30 lb. Because of the stability of baclofen, it is recommended that pump refills are done at least every 6 months (more frequently if the patient requires higher doses). Patients should always be instructed on the symptoms of overdose and withdrawal of baclofen in case of mechanical pump irregularities or failure. In case of pump failure, patients should also be given a prescription for oral baclofen to prevent acute withdrawal (a life-threatening event).

    www.apparelyzed.com/support/baclofen-pump/baclofen-pump.html

22. **Name some medications that have potentially deleterious implications for rehabilitation patients.**

    - **Amiodarone** has high iodine content, and patients must be monitored for development of hypothyroidism. It can cause pulmonary fibrosis, hepatotoxicity, peripheral neuropathy, and decreased vision (from corneal deposits) and has many drug interactions, most notably digoxin and warfarin.
    - **Meperidine (Demerol)** is metabolized to an active metabolite, **normeperidine**. Because of its long half-life, it accumulates with frequent and high-dose use and in patients with renal dysfunction. Normeperidine can provoke seizures, anxiety, tremors, and myoclonus.

23. **Many patients take a variety of "natural" supplements. Give some considerations when advising patients about these medications.**

    Herbal preparations, minerals, vitamins, botanical phytomedicines (including herbals), and nutraceuticals are commonly used by patients. These are not regulated by the FDA; therefore, the potency and consistency of the supplements may not be known. Some of these "natural" supplements can even have adverse effects and drug–herb interactions with commonly prescribed medications. A few examples include:

    - **St. John's Wort *(Hypericum perforatum)*** has a theoretical interaction with many antidepressants (increased risk of serotonin syndrome), warfarin (decreased INR), and digoxin (decreased effectiveness) among others.
    - **Ephedra (ma huang)** can cause hypertension, insomnia, arrhythmia, nervousness, tremor, headache, seizure, cerebrovascular event, myocardial infarction, and kidney stones and should be avoided with caffeine, decongestants, and stimulants.

- **Kava** can cause sedation and movement disorders and should be avoided with sleeping medications, antipsychotics, and alcohol.
- **Ginkgo biloba** should be avoided when taking any blood thinners, including aspirin, warfarin (Coumadin), ticlopidine (Ticlid), clopidogrel (Plavix), and dipyridamole (Persantine).
- Remember the rule of G's; many herbals that start with the letter G commonly interact adversely with **warfarin:** garlic, ginger, ginkgo, and green tea. There is a decrease in INR with ginseng.

www.mayoclinic.com/health/herbal-supplements/SA00039

CHAPTER 25

ASSISTIVE TECHNOLOGIES: CATALYSTS FOR ADAPTIVE FUNCTION

Michael L. Boninger, MD, Howard Choi, MD, MPH, Kurt Johnson, PhD, Mark A. Young, MD, MBA, Steven A. Stiens, MD, MS, and Andrew Sears, PhD

Any sufficiently advanced technology is indistinguishable from magic.

–Arthur C. Clarke (1917–)

1. **How is assistive technology (AT) employed as a therapeutic tool?**

   AT is a potent tool utilized to modify disablement. It may be used by people with disabilities to increase independent function and participation in preferred activities. AT can help to minimize disability and disablement by catalyzing activity and participation. A person with a disability benefits from AT in several important dimensions: within his or her own body (e.g., cochlear implant to enhance hearing), in direct contact (e.g., wheelchair to improve mobility), and in the intermediate environment (e.g., a ceiling-mounted track lift to facilitate transfers and propulsion from bed to toilet and surrounding space). Because rehabilitation physicians are often obligated to approve and sign off on AT prescriptions, a full understanding of the prescribed technology is essential.

   Stiens SA: Personhood, disablement, and mobility technology: Personal control of development. In Gry DB, Quatrano LA, Lieberman M (eds): Designing and Using Assistive Technology: The Human Perspective. Towson, MD, Paul Brookes, 1998, pp 29–49.

2. **Is there an official definition for "assistive technology"?**

   The U.S. government defines AT in Public Law 100-407 (Assistive Technology Act, 2004) as "Any item, piece of equipment or product system whether commercially off the shelf, modified, or customized that is used to increase or improve functional capabilities of individuals with disabilities." This definition highlights a most important point—that AT is used to improve function. Human function can be broken down into the broad categories of sensing, processing, and effecting. Each of these functions can either be augmented by, or substituted for, using AT. Examples of AT range from robotic arms and power wheelchairs to voice recognition software and eyeglasses. The legal definition of AT also includes those services necessary to effect implementation of AT, reflecting the importance of including these services in any AT prescription and/or plan and the concerns that without these services, AT will be abandoned.

   Young MA, Levi S, Tumanon RC, et al: Independence for people with disabilities: A physician's primer on assistive technology. Md Med 1(3):28–32, 2000.

3. **Provide three examples of accessible electronic and information technology?**

   Accessible electronic and information technology (E&IT) systems allow people with disabilities such as color blindness, learning disabilities, and limitations in arm and hand function, vision, and hearing to access everything from e-mail to distance learning courses and electronic shopping with or without their AT. Accessibility in the arena of IT can be considered analogous to building ramps in the environment. Examples of information systems include accessible Web portals and Internet sites. These sites employ accessibility features, including text equivalents for nontext features (e.g., audio, video, graphics). A blind person, with the help of a screen reader program (one form of AT), will be able to hear the textual description of a picture on an accessible website. (See Chapter 6 for more details about AT solutions for blindness.) Similar modifications work for multimedia products such as CDs, videotapes, and DVDs.

Access IT, Technical Assistance Project, University of Washington: www.washington.edu/accessit

4. **Are employers and schools required to provide AT?**
   Under the Americans with Disabilities Act and various state laws, employers are required to make reasonable accommodations for qualified employees with disabilities who are otherwise able to perform the essential functions of the job. AT is considered one kind of reasonable accommodation and may include assisted listening devices, specialized software, or other technology in addition to non–technology-based accommodations such as breaks for fatigue and modifications of desks. For children with disabilities, section 504 of the Rehabilitation Act requires that they receive reasonable accommodation so that they can participate in the least restrictive educational environment; and the Individuals with Disabilities Education Act (IDEA) requires that qualified students with disabilities receive those services necessary for them to proceed toward the goals of their individualized education plans. AT must be considered in plans under both Section 504 and IDEA.

5. **What is an environmental control unit (ECU)?**
   ECUs are a form of AT that controls an object or objects in a person's environment. Commonly used ECUs include controls for doors, house lights, televisions, home appliances, and hospital-type beds, among others. (Always remember that AT and ECUs refer to the disabled population only. The same types of devices employed by a nondisabled person are not referred to by these terms.) ECUs are comprised of five elements: the switch device, control device, connection, target device(s), and feedback device. The control device detects a signal from the switch, then transforms the signal and sends it through a connection to a target device to perform a function. The user is then alerted that the function has successfully been engaged or completed through feedback, such as the channel on the TV changing.

6. **When should an ECU be "prescribed"?**
   Simply put—as soon as possible. Early use (in the acute care hospital) of an ECU by a patient with a high spinal cord injury can reduce frustration by putting the patient back in control, reducing nurse workload, and teaching the patient that rehabilitation has functional rewards. Adaptive success with AT promotes future steps with other functional technologies after discharge. In the acute care setting, the ECU can control the nurse call, TV, and lights immediately by putting the patient into an "I can do it" paradigm. With the assistance of ECUs, many persons with severe mobility limitations and other disabilities have had the option to avoid institutionalization and live safely and comfortably in their own homes. Children, in particular, learn by doing with AT and therefore may have less dependent behavior or express less frustration. Geriatric patients at nursing homes also have been shown to benefit from access to an ECU. Outcome studies to demonstrate the expected cost savings are needed. Funding from medical insurance or public programs may be difficult to obtain, and support often comes from community groups, such as religious organizations or private foundations. Increasingly effective and adaptable ECUs are available for mainstream applications off the shelf in home improvement stores.

7. **Define augmentative and alternative communication (AAC).**
   AAC devices either augment or replace communication. For example, an individual unable to generate sufficient vocal volume might use a portable voice amplifier to augment communication. An individual on respiratory support who is temporarily unable to speak might use a vocabulary board to replace absent speech. For individuals with more persistent communication deficits, a variety of strategies are available depending on the individual's developmental stage, communication demands, communication context, and abilities. Examples

range from simple devices on which buttons with graphics/images are pressed to generate chunks of synthesized speech (e.g., "I am hungry") to elaborate devices that allow the individual to compose complex messages. Individuals who may be candidates for AAC include children and adults with cerebral palsy, individuals who have survived strokes or a head injury, and adults with progressive neuromuscular diseases such as amyotrophic lateral sclerosis (ALS).

8. **What is the problem with AAC devices?**
Unfortunately, for even the most proficient user, AAC is painfully slow. Individuals without impairment generate spoken speech at rates of 150–200 words per minute, whereas proficient AAC users may generate 10–12 words per minute and often must compose messages prior to speaking. Successful implementation requires significant support from a speech pathologist who can both program devices and train users and family members. Methods have been developed to increase the rate of word production (see question 12). These rate-enhancing systems can require considerable cognitive ability, and even with rate enhancement, word output rates remain low. As a result of this disparity, speaking individuals may dominate conversations; new rules of communication need to be learned by everyone.

9. **Give some examples of AT devices for persons with special sensory impairments (e.g., hearing and/or visually impaired).**
   - **Amplification devices:** Have been the mainstay for people who are hard of hearing. Advances in digital hearing aids have allowed users to manipulate the spectrum of sound to attenuate noise in public places and hook telephones/cell phones and other devices directly to their hearing aids. Also, there have been significant advances in large area amplification, such as classrooms and theaters.
   - **Telephone devices for the deaf** (TDD; commonly referred to by the historic initials TTY): Use QWERTY keyboards outfitted with text displays for incoming messages that connect to standard phone lines. Two TDD users can communicate with each other independently. A deaf user wishing to "speak" with any non-TTD user can do so using a voice carry-over relay service, which voices outgoing messages while textually displaying incoming messages. Relay services exist in each state, allowing TTD users and people who hear to communicate. Recently, there have been rapid advances in the use of cell phones enabled for text messaging as well as Blackberry and Sidekick technology. For many groups of people who are deaf, these flexible platforms have nearly replaced TTD.
   - **Low-tech vision aids:** There are a number of low-tech vision aids that may be useful to people with blindness, low vision, or difficulties with recognition (e.g., stroke). Examples include talking watches, calculators, and money identifiers. Kiosks, ATMs, and other public information systems increasingly offer accessibility features such as speech output. For people with low vision, there are closed circuit televisions (CCTVs), which magnify print material and allow control over contrast.
   - **Screen readers:** For visually impaired individuals incapable of reading text, there are screen readers that can read aloud electronic text, such as word documents and Web pages.

10. **How are AT devices such as ECUs and AAC controlled?**
The human operator controls the AT through movement, muscle activation, or voice. If a person can move it, AT can use it. The effectiveness of each control point is related not only to gross and fine motor control, but also to a person's cognitive and sensory ability. Movements interact with the AT device by way of switches. These switches or control interfaces can take numerous forms. Simple switches may vary dramatically in size to allow for problems with motor control. Each switch can have multiple positions or can be placed in series with another device, such as a scanner.
   One important example is the **sip-and-puff switch,** which involves blowing into and sucking on a straw to activate the switch. It is generally indicated for persons with unreliable head movements and profound loss of motor control of the body. It may also be indicated if repetitive

head movements are uncomfortable or cause overuse syndromes. Persons with C1 and C2 spinal cord injuries typically use sip and puff, whereas persons with C3 and C4 spinal cord injuries may opt to use chin controls or mouthsticks. Microswitches requiring minimal effort are increasingly popular, as are switches that can be activated by electromyography.

11. **How can AT be used to access a computer?**
Computers themselves may serve as AT. For example, a lightweight notebook computer may provide a mode for notetaking and remembering. There are a variety of ways to modify interactions with the computer. For example, input may be accommodated by using modified keyboards, substituting voice for keyboard, substituting sip-and-puff Morse code for keyboarding, using on-screen keyboards activated by eye gaze, or pointing devices manipulated with the mouth, a head-mounted laser, or trackable dot. The display can be manipulated to increase contrast, size of text, or even size of the display itself. For people who are easily distracted (e.g., those with attention deficit disorder, survivors of brain injury), the display environment may be simplified so that the focus is on salient tasks. Computer output can be modified so that the contents of the screen are sent to a Braille display employing electromechanically raised dots or speech output. Pointing devices can be accommodated so that a joystick or trackball replaces the mouse, or mouse buttons can be separated and activated by other types of switches. For people with very limited options, single switches and scanning of the computer desktop and/or on-screen keyboard can provide very slow access.

12. **How can speed of input be increased?**
For AAC devices and computer access, the rate of typing or ability to access the graphical interface is critical. For people with a disability who can only access a single switch, scan technology can be used to select letters or icons on a screen. The user is presented with rows of letters that are highlighted sequentially. The switch is hit when the row with the desired letter is highlighted. The individual letters are then scanned, and the switch is hit when the desired letter is highlighted. For icon selection, quadrants of the screens are sequentially highlighted and selected to isolate individual icons. For individuals who can use more than a single switch, it is possible to increase the rate of typing. A very fast way of typing for single switch users is Morse code; however, this strategy is not widely popular.

When input speed is below 10 words per minute, **word prediction** should be considered. Word prediction can also be useful for individuals with reading disabilities who have difficulty generating the correctly spelled word but can recognize the word in a list. In word prediction, as one starts typing, the system anticipates the word or phrase and proposes a series of choices in a list. Once the preferred choice appears, one clicks on the choice, and the word or phrase moves into the text.

13. **How is voice recognition used in AT?**
Voice recognition has improved dramatically. Under the best of circumstances, speakers who are fluent and use a standard voice can achieve dictation rates of well over 100 words per minute with nearly 100% accuracy after as little as 15 minutes of training the system to their voice. However, for most users, dictation rates are substantially lower, and error rates are much higher. Voice recognition systems can often be used entirely hands-free but are most effective when the user can incorporate some keyboard and mouse commands. With an expert programming the system, individuals on ventilators may be able to use voice recognition systems.

Voice recognition presents some unique cognitive challenges. It adds a cognitive load that may be difficult for patients with limited cognitive resources. Also, proofreading becomes an entirely different task because the errors are not in spelling but rather in word choice. The reliability of voice recognition decreases with fluctuations in voice quality and increases with background noise or when the user has a noticeable accent. Because voice recognition accuracy increases as the size of the vocabulary decreases, this technology can be very effective for applications that can be supported with a limited number of words or commands (e.g., an environmental control unit). This technology can be liberating or disabling and must be carefully and appropriately recommended. The demands of commercial industry and perpetual improvements in microprocessor technology will ensure that voice recognition technology continues to improve.

14. **How can the Internet aid AT?**
The Internet can be of profound importance to individuals with disabilities. It can provide a means to communicate with family members, participate in school, perform elements of jobs, talk with other people with disabilities, conduct research about their condition, or play games. For people with many disabilities, the Internet can be a "barrier-free" environment. People with disabilities can present themselves in written text, selected pictures, and music without displacing their adaptive reference to their disability, functional limitations, or AT. For example, e-mail in combination with appropriate AT allows deaf students and blind students to talk to each other on campus. For people with severe dysarthria, the disability can become irrelevant when e-mail is used to communicate. Providing patients with Internet access and the AT necessary to access the Internet should be a top priority for clinicians.

15. **Can robots be the perfect AT solution?**
Perhaps eventually, but not necessarily soon. Robotic technology has been developed that clearly can be of benefit for people with disabilities; however, high costs and difficulties with control limit its practicality. Past and present generation robots do not seem to perform well outside of very controlled environments and fail at some of the most basic tasks. Some will recall the experiments a few years ago when the most sophisticated research robots were pitted against two-year-old toddlers. The robots had great difficulty at tasks, such as picking up a red ball out of a group of other objects, whereas the feisty tykes accomplished the tasks with ease. In these days of cost cutting in medicine, cost-benefit analyses will have to demonstrate that routine use of advanced technologies such as robots is warranted. An alternative to consider for some limited tasks might be animal-assisted therapy.

KEY POINTS: ASSISTIVE DEVICES

1. ECUs consist of five elements: the switch device, control device, connection, target device(s), and feedback device.

2. Internet communication has enhanced the lives of people with disability.

3. Appropriate AT can significantly enhance a patient's ability to meaningfully participate in society. Knowledge of this important topic is a key tool for physiatrists.

4. Providing Internet/computer access is essential and possible through devices such as special keyboards or voice activation software for motor impairments and screen readers for sensory impairment.

16. **Are there devices that can help with cognitive problems such as memory loss?**
Low-tech devices such as **memory books** have been used for years to serve as compensatory tools for people with cognitive deficits. Recent advances in technology associated with **personal digital assistants** and **smart phones** make sophisticated reminding and cueing systems readily available. Unfortunately, because of the complexity of the interfaces, successful users are likely to be individuals who were proficient with the devices prior to disability. Rapidly

emerging technologies will combine these devices with ubiquitous computing, wearable sensors, and other technologies to provide highly flexible, context-driven tools to support memory, task performance, and appropriate social interaction.

17. Why do AT devices sometimes fail or their users abandon them?

A patient's motivation and potential for use of an assistive device (gadget tolerance) may be underestimated or overestimated by the caregiver(s) or rehabilitation team. Often, a potential user or the rehabilitation team will have unrealistic expectations about a device. The capabilities of, and the skills necessary to use, a device should be understood before committing to any specific solution. If possible, equipment trials with adequate provisions for training are helpful. Specialized centers often have sample devices that are adjustable for individual trials. They are also likely to have therapists or technicians familiar with the products who can train and comprehensively evaluate the device with the patient before a final commitment.

Patient preference and self-image should be considered high priorities. Frequently, a device's aesthetic appearance may be the sole reason it is not used. Items that draw adverse attention, such as loud alarms used as reminders for pressure relief, rapidly fall into disuse. Some devices simply do not accomplish their intended goals due to faulty design. Others can cause fatigue or overuse injury, even with optimal usage techniques. Devices can be unreliable or prone to mechanical breakdown. In general, the more complicated a gizmo, the more likely it will break down and the more it will cost to fix it. When possible, encouragement for use of the device should be provided. Reassessments should be made at appropriate intervals. It is also important not to provide too many items at once.

18. How is AT funding appropriated?

Funding of AT depends on the justification. Commercial insurance companies vary widely in their coverage, and many policies consider AT as durable medical equipment. Medicaid coverage varies from state to state depending on the exceptions approved for that state and local policies. Medicare and Medicaid have similar eligibility criteria, which require demonstration of medical necessity, "not experimental," and least costly alternative. State vocational rehabilitation agencies may purchase AT for clients when there is a potential vocational outcome, and K-12 schools may purchase AT as part of the students individualized education plan. For detailed information on funding, go to http://wata.org and click on "Funding."

WEBSITES

1. http://atto.buffalo.edu/

2. www.abilityhub.com/

3. www.resna.org/

4. www.dors.state.md.us/DORS/ProgramServices/AssistiveTech/

5. www.washington.edu/doit/

PHYSICAL AGENTS: DEVICES AND APPLICATIONS

CHAPTER 26

Jeffrey R. Basford, MD, PhD, and Veronika Fialka-Moser, MD

The important thing in science is not so much to obtain new facts as to discover new ways of thinking about them.

–Sir William Bragg (1862–1942)

1. **What is a modality?**
   A physical agent that uses physical forces to accomplish a therapeutic goal is a modality. In theory, any physical phenomenon (e.g., pressure, heat, cold, electricity, sound, light) may be utilized. In practice, all are used, but some (such as heat, cold, water, ultrasound, shortwaves, electricity, and pressure) are more common and more accepted than others (e.g., laser). These agents are, in essence, quite simple and, for the most part, produce only a limited number of effects: heating, cooling, analgesia, muscle movement, and tissue healing. The popularity of specific modalities fluctuates with time. Currently, although use of agents such as ultrasound has increased, heat and cold remain the basis of most treatments.

2. **Are physical agents used alone?**
   Physical agents are seldom used in isolation and are almost always an adjunct to a comprehensive therapy program that may also involve exercise, stretching, and education. As such, they may be viewed as a means to permit the patient to participate more fully and more rapidly in the program's other components.

3. **What are the limitations of the physical agents?**
   Although each agent has unique characteristics, many ultimately rely on heating or cooling to gain their effects. As a result, they share common restrictions in that temperatures above 45°C (100°F) or below 0°C (32°F) may injure tissue. In practice, treatments involving these temperatures are used for restricted portions of the body, but broader areas are treated less intensely.

HEAT AND COLD

4. **How do physical agents heat or cool tissue?**
   There are only three ways that tissue temperature can be altered:
   - **Conduction** is defined as the transfer of heat between two bodies in contact at different temperatures. Examples include hot packs and paraffin baths.
   - **Convection** also involves contact between two objects at different temperatures but also requires that one flow past the other. This flow maximizes the temperature gradient between the objects (e.g., a whirlpool bath), so more intense heating and cooling are possible than by conduction alone.
   - **Conversion** utilizes the conversion of another form of energy to heat. Heat lamps, radio waves, and ultrasound (US), for example, rely on the conversion of infrared light and sound to heat.

5. **What forms of heat therapy are available?**
Superficial and deep. Superficial agents (e.g., heat lamp) heat the skin and subcutaneous tissues. Deep heating agents (e.g., US, short waves), also known as diathermies, heat more deeply and can raise temperatures to therapeutic levels at depths of 3.5–7 cm.

6. **What forms of cold therapy (cryotherapy) are available?**
Cold is produced by the relative absence of thermal energy. Because a lack of energy cannot be projected, only superficial agents such as ice can be used. Conversive cooling is therefore not possible, and cooling therapies must rely on conduction and convection.

7. **List five general goals of heat and cryotherapy.**
See Table 26-1.

TABLE 26-1. GENERAL GOALS OF HEAT THERAPY AND CRYOTHERAPY

Heat Therapy	Cryotherapy
1. Analgesia	1. Analgesia
2. Muscle "spasm" relaxation	2. Muscle "spasm" relaxation
3. Hyperemia	3. Inflammation
4. Increased collagen extensibility	4. Spasticity
5. Acceleration of metabolic processes	5. Slowing of metabolic activity

8. **Name the major contraindications to therapeutic heat.**
- Acute hemorrhage, inflammation, or trauma
- Ischemia
- Insensitivity/inability to respond to pain
- Malignancy (poorly documented)
- Bleeding dyscrasias
- Atrophic or scarred skin

9. **List four common superficial heating agents.**
Hot packs, heat lamps, hot-water soaks/whirlpools, and paraffin baths.

10. **Describe the use of hot packs.**
Hot packs are typically maintained in water baths at 70–80°C (168–175°F). During use, the packs are taken from the baths and, after excess water is drained off, placed in an insulated cover and *laid on, not under,* the patient. Packs typically maintain therapeutically useful temperatures for 20–30 minutes. Mud packs contain materials that may have slightly different thermodynamic properties and purported medicinal benefits because of the nature of the filling material.

11. **What should I know about heat lamps?**
- There is no proof that special infrared (IR) heating elements are clinically more effective than standard incandescent bulbs.
- Most lamps act as "point" or "linear" sources; their heating effectiveness decreases with distance (d) by $1/d^2$ or $1/d$, respectively.
- Heat can produce reddish or brownish skin mottling (erythema ab igne), which may advance to permanent skin discoloration.
- In practice, many heat lamps use 100–150 W bulbs and are placed 50–75 cm from the body.

12. **How are paraffin baths used?**

Paraffin baths consist of 1:7 mixtures of mineral oil and paraffin maintained at about 52°C. Treatment commonly takes one of three forms. Dipping (the most common) involves placing the part to be treated in the bath, removing it, pausing briefly to let the wax harden, and then repeating the cycle 10 times. The treated area is then covered with a plastic sheet and an insulating mitt for about 20 minutes. Immersion provides more vigorous heating and entails dipping the area into paraffin several times and then keeping it immersed for about 20 minutes. The third method uses a brush to paint paraffin onto portions of the body that cannot be easily placed in a bath.

Paraffin baths are widely used to treat patients with rheumatoid arthritis of the hands who find simpler treatments, such as hot soaks or contrast baths, ineffective. These baths also are used to treat contractures, particularly in the hands and in those with scleroderma. Because paraffin baths are essentially filled with molten wax, bath temperatures must be monitored carefully to avoid burns.

13. **What are contrast baths? How are they used?**

Contrast baths consist of two reservoirs filled with water, one usually warm (43°C) and the other cool (16°C). Treatment usually is limited to the hands or feet and typically begins with a 10-minute soak in the warm bath and then cycles between the two baths. Soaking duration varies but is often about 4 minutes in the warm bath and 1–2 minutes in the cool bath.

14. **Why are contrast baths used?**

Contrast baths are used primarily for their purported desensitization and vasogenic reflex effects and are most often employed in patients with rheumatoid arthritis and neuropathic or autonomic pain (e.g., complex regional pain syndrome 1 [CRPS1]). Bath temperatures are adjusted to the patient; treatment of the feet and CRPS may require less extreme initial temperatures.

15. **Which superficial heating agent is the most beneficial?**

No agent is clearly the most beneficial, but a therapist or patient might prefer one (e.g., moist versus dry) over the other.

16. **When is cryotherapy appropriate? How is it performed?**

Ice is the most common form of cryotherapy and is enshrined in the RICE (rest, ice, compression, elevation) approach to the treatment of acute musculoskeletal injury. Ice massage is frequently used for intense treatment of localized areas of musculoskeletal pain such as lateral epicondylitis. Ice slushes and whirlpools are more aggressive and tend to be used mostly by motivated athletes who are willing to tolerate discomfort in the hope of a more rapid recovery. Chemical ice packs and vapocoolant sprays have varying levels of use, the former for acute injuries and the latter in the "spray and stretch" treatment of trigger points.

Knight KL: Cryotherapy: Theory, Technique and Physiology. Chattanooga, TN, Chattanooga Corp., 1985.

17. **What are some of the physiologic effects of cryotherapy?**

Cryotherapy may produce longer-lasting effects than heat. Analgesia, vasoconstriction, and control of the swelling associated with acute injury are the most obvious indications for longer duration (>3 min) cryotherapy, whereas shorter-term cooling has been reported to improve local circulation. Prolonged cooling reduces spasticity and slows both nerve conduction and metabolism.

18. **Name the contraindications of cryotherapy.**

The contraindications for cryotherapy, as for all physical agents, are often relative. Thus, ice massage of a diabetic with neuropathy and atherosclerotic disease might be appropriate for trochanteric bursitis but not for a foot condition. The most common contraindications for cryotherapy include ischemia, Raynaud's syndrome, insensitivity, inability to respond to pain, cryoglobulinemia, cold allergy, and cold-induced pressor responses.

HYDROTHERAPY

19. What do I need to know about whirlpools?

Whirlpools use agitated water to produce convective heating or cooling, massage, and gentle debridement. Unit size, water temperature, agitation intensity, and solvent properties may all be adjusted to meet treatment goals. Water temperature is determined by the amount of the body submerged, the patient's health, and goals of treatment. A hand or limited portion of a limb with intact sensation may tolerate temperatures up to 45°C, but as more of the body is submerged, temperature should decrease, commonly to 40–41°C for immersion to the waist and 38–39°C if most of the body is submerged. The condition of the patient is important; an elderly diabetic would be treated more cautiously than a young athlete.

20. How are wounds treated with hydrotherapy?

Wounds treated with hydrotherapy typically have open areas with necrotic debris, adherent dressings, or contaminated/irregular surfaces and can range from small hand cuts and abrasions to large, secondarily infected, abdominal wounds. Dehiscence is not a contraindication. For example, exposed omentum or intestinal tissues do not prevent treatment if bath temperature, osmolality, and agitation parameters are chosen carefully. Patients with large wounds may be fearful but can be reassured, as correctly adjusted baths are extraordinarily comfortable. Hand-held showerheads, sprays, and dental water jets may be used for more forceful debridement.

21. How can hydrotherapy solvent properties be manipulated? Why?

Warmed tap water (which is amazingly sterile) is usually used alone. Gentle detergents and antiseptic solutions may be added to improve debridement and wound cleansing. Salt can be dissolved in a bath to produce a normal saline (0.9% NaCl) solution to improve comfort and reduce concerns about hemolysis and water intoxication in patients with large open wounds. Carbodioxide baths can improve circulation.

22. List five common indications for hydrotherapy.

1. Open, contaminated wounds
2. Contractures
3. Muscle spasm
4. Burns
5. Morbidly obese, immobilized patients who cannot be cleansed in another manner

ULTRASOUND DIATHERMY

23. What is diathermy, and what are the diathermy agents?

Diathermy ("heating through") is available in three forms: ultrasound, shortwave/decimeter wave, and microwave. All heat tissue conversively. Shortwave diathermy is becoming less common; microwave diathermy, while used at times in a few areas of medicine (e.g., prostate surgery), is now seldom used in therapy.

Basford JR: Physical agents. In DeLisa JA, Gans BM (eds): Rehabilitation Medicine: Principles and Practice, 3rd ed. Philadelphia, Lippincott Williams & Wilkins, 1998, pp 483–504.

24. What are the important characteristics of therapeutic ultrasound?

Ultrasound has all the characteristics of audible sound but is limited to frequencies above the nominal 20,000-Hz limit of human hearing. As such, it requires a medium for transmission and can be focused, reflected, or refracted. Although frequencies between 0.3 and 3 MHz are used, many accept the 0.8–1.0 MHz frequency range as the best trade-off between focusing properties and tissue penetration.

25. **What effects does ultrasound have on the body?**
Heating is the most important effect. Nonthermal effects, such as cavitation, media motion, and standing waves, exist, but their risks/therapeutic benefits are poorly understood. Cavitation, for example, produces bubbles, which are capable of disrupting tissue by their forced oscillation and bursting. Small-scale media motion may occur from ultrasound exposure. Standing-wave patterns in a stationary ultrasound field produce fixed areas of elevated pressure and rarefaction shown to have physiologic effects.

26. **How deeply does ultrasound penetrate into tissue?**
The depth of clinically beneficial heating depends on the power applied, nature of the tissue, and direction/frequency of the beam. For example, 50% of an ultrasound beam may penetrate 7–8 cm of fat but less than 1 mm of bone. Direction may also be important: an ultrasound beam may penetrate 7 cm when traveling parallel to the fibers of a muscle but only 2 cm when traveling perpendicularly. Frequency also has striking effects. Beam penetration in tissue may fall by about 85% as its frequency increases from 0.3 to 3.3 MHz. In practice, therapeutic ultrasound sources with frequencies of 0.8–1.0 MHz can produce 4–5°C temperature elevations at depths of 8 cm.

27. **Where does the most intense heating take place during ultrasound treatment?**
Ultrasound can heat skin, fat, muscle, and bone with the most pronounced heating occurring at tissue interfaces. Bone soft tissue discontinuities produce the most intensive areas of heating. Most people are careful in these situations and avoid treatment in the vicinity of laminectomies.

28. **How is ultrasound applied?**
Acoustic gels or mineral oil are typically used to provide optimal acoustic coupling, with treatment performed with circular stroking of the applicator. Irregular body surfaces are sometimes submerged in degassed water, and an applicator is moved in a slightly offset manner over the surface. Ultrasound can produce intense heating and requires the constant attention of the therapist. Treatments are relatively brief, with durations of 7–15 minutes, and may be continuous or pulsed in nature. Dosage depends on location and goals. Treatments that emphasize tissue heating typically involve intensities of 0.5–1.5 W/cm^2, whereas those that focus on ultrasound's nonthermal properties tend to utilize much lower intensities.

29. **What is phonophoresis?**
Phonophoresis is a US technique in which medication is mixed with the acoustic-coupling medium in the expectation that the US beam will "drive" the pharmacologically active substance into the tissue. Penetration depths depend on the substance involved, and significant amounts of drug are absorbed by the subcutaneous circulation. Clinical studies with topical anesthetics, corticosteroids, phenylbutazone, and chymotrypsin have suggested benefits, but more work is needed to establish the advantage of phonophoresis over injection or US alone.

30. **What are the indications and contraindications for therapeutic ultrasound?**
Indications
Common
- Contractures
- Tendinitis
- Musculoskeletal pain
- Degenerative arthritis
- Carpal tunnel syndrome
- Subacute trauma

Less established
- Wound healing
- Herpes zoster
- Plantar warts

Contraindications
- All general contraindications for therapeutic heat
- Immature or acutely inflamed joints
- Laminectomy sites
- Tumors
- Gravid uterus, eyes and heart

SHORTWAVE AND MICROWAVE

31. What is shortwave diathermy?

Shortwave diathermy (SWD) conversively heats tissue by exposing it to radio waves. Although three frequencies—40.68, 27.12, and 13.56 MHz—have been allocated by the FCC for medical use in the United States, 27.12 MHz is the most commonly used frequency in both Europe and the United States. Typical treatments involve output powers of several hundred watts.

32. How is SWD administered?

Energy is delivered to the body in two ways. Capacitive coupling involves placing the tissue to be treated between two plates to which the shortwave output is applied, and the body thus acts as a dielectric in a series circuit. Heating is most marked in high-impedance, water-poor tissues, such as fat. On the other hand, inductive coupling uses the body as a receiver and induces eddy currents in the tissues in its field. The highest currents, and therefore the most intense heating, occur in low-impedance, water-rich tissues, such as muscle. In practice, intra-muscular temperature elevations of 4–6°C can be obtained at depths of 4–5 cm.

33. Discuss the limitations and contraindications of SWD.

Water and metal are excellent electrical conductors and potentially can cause burns if exposed to SWD. Therefore, patients must remove jewelry, and perspiration must be absorbed by toweling. In theory, metal implants and sutures might produce "hot spots," and their treatment with SWD should be avoided. SWD produces wide fields and precautions with varying degrees of support, including the avoidance of treating pregnant women, the menstruating uterus, or patients with implanted metal devices, pacemakers, defibrillators, pumps, or contact lenses.

34. What is microwave diathermy?

Microwave diathermy (MWD) is similar to SWD in that electromagnetic waves are used to heat tissue but at frequencies 30–100 times higher than those of SWD. MWD was once relatively common but now has, for the most part, been supplanted by ultrasound. In Europe, 2450 MHz MWD is used to provide heating for superficial musculoskeletal pain. MWD continues to have some use for localized hyperthermia in specific surgical and oncologic applications.

35. What are the characteristics/contraindications of MWD?

Microwave beams, because of their higher frequencies, are much more directable than SWD; however, they attenuate more rapidly and often deliver much of their energy to subcutaneous tissue. The contraindications of heat and SWD apply. In particular, microwaves produce cataracts, selectively heat fluid-filled cavities, and may affect the growth plates of immature bones.

ELECTRICAL STIMULATION

36. What is TENS?

Transcutaneous electrical nerve stimulation (TENS) is a form of analgesia that applies small electrical signals to the body with superficial skin electrodes. Electrodes may be placed over peripheral nerves, nerve roots, and acupuncture points, as well as proximal to, distal to, over, and (more controversially) contralateral to the areas of pain. (See Chapter 28, Electrotherapy.)

37. How does TENS produce analgesia?

A uniform mechanism is not established. The "gate theory," in which stimulation of large myelinated afferent fibers blocks the transmission of pain by small unmyelinated fibers at the level of the spinal cord, is often mentioned. Although it seems plausible in many ways, this theory does not explain all aspects of TENS analgesia (e.g., prolonged pain relief following use). Alteration of cerebrospinal endorphin concentrations is also reported following treatment (particularly for high-intensity TENS) but is difficult to correlate with therapeutic response.

38. What is iontophoresis?

Iontophoresis uses charged electrodes (positive or negative) to drive medically active, electrically charged, or polar substances into the skin. Any charged or polar substance can theoretically be phoresed, and medications have included lidocaine, iodine, salicylate, gentamicin, cefoxitin, and silver.

39. What is iontophoresis used for?

Iontophoresis with tap water (referred to as *galvanization* in Europe) is an effective treatment of hyperhidrosis. It has also been used to deliver antibiotics to poorly vascularized tissue, to produce local anesthesia, to speed wound healing, and to treat musculoskeletal pain. Although iontophoresis can be effective, many feel that an injection can provide higher concentrations of an active medication with more speed and less difficulty.

KEY POINTS: PHYSICAL AGENTS

1. Physical agents are essentially quite simple and, for the most part, produce only a limited number of effects, such as heating, cooling, analgesia, and neuromuscular stimulation.

2. Tissue temperatures can be altered in only three ways: by conduction, convection, or conversion of another form of energy to heat.

3. Major contraindications to therapeutic heat include acute hemorrhage, inflammation, or trauma; ischemia; insensitivity/inability to respond to pain; bleeding dyscrasias; atrophic or scarred skin; and malignancy (poorly documented).

4. Ultrasound requires a medium for transmission and can be focused, reflected, or refracted. Although frequencies between 0.3 and 3 MHz are used, many accept the 0.8–1.0 MHz frequency range as the best therapeutic trade-off between focusing properties and tissue penetration.

5. There are three common choices for TENS parameters: high ("conventional") TENS with barely perceptible signal intensities with frequencies of 60–80 Hz; low TENS that uses larger-amplitude, low-frequency (<4–8 Hz) signals; and burst stimulation that uses varying frequencies.

40. **What is low-intensity electrical stimulation?**

TENS is one form of low-intensity electrical stimulation. In addition, a variety of milliampere- and even microampere-current generators have been studied for more than 30 years. Benefits are well established in the treatment of nonhealing fractures, and their use in diabetic ulcers appears promising.

Baker LL, Chambers R, DeMuth SK, Villar F: Effects of electrical stimulation on wound healing in patients with diabetic ulcers. Diabetes Care 20(3):405–412, 1997.

Peters EJ, Lavery LA, Armstrong DG, Fleischli JG: Electric stimulation as an adjunct to heal diabetic foot ulcers: a randomized clinical trial. Arch Phys Med Rehabil 82:721–725, 2001.

41. **Can electrical stimulation increase muscle strength?**

Yes. Electrical stimulation can be used to maintain and increase muscle bulk and strength in immobilized limbs and paretic muscles. Recent research shows that effects in neurologically intact individuals approach those of conventional resistive exercises.

Nuhr MJ, Pette D, Berger R, et al: Beneficial effects of chronic low-frequency stimulation of thigh muscles in patients with advanced chronic heart failure. Eur Heart J 25:136–143, 2004.

Yanagi T, Shiba N, Maeda T, et al: Agonist contractions against electrically stimulated antagonists. Arch Phys Med Rehabil 84(6):843–848, 2003.

42. **What is functional neuromuscular stimulation?**

Functional neuromuscular stimulation, also known as functional electrical stimulation, utilizes electrical stimulation to provide functional movement of paretic muscles. Stimulation may be done in conjunction with orthoses and may involve coordinated stimulation of multiple muscles. Limitations due to complexity, cost, reliability, and safety have restricted its use. Exercise devices for patients with spinal cord injury are the best-known applications of this approach.

43. **What is interferential current (IFC)?**

Electrical waves that differ slightly in frequency can interact with each other and produce product waveforms with frequencies equal to the sum or differences of the original waves. IFC machines take advantage of this phenomena and generate waves at different frequencies (e.g., 2000 and 2040 Hz), which can penetrate tissue without discomfort. Pairs of electrodes associated with each wave are placed so that their waves *interfere* at the site of treatment; in the clinical situation, only the low-frequency "difference" waves are important. IFC can be used to produce TENS effects or stimulate muscle contraction.

PRESSURE

44. **How are pneumatic pumps used?**

Numerous pneumatic devices are available with varying cycling modes and construction. These pumps are often effective in controlling edema but should be used only if elevation and compressive wraps alone are ineffective. Pressure settings depend on the application but are often set between the venous and arterial pressures. Treatment durations are prolonged, and the limb is kept elevated and wrapped in compressive dressings between sessions. Pneumatic pumping is used to improve arterial perfusion in the distal extremities, but its effectiveness is still under investigation.

45. **List four contraindications to pneumatic pumping.**

- Acute deep venous thrombosis
- Cellulitis
- Compromised perfusion
- Severely impaired sensation

46. **What do I need to know about using compressive garments?**
Compressive garments are measured and applied once limb edema has been minimized. Pressures are maximal at the wrist or ankle and lessen proximally in a graduated manner. Garment pressures and style (e.g., calf-high, thigh-high, leotard) are dictated by edema severity and the patient's ability to tolerate and put on the garment. Lower-extremity stockings are typically in the 30–40 mmHg range, with allowances made for sensation, perfusion, and patient compliance. Off-the-shelf garments are usually suitable, although custom-measured garments may be necessary for people who are obese, difficult to fit, or need compression over irregularly shaped locations.

47. **List six common indications for compression garments.**
   - Treated deep venous thrombosis
   - Lymphedema
   - Edema due to congestive heart failure
   - Venous incompetence
   - Postmastectomy edema
   - Orthostatic hypotension (abdominal compression may be helpful; garments must be thigh-length to be effective)

48. **What are some simple rules of thumb about compressive garments?**
   - Use the shortest garment possible.
   - Thigh-length garments slide down the leg without the use of straps or adhesive.
   - Men tend to resist leotards.
   - Garments are more effective and better tolerated with slender people.

ALTERNATIVE AND NEW PHYSICAL AGENTS

49. **How is laser therapy used in physical medicine?**
Low-intensity (also known as "cold" or "low level") laser and monochromatic irradiation have been used for more than 35 years to promote wound healing, to lessen pain, and to speed recovery from musculoskeletal injury. Many devices have been used, but most have powers <100 mW and utilize red (0.6 μm) or infrared (0.82–1.06 μm) wavelengths. Irradiation produces striking effects on cellular processes, immune function, and collagen formation in the laboratory. Proof of efficacy and the choice of optimal clinical parameters remain controversial, but use is widespread; about 20 devices are approved for clinical use in the United States.

   Basford JR: Low intensity laser therapy: still not an established clinical tool. Lasers Surg Med 16:31–42, 1995. www.walt.nu/dose/index.html

50. **Are there other new physical agents or new applications of older agents?**
Yes. Laser therapy perhaps has had the most attention, but other agents and old agents with new uses exist. For example, ultrasound and low-intensity electromagnetic fields accelerate fracture healing. In addition, there are a number of newer agents with, thus far, limited proof of effectiveness. Among these are the use of transcortical electrical stimulation to enhance learning and recovery from brain injury, dynamic magnetic field stimulation to treat painful musculoskeletal conditions, and the use of "micro"-electromagnetic fields to treat a variety of wound and painful conditions.

WEBSITES

1. http://physicaltherapy.about.com/od/abbreviationsandterms/p/Modalities.htm

2. www.aaos.org/wordhtml/papers/advistmt/1010.htm

CHAPTER 27

MANIPULATION, MASSAGE, AND TRACTION: AN OVERVIEW

Steven R. Hinderer, MD, MS, PT, and Peter E. Biglin, DO

It seems a universal human impulse to put our hands to areas of pain or injury.
—Janet R. Kahn, PhD, LMT

1. **Are traction, manipulation, and massage considered important rehabilitative physical modalities?**
   Yes. Traction, manipulation, and massage are considered essential adjunctive healing modalities and are used extensively in physiatric practice. According to the National Center for Complementary and Alternative Medicine (NCCAM), manipulation, massage, and traction are modalities that fall under the umbrella of "manipulative and body-based techniques." This category of treatment is one of five established modes of complementary and alternative medicine (CAM), along with "biological based practices," "energy medicine," "mind body medicine," and "whole medicine systems," that have come to play an important role in physical medicine and rehabilitation (PM&R).

   http://nccam.nih.gov/health/

2. **What techniques are available for applying traction?**
   1. **Manual**—cervical traction performed by the physician or therapist, usually to gauge the effectiveness of mechanical or motorized methods of application
   2. **Mechanical**—administered using a pulley and free weight system
   3. **Motorized**—mechanical traction applied by a motorized system, administered in continuous or intermittent periods
   4. **Gravity**—hanging upside down
   5. **Autotraction**—uses a specially designed device that self-administers lumbar traction by pulling with the arms

3. **What are the physiologic effects of traction?**
   While many studies have shown that elongation of the cervical spine by 2–20 mm can be achieved with 25 lb or more of tractive force, 10 lb are needed to counterbalance the weight of the head (less in some persons, more in others). Prolonged pull on the cervical spine with adequate force may lead to cervical paraspinal muscle fatigue, which may alleviate muscle spasm.

   Although lumbar traction has not been studied as extensively, it promotes elongation when the effects of friction are overcome by adequate pull or a split table. Retraction of herniated disc material is another potential effect of lumbar traction.

4. **What advantages does home mechanical traction have over a clinic-based traction program?**
   Mechanical traction can be administered at home using a pulley and free weight system. Home cervical traction units typically consist of a bag filled with 20 lb or more of water or sand and a pulley system mounted on top of a door. Improper head or neck position and inadequate weight (<20 lb) are the most common reasons home cervical traction fails. Initial instruction and weekly follow-ups by the therapist or physician greatly improve the chances for success.

Administration of continuous or intermittent (timed on-and-off periods) mechanical traction applied with a motorized device is commonly limited to physical therapy clinics because of the need for close monitoring of position and its effect on symptoms. Most patients tolerate greater forces of pull with intermittent administration. Mechanical traction is often prescribed early on in the treatment course and later continued with home traction.

5. **Is there a role for gravity traction?**
Gravity (inversion) traction was touted extensively a few years ago. Its theoretical basis is that body weight, when inverted (by hanging upside down), will distract the lumbar spine. Numerous side effects have been reported, including persistent headaches, blurred vision, petechiae, and numerous musculoskeletal complaints. Along with the potential implications of contraindications associated with these symptoms, one should probably reserve this method for use only with nonhuman primates having back pain.

6. **When prescribing traction, what parameters should be specified?**
   - Positioning
   - Intermittent or continuous administration
   - Amount of pull
   - Duration

   Other modalities to be used concurrently with traction also should be specified and may include methods to facilitate muscle relaxation, which is essential to maximize the therapeutic effects of traction. Hot packs are most commonly prescribed.

7. **Discuss positioning.**
Positioning is a key element of a traction prescription. For **cervical traction,** specification of sitting or supine position should be based on patient comfort. If cervical traction is being administered to relieve symptoms of nerve root compression, 20–30 degrees of flexion will optimally open the intervertebral foramina. Less flexion is required for treatment of muscle spasm in the absence of radicular symptoms.

The supine position with 90 degrees of hip and knee flexion is the most common position for **lumbar traction**. In this position, the lumbar lordosis is maximally reduced with the lower back well supported on the traction table and the spine in a relatively flexed position to facilitate optimal vertebral separation.

8. **What is the difference between intermittent and continuous traction?**
It is thought that a greater force of pull can be tolerated with intermittent, as opposed to continuous, administration. Selection is based on the desired therapeutic effect. If distraction of the spine is desired to open neural foramina or retract herniated disc material, then the greater forces of pull that can be tolerated by intermittent application are more desirable. If the goal is muscle relaxation, then it may be more beneficial to provide the prolonged stretch of continuous traction.

9. **How much pull is usually used and for how long?**
The amount of pull should be specified in the traction prescription. For cervical spine distraction, forces >25 lb need to be achieved, but forces >50 lb probably do not provide any additional advantage. Forces above >50 lb are required with lumbar traction to achieve posterior vertebral separation, and forces >100 lb are required for anterior separation. The countertraction on the chest and shoulders to provide tractive forces over 100 lb is often poorly tolerated by patients.

The duration of a treatment session is usually specified as 20 minutes. Studies seem to support that therapeutic effects are achieved over this time period.

10. **What are the contraindications to traction?**
The potential for cervical ligamentous instability, as might occur with rheumatoid arthritis, Down's syndrome, achondroplastic dwarfism, Marfan syndrome, or previous trauma, are

absolute contraindications. Cervical extension during traction should be avoided, especially in the presence of vertebrobasilar insufficiency. Documented or suspected tumor in the region of the spine, osteopenia, infectious process of the spine or surrounding soft tissue, and pregnancy are also absolute contraindications. Old age is a relative contraindication due to degenerative spine changes.

KEY POINTS: FUNDAMENTALS OF MANUAL TECHNIQUES

1. Manipulation and related manual techniques are modalities recognized by the NCCAM.

2. The goals of manipulation are to optimize motion, relieve pain, promote symmetry, and enhance physical function.

3. Traction N.O. prescriptions must specify precise parameters.

4. The clinician must be aware of potential, absolute, and relative contraindication to traction.

5. Effleurage, pétrissage, and tapotement are the classical types of massage.

11. **What is manipulation?**
Manipulation is defined as the use of hands in the patient management process using instructions and maneuvers to maintain maximal, painless movement of the musculoskeletal system in postural balance.

12. **What are the goals of manipulation?**
The primary goal is to optimize physical function in areas such as gait, activities of daily living, and transfers by maintaining body symmetry, improving motion in restricted areas, and enhancing pain-free motion.

13. **When do you use manipulation?**
Manipulation is used in the presence of a **somatic dysfunction,** which is defined as impaired or altered function of related components of the somatic system, including skeletal, ligamentous, myofascial, related vascular, neural, and lymphatic elements. Somatic dysfunction can be detected on physical exam, as summarized by the acronym
TART:
- **T** = **T**enderness
- **A** = **A**symmetric structure
- **R** = **R**ange of motion abnormalities
- **T** = **T**issue texture changes

14. **In which conditions might manipulation prove helpful?**
Manipulation can be helpful, when appropriate, in the following conditions:
- Acute or chronic back and neck pain
- Rib pain
- Bulging intervertebral discs
- Facet syndrome
- Piriformis syndrome
- Sciatica
- Headaches
- Sacroiliac syndrome

15. **When is a massage medium required?**
A massage medium is used to reduce friction over the skin. Examples include mineral oil, glycerin, coconut oil, cocoa butter, Nivea® cream, and baby powder. Such media are used when the massage is intended for edema reduction, relaxation/sedation, or relief of muscle spasm/tightness. When the massage is used to loosen or stretch scar tissue, fascia, or subcutaneous tissue, no medium is used, allowing the therapist to gain purchase on and move appropriate tissue structures.

16. **What are commonly used techniques of therapeutic massage?**
Classical massage involves stroking and gliding movements **(effleurage),** kneading **(pétrissage),** and percussion **(tapotement)**. Stroking, gliding, and friction movements are helpful for locating areas of muscle spasm or focal pain. Stroking can help produce muscle relaxation in locations where spasm exists. Kneading techniques are performed on muscle and subcutaneous tissue for the purposes of muscle relaxation, improving circulation, and reducing edema. Percussion is primarily used for chest therapy in conjunction with postural drainage.

17. **What physical parameters of massage can be altered, depending on the desired therapeutic effect?**
- **Myofascial release** has been defined as "a hands-on technique that applies prolonged light pressure in specific directions into the fascia system." It is applied in conjunction with passive range of motion with the purpose of stretching focal areas of muscle or fascial tightness.
- **Deep friction massage** is used to prevent adhesions in acute muscle injuries and to break up adhesions in subacute and chronic injuries. Deep friction is applied transversely across the muscle fiber, tendon, or ligament.
- **Soft-tissue mobilization** is a forceful massage of the muscle-fascial system element and differs from most massage in that it is done with fascia and muscle in a stretched position rather than relaxed or shortened. It is particularly effective as an adjunct to passive stretching for reduction of contractures.
- **Acupressure** is the application of sustained deep pressure over trigger points, as defined by Travell. Acupressure is often done in conjunction with application of other therapeutic modalities (e.g., ice, ultrasound, electrical stimulation) to the trigger points.

18. **Are there any contraindications to massage?**
Yes—there can be potential harm from massage. It is contraindicated over malignancies, open wounds, thrombophlebitis, and infected tissues. Peripheral nerve compression from hematoma formation has been reported when acupressure was applied too vigorously.

WEBSITES

1. European Teaching Group of Orthopaedic Medicine Cyriax
   http://www.om-cyriax.com/info.asp?language=EN&pagina=Literature

2. Massage, Traction, Manipulation: Wieting and Cuglij
   http://www.emedicine.com/pmr/topic200.htm

3. National Center for Complementary and Alternative Medicine
   http://nccam.nih.gov/

4. NCCAM Backgrounder: Manipulative and Body Based Practices: An Overview
   http://nccam.nih.gov/health/backgrounds/manipulative.htm

5. Overview of Manual Medicine Use in the United States
   http://nccam.nih.gov/news/upcomingmeetings/abstracts_mt/overview_US.htm

BIBLIOGRAPHY

1. Atchinson JW, Stoll ST, Cotter AC: Traction, manipulation, and massage. In Braddom RL (ed): Physical Medicine and Rehabilitation, 2nd ed. Philadelphia, W.B. Saunders, 2000, pp 413–439.

2. Braddock EJ, Greenlee J, Hammer RE, et al: Dec 1. Manual medicine guidelines for musculoskeletal injuries. California: Academy for Chiropractic Education; 2004 Dec 1. http://www.guideline.gov/summary/summary.aspx?ss=15&doc_id=6423&nbr=4054.

3. Bridger RS, Ossey S, Gourie G: Effect of lumbar traction on stature. Spine 14:82–90, 1989.

4. Cyriax JH: Textbook of Orthopaedic Medicine: Treatment by Manipulation, Massage and Injection, 10th ed. London, Bailliere-Tindall, 1982.

5. Gianakopoulos G, Waylonis GW, Grant PA, et al: Inversion devices: Their role in producing lumbar distraction. Arch Phys Med Rehabil 66:100–102, 1985.

6. Greenman PE: Principles of Manual Medicine. Baltimore, Williams & Wilkins, 1989.

7. Onel D, Tukzlaci M, Sari H, Demir K: Computed tomographic investigation of the effect of traction on lumbar disc herniations. Spine 14:82–90, 1989.

8. Rechtien JJ, Andary M, Holmes TG, Wieting JM: Manipulation, massage, and traction. In DeLisa JA, Gans BM (eds): Rehabilitation Medicine: Principles and Practice, 3rd ed. Philadelphia, Lippincott-Raven, 1998, pp 521–552.

9. Travell J: Myofascial Pain and Dysfunction. Baltimore, Williams & Wilkins, 1999.

CHAPTER 28

MANUAL MEDICINE: MANIPULATION, MOBILIZATION, AND MYOFASCIAL BODY WORK

Neil Cohen, DC, Tyler Childs Cymet, DO, Abner Salas, DC, and Jeffrey Meyers, MD, LAc

Healing, Papa would tell me, "is not a science, but the intuitive art of wooing nature."
—WH Auden (1907–1973)

1. **What is manual medicine?**

   Manual medicine and manual therapies encompass a variety of techniques that target bodily structures and systems, including the joints, bones, and circulatory, lymphatic, and soft tissue systems. Examples of manual therapies include osteopathic manipulation, massage therapy (discussed in previous chapter), and chiropractic intervention. The National Center of Complementary and Alternative Medicine recognizes manipulative and body-based practices, which are currently the subject of scientific investigation.

2. **What is manipulation?**

   Manipulation refers to the therapeutic application of a force with the goal of restoring normal tissue integrity and normal motion and the elimination of biomechanically based pain. Often manipulation is described by the manner, speed, intensity, and direction of the force applied. Variations include low-velocity, high-amplitude and high-velocity, low-amplitude manipulation (describing speed and amplitude of the thrust). Long-lever and short-lever manipulations vary the specificity of the vertebral level(s) being manipulated. A direct technique is a manipulative force applied in the direction of greatest resistance to overcome motion restriction. An indirect technique involves application of force in a direction opposite to where the musculoskeletal restriction exists.

   Manipulative techniques are a diverse group of body-based practices and may include osteopathic and chiropractic manipulations, Trager body work, Alexander technique, Bowen technique, Rolfing, reflexology, Feldenkrais method, massage, and Tui Na (Box 28-1).

   NCCAM information site: http://nccam.nih.gov/health/backgrounds/manipulative.htm

3. **What is somatic dysfunction?**

   Somatic dysfunction is the "impaired or altered function of related components of the somatic (body framework) system" that are addressed by manual medicine techniques. The anatomic components include joint, skeletal, and myofascial structures, along with their related vascular, lymphatic, and neural components.

   Atchison JW, Stoll ST, Cotter A: Manipulation, traction, and massage. In Braddom J (ed): Physical Medicine and Rehabilitation, 2nd ed. Philadelphia, W.B. Saunders, 2000, pp 413–439.

4. **What are direct and indirect techniques?**

   - **Direct** techniques use force in the direction of the barrier with the goal of moving through the barrier to restore normal motion.
   - **Indirect** techniques use movement and forces away from the barrier using the path of least resistance.

BOX 28-1. GLOSSARY OF TECHNIQUE DEFINITIONS

Alexander technique: Patient education/guidance in ways to improve posture and movement and to use muscles efficiently.

Bowen technique: Gentle massage of muscles and tendons over acupuncture and reflex points.

Chiropractic manipulation: Adjustments of the joints of the spine, as well as other joints and muscles.

Feldenkrais method: Group classes and hands-on lessons designed to improve the coordination of the whole person in comfortable, effective, and intelligent movement.

Massage therapy: Assortment of techniques involving manipulation of the soft tissues of the body through pressure and movement.

Osteopathic manipulation: Manipulation of the joints combined with physical therapy and instruction in proper posture.

Reflexology: Method of foot (and sometimes hand) massage in which pressure is applied to "reflex" zones mapped out on the feet (or hands).

Rolfing: Deep tissue massage (also called structural integration).

Trager body work: Slight rocking and shaking of the patient's trunk and limbs in a rhythmic fashion.

Tui Na: Application of pressure with the fingers and thumb and manipulation of specific points on the body (acupoints).

From http://nccam.nih.gov/health/backgrounds/manipulative.htm

---

5. **What is the crack you hear during a manipulation?**
The noise heard when a joint is manipulated is the result of cavitation and is the breaking of the surface tension of the synovial fluid and the release of gases into the fluid from pressure changes in the joint capsule. Generally referred to as an "audible release," it is heard more often when the manipulation is a high-velocity, low-amplitude technique and is not needed for a successful manipulation.

Flynn TW, Fritz JM, Wainner RS, Whitman JS: The audible pop is not necessary for successful spinal high-velocity thrust manipulation in individuals with low back pain. Arch Phys Med Rehabil 84:1057–1060, 2003.

Reggars JW: The therapeutic benefit of the audible release associated with spinal manipulative therapy: A critical review of the literature. Aust Chiropract Osteopath 7:80–85, 1998.

6. **What are the indications for manipulation?**
A diagnosis of somatic dysfunction or subluxation is the usual indication. Referral for manipulation is common when there is restricted quality of range of motion or limitation of motion because of pain.

7. **What are the contraindications to mobilization and manipulation?**
Although no studies measure the risks associated with manipulation of patients with various comorbidities, case studies have provided guidance. Low-velocity techniques have greater safety than high-velocity (thrust) techniques and therefore have a lower threshold of

contraindication. Absolute contraindications to manipulation include vertebral malignancy, active inflammatory arthropathy, acute spondyloarthropathy, ligamentous instability (Marfan's, Ehlers-Danlos), tumor or metastasis, active spinal infection or osteomyelitis, acute fracture or dislocation, severe osteoporosis, acute myelopathy, and cauda equina syndrome. Relative contraindications include poor outcome to prior manipulation, prior tracheostomy, ankylosing spondylitis or spondyloarthropathy, symptoms of vertebrobasilar insufficiency or vertebral artery disease, severe spondylosis, systemic anti-coagulation (either pathologic or pharmacologic), and history of spinal surgery.

Although reports of complications from cervical spine manipulation have gained attention in recent years, literature reviews have noted the incidence to be rare.

Haldeman S, Kohlbeck FJ, McGregor M: Unpredictability of cerebrovascular ischemia associated with cervical spine manipulation therapy: A review of sixty-four cases after cervical spine manipulation. Spine 27:49–55, 2002.

8. Can every patient in rehabilitation benefit from manipulation?

No. Although certain conditions have been studied and have shown definite benefit, such as acute low back pain or subchronic low back pain, there are also places where it has shown no benefit, such as in post-knee or hip arthroplasty patients.

9. How long does a course of manipulative treatment last?

Like all treatments, manipulation frequency and duration of treatment depend on several factors, including the treated condition, the severity and duration of the current and prior painful episodes, the presence of complicating factors, patient motivation, and practitioner training. Patients receiving these treatments may have comorbidity or other complicating factors. Like most treatments, there are no hard and fast rules regarding spinal manipulative treatment frequency or duration. Literature suggests that treatment with the correct diagnosis usually produces objective improvement in 2–4 weeks. Manipulation by itself is rarely appropriate.

Maitlin GD: Maitlin Vertebral Manipulation, 6th ed. Woburn, MA, Butterworth-Heinemann, 2000.

10. What treatment modalities can complement manipulative therapy?

Therapeutic exercises and other manual techniques and physical modalities should be combined with manipulation. Medication may be appropriate. Although research suggests the efficacy of combining manipulation with other modalities, including general anesthesia, epidural steroid injection, epidural and joint anesthesia, and manipulation with injectants such as steroids and proliferative agents, these practices have not become mainstream.

Kohlbeck FJ, Haldeman S, Hurwitz EL, Dagenais S: Supplemental care with medication-assisted manipulation versus spinal manipulation therapy alone for patients with chronic low back pain. J Manipulative Physiol Ther 28:245–252, 2005.

11. If a patient brings in an x-ray done by a chiropractor, can it be read just like the x-rays that are done in allopathic institutions?

The x-ray can be used to look for cancer, infection, or signs of trauma. But chiropractic x-rays are typically weight-bearing, so they provide better functional information about joints. Allopathic x-rays are meant to give anatomic and pathologic information, so they are typically done in a non–weight-bearing manner.

Taylor JA, Clopton P, Bosch E, et al: Interpretation of abnormal lumbosacral spine radiographs: A test comparing students, clinicians, radiology residents, and radiologists in medicine and chiropractic. Spine 20:1147–1153, 1995.

12. **Is the "biology" of manual medicine techniques understood?**
An understanding of the complex mechanisms of action underlying manual therapies has not yet been achieved. Research exploring the efficacy and safety of these techniques has been hampered by the following impediments:
- Scarcity of cross-disciplinary collaboration
- Lack of suitable animal models
- Inadequate use of state-of-the-art scientific technologies

http://nccam.nih.gov/health/backgrounds/manipulative.htm

13. **When is a massage medium required?**
A massage medium is used to reduce friction over the skin. Examples include mineral oil, glycerin, coconut oil, cocoa butter, Nivea® cream, and baby powder. Such media are used when the massage is intended for edema reduction, relaxation/sedation, or relief of muscle spasm/tightness. When the massage is used to loosen or stretch scar tissue, fascia, or subcutaneous tissue, no medium is used.

KEY POINTS:

1. Manual therapies include osteopathic manipulation, massage therapy, and chiropractic manipulation.

2. Referral for manipulation is common when there is restricted quality of range of motion or limitation of motion because of pain.

14. **What are commonly used techniques of therapeutic massage?**
Classical massage involves stroking and gliding movements (effleurage), kneading (pétrissage), and percussion (tapotement). Stroking, gliding, and friction movements are helpful for locating areas of muscle spasm or focal pain. Stroking can help produce muscle relaxation in locations where spasm exists. Kneading techniques are performed on muscle and subcutaneous tissue for the purposes of muscle relaxation, improving circulation, and reducing edema. Percussion is primarily used for chest therapy in conjunction with postural drainage.

15. **What physical parameters of massage can be altered depending on the desired therapeutic effect?**
Deep friction massage is used to prevent adhesions in acute muscle injuries and to break up adhesions in subacute and chronic injuries. Deep friction is applied transversely across the muscle fiber, tendon, or ligament.

Soft-tissue mobilization is a forceful massage of the muscle-fascial system element and differs from most massage in that it is done with fascia and muscle in a stretched position rather than relaxed or shortened. It is particularly effective as an adjunct to passive stretching for reduction of contractures.

Myofascial release has been defined as "a hands-on technique that applies prolonged light pressure in specific directions into the fascia system." It is applied in conjunction with passive range of motion with the purpose of stretching focal areas of muscle or fascial tightness.

Accupressure is the application of sustained deep pressure over trigger points, as defined by Travell. Accupressure is often done in conjunction with application of other therapeutic modalities (e.g., ice, ultrasound, electrical stimulation) to the trigger points.

Travell JG, Simmons DG: Myofascial Pain and Dysfunction, the Trigger Point Manual. Vol 4–20. Baltimore, Williams & Wilkins, 1983.

16. Are there any contraindications to massage?
Yes, there can be potential harm from massage. It is contraindicated over malignancies, open wounds, thrombophlebitis, and infected tissues. Peripheral nerve compression from hematoma formation has been reported when accupressure was applied too vigorously.

BIBLIOGRAPHY

1. Anderson GBJ, Lucente T, Davis A, et al: A comparison of osteopathic spinal manipulation with standard care for patients with low back pain. N Engl J Med 341:1426–1431, 1999.

2. Atchison JW, Stoll ST, Cotter A: Manipulation, traction, and massage. In Braddom J (ed): Physical Medicine and Rehabilitation, 2nd ed. Philadelphia, W.B. Saunders, 2000, pp 413–439.

3. Flynn TW, Fritz JM, Wainner RS, Whitman JS: The audible pop is not necessary for successful spinal high-velocity thrust manipulation in individuals with low back pain. Arch Phys Med Rehabil 84:1057–1060, 2003.

4. Haas M, Groupp E, Kraemer DF: Dose-response for chiropractic care of low back pain. Spine 25:574–583, 2004.

5. Haldeman S, Chapman-Smith D, Petersen DM (eds): Guidelines for Chiropractic Quality Assurance and Practice Parameters: Proceedings of the Mercy Center Consensus Conference. New York, Aspen Publishers, 1992.

6. Haldeman S, Kohlbeck FJ, McGregor M: Unpredictability of cerebrovascular ischemia associated with cervical spine manipulation therapy: A review of sixty-four cases after cervical spine manipulation. Spine 27:49–55, 2002.

7. Licciardone JC, Stoll ST, Cardarelli KM, et al: A randomized controlled trial of osteopathic manipulative treatment following knee or hip arthroplasty. J Am Osteopath Assoc 104:193–202, 2004.

8. Michaelsen M, Dreyfuss P: MUJA: Manipulation under joint anesthesia/analgesia: A proposed interdisciplinary treatment approach for recalcitrant spinal axis pain of synovial joint origin. Advances in Chiropractic, Yearbook Series, Vol. 4.

9. Protopapas MG, Cymet TC: Joint cracking and popping: Understanding noises that accompany articular release. J Am Osteopath Assoc 102:283–287, 2002.

10. Reggars JW: The therapeutic benefit of the audible release associated with spinal manipulative therapy: A critical review of the literature. Aust Chiropract Osteopath 7:80–85, 1998.

11. Sheckelle PG, Adams AH, Chassin MR, et al: Spinal manipulation for low back pain. Ann Intern Med 117:590–598, 1992.

12. Taylor JA, Clopton P, Bosch E, et al: Interpretation of abnormal lumbosacral spine radiographs: A test comparing students, clinicians, radiology residents, and radiologists in medicine and chiropractic. Spine 20:1147–1153, 1995.

13. Wieting JL, Andary MT, Holmes TG, et al: Manipulation, massage, and traction. In DeLisa JA, Gans BM (eds): Physical Medicine and Rehabilitation: Principles and Practice, 4th ed. Philadelphia, Lippincott-Raven, 2005, pp 285–310.

CHAPTER 29

ELECTROTHERAPY: MEDICAL TREATMENT USING ELECTRICAL CURRENTS

Peter H. Gorman, MD, MS, Gad Alon, PhD, PT, and
Stanley H. Kornhauser, PhD

*Listening is a magnetic and strange thing, a creative force. When we really listen to people
there is an alternating current, and this recharges us so that we never get tired of each other.
We are constantly being recreated.*

—Brenda Ueland (1891–1986)

1. **What is functional electrical stimulation (FES)?**
   FES is the method of applying safe levels of electric current to activate the damaged or
   disabled nervous system. FES can be completely or partially (i.e., percutaneously) implanted,
   or it can be applied over the skin (transcutaneously). FES is sometimes referred to as **functional
   neuromuscular stimulation (FNS)** or **neuromuscular electrical stimulation (NMES)**.
   Depending on one's perspective, NMES may be considered a more general or more specific term
   because it includes both therapeutic and functional purposes. Stimulation that is exclusively
   limited to sensory nerves only, such as cochlear prostheses or implanted spinal cord
   stimulators, are known collectively as **neuromodulation systems** and are distinctive from FES.

2. **What are the differences between NMES and FES?**
   The term NMES is used when the treatment objectives are set to improve physical impairments
   (e.g., atrophy, edema), whereas FES is used when the treatment objectives are to achieve
   functional activity (tasks) such as walking, standing from a sitting position, and upper extremity
   grasping, holding, and manipulating of objects.

   FES Information Center, 11000 Cedar Avenue, Cleveland, OH 44106-3052. Telephone: (800) 666-2352 or
   (216) 231-3257. Website: http://fescenter.case.edu

3. **Do FES systems directly stimulate nerves or muscle?**
   Motor units are activated electrically by depolarization of motor axons at the mixed nerves or
   their terminal nerve branches at the neuromuscular junction. A muscle can be directly
   depolarized by electrical current, but the amount of current necessary (threshold) for this to
   occur is considerably greater than that for the nerve. Therefore, for practical purposes, FES
   systems stimulate nerves, not muscles.

4. **What happens to FES-stimulated muscles over time?**
   Similar to muscles undergoing voluntary exercise, FES-stimulated muscles will change
   morphologically and physiologically. Some, but not all, type II glycolytic fibers will convert to
   type I oxidative fibers over weeks to months, depending on the intensity and frequency of
   stimulation. This phenomenon is associated with changes in vascular supply and increases the
   fatigue resistance of the muscle.

5. **What conditions may benefit from FES technology?**
   - Paralysis, joint contractures, loss of motor control, spasticity, disuse atrophy, and
     cardiovascular deconditioning

- Neurogenic bowel, bladder, and sexual dysfunction resulting from spinal cord injury (SCI), stroke, or multiple sclerosis
- Pain control, wound healing
- Epilepsy, scoliosis, tremor, restoration of hearing, and restoration of vision (beyond the scope of this chapter)

6. **What are the clinical applications of FES in rehabilitation?**
   - Muscle strengthening
   - Improvement in range of motion (ROM)
   - Facilitation and relearning of voluntary and functional motor control
   - Orthotic training, restoration of functional movement or activity
   - Partial and temporary inhibition of spasticity or muscle spasm
   - Augmentation of arterial, venous, and lymphatic blood flow

   Baker LL, Wederich CL, McNeal DR, et al:. Neuromuscular Electrical Stimulation: A Practical Guide, 4th ed. Downey, CA, Rancho Los Amigos Medical Center, 2000.

7. **What are the contraindications to FES?**
   Although there are **no absolute contraindications** for use of FES, patients with a cardiac demand pacemaker should be approached with extreme caution. Electrical stimulation applied anywhere on the body has the potential to interfere with the sensing portion of the demand pacemaker. **Significant precautions** include patients with cardiac arrhythmias, congestive heart failure, pregnancy, electrode sensitivity, or healing wounds (muscle stimulation may adversely move healing tissues). For the most part, implantable FES devices are MRI compatible, but each device must be assessed individually before imaging is performed.

8. **What are the uses of FES in spinal cord injury?**
   - **Therapeutic uses:** Muscle strengthening and cardiac conditioning. Possible other benefits include improvement in venous return from the legs, reduction of osteoporosis, improvement in bowel function, and psychological benefits.
   - **Functional uses:** Standing, walking, hand grasp (and release), bladder, bowel and sexual function, respiratory assist, and electroejaculation for fertility.

   Peckham PH, Gorman PH: Functional Electrical Stimulation in the 21st Century. Top Spinal Cord Rehabil 10(2):126–150, 2004.

9. **Explain the rationale behind the use of FES-induced exercise in patients with spinal cord injury.**
   Persons with SCI are generally forced to become more sedentary. Paralysis is compounded by impaired autonomic nervous system function, which limits the cardiovascular response to exercise, especially in individuals with lesions at T6 or above. Muscle mass, strength, and endurance all decrease after SCI, and muscle fibers convert primarily to anaerobic metabolism after injury. Paralysis of intercostal musculature reduces vital capacity and cough efficiency. In addition, there is reduced peripheral circulation, lean body mass, and bone density and an altered endocrine response. All of the above mentioned debilitating conditions can be partially reversed by FES.

10. **What systems are available for therapeutic electrical stimulation in persons with SCI?**
    The most common system for lower-extremity FES exercise is the bicycle ergometer. One commercially available ergometer is the ERGYS2 Clinical Rehabilitation System made by Therapeutic Alliances, Inc. (Fairborn, OH). This computer-controlled FES exercise ergometer used six channels and surface electrodes to sequentially stimulate quadriceps, hamstring, and glutei bilaterally. A newer, more compact bicycle ergometer for use with persons sitting

in their own wheelchair is the RTS-300S device made by Restorative Therapies, Inc. (Baltimore, MD). Some systems also include the capacity for simultaneous voluntary arm-crank exercise by paraplegics, permitting hybrid exercise.

For ERGYS2: http://www.musclepower.com/ and RTS-300S: http://www.restorative-therapies.com/

11. **What benefits can be anticipated in subjects involved in FES bicycle ergometry?**
Cardiac output and muscle oxidative capacity both improve with FES ergometry. Some patients can train with FES ergometry up to a similar aerobic metabolic rate (measured by peak VO_2), as is achieved in people without disabilities. Electrical exercise also increases peripheral venous return and fibrinolysis, and, in one study, FES in conjunction with heparin therapy was more effective in preventing deep venous thrombosis than heparin alone. There are limits to the cardiovascular benefits of FES ergometry, however, especially in those with lesions at or above T5. In those patients, there is loss of supraspinal sympathetic control, which, in turn, limits the body's ability to increase heart rate, stroke volume, and cardiac output.

Glaser RM: Physiology of functional electrical stimulation-induced exercise: Basic science perspective. J Neurol Rehabil 5:49–61, 1991.

12. **What are the applications of FES for standing and walking in paraplegia?**
Several different approaches to the use of FES for lower-extremity standing and walking in paraplegia are being researched. Hybrid approaches, such as the **reciprocating gait orthosis** (RGO), use both mechanical bracing and surface FES. Specifically, FES hip extension on one side provides contralateral leg swing through the RGO mechanism. Quadriceps stimulation then provides knee lock.

Only one surface FES walking system is Food and Drug Administration (FDA) approved for use in the United States. The Parastep System (Sigmedics, Inc.) uses the triple flexion response elicited by peroneal nerve stimulation, as well as knee and hip extensor surface stimulation, to construct the gait cycle. The patient controls the gait with switches integrated into a rolling walker, which is also needed for stability and safety. Implantable lower-extremity FES has also been developed to aid in activating deep musculature. Both percutaneous electrodes and implantable stimulator-receivers with epimysial or intramuscular electrodes have been tested, although neither is currently available commercially.

Agarwal S, Triolo RJ, Kobetic R, et al: Long-term user perceptions of an implanted neuroprosthesis for exercise, standing, and transfers after spinal cord injury. J Rehabil Res Dev 40(3):241–252, 2003. http://www.sigmedics.com/

13. **What about FES for restoration of hand grasp in tetraplegia?**
Tetraplegic hand grasp systems have focused on people with C5- and C6-level SCI. Subject data with C4-level injury are limited. Those injured at the C7 and lower levels have multiple voluntary active forearm muscles (e.g., brachioradialis, extensor carpi radialis longus and brevis, pronator teres), which can be used in many activities, making tendon transfer and FES minimally beneficial. The best FES results are achieved with motivated people who have goals for the activity and social support system to reinforce use.

14. **What are the components of the implantable FES hand grasp system? How does it work?**
The Neuroprosthetic Hand Grasp System, commercially known as the Freehand System, initially developed at Case Western Reserve University, consists of (1) an external joint position transducer/controller, (2) a rechargeable, programmable external control unit (ECU), and (3) an implantable eight-channel stimulator/receiver attached via flexible wires to epimysial disc electrodes. The user controls the system through small movements of either the shoulder or wrist. The joint position transducer, which operates somewhat like a computer joystick, typically is mounted on the skin from sternum to contralateral shoulder or across the ipsilateral

wrist and senses these movements. The ECU uses this signal to proportionally control hand grasp and release. Communication between the ECU and the implantable stimulator, which is located in a surgical pocket created in the upper chest, occurs through radio frequency coupling. The system can be programmed through a personal computer interface by a trained therapist to individualize the grasps as well as the shoulder control for each patient. Unfortunately, the device, although FDA approved, is no longer commercially available, but efforts are being made to reintroduce it into the market in the next few years.

Peckham PH, Keith MW, Kilgore KL, et al, for the Implantable Neuroprosthesis Research Group: Efficacy of an Implanted Neuroprosthesis for Restoring Hand Grasp in Tetraplegia; A Multicenter Study. Arch Phys Med Rehabil 82:1380–1388, 2001.

15. How do bladder stimulation systems work in spinal cord injury?

Electrical stimulation to control bladder function after supra-sacral SCI is now FDA approved in the United States and commercially available in Europe. The most experience and success has occurred with a device termed the **Vocare System** (in the United States), which provides S2–S4 anterior sacral nerve root stimulation. This system is surgically implanted through lumbar laminectomy, employs either epidural or intradural electrodes, and usually is done in conjunction with a dorsal rhizotomy (to prevent detrusor-sphincter dyssynergia). The electrodes are connected via cable to an implanted radio receiver, which couples to an external stimulator/transmitter. Pulsed stimulation is used to take advantage of the differences between activation of the slow-response smooth musculature of the detrusor and activation of the fast-twitch striated sphincter musculature. This produces short spurts of urination, but can result in nearly complete bladder emptying. The sacral anterior root stimulators have also been shown to improve bowel care (i.e., increased defecation efficiency, reduced constipation) in those patients using them. Approximately 60% of men can also produce penile erection with the device.

Creasey GH, Grill JH, Korsten M, et al: Implanted Neuroprosthesis Research Group. An implantable neuroprosthesis for restoring bladder and bowel control to patients with spinal cord injuries: a multicenter trial. Arch Phys Med Rehabil 82(11):1512–1519, 2001.

16. What is the role of FES in respiratory assistance?

In a high-level tetraplegic individual injured at C1 or C2, the use of the **phrenic pacemaker** has become a standard part of the clinical armamentarium and an alternative to chronic ventilator dependence. Those with spinal cord damage at C3 and C4 often have damaged the anterior horns of those segments, resulting in Wallerian degeneration of the phrenic nerves. Therefore, phrenic nerve conduction studies must be performed before considering this type of FES device.

Glenn WWL, Brouillette RT, Dentz B, et al: Fundamental considerations in pacing of the diaphragm for chronic ventilatory insufficiency: A multi-center study. Pacing Clin Electrophysiol 11:2121–2127, 1988.

17. What are the common uses of noninvasive (surface) electrical stimulation?

- Temporary management of acute (postoperative, post-trauma), chronic, musculoskeletal, and ischemic pain through the use of TENS
- Strengthening of weak and atrophied skeletal muscles
- Maintaining or improving joint mobility
- Enhancing peripheral arterial, venous, and lymphatic blood flow
- Enhancing the recovery of motor control, upper limb function, and ambulation ability following damage to the central nervous system, such as after stroke, traumatic brain injury, and cerebral palsy
- Enhancing the healing of slow-to-heal wounds such as pressure and neuropathic wounds

Nelson RM, Hayes KW, Currier DP: Clinical Electrotherapy, 3rd ed. Appleton & Stamford, Connecticut, Lange, 1999.

18. **What are the similarities and differences between TENS and NMES?**
Both are electrical pulse generators that can put out a current with a monophasic, biphasic, or multiphasic waveform. If the **waveform is monophasic,** the output pulse exhibits polarity (unidirectional current flow) so that one electrode is negative (−) and the other is positive (+). If the **waveform is biphasic,** the output pulse reverses polarity with each phase of each pulse, so designation of the electrodes as negative or positive is no longer valid or meaningful.
In both TENS and NMES, the clinician can usually control the duration of the pulse, the pulse rate (frequency), and the intensity of the stimulus. Both TENS and NMES depolarize the peripheral sensory and motor nerves. In TENS, there is no option to interrupt the pulses, so the excitation of the peripheral nerves continues as long as the intensity of the stimulus remains ON (known as **continuous** or **uninterrupted mode** or **continuous train** of pulses). In contrast, NMES provides an option of interrupted pulses where the clinician can set the stimulator to deliver the pulses for a finite number of seconds, followed by a period of a few seconds of no current (pulses) flow. This is known as **interrupted pulses mode** or ON-OFF time setting. If the clinician decides to set the OFF time at zero (0) seconds, the pulses become continuous, exactly like in TENS. The strength of TENS or NMES stimulus is a function of the maximal phase charge (measured in microcoulombs). TENS are typically weaker than NMES (15–18 versus 25–30 microcoulombs). Finally, some clinical indications require monophasic waveform (wound healing and acute inflammation). All other clinical indications do not require that polarity, and biphasic pulses are typically used. Any clinical condition that requires contraction and relaxation of muscles can be treated with NMES but not with TENS.

19. **Is there an optimal waveform employed in the use of TENS for pain management?**
Some studies claim that there is a stronger endorphin release at low-frequency (<10 Hz), high-amplitude stimulation than with higher-frequency (60–100 Hz), lower-intensity stimulation ("conventional" TENS); however, experimental findings are mixed.

20. **What applications are commonly used for TENS in pain management?**
TENS is appropriate in the treatment of both acute and chronic musculoskeletal, neurovascular, and even ischemic cardiac (angina) pain. Success rates vary, from placebo rates to approximately 30–95%. The difference in outcomes probably results from differences in stimulating parameters, electrode placement, type and duration of pain, concurrent medication, previous treatment, choice of controls, length of follow-up, and patient expectations. TENS is likely to be effective during stimulation, but it is unlikely to produce long-lasting (post-treatment) pain relief. Whether the mechanism of action is the **gate theory** or the release of endogenous opiates (neuropeptides), it is not likely to be sustainable.

Lampl C, Kreczi T, Klingler D: Transcutaneous electrical nerve stimulation in the treatment of chronic pain: predictive factors and evaluation of the method. Clin J Pain 14(2):134–142, 1998.

21. **What is the key to successful use of TENS?**
If TENS is to be successful, it directly reflects the patience, time, and anatomic knowledge of the clinician. Electrode placement is imperative. TENS should never be employed solely in the treatment of low back pain or other musculoskeletal disorders. The Quebec Task Force concluded that decreased pain relief in the low back has been demonstrated, but the sole use of TENS has not been shown to accelerate return to work or return to a normal level of function. TENS contributes most effectively to a carefully developed comprehensive rehab program with close rehabilitation physician monitoring.

22. **Is TENS used continuously for pain management when it has been determined to be beneficial in a subject?**

No optional utilization time of TENS has been determined. Usage is individualized and usually determined with an adequate trial-and-error period. High-frequency TENS ("conversational" TENS, 60–100 Hz) is applied at barely perceptible levels to two to three times the sensory threshold and can usually be tolerated for many hours daily. Low-frequency TENS ($\sim$0.5–10 Hz) usually involves stronger intensities at three to five times the sensory threshold. It is comfortably tolerated for 20–30-minute periods for several short sessions daily. An often-used approach is to initiate TENS therapy at high-frequency levels and then switch to low frequency only if the higher frequency is not effective. Most patients find the low frequency uncomfortable and complain of the annoying perception of "beating."

23. **NMES is now routinely used to strengthen weak and atrophic muscles. What clinical conditions have indication to add NMES to the rehabilitation program?**

- Post–knee reconstruction such as anterior cruciate ligament (ACL) repair
- Post–knee joint replacement
- Chronic low back pain
- Rheumatoid arthritis of the hand
- Stress and urge incontinence (covered by Medicare)

Fitzgerald GK, Piva SR, Irrgang JJ: A modified neuromuscular electrical stimulation protocol for quadriceps strength training following anterior cruciate ligament reconstruction. J Orthop Sports Phys Ther 33(9): 492–501, 2003.

Snyder-Mackler L, Delitto A, Bailey SL, Stralka SW: Strength of the quadriceps femoris muscle and functional recovery after reconstruction of the anterior cruciate ligament. A prospective, randomized clinical trial of electrical stimulation. J Bone Joint Surg 77A:1166–1173, 1995.

Stevens JE, Mizner RL, Snyder-Mackler L: Neuromuscular electrical stimulation for quadriceps muscle strengthening after bilateral total knee arthroplasty: a case series. J Orthop Sports Phys Ther 34(1):21–29, 2004.

24. **Is there credible medical evidence to delay initiation of FES in the management of stroke or traumatic brain injury survivors?**

Not at all. A number of clinical trials, some randomized, have reported specific benefits, including minimizing shoulder subluxation and shoulder pain, improving active ROM, reducing spasticity, and gaining hand function and ability to walk. None of these studies reported any increased risk of recurrent stroke, transient ischemic attack, seizures, shoulder-hand syndrome, or edema.

Chantraine A, Baribeault A, Uebelhart D, Gremion G: Shoulder pain and dysfunction in hemiplegia: effects of functional electrical stimulation. Arch Phys Med Rehabil 80(3):328–331, 1999.

Popovic MB, Popovic DB, Sinkjaer T, et al: Clinical evaluation of functional electrical therapy in acute hemiplegic subjects. J Rehabil Res Dev 40(5):443–453, 2003.

25. **Can FES training benefit patients with chronic stroke, TBI, or multiple sclerosis?**

There are numerous clinical studies of varying quality that support the use of NMES/FES to minimize spasticity. Although the majority of studies report statistically significant reduction of spasticity, the clinical significance is not clear because the amount of spasticity reduction (as routinely assessed by the Ashworth scale) is typically small. In contrast, strengthening of paretic muscles, improving joint ROM, and enhancing motor control in chronic stroke is repeatedly reported in clinical literature. Transcutaneous electromyography (EMG) detection can be utilized to trigger stimulation of a muscle that is being rehabilitated after a central nervous system (CNS) insult. An active effort to contract the muscle is detected and reinforced with FES stimulation to complete the contraction. Toe drag during swing phase of hemiplegic gait can be improved with FES stimulation of the ankle dorsiflexors triggered by a switch soon after heel off. Regaining better hand function and walking ability have been reported by some investigators, but the degree and diversity of improving daily functions remain unknown at this time.

Alon G, Stibrant-Sunnerhagen K, Geurfs AC, Ohry A: A home-based, self-administered stimulation program to improve selected hand functions of chronic stroke. NeuroRehabilitation 18:215–225, 2003.

Cauraugh JH, Kim SB: Stroke motor recovery: active neuromuscular stimulation and repetitive practice schedules. J Neurol Neurosurg Psychiatry 74(11):1562–1566, 2003.

26. **What is the evidence in support of using electrical stimulation to accelerate healing of open wounds/ulcers?**

Numerous clinical reports, including some randomized placebo-controlled trials, pre-post comparison trials, and many case reports, support the use of electrical stimulation in the management of slowly healing pressure ulcers, diabetic neuropathic ulcers, and, to a lesser degree, venous stasis ulcers. In most studies, a monophasic waveform has been used, placing the sterile and biocompatible anode or cathode electrode directly onto the wound. The rate of healing and the percentage of completely healed wounds have been shown to be statistically and clinically better than standard wound care. Any TENS device having monophasic waveform, very short (5–100 microsecond) pulse duration, and a pulse rate of 100–120 pulses per second can be used. The proposed mechanism of healing may be based on the electrically mediated increase of microcirculation via the activation of vasoactive peptides, such as calcitonin gene-related peptide or vasoactive intestinal polypeptide. Another, possibly concurrent, mechanism of action is the electrically induced synthesis of protein leading to collagen fiber regeneration.

Kloth LC: Electrical stimulation for wound healing: A review of evidence from in vitro studies, animal experiments, and clinical trials. Int J Low Extrem Wounds 4(1):23–44, 2005.

KEY POINTS: USES OF ELECTRICAL STIMULATION

1. Neuromuscular electrical stimulation improves physical impairments such as muscle atrophy.

2. Functional electrical stimulation produces functional movement that contributes to completion of a task.

3. Transcutaneous electrical nerve stimulation is helpful in reducing acute and chronic musculoskeletal pain and ischemic pain.

BIBLIOGRAPHY

1. FES Information Center, 11000 Cedar Avenue, Cleveland, Ohio 44106-3052. Telephone: (800) 666-2352 or (216) 231-3257. Website: http://fescenter.case.edu

2. Pape KE, Chipman ML: Electrotherapy in Rehabilitation. In DeLisa JA, Gans BM (eds): Physical Medicine and Rehabilitation: Principles and Practice, 4th ed. Philadelphia, Lippincott Williams & Wilkins, 2005, pp 435–464.

INJECTIONS OF PERIPHERAL JOINTS, BURSAE, TENDON SHEATHS, AND TENDON INSERTIONS

Gerard P. Varlotta, DO, and William Gibbs, MD

CHAPTER 30

Pain is no evil; unless, it conquers us.

–Charles Kingsley (1819–1875)

INJECTION MEDICATIONS: ANESTHETICS

1. **How do local anesthetic medications work in peripheral joint and soft tissue injections?**
   Local anesthetics reversibly block nerve transmission by inhibiting ion flux through sodium channels of the axon. As a result, the action potential does not reach threshold and nerve transmission ceases, resulting in anesthesia. The speed of onset, depth, and duration of anesthesia are based on multiple factors, including characteristics of the nerve, anesthetic dosage, tissue site injected, and structure of the anesthetic module. Once injected, anesthetics are transported within the body by simple mechanical bulk flow, diffusion, and vascular transport. The location of injection, especially in highly vascular areas, affects the drug's absorption, duration of action, and toxicity.

2. **How do I choose a local anesthetic?**
   The choice of local anesthetic depends on the duration of the desired anesthetic effect. Chloroprocaine has a short duration of action. Lidocaine and mepivacaine have an intermediate duration of action, and bupivacaine, ropivacaine, and etidocaine have the longest durations of action. Duration of action is determined by the amount of drug bound to plasma proteins. Local anesthetics with a high protein-binding capacity have a longer duration of action. Adding vasoconstrictors such as phenylephrine, epinephrine, or norepinephrine also will prolong the effect of local anesthetics by decreasing the local absorption of the drug.

3. **Which local anesthetics should be used and in what quantity?**
   The anesthetic of choice for most musculoskeletal injections is usually 1% lidocaine without epinephrine. Bupivacaine 0.25% or 0.5% is useful in providing a longer analgesic effect. Longer-acting anesthetic agents should not be used in weight-bearing joints to minimize the potential destruction of an insensate joint. The amount injected depends on the size of the joint. The acromioclavicular, sternoclavicular, and elbow joints can take 1–2 mL of 1% lidocaine combined with the corticosteroid. The glenohumeral, knee, and hip joints can take 2–4 mL. Bupivacaine is often preferable for non–weight-bearing joints.

4. **What are the complications related to local anesthetic use?**
   Toxicity from local anesthetics is usually dose-related and is cumulative. It often results from rapid absorption from the injection site or from inadvertent intravascular injection. Peak plasma concentration occurs within 5–25 minutes.

5. **What are the two organ systems and symptoms affected by local anesthetic toxic effects?**
These two organ systems are the central nervous system (CNS) and cardiovascular system. The CNS effects initially include dizziness, circumoral numbness, tinnitus, and blurred vision. Excitatory symptoms such as agitation, muscular twitching, or tremors precede CNS depression. Ultimately, convulsions, respiratory depression, and cardiac arrest can occur. The cardiovascular system symptoms include peripheral vasodilatation, myocardial depression, angina, bradycardia, arrhythmias, and cardiac arrest.

INJECTION MEDICATIONS: STEROIDS

6. **How do glucocorticoids work?**
Glucocorticoids exert their action by blocking prostaglandin and leukotriene synthesis. They bind to specific intracellular receptors upon entering target cells and alter gene expression that regulates many cellular processes. The anti-inflammatory effect of glucocorticoids is due to its immunosuppressive action on leukocyte function and availability. The proposed mechanisms of action of corticosteroids are:
- Decrease synovial fluid complement
- Decrease neutrophil number
- Decrease synovial membrane/vascular permeability
- Decrease synovial fluid acid hydrolases
- Stimulation of synovial lining cell lysosomes
- Decrease number of mast cells in synovium

7. **What glucocorticoids are available for use in peripheral joints, bursae, and tendon sheaths?**
The most widely used corticosteroids are listed in Table 30-1. These compounds were developed to reduce undesirable hormonal side effects with less rapid dissipation from the joint. None of these corticosteroid derivatives appears to have any superiority over another;

TABLE 30-1. COMPARISON OF COMMONLY USED GLUCOCORTICOID STEROIDS

Agent	Anti-Inflammatory Potency*	Plasma Half Life (minutes)	Duration of Action
Hydrocortisone (Cortisol®)	1	90	Short
Cortisone	0.8	30	Short
Prednisone	4–5	60	Intermediate
Prednisolone	4–5	200	Intermediate
Methylprednisolone (Depo-Medrol®)	5	180	Intermediate
Triamcinolone (Kenalog®)	5	300	Intermediate
Betamethasone (Celestone®)	25–35	100–300	Long
Dexamethasone (Decadron®)	25–30	100–300	Long

*Relative to hydrocortisone.

however, triamcinolone hexacetonide is the least water-soluble preparation and thus provides the longest duration of effectiveness within the peripheral joint space.

8. **List the absolute and relative contraindications for intra-articular and extra-articular corticosteroid injections.**

Absolute contraindications	Relative contraindications
■ Infectious arthritis	■ Juxta-articular osteopenia
■ Bacteremia	■ Anticoagulant therapy
■ Peri-articular cellulitis	■ Joint instability
■ Acute injury	■ Hemarthrosis
■ Osteochondral fracture	■ Joint prosthesis
■ Adjacent osteomyelitis	■ Questionable therapeutic benefit from prior injections
■ Uncontrolled bleeding or clotting disorder	

9. **What are the potential adverse effects of corticosteroid injection?**
   1. **Systemic absorption** (more common with repeated injections)
      - Suppression of the hypothalamic-pituitary-adrenal axis
      - Iatrogenic Cushing's syndrome
      - Transient hyperglycemia and glucosuria
      - Glucocorticoid-induced osteoporosis
   2. **Local effects**
      - Iatrogenic joint infection occurs at a rate of 0.0001% in properly prepared joints.
      - Steroid-induced arthropathy
      - Destructive arthropathy may occur from post-injection pain relief and overuse of the joint rather than steroid-induced cartilage injury.
   3. **Other rare local effects**
      - Iatrogenic joint inflammation may occur if the site is prepared with alcohol solution and disposable needles are used.
      - Tendon and ligament rupture can occur with systemic steroid use, frequent injection of weight-bearing joint or periarticular soft tissue, injections directly into tendon or ligament, or injection of a high dose of corticosteroids.
      - Post-injection flare or true crystal-induced arthropathy can occur in the presence of certain paraben preservatives used in local anesthetic preparations. The acute synovitis is self-limiting and responds well to ice, rest, and nonsteroidal anti-inflammatory drugs (NSAIDs). It can be avoided by using single-dose vials of lidocaine or by using longer-acting bupivacaine that does not contain the paraben preservative. It is more common after use of microcrystalline steroid preparations (triamcinolone hexacetonide).
      - Skin hypopigmentation and subcutaneous atrophy can occur if the depth of injection is less than 5 mm or the steroid is deposited along the needle tract during withdrawal.

10. **What constitutes proper informed consent prior to the performance of injections?**
    Informed consent is an independent action by a patient authorizing medical personnel to initiate a treatment plan. Three key elements are necessary in obtaining proper informed consent: (1) disclosure of information, (2) comprehension of the information by a competent patient, and (3) decision making free of coercion. The act of signing a consent form does not negate the need for proper informed consent for the performance of a procedure.

11. **What forms of treatment are used to compliment corticosteroid injections?**
The proper implementation of procedures results in good patient care, providing safety to the physician and, most importantly, the patient. The safety of the patient is directly related to the physician's technical skills, knowledge of drug pharmacology, and his or her ability to recognize potential complication. The procedure should not be in isolation but rather integrated into a comprehensive treatment plan including modalities, activity modification, bracing, oral medications, and physical therapy directed by the physiatrist.

12. **What are the indications for intra-articular steroid injections?**
The most common indications for intra-articular injections of steroids are for articular and periarticular inflammatory conditions and painful arthritic conditions. These include synovitis related to rheumatoid arthritis, osteoarthritis, adhesive capsulitis, meniscal derangement or tears, chondral defects, labral tears, and shearing damage of the articular cartilage as seen in maltracking of a joint.

13. **How much methylprednisolone acetate (Depo-Medrol®) should be injected into a joint and in what frequency?**
Commonly larger joints (hip, knee, and shoulder) require injection of 40 mg, whereas medium-sized joints (wrist, elbow, and ankle) require 20–30 mg and small joints (acromioclavicular, finger, and toe) require 10–20 mg. Larger joints can accommodate a volume of 2–4 mL, whereas smaller joints accommodate 1–2 mL. The most common frequency of injections is every 4–6 weeks, with a maximum of three injections. Arthroscopic debridement may be necessary if the patient's pain continues.

14. **Are there harmful effects of intra-articular injections of steroids?**
Since the introduction of hydrocortisone in 1951, there have been anecdotal reports of the deleterious effects of corticosteroid injections, including articular surface damage, osteonecrosis, and periarticular problems. These reports have been disputed, and the reported deleterious effects are transient when the injections are performed under accepted guidelines. Multiple injections beyond the recommended dosage or frequency can interfere with normal cartilage protein synthesis.

INJECTION TECHNIQUES

15. **What is the most common technique for intra-articular injections of peripheral joints?**
Most commonly a 25- or 22-gauge 1.5-inch needle is used. The clinician should use slow, directed needle placement, avoiding forceful, sudden thrusts. Aspiration should be performed prior to injection to ensure that there is no blood return that may indicate an intravascular injection. Once the needle is placed in the appropriate location, the injectate should be delivered with a slow and steady force. If there is resistance to the introduction of the solution, the needle should be adjusted prior to continuing the injection. If a larger bore needle is necessary, a lidocaine wheal should be performed prior to the injection. A small amount of lidocaine should be used to flush the corticosteroids prior to its removal as to avoid the introduction into the subcutaneous skin. Pressure should be applied to the area after injection.

16. **When should I apply a vapocoolant spray?**
Local application of vapocoolant to the skin may be necessary in apprehensive patients to provide superficial anesthesia. The vapocoolant should be applied prior to the use of a cleansing agent, as the contents are aseptic but not sterile. The delivery is under pressure and should be applied with movement of the stream as to not cause a cryo-burn to the skin.

JOINTS

17. **In which disorders of the shoulder should anterior, superior, lateral, and posterior approaches be used?**

    The anterior approach is most commonly used in bicipital tendinitis. The superior approach can be used to enter the acromioclavicular joint and, with further advancement, into the subacromial space. Care should be taken as to not advance the needle into the supraspinatus tendon. If resistance is met with the injection, the needle should be withdrawn until the resistance is eliminated. The lateral injection can be used when treating supraspinatus tendinitis, especially when there is an enthesopathy or insertional pathology. Once again, care must be taken not to inject into the substance of the tendon. Most commonly, the posterior approach is used to treat supraspinatus tendinitis, subacromial bursitis, labral tears, adhesive capsulitis, and glenohumeral osteoarthritis.

18. **What structures are of concern and should be avoided when injecting the sternoclavicular joint?**

    When injecting the sternoclavicular joint, the needle should be placed superficially in the joint to avoid penetration of the brachiocephalic veins.

19. **What is the safest injection technique when performing an intra-articular elbow injection?**

    Injection of the elbow is safest when performed from the posterolateral approach. This avoids the major vessels and nerves in the medial and anterior aspect of the elbow.

20. **What specific disorders of the wrist require an intra-articular injection of corticosteroids? How should the injection be performed?**

    Rheumatoid arthritis and osteoarthritis are the most common reasons for intra-articular wrist injections. Other wrist pathology includes scapholunate ligament and triangular fibrocartilage complex tears. All injections should be performed from the dorsal aspect of the joint. Because most of the wrist joints have interconnecting synovial spaces, the injection should be placed in the area of maximal tenderness or in the region of the most severe pathology.

21. **When is it necessary to inject the sacroiliac joints? How should the injection be performed?**

    Synovitis and dysfunction of the sacroiliac joint may cause pain. The sacroiliac joint is composed of fibrous and synovial portions of the joint. With the patient prone, the fibrous portion can be injected medial to the posterior superior iliac crest. The synovial portion of the joint requires fluoroscopic guidance, with needle placement in the inferior portion of the joint. The results of injections may yield diagnostic information, and the therapeutic benefits are variable.

22. **What are the different approaches when injecting the hip?**

    The best approach is the anterior approach performed under radiographic guidance. The anatomic landmarks are 2 cm distal to the anterior superior iliac spine and 3 cm lateral to the femoral artery. The needle is advanced at a 60 degree angle posteromedially until it enters the joint. When performing a hip injection from the lateral approach, a 3–4 inch needle needs to be used. Needle placement is just anterior to the greater trochanter.

23. **What are the most common axial joints that can cause a referred pain, mimicking peripheral joint pain?**

    The most common axial joints are the facet (zygapophyseal) joints and costovertebral joints. Adjacent pathology should be investigated if the patient's peripheral joint pain is refractory to direct treatment.

24. **When should fluoroscopically guided injections be used when injecting a joint?**
Many small joints require the use of fluoroscopic guidance to ensure accurate placement of the corticosteroids into the joint. The intercarpal joints of the wrist, midfoot (Lisfranc and Chopart) joints, subtalar joints, and interphalangeal joints of the hand and foot may require the use of fluoroscopy. Fluoroscopic guidance of larger and deeper joints such as the hip and glenohumeral joints may be needed to confirm placement of the medication in the intended location.

25. **Describe the different visco-supplementation that can be used in osteoarthritis of the knee and their intended benefits.**
Three visco-supplementation products are available: sodium hyaluronate (Hyalgan®), hyaline G-F 20 (Synvisc®), and sodium hyaluronate (Supartz®). Hyaluronate is a component of synovial fluid, which is responsible for its viscoelasticity. The source of hyaluronate is rooster combs. Clinical studies demonstrate that injections of visco-supplementation substances into the joints of osteoarthritic knees result in a reduction of pain and improvement of function in the majority of patients. Prospective clinical data in knee osteoarthritis patients have shown benefit of treatment up to 52 weeks following a single course of injections. Additional injection may be needed every 6–12 months depending on the duration of benefit. A comparison of the products is found in Table 30-2.

TABLE 30-2. VISCO-SUPPLEMENTATION PRODUCTS

Trade Name	Supartz	Synvisc	Hyalgan	Orthovisc	Euflexxa
Active ingredient	1% Sodium hyaluronate (25 mg)	0.8% Sodium hyaluronate (16 mg)	1% Sodium hyaluronate (20 mg)	1% Sodium hyaluronate (30 mg)	1% Sodium hyaluronate (20 mg)
# of injections per series	5 weekly	3 weekly	5 weekly	3 weekly	3 weekly
Hyaluronan per series	125 mg	48 mg	120 mg	90 mg	60 mg

BURSAE

26. **Describe the structure and function of bursae.**
Bursae are synovial-lined fluid sacs that are located adjacent to joints. Inflammation within the bursa results from direct trauma or indirectly due to repetitive activities resulting in muscular weakness, musculotendinous contractures, and muscular imbalances altering joint mechanics. Bursae function to reduce friction between muscles, tendon skin, and bone. Most bursae are named by the anatomical structure that they are closest to and protect.

27. **What treatments are required to prevent chronic inflammation of the bursae?**
In addition to injections, other treatments used in bursitis include nonsteroidal anti-inflammatory drugs (NSAIDs), therapeutic modalities, stretching, and strengthening exercises. Correction of the improper postural mechanics is essential to avoid chronic bursal inflammation.

28. **What is the most common bursitis in the shoulder? What are the causes?**
Subacromial (subdeltoid) bursitis is the most common bursitis of the shoulder. The bursa is located superior to the supraspinatus tendon, inferior to the acromion, behind the coracoacromial ligament, and beneath the deltoid muscle. Subacromial bursitis is secondary

to rotator cuff tendinitis, impingement syndrome, cervical radiculitis/radiculopathy, suprascapular neuropathy, and repetitive strain disorders of the periscapular muscles that result in scapular rotation with acromial depression.

29. **Which approach is most commonly used in injection of subacromial bursitis?**
The most common and easiest approach is a posterolateral approach. The needle placement is in the depression below the acromion, with the needle directed in an anterior, medial, and superior direction aiming toward the acromioclavicular joint. The total volume accepted by the bursa is 4–6 mL.

30. **What is the most common bursitis around the elbow? What are its causes and treatment?**
The most common bursitis around the elbow is olecranon bursitis, or Draftsman's elbow. It is usually secondary to direct trauma to the olecranon process of the ulnar bone but can also be seen in rheumatologic disorders such as gout. Aspiration with a larger needle (18 gauge), injection with corticosteroids, and application of a compression dressing are the recommended treatments. The needle insertion point should be proximal to the bursal swelling, as direct injection into the bursa may lead to the development of a chronically draining sinus tract.

31. **What are the three most common types of bursitis around the hip?**
Greater trochanteric, iliopsoas (iliopectineal), and ischial (Tailor's or Weaver's bottom) bursitis are seen around the hip. In greater trochanteric bursitis, the pain is lateral over the greater trochanteric prominence of the femur bone. The greater trochanteric bursa is located in the lateral, proximal thigh. The iliopsoas bursa is located interior to the hip joint. The ischial bursa is located over the ischial prominence.

32. **What is most commonly associated with greater trochanteric bursitis?**
The most common etiology of greater trochanteric bursitis is gluteus medius weakness. Pain is localized lateral but also proximal to the greater trochanter. Weakness is found in hip abduction on manual muscle testing in a side lying position and on single leg standing (Trendelenburg sign). Visual gait analysis reveals a truncal tilt to the affected side (compensated) or tilt to the contralateral side (uncompensated), Trendelenburg gait pattern. Additionally, internal rotation of the hip seated and supine should be tested to determine if limitations are present, indicating a hip osteoarthritis. Observation of leg length discrepancies and scoliosis should be noted and treated. Testing for iliotibial band (ITB) contracture with the performance of an Ober maneuver should be done. Injections in isolation without resolution of the gluteus medius tendinitis, ITB contracture, leg length discrepancy, and pronation may lead to a return in pain.

33. **What structure can cause medial knee pain that is located inferior to the knee joint line?**
The pes anserinus bursa is located on the medial aspect of the knee inferior to the joint line. It is found below the conjoined tendons of the semitendinosus, sartorius, and gracilis muscles. It is found in osteoarthritis, increased femoral anteversion of the hip, excessive pronation, and genu valgum deformities. There is an associated medial hamstring weakness on manual muscle testing of knee flexion seated or prone. An injection of corticosteroids into the bursa combined with heating modalities and a hamstring stretching and strengthening program are most effective in treatment of pes anserinus bursitis.

34. What bursitis is found in patients who perform excessive kneeling?
Prepatellar bursitis (housemaid's knee) is found in patients who perform kneeling activities, usually associated with employment (e.g., carpenters). Treatment can include NSAIDs, therapy modalities, and quadriceps stretching. Injection is performed from the superior and medial approaches. Avoidance of kneeling and the use of knee pads are effective in preventing a return in pain.

35. When is Achilles pain not Achilles tendinitis?
The retrocalcaneal (subtendinous) bursa is located between the posterior calcaneus and the Achilles tendon. The subcutaneous (Achilles) bursa is located superficial to the Achilles tendon. Inflammation of the subcutaneous bursa is found from direct pressure from the heel counter, especially with high-heeled shoes that cause plantar flexion of the ankle. The inflammation of the retrocalcaneal bursa occurs with pressure from tight heel counters, Achilles contractures, and in runners overtraining with a sudden increase in mileage. The diagnostic differentiation is made on clinical examination, with no tenderness of the Achilles tendon or the enthesis but tenderness below the Achilles in retrocalcaneal bursitis and superficial to the tendon in subcutaneous bursitis. Treatment consists of avoidance of direct pressure, training modification, anti-inflammatory medications, and physical therapy modalities. For refractory cases, an injection is helpful. Care needs to be taken not to perform the injection into the Achilles tendon, and the angle of the needle should be 15–20 degrees anteriorly from a lateral approach.

36. What bursa is found on the plantar aspect of the heel?
Calcaneal bursitis is a common cause of heel pain that mimics plantar fascitis. It occurs after prolonged walking or running, especially in footwear with poor shock absorption. It is diagnosed by tenderness over the calcaneus without pain on toe-walking or plantar fascial stretch. Shock-absorbing heel cups, Achilles stretching, modalities, and injections are helpful in resolving the pain. Injection into the bursa located more superficially than the plantar fascia is recommended for patients refractory to other treatments.

KEY POINTS: COMMON CAUSES OF BURSITIS AND TENDINITIS

1. Abnormal mechanics of the adjacent joint

2. Muscular weakness

3. Overuse/repetitive strain

4. Poor postural control

5. Proximal problem manifesting its effects distally (i.e., cervical radiculopathy resulting in weakness of the muscle group adjacent to the bursa)

TENDONS/ENTHESOPATHIES

37. What are the function and construct of tendon and tendon sheath? How do they compare to a coaxial cable television cable?
The tendon's function is to transmit the force of muscular contraction to the bone, thereby moving a joint. The organizational unit in a tendon is the collagen fibril, which together form

fascicles and as a group compose the tendon itself. Some tendons, especially long ones, are guided and lubricated along their paths by sheaths. The tendon is held close to the bone by a pulley system or fibrous arches. The copper inner core of the cable is the tendon, the white outer covering is the fluid in the sheath, and the tacks that hold the cable to the edge of the baseboard are the pulleys.

38. What is an enthesopathy?
The enthesis is the portion of the tendon as it inserts into the bone. Inflammation can occur in this attachment site, resulting in tendinitis pain and weakness of the corresponding muscle.

39. In which tendon regions should injections be avoided?
Injection should be avoided into the region of large weight-bearing tendons, including the patellar tendon, quadriceps tendon, and Achilles tendon.

40. Why are patients prone to tendinitis in the shoulder joint?
The shoulder is susceptible to the development of tendinitis for three basic reasons. First, the joint is subjected to a wide range of repetitive motions. Second, the space in which the musculotendinous unit functions is restricted by the coracoacromial arch, making impingement a likely possibility with extreme abduction with internal and external rotation. Third, the blood supply to the middle of the tendon is poor, thus making the healing of microtrauma more difficult.

41. What are the causes of tendinitis in the shoulder?
The primary cause of shoulder tendinitis is from impingement of the supraspinatus tendon as it traverses under the acromial arch. With the arm at elevated positions, internal and external rotation causes an abrasion of the supraspinatus tendon. Partial-thickness, full-thickness, and complete tears of the supraspinatus tendon can occur. The cause of bicipital tendinitis is impingement on the biceps tendons at the coracoacromial arch. The onset is usually acute, occurring after over-use or misuse of the shoulder. Impingement can be caused by weakness, laxity or contracture of the trapezius, and periscapular musculature from repetitive use or cervical radiculopathy.

42. What are the different tests used to diagnosis an impingement syndrome?
The Neer and Hawkins tests are the most commonly used tests for the diagnosis of impingement.

43. How is bicipital tendinitis diagnosed?
The pain of bicipital tendinitis is constant, severe, and is localized in the anterior shoulder over the bicipital groove. Diagnosis is made by palpating the proximal and anterior aspect of the shoulder. Tenderness is found when the arm is externally rotated, bringing the bicipital groove under the clinician's finger. When the arm is internally rotated with continued pressure, the pain is absent. A catching with range of motion of the shoulder may accompany the pain and is usually indicative of subluxation of the tendon out of the groove. A positive Yergason's sign can also be found. Speed's test is a more dynamic test to reproduce the patient's symptoms as the tendon glides through the bicipital groove.

44. Where do I inject to relieve the symptoms?
The injection of the biceps tendon sheath is performed with the patient seated. The bicipital groove is palpated with internal and external rotation. The needle direction should be at a 45 degree angle. The tendon sheath is able to accommodated approximately 2 mL of the corticosteroid/lidocaine preparation.

KEY POINTS: MEDICATIONS AND INJECTIONS

1. Avoid injection into Achilles, patellar, and quadriceps tendons.

2. "Say Grace before Tea" is a way to remember the components of the conjoined tendons on the medial aspect of the knee (S = Sartorius, G = Gracilis, T = semiTendinosis).

3. The *watershed area* is the region of the tendon that is most susceptible to the development of tendinitis due to the poor blood supply.

4. An injection of plantar fasciitis always should include a stretching of the Achilles in a subtalar neutral position.

---

45. **What is tennis elbow?**

Tennis elbow, or lateral epicondylitis, is an inflammation of the fibrous origin of the extensor digitorum and extensor carpi radialis brevis muscles (the longus portion of the muscle inserts above the elbow). It occurs at the lateral aspect of the elbow usually secondary to excessive or repetitive dorsiflexion forces of the extensor group.

Tenderness over the lateral epicondyle and pain with resisted dorsiflexion are diagnostic of lateral epicondylitis. Cozen's test is done with the elbow in full extension with a passive stretch of the wrist extensors.

Injections of corticosteroids into the lateral epicondylar region are very helpful in pain reduction. Additional treatment, including NSAIDs, relative rest, physical modalities (heat, ultrasound, and electrical stimulation), extensor stretching, and wrist extension strengthening, is necessary to prevent recurrences. The use of a tennis elbow band or strap is helpful in deflecting the wrist extension forces from the insertional site. The location of the brace pressure should be 1 inch below the point of maximum tenderness. In patients playing tennis, reduction in string tension and enlargement of the grip of the racket are helpful in preventing recurrences. Surgery is necessary in cases refractory to the above-mentioned treatment and usually is associated with tears.

46. **What is the difference between little leaguer's elbow and golfer's elbow?**

The difference is the age of the participants. Little leaguer's elbow/golfer's elbow, also known as medial epicondylitis, is an inflammation of the origin of the flexor carpi radialis and flexor digitorum group. It occurs on the medial aspect of the elbow and is usually secondary to excessive or repetitive volar flexion forces of the wrist. Tenderness over the medial epicondyle and pain with resisted wrist flexion are diagnostic of medial epicondylitis. Injections of corticosteroids into the medial epicondylar region are very helpful in pain reduction. Additional treatment, including NSAIDs, relative rest, physical modalities (heat, ultrasound, and electrical stimulation), flexor stretching, and wrist flexion strengthening, is necessary to prevent recurrences. The use of a tennis elbow band or strap is helpful in deflecting the wrist flexor forces from the insertional site. In children involved in throwing sports, modification of pitching/throwing technique, a reduction of the amount of pitching, and strengthening of the rotator cuff and lower extremities are recommended. In golfers, modification of technique to prevent repetitive wrist motion is recommended. Surgery is necessary in cases refractory to the previously mentioned treatment, and it is usually associated with tears.

47. **What should I look for in patients with reported numbness and/or tingling in the hand in the patient with medial or lateral epicondylitis?**

In lateral epicondylitis, excessive strain on the extensor mechanism results in irritation of the posterior interosseous nerve as it traverses through the extensor muscle group. In medial epicondylitis, inflammation of the anterior interosseous nerve can occur as it traverses through the flexor group. Tenderness is found within the muscle distal to the insertion of the flexor or extensor group and can reproduce the distal symptoms.

48. **Can cubital tunnel syndrome be found with medial epicondylitis?**
Yes, it can. Cubital tunnel syndrome is an inflammation of the ulnar nerve that occurs with excessive stretching or crimping of the nerve as it traverses the ulnar groove behind the elbow. Weakness of hand intrinsics, tenderness, and a positive Tinel sign on palpation of the ulnar nerve in the groove (with or without subluxation) are diagnostic of an ulnar neuropathy. Electrodiagnostic testing (nerve conduction studies and needle electromyography) of the ulnar nerve above and below the elbow should be obtained in pitchers with neurogenic symptoms into the 4th or 5th fingers or hand intrinsic weakness. Surgery may be necessary if there is an associated laxity of the medial collateral ligament of the elbow or if there is persistence of neurologic symptoms.

49. **What is de Quervain's stenosing tenosynovitis?**
De Quervain's stenosing tenosynovitis is caused by an inflammation and swelling of the tendons of the abductor pollicis longus and extensor pollicis brevis at the level of the radial styloid process. This inflammation and swelling is usually the result of trauma to the tendon from repetitive twisting motions of the wrist. It is commonly seen in pregnant women due to weight gain and swelling within the first dorsal wrist compartment.

50. **What test is diagnostic of de Quervain's stenosing tenosynovitis?**
The diagnostic test for this syndrome is Finkelstein's maneuver. The thumb is placed inside the closed hand, and the wrist is passively ulnar deviated with a reproduction of pain.

51. **What are the treatments for de Quervain's stenosing tenosynovitis?**
Treatment should include NSAIDs, relative rest, physical modalities (heat, ultrasound, and electrical stimulation), thumb spica splinting, and exercises in a wrist-neutral position. Injections of corticosteroids can be performed into the first dorsal wrist compartment at the level of the radial styloid. Surgery is recommended for cases refractory to conservative care.

52. **What is the treatment for stenosing flexor tenosynovitis?**
The primary treatment is injection into the tendon sheath. Avoidance of gripping hard items should be encouraged post-injection. Surgical release is recommended in refractory cases and in patients with locking. Rupture of the tendon is rare and requires primary repair in acute cases and tendon grafting in chronic cases. Patients performing repetitive gripping require the use of padded gloves.

53. **What are the treatments for piriformis syndrome?**
The piriformis traverses the posterior pelvis from the sacrum to the posterolateral greater trochanter. Tenderness is found in the muscle belly, with weakness in hip abduction and extension. The most common location of tenderness is 3 cm caudal and lateral to the midpoint of the sacrum's lateral border. It can be associated with sciatica. The muscle functions as an internal rotator of the hip. Treatment includes NSAIDs, relative rest, physical modalities (heat, ultrasound, and electrical stimulation), piriformis stretching, and hip abduction and extension strengthening. In refractory cases, injection and orthotics may be necessary. Rarely, and in the presence of a taut band, surgery may be necessary.

54. **Where do you inject for iliopsoas tendinitis?**
The injection is performed in the proximal and medial aspect of the thigh at the insertion of the iliopsoas onto the lesser tuberosity. Fluoroscopy is usually necessary for the accurate localization of the injection.

55. **How is hamstring tendinitis acquired?**
The knee is subjected to significant repetitive motion under weight-bearing conditions. The relatively poor blood supply of the musculotendinous insertions make it susceptible to the development of tendinitis. Inciting factors may include long-distance running, dancing injuries, or vigorous use of lower extremity strengthening exercise equipment. A contracture and weakness of the hamstring is usually found on the ipsilateral side of the tendinitis.

56. **What are the symptoms of hamstring tendinitis?**
Evaluation of patients with constant and severe pain reveals a lurch-type antalgic gait. There is severe pain to palpation over the tendinous insertion onto the tibia, with the medial portion of the tendon more commonly affected than the lateral portion. Crepitus and pain usually are elicited when palpating the tendon while the patient flexes the affected knee. There is usually an associated contracture and weakness of the affected hamstring.

57. **What is the recommended treatment for hamstring tendinitis?**
Treatment should include NSAIDs, relative rest, physical modalities (heat, ultrasound, and electrical stimulation), hamstring stretching, and open and closed chain hamstring strengthening. Plyometrics and sport-specific exercises should be included prior to return to full activities. Occasionally, foot orthotics with medial posting can be used to reduce stress on the medial hamstring. Rarely, injection of the region around the hamstring tendon is necessary to reduce inflammation.

58. **Identify the two locations of ITB tendinitis.**
The ITB can become inflamed proximally as it traverses the greater trochanter and distally over the lateral femoral condyle.

59. **What test is diagnostic of an iliotibial band contracture?**
How is it performed?
The Ober test is diagnostic for iliotibial band contracture. It is performed with the patient in the side lying position with the hip and knee flexed to 90 degrees. The hip is abducted then extended with the knee maintained in a flexed position. A leg then is allowed to go toward an adducted position. If the knee remains above horizontal, then there is an ITB contracture.

60. **What functional changes are seen in a visual gait analysis of someone with ITB tendinitis?**
Excessive internal rotation of the entire lower extremity is found and results as a tight ITB passes over the greater trochanter and of the distal ITB when there is internal rotation of the tibia on the femur. Pronation, excessive femoral anteversion, torsional abnormalities, and gluteus medius weakness are some of the causes of ITB tendinitis.

61. **What causes posterior tibial tendinitis?**
Posterior tibial tendinitis is seen most commonly in athletes and elderly women. Excessive pronation is the usual cause of an excessive stretch to the tendon. Running on soft or uneven surfaces and improper shoe wear has been implicated in the development of chronic stretching of the posterior tibial tendon.

62. **What is the treatment for posterior tibial tendinitis?**
Treatment should include NSAIDs, relative rest, physical modalities (heat, ultrasound, and electrical stimulation), Achilles stretching in subtalar neutral, and inversion strengthening. Foot orthoses are necessary in chronic cases or in patients exerting excessive pronation forces. Rupture is rare, but when it occurs, the only treatment is shoewear accommodation or subtalar fusion.

63. **What is plantar fasciitis?**

Plantar fasciitis is an inflammation of the tight fibrous band on the plantar aspect of the foot, usually at the insertion onto the calcaneus. It can be found in patients with excessive pronation and Achilles contractures. Treatment should include NSAIDs, relative rest, physical modalities (heat, ultrasound, and electrical stimulation), Achilles stretching, and gastrocnemius strengthening. The use of foot orthotics and a night dorsiflexion splint may be helpful in pain reduction. The use of padded or gel heel pads is usually not effective. Injections of corticosteroids into the site of the insertion of the plantar fascia are helpful in refractory cases. Correction of other intrinsic or extrinsic biomechanical factors is helpful in pain reduction.

KEY POINTS: REHABILITATION

1. Proximal lateral thigh pain that does not resolve with an injection into the greater trochanteric bursa injection usually indicates gluteal tendinitis (in the presence of a positive Trendelenburg sign and hip abduction weakness) or hip arthritis (in the presence of reduced internal rotation of the hip).

2. Heel pain in the absence of tenderness of the Achilles enthesis may represent an injectable pain emanating from the retrocalcaneal bursa.

3. Periscapular pain and weakness are usually a secondary cause of posterior shoulder pain resulting from rotator cuff tendinitis, subacromial bursitis, acromioclavicular arthropathy, subacromial impingement, or cervical radiculopathy but also from a pectoral contracture that needs resolution with a focused physical therapy program.

4. In the diagnosis of anterior knee joint pain, the presence of patellar tendinitis usually represents a rotational malalignment of the lower extremity (femoral anteversion, patellar angle, increased tibial torsion, or excessive pronation), contracture of the thigh musculature (quadriceps and/or hamstring), proximal gluteal weakness, or a combination of the above that needs to be resolved with a combination of treatments (physical therapy, injections, and bracing).

BIBLIOGRAPHY

1. Balch HW, Gibson JMC, el Ghobarey AF, et al: Repeated corticosteroid injections into knee joints. Rheumatol Rehabil 16:137–140, 1997.

2. Dreyfuss P, Cole AJ, Pauza K: Sacroiliac joint injection techniques. Phys Med Rehabil Clin North Am 6:785–813, 1995.

3. Finkelstein D, Smith MK, Faden R: Informed consent and medical ethics. Arch Ophthalmol 111:324–326, 1993.

4. Geiringer SR, Bowyer BL, Press JM: Sports medicine. The physiatric approach. Arch Phys Med Rehabil 74:S428–S432, 1993.

5. Gray RG, Gottlieb NL: Intra-articular corticosteroids. An updated assessment. Clin Orthop 177:235–263, 1983.

6. Gray RG, Gottlieb NL: Intra-articular corticosteroids, basic science and pathology. Clin Orthop Rel Res 177:235–263, 1983.

7. Lennard TA (ed): Pain Procedures in Clinical Practice, 2nd ed. Philadelphia, Hanley & Belfus, 2000.

8. Marks MR, Gunther SF: Efficacy of cortisone injection in treatment of trigger fingers and thumbs. J Hand Surg 14A:722–727, 1989.

9. Mazanec DJ: Pharmacology of corticosteroids in synovial joints. Phys Med Rehabil Clin North Am 6:815–821, 1995.

10. Micheo WF, Rodriques RA, Amy E: Joint and soft-tissue injections of the upper extremity. Phys Med Rehabil Clin North Am 6:823–840, 1995.

11. Millard RS, Dillingham MF: Peripheral joint injections: Lower extremity. Phys Med Rehabil Clin North Am 6:841–849, 1995.

12. Nirschl RP: Elbow tendinosis/tennis elbow. Clin Sports Med 11:851–870, 1992.

13. Pfenninger JL: Injections of joints and soft tissues: Part II. Guidelines for specific joints. Am Fam Physician 44:1690–1701, 1991.

14. Price R, Sinclair H, Heinrich I, et al: Local injection treatment of tennis elbow—hydrocortisone, triamcinolone and lidocaine compared. Br J Rheumatol 30:39–44, 1991.

15. Stefanich RJ: Intra-articular corticosteroids in treatment of osteoarthritis. Orthop Rev 15:65–71, 1986.

16. Strichartz GR: Neural physiology and local anesthetic action. In Cousins MJ, Bridenbaugh PO (eds): Neural Blockade in Clinical Anesthesia and Management of Pain, 2nd ed. Philadelphia, JB Lippincott, 1988, pp 25–45.

17. Young ER, MacKenzie TA: The pharmacology of local anesthetics—A review of the literature. J Can Dent Assoc 58:34–42, 1992.

CHAPTER 31

SPINE: INTERVENTIONAL PHYSIATRIC CARE

Michael B. Furman, MD, MS, Ninad D. Sthalekar, MD, Leland Berkwits, MD, and Frank J.E. Falco, MD

Grant me the courage and skill to aggressively treat those patients that I can improve,
…the strength and serenity to be conservative with those I cannot,
…and the wisdom to know the difference.
                    —Adapted by Michael Furman from Reinhold Niebuhr's *Serenity Prayer*

1. **What is interventional physiatry?**

   Interventional physiatry integrates a thorough musculoskeletal evaluation with diagnostic and therapeutic spinal procedures and appropriate rehabilitation for comprehensive spine care. These diagnostic and therapeutic spinal procedures include sympathetic blocks, epidural injections, sacroiliac joint injections, diagnostic nerve blocks, intra-articular injections, nerve ablations, discography, intradiscal electrothermal annuloplasty, percutaneous disc decompression, vertebroplasty, and kyphoplasty.

2. **How does one differentiate among disc bulge, herniation, protrusion, extrusion, and sequestration?**

   Disc bulge, herniation, protrusion, extrusion, and sequestration are varying types of disc displacements (Table 31-1; Fig. 31-1). Bulges and herniations can be further described based on the degree of displacement, and herniations can be described by their size (Table 31-2; Fig. 31-2).

   Fardon DF, Milette PC: Nomenclature and classification of lumbar disc pathology: Recommendations of the Combined Task Forces of the North American Spine Society, American Society of Spine Radiology, and American Society of Neuroradiology. Spine 26(5):E93–E113, 2001.

TABLE 31-1.   TYPES OF DISC DISPLACEMENTS

Disc Displacement	Definition
Bulge	Nuclear material extending beyond the vertebral margin but with no annulus defect
Herniation	Localized displacement of disc material beyond the limits of the intervertebral disc space into or through an annulus defect
■ Protrusion	When the distance between the edges of the disc material beyond the disc space is **less** than the distance between the edges at its base
■ Extrusion	When the distance between the edges of the disc material beyond the disc space is **greater** than the distance between the edges at its base; this can be described as a "**pinch.**"
■ Sequestration	A type of extrusion when no disc tissue bridges the displaced portion and the tissues of the disc of origin; this can be described as a "**free fragment.**"

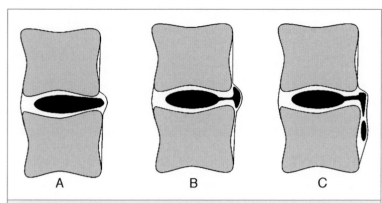

Figure 31-1. Sagittal drawings of the three types of disc herniations: *A,* Protrusion; *B,* Extrusion; *C,* Sequestration. (Adopted from Fardon DF, Milette PC: Nomenclature and classification of lumbar disc pathology: Recommendations of the Combined Task Forces of the North American Spine Society, American Society of Spine Radiology, and American Society of Neuroradiology. Spine 26[5]:E93–E113, 2001.)

TABLE 31-2. CLASSIFICATION OF DISC BULGES AND HERNIATIONS

Description	Degree of Displacement (% of Disc Circumference)
Localized/focal	<25
Broad-based	25–50
Generalized	>50

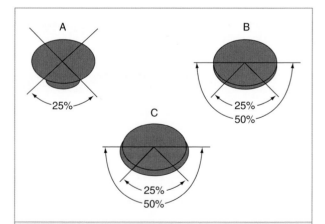

Figure 31-2. Bulges and herniations can be further described based on the degree of displacement: *A,* Localized protrusion; *B,* Broad-based protrusion; *C,* Generalized protrusion. (Adopted from Fardon DF, Milette PC: Nomenclature and classification of lumbar disc pathology: Recommendations of the Combined Task Forces of the North American Spine Society, American Society of Spine Radiology, and American Society of Neuroradiology. Spine 26[5]:E93–E113, 2001.)

3. **In a right extraforaminal herniation of the L4–L5 disc, what spinal nerve is involved and should be treated with a more specific selective injection?**
The direction of disc herniations in the axial plane can be more precisely identified by their occurrence in different zones. These zones can be defined as central, subarticular, foraminal, and extraforaminal (Fig. 31-3). Older texts may define these areas as posterior-lateral, paracentral, or far-lateral.

At each disc level, a nerve either exits slightly superior to the level or traverses centrally and exits inferior to the level. **Central herniations** (more common) affect the traversing nerve roots before they exit inferior to that level. Therefore, a central L4–L5 disc herniation would affect the L5 nerve prior to its exit through the L5 neural foramen inferior to the disc (Fig. 31-4).

An **extraforaminal herniation** (less common) contacts the nerve root superior to that level after it exits (laterally) and descends past the disc. Because the L4 nerve root exits slightly superior to the L4–L5 disc, an extraforaminal herniation would affect the nerve root superior to that level. Therefore, in a right L4–L5 extraforaminal disc herniation contact, the L4 spinal nerve would be affected (Table 31-3).

Fardon DF, Milette PC: Nomenclature and classification of lumbar disc pathology: Recommendations of the Combined Task Forces of the North American Spine Society, American Society of Spine Radiology, and American Society of Neuroradiology. Spine 26(5):E93–E113, 2001.

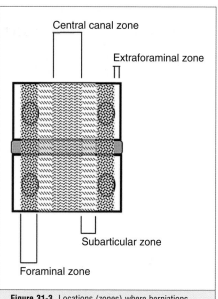

Figure 31-3. Locations (zones) where herniations occur.

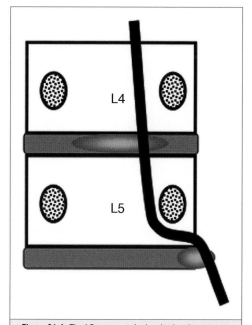

Figure 31-4. The L5 nerve can be involved as it traverses centrally past the L4–L5 disc or laterally as it exits the L5–S1 disc.

TABLE 31-3. SEGMENTAL NERVE INVOLVED WITH LUMBAR HERNIATED NUCLEUS PULPOSUS (HNP)

Herniated Disc	Nerve Involved in Central HNP	Nerve Involved in Extraforaminal HNP
L1–L2	L2	L1
L2–L3	L3	L2
L3–L4	L4	L3
L4–L5	L5	L4
L5–S1	S1	L5

4. **In a C4–C5 disc extraforaminal herniation, what spinal nerve is involved and should be treated with a more selective injection?**

As described above for the lumbar spine, an exiting cervical nerve traverses centrally and exits inferior to the level. In the cervical spine, however, the nerves exit more horizontally than in the thoracic and lumbar spine. Hence, an extraforaminal cervical herniation also contacts the traversing nerve as it exits (laterally). Therefore, both a right C4–C5 central and extraforaminal disc herniation contacts the C5 spinal nerve.

Above C8, a central and extraforaminal herniation would always contact the nerve that exits between the two levels. For example, in a C6–C7 herniation, the traversing C7 nerve root would be affected. In a C7–T1 herniation, the traversing C8 root would be affected (Table 31-4).

Fardon DF, Milette PC: Nomenclature and classification of lumbar disc pathology: Recommendations of the Combined Task Forces of the North American Spine Society, American Society of Spine Radiology, and American Society of Neuroradiology. Spine 26(5):E93–E113, 2001.

TABLE 31-4. SEGMENTAL NERVE INVOLVED WITH CERVICAL (HNP)

Herniated Disc	Nerve Involved in Central HNP	Nerve Involved in Extraforaminal HNP
C2–C3	C3	C3
C3–C4	C4	C4
C4–C5	C5	C5
C5–C6	C6	C6
C6–C7	C7	C7
C7–T1	C8	C8

5. **Describe the innervation of the lumbar intervertebral disc.**

The sinuvertebral nerve, gray rami communicans, and ventral rami innervate the lumbar intervertebral discs. The gray ramus communicans from the sympathetic trunks supplies the ipsilateral anterior, lateral, and posterolateral annulus. The ventral ramus directly branches as it exits the intervertebral foramen to supply the ipsilateral outer third to half of the lateral annulus. The sinuvertebral nerve, formed by the gray ramus communicans and a branch from the segmental ventral ramus, innervates the posterior annular fibers of the segmental and cephalad intervertebral discs.

Groen GJ, Baljet B, Drukker J: Nerves and nerve plexuses of the human vertebral column. Am J Anatomy 188(3):282–296, 1990.

6. **Which nerves innervate the L4–L5 and L5–S1 zygapophyseal joints (Z-joints)?**

All Z-joints are innervated by two nerve branches: one from the posterior ramus above and one at the same segmental level. In the cervical spine (above C7–T1), the numbering is intuitive. For C7–T1 and inferiorly, the innervation is a bit more challenging, as demonstrated in Table 31-5.

The L4 medial branch and the L5 dorsal ramus innervate the L5–S1 Z-joint. (Incidentally, older papers cite S1 as innervating the joint; however, this has been shown not to be true.) The L4–L5 Z-joint is innervated by the L3 and L4 medial branches of the dorsal rami nerves. Therefore, when performing a single Z-joint block, two nerves need to be anesthetized.

If two consecutive Z-joints are treated ipsilaterally, then three nerves need to be anesthetized. If one were to treat the L4–L5 and L5–S1 Z-joints, then the nerves to be anesthetized would be the L3 and L4 medial branches and the L5 dorsal ramus. For "n" consecutive, ipsilateral Z-joints, n + 1 nerves should be blocked.

Bogduk N: The innervation of the lumbar spine. Spine 8(3):286–293, 1983.

TABLE 31-5.   INNERVATION OF THE ZYGAPOPHYSEAL (FACET) JOINTS

Zygapophyseal Joint	Innervation
C2–C3	C2/3 (third occipital nerve) and C3
C3–C4	C3 and C4 medial branches
C4–C5	C4 and C5 medial branches
C5–C6	C5 and C6 medial branches
C6–C7	C6 and C7 medial branches
C7–T1	C7 and C8 medial branches
T1–T2	C8 and T1 medial branches
⋮	⋮
T2–T3	T1 and T2 medial branches
L3–L4	L2 and L3 medial branches
L4–L5	L3 and L4 medial branches
L5–S1	L4 medial branch and L5 dorsal ramus

7. **What should be considered prior to performing a radiofrequency denervation procedure of a lumbar zygapophyseal (facet) joint?**

Patients should have an absolute diagnosis of facet Z-joint pain. This cannot be validly diagnosed by clinical impression, physical exam, or radiographic imaging alone. The recommended method of making this diagnosis and minimizing the large percentage of placebo responders (approximately 30% false-positive rate) is to use a double block paradigm. A comparative blockade of the medial branch nerves on two different visits using two different anesthetic agents significantly reduces the false-positive response. The patient should have at least 50–80% relief following both medial branch blocks to be considered a positive response.

Dreyfuss P, Halbrook B, Pauza K, et al: Efficacy and validity of radiofrequency neurotomy for chronic lumbar *zygapophyseal* joint pain. Spine 25(10):1270–1277, 2000.

8. **What is the prevalence of discogenic axial low back pain? What are its symptoms?**

Annular fiber deterioration can lead to radial fissuring, which can extend into the outer innervated disc margin, resulting in axial low back pain. Discogenic axial low back pain prevalence is approximately 40% in low back pain sufferers.

Pain is typically described as centralized, nonradicular pain produced by certain activities. Patients can also have diffuse nondermatomal lower limb pain associated with axial low back pain, but not typically in isolation. Symptoms are increased with axial loading activities such as sitting, lifting, or standing. Physical examination findings are usually unremarkable except for restricted range of motion, pain with flexion or extension, and discogenic segmental mobilization tenderness.

Schwarzer AC, Aprill CN, Derby R, et al: The prevalence and clinical features of internal disc disruption in patients with chronic low back pain. Spine 20:1878–1883, 1995.

9. **When is provocation lumbar discography used?**

No radiologic studies alone can definitively identify the disc as the pain source. Lumbar discography's primary indication is to identify the pain generator in a patient with chronic low back pain without radicular pain or magnetic resonance imaging (MRI)-documented neural compression.

Discography can also be used for identifying disc lesions when MRIs are equivocal (or unreadable) and when evaluating discs adjacent to previously fused lumbar segments. It also can be used to evaluate discs that are adjacent to clearly pathologic levels considered for fusion or intradiscal therapies.

Discography can also be useful in patients who have undergone partial posterolateral lumbar fusion in which a posterior lumbar interbody fusion has not been performed. Discography also may be indicated to assist in the diagnosis of pseudoarthrosis. Post-discography computed tomography (CT) scans can also visualize extra-foraminal herniations, which cannot be visualized by traditional CT-myelograms. This may be helpful when MRI is contraindicated (post-pacemaker or spinal cord stimulator).

Gevirtz C: A critical evaluation of discography. Top Pain Manage 21(2):1–6, 2005.

10. **When performing a discogram, how are findings and intradiscal tears classified and graded under fluoroscopy?**

1. Clinical rating of pain
   - **Subjective scale 1–10**
   - **Type of pain:** Pressure, dissimilar, exact reproduction (concordant)
2. Volume of contrast injected
3. Manometry
4. Nucleogram
   - **Cottonball:** No sign of disc disruption. Contrast collects uniformly within the nucleus.
   - **Lobular:** No sign of disc disruption. Contrast is contained within the nucleus and coalesces into fibrous lumps.
   - **Irregular:** Contrast disperses into fissures and clefts and penetrates the inner annulus.
   - **Fissured:** Contrast extends through radial fissures to the outer edge of the annulus.
   - **Ruptured:** Contrast extends through radial fissures and leaks beyond the outer edge of the annulus.
5. Other information thought to be important (e.g., end-plate penetration, Schmorl's nodes)

Aprill C, Bogduk N: High-intensity zone: A diagnostic sign of painful lumbar disc on magnetic resonance imaging. Br J Radiol 65:361–369, 1992.

Sachs BL, Vanharanta H, Spivey MA, et al: Dallas discogram description. A new classification of CT/discography in low-back disorders. Spine 12(3):287–294, 1987.

Windsor RE, Falco FJE, Dreyer SJ: Lumbar discography. In Weinstein S (ed): Physical Medicine and Rehabilitation. Injection Techniques. Philadelphia, W.B. Saunders, 1995, pp 743–770.

11. **What is visualized on a post-discogram CT scan?**

A post-discogram CT scan be done to determine if the contrast is internuclear and to better visualize its dispersal pattern. This can be classified in two ways in the axial view:

1. **General degeneration:** Based on the annular appearance of the axial contrast-enhanced view of the disc
   - **Grade 0:** No change
   - **Grade 1:** Local (<10% quadrant distribution)
   - **Grade 2:** Partial (<50% quadrant distribution)
   - **Grade 3:** Total (>50% quadrant distribution)
2. **Annular disruption:** The degree of protrusion and location of annular contrast
   - **Grade 0:** None
   - **Grade 1:** Into the inner annulus
   - **Grade 2:** Into the outer annulus
   - **Grade 3:** Beyond the outer annulus
   - **Grade 4:** Beyond the outer annulus extending into a 30-degree circumferential arc
   - **Grade 5:** Full-thickness tear with extension of contrast outside the annulus

Aprill C, Bogduk N: High-intensity zone: A diagnostic sign of painful lumbar disc on magnetic resonance imaging. Br J Radiol 65(773):361–369, 1992.

Sachs BL, Vanharanta H, Spivey MA, et al: Dallas discogram description: A new classification of CT/discography in low-back disorders. Spine 12(3):287–294, 1987.

Schellhas KP, Pollei SR, Gundry CR, et al. Lumbar disc high-intensity zone: Correlation of magnetic resonance imaging and discography. Spine 21(1):79–86, 1996.

12. **What complications are associated with lumbar discography?**

The risk of complications from lumbar discography is low. They are infrequent and include discitis, subarachnoid puncture, nerve root injury, meningitis, bleeding, and allergic reaction. Risks can be minimized by excluding individuals with contrast dye allergies, using nonionic contrast, and sterile technique.

Bogduk N, Aprill C, Derby R: Discography. In White AH (ed): Spine Care, Vol 1. St Louis, Mosby, 1995, pp 219–238.

13. **What is discitis?**

Discitis is the most concerning complication of lumbar discography, with a reported incidence of 0.05–1.3% for each evaluated disc level. The most common pathogen is *Staphylococcus epidermidis*. Prophylactic and intradiscal antibiotics may decrease the risks.

Individuals who develop discitis typically present with severe back pain and spasms 2–4 weeks after the procedure. Back pain is increased by any activity and relieved by rest. Patients may report fever and chills. The erythrocyte sedimentation rate (ESR) is usually increased at an average of 20 days, followed by a positive bone scan at an average of 33 days. C-reactive protein (CRP) and temperature have also been shown to be increased. Although ESR and CRP are highly sensitive, MRI with gadolinium is considered the best means for definitive diagnosis (higher specificity). It may show retrodiscal infection and spondylodiscitis. In cases of retrodiscal infection or discitis, conservative treatment with IV antibiotics is sufficient. In cases of retrodiscal abscess, operative intervention should be considered.

Bogduk N, Aprill C, Derby R: Discography. In White AH (ed): Spine Care, Vol 1. St Louis, Mosby, 1995, pp 219–238.

Fraser RD, Osti AI, Vernon-Roberts B: Discitis after discography. J Bone Joint Surg 69B:26–35, 1987.

Guyer RD, Collier R, Stith WJ, et al: Discitis after discography. Spine 13(12):1352–1354, 1988.

Schulitz KP, Assheuer J: Discitis after procedures on the intervertebral disc. Spine 19(10):1172–1177, 1994.

14. **What findings on physical exam provide conclusive evidence of sacroiliac joint pathology?**

None. There are a number of physical exam maneuvers that can help to lead to a suggestive diagnosis of sacroiliac joint pathology. These include the Gillet test, the Gaenslen test, the Patrick or flexion abduction and external rotation (FABER) test, the posterior shear (POSH) or thigh thrust test, the resisted abduction (REAB) test, and the Yeoman test. Patients may also point to within 2 inches of the posterior superior iliac spine (PSIS) to indicate the site of maximal pain.

Despite providing a high predictive value, it is widely accepted that physical examination gives valuable but not conclusive information concerning the presence of sacroiliac joint syndrome (SIJS) and that confirmation of SIJS requires a positive sacroiliac joint block.

Dreyfuss P, Michaelsen M, Pauza K, et al: The value of medical history and physical examination in diagnosing sacroiliac joint pain. Spine 21(22):2594–2602, 1996.

Slipman CW, Sterenfeld EB, Chou LH, et al: The value of radionuclide imaging in the diagnosis of sacroiliac joint syndrome. Spine 21(19):2251–2254, 1996.

Zelle BA, Gruen GS, Brown S, et al: Sacroiliac joint dysfunction: Evaluation and management. Clin J Pain 21(5):446–455, 2005.

15. **In a lumbar transforaminal epidural steroid injection, what is the "safe triangle"? What structures delineate its borders?**

When performing lumbar transforaminal epidural steroid injections, it is best to avoid directly contacting dura or spinal nerve. By targeting the safe triangle, the area where the needle tip should be introduced, direct contact with these structures is rare. The safe triangle contains only the sinuvertebral nerve and its accompanying vessels. A needle may typically be introduced into the triangle without damaging other structures. In a two-dimensional anteroposterior (AP) view, the superior border is the pedicle, the medial border is the nerve root/dural sleeve, and the lateral border is the vertical portion of the vertebral body (Fig. 31-5).

Derby R, Bogduk N, Kine G: Precision percutaneous blocking procedures for localizing spinal pain. Part 2: The lumbar neuroaxial compartment. Pain Digest 3:175–188, 1993.

16. **When performing a cervical transforaminal epidural steroid, what structures should be avoided? What are the potential complications associated with these structures?**

The incidence of fluoroscopically confirmed intravascular uptake of contrast has been shown to be as high as 19.4% in cervical transforaminal injections. There are two major vascular structures to be avoided when performing the procedure:

- The **anterior spinal artery**, which receives supply from the cervical radicular arteries. When injecting a steroid solution such as depot preparations, the particulate material can act as an embolus and theoretically lead to spinal cord infarction or cerebrovascular accident.
- The **vertebral artery**, which lies adjacent and ventral to the spinal nerve. Local anesthetic injected into the vertebral artery can lead to seizure. Injection of particulate matter could lead to vertebrobasilar thrombosis and brain stem infarction.

Baker R, Dreyfuss P, Mercer S, Bogduk N: Cervical transforaminal injection of corticosteroids into a radicular artery: A possible mechanism for spinal cord injury. Pain 103(1–2):211–215, 2003.

Brouwers PJ, Kottink EJ, Simon MA, Prevo RL: A cervical anterior spinal artery syndrome after diagnostic blockade of the right C6-nerve root. Pain 91(3):397–399, 2001.

Furman MB, Giovanniello MT, O'Brien EM: Incidence of intravascular penetration in transforaminal cervical epidural steroid injections. Spine 28(1):21–25, 2003.

17. **What is the most common potential complication associated with an interlaminar epidural steroid injection?**

The most common complication is thecal sac puncture, occurring in 1–2% of lumbar epidurals. The most notable effect is spinal headache, with incidence of 1–4%. Infection, direct trauma

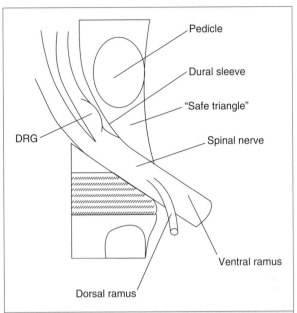

Figure 31-5. Needle placement for a lumbar transforaminal ESI typically targets the "safe triangle." (Modified from Derby R, Bogduk N, Kine G: Precision percutaneous blocking procedures for localizing spinal pain. Part 2: The lumbar neuroaxial compartment. Pain Digest 3:175–188, 1993.)

to the spinal cord, and epidural hematomas (extremely rare) may occur. Severe cases of epidural hematomas present with profound weakness and usually occur in the immediate postprocedural period. These complications may result in devastating sequelae in the cervical or thoracic spine.

Bogduk N, Christophidus N, Cherry D, et al: Epidural use of steroids in the management of back pain and sciatica of spinal origin. Report of the Working Party on Epidural Use of Steroids in the Management of Back Pain. National Health and Medical Research Council, Camberra, 1993.

18. **After a lumbar epidural steroid injection, a patient reports headache that does not change with position. Would you consider doing a blood patch?**
This scenario is not consistent with a spinal headache. Spinal headaches are much more severe when the person is in an upright position and improve when the person lies down. These headaches occur secondary to an inadvertent puncture of the dura during a spinal procedure. They may begin within an hour to several days after the procedure based on the triggering mechanism. The mechanism of cerebrospinal fluid (CSF) leakage led to the rationale for the several therapeutic methods currently used in the conservative management of spinal headache. Hydration is instituted with the intent of increasing the production of CSF such that it exceeds its loss through the puncture site, thus restoring the CSF pressure to normal. Caffeine is an optional supplement that seems to be effective because of its vasoconstrictor effect.

If a spinal headache persists after 24 hours of conservative treatment consisting of rest, IV fluids, and analgesic therapy, an epidural blood patch can be performed. This is done by placing a needle in the epidural space in the vicinity of the dural puncture and aseptically injecting autologous blood. The blood clots and seals the punctured region of the dura.

Elkersh MA, Simopoulos TT, Bajwa ZH: Fundamentals of interventional pain medicine. Neurologist 11(5):285–293, 2005.

Safa-Tisseront V, Thormann F, Malassine P, et al: Effectiveness of epidural blood patch in the management of post-dural puncture headache. Anesthesiology 95(2):334–339, 2001.

19. **A patient presents for evaluation for a lumbar epidural steroid injection. The patient complains of lateral right thigh pain and denies numbness or weakness. Reflexes are normal. What must be ruled out?**
Trochanteric bursitis is characterized by chronic, intermittent aching pain over the lateral aspect of the hip. Occasionally, the onset of pain is acute or subacute, and the quality of pain can be sharp and intense. The pain extends into the lateral aspect of the thigh in 25–40% of cases; however, it rarely extends into the posterior aspect of the thigh or distal to the knee. In a minority of patients, pain initially may be perceived in the *low-back* area or around the knee, but the typical pain pattern usually emerges. Patients may report numbness and paresthesia-like symptoms in the upper thigh, which typically do not follow a dermatomal segment.

Shbeeb MI, Matteson EL: Trochanteric bursitis (greater trochanter pain syndrome). Mayo Clin Proc 71:565–569, 1996.

20. **What are the indications for implantation of a spinal cord stimulator (SCS)?**
Indications for SCS placement are complex regional pain syndrome, failed back surgery syndrome, severe peripheral vascular disease, and ischemic heart disease. In contrast, paraplegic pain, stump pain, phantom limb pain, primary bone pain, and joint disease pain have demonstrated a poor response to SCSs. It must also be confirmed that the patient's pain is mostly appendicular and that there are no treatable causes of the patient's pain as described on imaging or electrodiagnostic studies. Absolute contraindications for SCS placement are infection, drug abuse, and severe psychiatric illness. Prior to implantation of an SCS, a psychological evaluation is recommended.

Kumar K, Toth C, Nath RK, Laing P: Epidural spinal cord stimulation for treatment of chronic pain—some predictors of success. A 15-year experience. Surg Neurol 50(2):110–120; discussion 120–121, 1998.

KEY POINTS: INTERVENTIONAL PHYSIATRIC PEARLS

1. The L4 spinal nerve exits laterally between the L4 and L5 vertebral body. The L5 spinal nerve exits laterally between the L5 and S1 vertebral body. In the cervical spine, because eight cervical spinal nerves exit more horizontally, the C7 nerve exits between the C6 and C7 vertebral bodies. The C8 nerve exits between the C7 and T1 vertebral bodies, etc.

2. The major risk associated with cervical transforaminal epidural steroid injections is an advertent injection of the vertebral artery.

3. Trochanteric bursitis can present with lateral thigh pain mimicking the proximal symptoms of an L5 radiculopathy.

4. The most common indication for vertebroplasty or kyphoplasty is painful vertebral compression fracture secondary to osteoporosis.

5. Intradiscal electrothermal annuloplasty (IDET) is indicated for axial pain, and percutaneous disc decompression is indicated for radicular pain.

21. **What is vertebroplasty? What are its indications?**
Percutaneous vertebroplasty is the injection of polymethylmethacrylate into the vertebral body. It is indicated for the treatment of painful vertebral compression fractures caused by osteoporosis, some primary bone tumors, and metastatic disease. The most common cause of vertebral compression fractures is osteoporosis. These fractures most commonly occur at the thoracolumbar junction.

Diagnosis can be made by bone scan or MRI. Acute or subacute fractures less than 30 days old appear hypointense on T1-weighted images and hyperintense on T2 images secondary to edema.

The procedure is less likely to be successful if the fracture is greater than 6 months old or if the vertebral body has lost more than 70% of its height. If the lesion lies above T6, the approach is usually transpedicular, therefore making it more technically challenging.

No more than two to three levels should be done at one time because of the increased incidence of complications related to venous extravasation of cement, increased risk of fat embolization, as well as transient arterial hypotension thought to be caused by the methylmethacrylate.

Stallmeyer B, Zoarsk GH, Obuchowski AM: Optimizing patient selection in percutaneous vertebroplasty. J Vasc Intervent Radiol 14(6):683–696, 2003.

22. **What is kyphoplasty? What are its indications?**
A compression fracture in the osteoporotic spine may lead to a kyphotic deformity, which creates a biomechanical environment favoring additional fractures. Kyphoplasty is a minimally invasive procedure designed to address the kyphotic deformity as well as fracture pain. It involves the percutaneous placement of an inflatable bone tamp into a fractured vertebral body. Inflation of the bone tamp will result in a cavity being created within the vertebral body, thereby restoring vertebral height and improving sagittal alignment.

Kyphoplasty may improve pulmonary mechanics, decrease pain, and reduce the risk of adjacent level vertebral fractures; however, long-term studies confirming these opinions are lacking since the procedure was first reported in 2000.

The risks and contraindications associated with the procedure are similar to those associated with vertebroplasty. Because kyphoplasty involves the creation of an intervertebral cavity, however, it allows application of more viscous cement, which may reduce the risk of extravertebral cement extravasation.

Frank M: Minimally invasive treatments of osteoporotic vertebral compression fractures. Spine 28(Suppl 15):S45–S53, 2003.

23. **What is intradiscal electrothermal annuloplasty (IDET)? What are its indications?**
IDET® (Smith and Nephew, London) is used to treat unremitting lumbar axial pain caused by internal disc disruption that has failed conservative treatment. This diagnosis is usually confirmed with provocation discography. The percutaneous procedure involves the insertion of a catheter via a large bore needle into the nuclear/annular interface. The distal portion of the catheter incorporates an active electrothermal tip. Its proposed mechanism of action is to "shut off" intervertebral disc pain fibers by coagulating the nociceptors and by "strengthening" the disc by modifying its collagen structure. The procedure is typically not indicated for discs with greater than a 50% collapse or for patients with predominantly radicular pain.

Derby R, Eek B, Chen Y, et al: Intradiscal electrothermal annuloplasty (IDET): A novel approach for treating chronic discogenic low back pain. Neuromodulation 3:82–88, 2000.

Kleinstueck FS, Diederich CJ, Nau WH, et al: Acute biomechanical and histological effects of intradiscal electrothermal therapy on human lumbar discs. Spine 26(20):2198–2207, 2001.

Lutz LJ, Rodeo CD, Wright T: Stability of the lumbar spine after intradiscal electrothermal therapy. Arch Phys Med Rehabil 82(1):120–122, 2001.

24. **Describe the different methods of percutaneous disc decompression and their indications.**
Disc decompression is used to treat patients with predominantly radicular type pain caused by small contained disc herniations that produce pressure on adjacent spinal nerves. The

procedure involves decompressing the center of the disc and collapsing a contained herniation, thereby relieving pressure on the spinal nerve. Removal of disc material can be accomplished percutaneously through a chemical reaction, mechanical removal, or by the use of a laser.

Chymopapain depolymerizes the proteoglycan and glycoprotein macromolecules of the nucleus pulposus, leading to reductions in intervertebral disc height and disc bulge. Chymopapain may also act by reducing the inflammatory response in the affected nerve root or by direct effects on the nerve root itself.

Suction discectomy uses the reciprocating action of a cutting tool and aspiration of macerated disc material through a small cannula that is introduced into the disc.

Dekompressor® (Stryker, Kalamazoo, MI) involves extracting nuclear material by an auger within a cannula, which is positioned inside the nucleus. Extracted nuclear material can be examined pathologically and quantified. The possible mechanism of action of intervertebral disc decompression using the Dekompressor involves volume reduction within an enclosed hydraulic space by the device, which, in turn, leads to significant change in intradiscal pressure and a decrease to the annular wall stress.

Laser decompression involves percutaneous placement of a single needle in the disc space and transmitting laser energy in short bursts that vaporize disc material.

Nucleoplasty® (ArthroCare, Sunnyvale, CA) utilizes coblation technology to decompress contained herniated discs percutaneously. Coblation is a radiofrequency-based technology that ablates and coagulates soft tissue. During coblation, a ***Perc-D** LR Spine Wand* is inserted into the disc via an introducer. An ionized vapor layer, or plasma field, is generated at the tip of the device. The ionized plasma field cleaves covalent bonds, resulting in molecular dissociation and therefore decreasing the volume within the disc. Because this effect is typically achieved at temperatures of approximately 40–70°C, thermal damage to surrounding tissue is minimized.

Acutherm® (Smith and Nephew, London) is used for targeted disc decompression. A catheter is inserted into the outer rim of the nucleus pulposus via a large bore needle. The catheter is then positioned over the area of disc herniation. Acutherm uses heat energy to coagulate the collagen in the disc, causing tissue contraction and a reduction in the herniation. It is different from other forms of percutaneous disc decompression because the catheter is positioned over the herniation rather than being inserted into the center of the disc.

Although success has been described for these procedures, the outcomes from these procedures have not been compared to each other. There have been high success rates in improved function and patient satisfaction with these procedures; however, open discectomy remains the gold standard for treatment of radicular pain secondary to lumbar disc herniation.

Atlas SJ, Keller RB, Wu YA, et al: Long-term outcomes of surgical and nonsurgical management of sciatica secondary to a lumbar disc herniation: 10-year results from the Maine Lumbar Spine Study. Spine 30(8):927–935, 2005.

Jaikumar S, Kim DH, Kam AC: History of minimally invasive spine surgery. Neurosurgery 51(Suppl 2): S212–S214, 2002.

Kapural L, Goldner J: Interventional pain management: When/what therapies are best for low back pain. Curr Opin Anesthesiol 18(5):569–575, 2005.

www.EndoPoints:smith-nephew.com

WEBSITES

1. International Spinal Intervention Society
   http://www.spinalinjection.com/
2. American Society of Interventional Pain Physicians
   http://www.asipp.org/
3. American Society of Regional Anesthesia and Pain Medicine
   http://www.asra.com/

CHAPTER 32

MEDICAL ACUPUNCTURE: FUNDAMENTALS AND CLINICAL APPLICATIONS

John Giusto, MD, and Joseph M. Helms, MD

Obviously, we need much more research, but we did find there was sufficient evidence to show a relationship between this technique (acupuncture) and things that happen physiologically.... I think this is a very exciting beginning, because this is a promising treatment that is less invasive, with fewer side effects, than much of what's available in conventional medicine in this country. It's time to take acupuncture seriously.

–David Ramsay, president of the University of Maryland and chairman of the conference, NIH Consensus Development Conference on Acupuncture, November 3–5, 1997

1. **What is acupuncture?**

   Acupuncture is the use of fine needles inserted through the skin at specific points on the body to treat illness. The basic premise is that the stimulation from the needles assists the body's mechanisms of physiologic regulation and repair.

2. **When and where did acupuncture begin? How long has it been used in Western medicine?**

   Acupuncture is a traditional treatment that dates back over 2,000 years in China. As a tradition, it has spread to other cultures, being adapted to local needs and customs. As a medical art, it has evolved with the passage of time. Acupuncture has been used for 1,500 years in Japan and 200 years in Europe, but it has only been prominent in the United States for 30 years. Comparatively, recent developments include the use of electrical stimulation and treatments solely based on neuroanatomic principles. **Medical acupuncture** is a hybrid approach that "respects our contemporary understanding of neuromuscular anatomy and pain physiology while embracing the classical Chinese perception of a subtle circulation network of a vivifying force called *qi*."

3. **Explain the classical Chinese conception of acupuncture.**

   Acupuncture is one discipline extracted from a complex heritage of Chinese medicine—a tradition that also includes massage and manipulation, stretching and breathing exercises, and herbal formulae, as well as exorcism of demons and magical correspondences.
   The language in classical Chinese medicine texts reflects nature and agrarian village metaphors and describes a philosophy of man functioning harmoniously within an orderly universe. The models of health, disease, and treatment are presented in terms of patients' harmony or disharmony within this larger order and involve their responses to external extremes of wind, heat, damp, dryness, and cold, as well as to internal extremes of anger, excitement, worry, sadness, and fear. Illnesses, likewise, are described and defined poetically by divisions of the yin and yang polar opposites (interior or exterior, cold or hot, deficient or excessive), by descriptors attached to elemental qualities (wood, fire, earth, metal, and water), and by the functional influences traditionally associated with each of the internal organs. The classical anatomy of acupuncture consists of energy channels traversing the body. The principle energy pathways are named for the organs whose realms of influence are expanded from their

conventional biomedical physiology to include functional, energetic, and metaphorical qualities (e.g., kidney supervises bones, marrow, joints, hearing, head hair, will, and motivation).

4. **What disorders can acupuncture treat?**
   The clinical literature of **controlled trials** includes treatment of low back pain, headaches, arthritic pain, extremity pain, postoperative pain, respiratory problems, urologic problems, and substance abuse. **Uncontrolled reports** include claims of effective application in almost every discipline of medicine. The World Health Organization maintains a list of conditions recommended for treatment by acupuncture and, in 1997, the National Institutes of Health issued a consensus statement dealing with the rational basis for acupuncture treatment. Both reports are available online.

5. **How big are the needles? How deep do they go?**
   Acupuncture needles are much thinner than needles to draw blood or give injections. They are available in sizes from 30–36 gauge. The needles are usually 1–1.5 inches long but range from 0.5–5 inches for special applications. The depth of insertion depends on the type of treatment and point location as well as the patient's size. Most points on the extremities are needled to a depth of 0.25–0.5 inch, whereas points on the low back are routinely needled 1–1.5 inches. Points on the buttocks may require insertion of 3 inches or more.

6. **How many needles are used in a treatment?**
   The usual range is 10–20 needles in any given treatment. Often fewer needles (5–10) are used in the initial treatment of someone who has not had acupuncture before. Many needles (25–40) may be used when superficial (<1/8 inch) needling techniques are employed to treat diffuse chronic myofascial pain.

7. **Does it hurt?**
   There may be a pinching sensation when the needle first breaks the skin. This sensation is minimized through the use of proper insertion techniques or guide tubes. Most patients report a mild but deep ache lasting for several seconds when the acupuncture needle reaches the depth of the point. Occasionally, fleeting, sharp, or electric sensations occur when a sensory nerve is stimulated. These are not dangerous and do not last.

8. **How many treatments are needed? How often are they given?**
   A typical course of treatment will number 6–12 sessions, with the first 2–4 treatments done twice weekly, the next 4–6 done weekly, and the remainder at 2–4-week intervals. Whereas some problems <3 months' duration can be resolved in as few as three visits, most long-standing conditions (>1 year's duration) need a full course of 10–12 sessions. Chronic neuromusculoskeletal pain problems commonly require maintenance treatments at 4–6 week intervals for a protracted period. A reasonable clinical trial would be six treatments; it is unlikely that significant results will be obtained if an initial response has not occurred in this period.

9. **What effects can one expect after receiving acupuncture?**
   The most common effect after the first few treatments is a global feeling of euphoria and mild disorientation that can last several hours. It is more pronounced after the use of electrical stimulation and is attributed to endorphin release. At times, patients experience intermittent residual **achiness** at the points that were needled. This achiness rarely lasts > 12 hours and can be relieved with nonprescription analgesics.

   With respect to the underlying condition, there are three possible *treatment outcomes*—no response, improvement, or worsening. The last response, treatment aggravation, is not necessarily a bad sign. Often, it is simply the result of too vigorous or too extensive an input.

It should not last >3 days and may be addressed with anti-inflammatory or analgesic medications, including prescription-strength drugs.

10. **Have studies been done to show the analgesic effects of acupuncture?**
Acupuncture analgesia is one of the most thoroughly researched areas in medicine. Animal and human experiments that started in China in the 1960s have been pursued in Europe and the United States. Two types of analgesia have been identified:
- **Endorphin-dependent** analgesia is induced by manual twirling of the needle or electrical stimulation that is of low frequency (2–4 Hz) and high intensity (>10 mA). Characteristics of this response include slow onset with peak response at 30 minutes; long duration with effects usually lasting many hours; potentiation, with a second treatment in a few hours having a greater effect than the first one; cumulative effects after several treatments; and systemic reactions.
- **Monoamine-dependent** analgesia is induced by electrical stimulation that is high frequency (>70 Hz) and low intensity (<10 mA). Its characteristics include rapid onset and local/segmental effects only.

11. **How is the brain stimulated by acupuncture?**
According to B. Pomeranz in Scientific basis of acupuncture. In Stux G, Pomeranz B: Acupuncture: Textbook and Atlas. Heidelberg, Springer-Verlag, 1987, pp 1–34,

> Acupuncture actuates nerve fibers (type II and type III) in the muscle which send impulses to the spinal cord and activate three centers (spinal cord, midbrain, and hypothalamus-pituitary) to cause analgesia. The **spinal** site uses enkephalin and dynorphin to block incoming messages with stimulation at low frequency, and other transmitters (perhaps GABA) with high-frequency stimulation. The **midbrain** uses enkephalin to activate the raphe descending system, which inhibits spinal cord pain transmission by a synergistic effect of the monoamines, serotonin, and norepinephrine. The midbrain also has a circuit which bypasses the endorphinergic links at high-frequency stimulation. Finally, at the third center, the **hypothalamus-pituitary,** the pituitary releases beta-endorphin into the blood and CSF to cause analgesia at a distance (e.g., the midbrain). Also, the hypothalamus sends long axons to the midbrain and via beta-endorphin activates the descending analgesia system. This third center is not activated at high frequency, only a low-frequency stimulation.

12. **Has research shown any other effects?**
Research has investigated the circulatory and autonomic influences of acupuncture. Needle insertion into a muscle in spasm dilates blood vessels in the muscle via a reflex action involving sympathetic nerve fibers. Needles inserted into paravertebral muscles result in dilatation of blood vessels in peripheral spastic ischemic muscles at the same segmental level through a somato-autonomic reflex whose center is located in the contralateral anterior hypothalamus. Both the local and segmental needling result in decreased muscle spasm in the symptomatic area. A generalized decrease in peripheral sympathetic tone also has been noted after acupuncture. The above findings may help explain thermographic studies that show a normalizing increase in the temperature of chronic pain areas from acupuncture treatments given locally or distant to the painful site.

Studies on tissue healing have found a measurable current of injury emanating from acupuncture points after needling. This current has been shown to modulate neurohormonal activity and activate tissue-repair mechanisms. An area of intense speculation is whether acupuncture has its main effect on an electromagnetic bioinformational system in the body.

13. **How effective is acupuncture?**
See Table 32-1.

TABLE 32-1. EFFECTIVENESS OF ANALGESIA FOR CHRONIC PAIN	
Treatment	Effectiveness
Placebo	30–35%
Sham acupuncture (needles inserted in wrong location)	33–50%
True acupuncture	55–85%
Morphine	70%

14. Is acupuncture safe? What are the risks?
- **Infection** is an uncommon consequence of acupuncture treatment, although bacterial skin abscesses and ear chondritis can occur. Hepatitis B transmission is extremely rare, and the only reported incidences in the United States literature involve non-physicians re-using unsterilized needles. There have been no responsible reports of HIV transmission.
- **Pneumothorax** is an infrequent complication. Deep needling of the thoracic cage and hilar areas is discouraged. The small size of the acupuncture needles makes a significant pneumothorax unlikely in any case.
- While **ecchymoses** occasionally occur, significant **hematomata** do not. This is probably because of the torpedo shape of an acupuncture needle, as opposed to the beveled cutting edge of a hypodermic needle. The needle shape is also probably responsible for the lack of enduring damage to nerves or other tissues and structures.
- One phenomenon to be aware of is "**needle shock,**" which is a vasovagal response to needling that may occur in initial treatments that responds readily to standard maneuvers.

15. Are there any contraindications to acupuncture?
Contraindications are similar but less restrictive than those for injection techniques: overlying cellulitis, severe coagulopathy, and uncontrolled anticoagulation. Therapeutic anticoagulation does not, in general, present any difficulties, although ecchymoses are more common. Vigorous or deep needling and repetitive needle-pecking techniques should be avoided. Pregnancy is not a contraindication to acupuncture. Certain points, however, are avoided on practical or theoretical grounds, such as points overlying the pregnant uterus and those stimulating the lumbosacral nerve plexuses.

Contraindications to **electrical stimulation** of acupuncture needles are the same as those for electrical stimulation in general: stimulation of the thorax in patients with pacemakers, pregnancy (safety not established), and carcinoma (unknown effects).

16. Is there any standardized training in acupuncture?
There are not yet nationally recognized standards for physician training in acupuncture. Each state establishes its own requirements for licensure, and those requirements vary widely. The most comprehensive training available for physicians has been developed by the Helms Medical Institute, which is cosponsored with the Office of Continuing Medical Education (CME) at the UCLA School of Medicine and Stanford University School of Medicine. It is a 300-hour CME I program entitled Medical Acupuncture for Physicians. Shorter courses are offered at other teaching centers. It should be noted that licensed nonphysician acupuncturists are not generally familiar with the principles and techniques of medical acupuncture.

17. **Where does one get more information and find a qualified practitioner?**
   The most important resource for general information and referrals to qualified practitioners is:
   American Academy of Medical Acupuncture (AAMA)
   4929 Wilshire Boulevard
   Los Angeles, CA 90010
   Tel: 323–937–5514 (general information) or 800–521–5016 (referrals)
   Fax: 323–937–0959
   Internet: www.medicalacupuncture.org

18. **How many acupuncture points are there? Where are they located?**
   There are 361 classically described channel points and almost as many nonchannel points.
   General anatomic characteristics of acupuncture points include:
   - Proximity to the neurovascular hilus of the muscle, probably equivalent to motor or trigger points
   - Passage of peripheral nerves through bone foramina
   - Penetration of deep fascia by peripheral nerves
   - Bifurcation points of peripheral nerves
   - Nerve plexuses
   - Sagittal plane where superficial nerves from both sides of the body meet
   - Areas of dense fibrous connective tissue that are richly innervated
   - Suture lines of the skull

   As all of the above points generally show a decrease in electrical resistance when compared to the surrounding tissue, especially when they are tender to palpation, any point of lowered electrical resistance can be considered a potential acupuncture point.

19. **What are the most common problems treated by acupuncture in outpatient pain management?**
   The most common problem is pain of >3 months' duration that has not responded to pharmacologic, surgical, or traditional physical therapies. By location, low back and neck/shoulder pain are the most common, followed by appendicular joint pains and headaches. By physiologic pathology, myofascial mechanisms are the most common, followed by neurologic, degenerative, and inflammatory processes.

KEY POINTS: MEDICAL ACUPUNCTURE

1. Acupuncture uses fine needles inserted through the skin at anatomical points on the body to treat illness.

2. The basic premise is that stimulation from the needles assists the body's mechanisms of physiologic regulation and repair.

3. The Chinese classical model of acupuncture postulates that acupuncture works through affecting energy pathways (meridians or channels) that traverse the body and circulate a vital force called *qi*.

4. Acupuncture analgesia has been shown to work through endorphin-dependent and monoamine-dependent pathways.

5. Controlled trials have supported acupuncture to be useful in treating arthritis, low back pain, headaches, extremity pain, post-operative pain, respiratory and urologic problems, and substance abuse.

20. **Are there specialized needle techniques used with musculoskeletal problems?**
    Apart from the use of electrical stimulation and obtaining needle grasp in the classical
    acupuncture points, there are three major techniques for musculoskeletal problems. They are
    distinguished by the location and depth of needle insertion:
    - In the **surface technique,** many needles are employed, and a repetitive pecking motion is
      utilized to free up palpable restrictions in the superficial fascia of entire zones of the body.
    - **Intramuscular needling** is used for treating trigger points anywhere in the body and
      generally makes use of a four-quadrant fanning technique.
    - **Deep needling** of fascia or even periosteum is used when these tissues or adjacent
      neurovascular structures are implicated in the pain syndrome (e.g., by tenderness to
      palpation, analysis of pain distribution patterns).

    One highly effective method for treating recalcitrant chronic pain combines elements from
    all three techniques for its local treatment. In its purest form, these local (symptomatic) points
    are accompanied by paravertebral points to address the spinal segments responsible for
    dermatomal (skin), myotomal (muscle), sclerotomal (bone), and even sympathetic nervous
    system pain-referral zones.

21. **How is electrical stimulation used?**
    Electrical stimulation can be used with intramuscular or deep needling techniques. For most
    chronic pain problems, treatment is begun at low frequencies (2–4 Hz) at an intensity that is
    strong enough to be felt but is not uncomfortable. If there is no satisfactory response after
    two to three treatments, intermediate (10–30 Hz) and then high (75–200 Hz) frequencies may
    be tried. More acute problems or flare-ups of chronic conditions may be treated solely with
    high-frequency stimulation, a combination of low- followed by high-frequency stimulation, or
    alternating low- and high-frequency stimulation.

22. **What is the role of ear acupuncture?**
    The ear is considered an acupuncture microsystem, or somatotopic system, an area of the
    body that registers and can be used to treat pathology occurring anywhere in the body.
    The other popular microsystem approaches are Korean hand acupuncture and scalp
    acupuncture. (For justification of the somatotopic claim for the ear, see Helms and Oleson in the
    bibliography.) Clinically, the ear can be needled as an entire treatment in itself, especially in
    needle-sensitive patients, or used to reinforce the body acupuncture treatment. Points on the ear
    generally are located with the aid of a point-locating device that detects areas of decreased
    resistance (increased conductivity) with respect to the surrounding skin. Ear points commonly
    are used in treatment protocols for substance abuse management.

23. **How can acupuncture be integrated into the therapeutic armamentarium of the
    physiatrist?**
    Acupuncture is on a continuum of available treatment options. In terms of increasing
    invasiveness, consider the following order: conventional physical therapy modalities,
    acupuncture, therapeutic injections, and then surgery. For electrical stimulation procedures,
    the following breakdown may be useful: transcutaneous electrical nerve stimulation,
    interferential current, neuromuscular stimulation, and then electro-acupuncture.

    One method of integration is simply to proceed across the spectrum, increasing the
    invasiveness if the starting treatment regimen is not successful. Another method is to follow
    the continuum in the opposite direction as part of an effort at progressive rehabilitation and
    decreased reliance on invasive procedures. Perhaps the best method is to gain experience
    with acupuncture and apply it where it seems most effective (e.g., myofascial pain of
    neuropathic origin).

WEBSITES

1. American Academy of Medical Acupuncture
   www.medicalacupuncture.org

2. CAM on PubMed
   www.nlm.nih.gov/nccam/camonpubmed.html

3. ClinicalTrials.gov
   www.clinicaltrials.gov

4. Helms Medical Institute
   www.HMIacupuncture.com

5. National Center for Complementary and Alternative Medicine: Acupuncture
   http://nccam.nih.gov/health/acupuncture

6. NIH Acupuncture Consensus Statement
   http://consensus.nih.gov/1997/1997Acupuncture107html.htm

BIBLIOGRAPHY

1. Greenman PE: Principles of Manual Medicine. Baltimore, Williams & Wilkins, 1989.

2. Gunn CC: Treating Myofascial Pain: Intramuscular Stimulation (IMS) for Myofascial Pain Syndromes of Neuropathic Origin. Seattle, WA, University of Washington, 1989.

3. Helms JM: Acupuncture Energetics: A Clinical Approach for Physicians. Berkeley, CA, Medical Acupuncture Publishers, 1995.

4. Helms JM: An overview of medical acupuncture. In Jonas WB, Levin JS (eds): Essentials of Complementary and Alternative Medicine. Baltimore, Williams & Wilkins, 1999, pp 340–354.

5. Lee MHM, Liao SJ: Acupuncture in physiatry. In Kottke FJ, Lehmann JF (eds): Krusen's Handbook of Physical Medicine and Rehabilitation. Philadelphia, W.B. Saunders, 1990, pp 402–427.

6. Ng LKY, Katims JJ, Lee MHM: Acupuncture: A neuromodulation technique for pain control. In Aronoff GM (ed): Evaluation and Treatment of Chronic Pain, 2nd ed. Baltimore, Williams & Wilkins, 1992, pp 291–298.

7. Oleson TD, Kroening RJ, Bresler DE: An experimental evaluation of auricular diagnosis: The somatotopic mapping of musculoskeletal pain at ear acupuncture points. Pain 8:217–229, 1980.

8. Pomeranz B: Scientific basis of acupuncture. In Stux G, Pomeranz B: Acupuncture: Textbook and Atlas. Heidelberg, Germany, Springer-Verlag, 1987, pp 1–34.

9. Rotchford JK: Overview: Adverse events of acupuncture. Medical Acupuncture 11(2):32–35,1999.

10. Seem M: The New American Acupuncture: Acupuncture Osteopathy: The Myofascial Release of the Bodymind's Holding Patterns. Boulder, CO, Blue Poppy Press, 1993.

11. Travell JG, Simons DG: Myofascial Pain and Dysfunction: The Trigger Point Manual. The Lower Extremities Vol 2. Baltimore, Williams & Wilkins, 1992.

12. Walsh NE, Dumitru D, Ramamurthy S, et al: Treatment of the patient with chronic pain. In DeLisa J (ed): Rehabilitation Medicine: Principles and Practice. Philadelphia, J.B. Lippincott, 1988, pp 708–725.

AMPUTATION REHABILITATION: EPIDEMIOLOGY, PREPROSTHETIC MANAGEMENT, AND COMPLICATIONS

CHAPTER 33

Kevin Hakimi, MD, Nasser Eftekhari, MD, and Joseph Czerniecki, MD

In every walk with nature one receives far more than one seeks.

–John Muir (1838–1914)

1. **How common is limb loss in the United States?**
   The incidence (new cases annually) of all amputations is estimated to be 140,000 based on hospital discharge statistics. There are 1.2 million people (prevalence) living with limb loss in the United States.

2. **What are the major reasons for amputation in the United States?**
   See Table 33-1.

TABLE 33-1. CAUSES OF AMPUTATION		
Cause	Percent	Trend Over Past 30 Years
Dysvascular (includes PVD and DM)	82%	Increased by 27%
Trauma	16.4 %	Down 50%
Cancer	0.9 %	Down 50%
Congenital	0.8 %	Stable

PVD = peripheral vascular disease, DM = diabetes mellitus.

3. **Which limb is amputated more often, the upper or lower?**
   It depends on the cause:
   - **Dysvascular:** 97% lower extremity
   - **Trauma:** 69% upper extremity
   - **Congenital:** 59% lower extremity
   - **Cancer:** 76% lower extremity

   Dillingham TR, Pezzin LE, Mackenzie EJ: Limb amputation and limb deficiency: Epidemiology and recent trends in the U.S. South Med J 95:875–879, 2003.

4. **Outline some statistical trends and prognostic implications pertinent to elderly patients undergoing amputation.**
   Geriatric amputation deserves special attention because of the higher incidence of diabetes and peripheral vascular diseases.
   - Elderly patients are more likely to require higher levels of amputation. About 80% of all amputations performed at age 80 or later are above the knee.

- Long-term survival for elderly amputees has been increasing in the past few decades, but elderly amputees continue to remain at considerable risk. In most major series, the 2-year survival rate after bilateral amputation is <50% and decreases steadily with age at the time of amputation.
- As expected, the common causes of death are cardiac complications, stroke, and malignancy.
- The more proximal the amputation, the higher the mortality rate.

5. **How does the prevalence of diabetes affect overall amputation rates? What are the prognostic implications of a slowly healing diabetic foot ulcer?**
The prevalence of patients with diabetes mellitus in the general U.S. population is 7% (around 20.8 million people); however, in those over 60 years of age, the prevalence increases to 18.3%. An estimated 15% of diabetic patients will develop an ulcer on the feet or ankles at some time during the disease course; furthermore, 85% of all amputations in diabetics are preceded by a foot ulcer.

Boulton AJ, Kirsner RS, Vileikyte L: Neuropathic foot ulcers: N Engl J Med 351:48–55, 2004.
National Institute of Diabetes and Digestive and Kidney Diseases: National diabetes statistics fact sheet: General information and national estimates in the United States, 2005. U.S. Department of Health and Human Services, National Institutes of Health, Bethesda, MD, 2005.

6. **What important triad is seen in two-thirds of patients who develop foot ulcers?**
   1. Peripheral neuropathy, which leads to loss of protective sensation
   2. Claw foot deformity, which leads to three areas of ulceration:
      - Metatarsal heads (migration of fat pad leaves metatarsal heads exposed)
      - Dorsal aspect of proximal interphalangeal (PIP) (rubs against top of shoe)
      - Tip of distal phalanx (rubs against bottom of shoe)
   3. Often only a minor trauma may lead to infection. Poor footwear can also be a source of trauma.

KEY POINTS: DIABETIC FOOT EXAM

1. Perform exam at least annually.

2. Evaluate protective sensation with a Semmes-Weinstein 5.07 (10 gm) monofilament.

3. Evaluate vascular status by assessing pedal pulses and skin temperature.

4. Assess skin integrity, especially the metatarsal heads and between toes.

5. Evaluate for foot deformities and limitations in range of motion.

7. **Is there a link between glycemic control and amputation risk in diabetics?**
The relationship between glycemic control and amputation was addressed by West, who found a twofold increased risk for leg lesions, including gangrene, among patients with diabetes and higher blood glucose levels than in those with lower blood glucose concentrations. In the population-based Rochester study, amputation risk was higher for non–insulin-dependent diabetics than for insulin-dependent diabetics (35.6 versus 28.3 per 10,000 patients).
There has also been more recent evidence that tight glycemic control delays or prevents diabetic polyneuropathy, which is a major risk factor in development of lower extremity ulcers.
Diabetes Control and Complications Research Group: The effect of intensive treatment of diabetes on the development and progression of long-term complications in insulin-dependent diabetes mellitus. N Engl J Med 329:977–986, 1993.

8. **What is the risk categorization for injury prevention of an insensate foot?**
   See Table 33-2.

TABLE 33-2. FOOT COMPLICATIONS RISK CATEGORIES FOR PATIENTS WITH DIABETES

Risk Category	Definition	Management Guidelines
Low risk	None of the five high-risk characteristics below	Conduct an annual foot screening exam. Assess/recommend appropriate footwear. Provide patient education for preventive self-care.
High risk	One or more of the following:	Conduct foot assessment every 3 months.
	■ Loss of protective sensation	Demonstrate preventive self-care of the feet.
	■ Absent pedal pulses	Refer to specialists and a diabetes educator as indicated. (Always refer to a specialist if Charcot joints are suspected.)
	■ Severe foot deformity	Assess/prescribe appropriate footwear.
	■ History of foot ulcer	Certify Medicare patients for therapeutic shoe benefits.
	■ Prior amputation	Place "high risk feet" sticker on medical record.

From the National Institutes of Health (NIH) National Diabetes Education Program.

9. **Name the most significant signs and symptoms of acute arterial occlusion.**
   The signs and symptoms of acute arterial occlusion are commonly referred to as the **five Ps**:
   1. **P**ain (sudden onset)
   2. **P**allor (waxy)
   3. **P**aresthesia (numbness)
   4. **P**ulselessness (no pulse below the block)
   5. **P**aresis (sudden weakness)

10. **What are the major factors in prognosis of a dysvascular limb?**
    See Table 33-3.

11. **Name the major vascular complications of smoking.**
    - Acceleration of atherosclerosis
    - Increased blood viscosity and clotting factors
    - Inhibition of prostacyclin production
    - Increased very low density lipoprotein and decreased high-density lipoprotein (HDL) cholesterol
    - Increased platelet aggregation, fibrinogen, and von Willebrand factor
    - Decreased plasminogen
    - Increased carboxyhemoglobin and carbon monoxide

TABLE 33-3. MAJOR FACTORS IN PROGNOSIS OF DYSVASCULAR LIMB		
Symptoms	Better Prognosis	Poor Prognosis
Pain	Slow onset	Rapid onset
Vibratory sensation	Present	Absent
Deep tendon reflexes	Present	Absent
Gangrene	Slow onset	Rapid onset
Infection	Absent	Present and spreading
Edema	Absent	Present
Diabetes	Absent or well-controlled	Present
Smoking	Nonsmoker	Smoker

12. **What is the ankle-brachial index?**
The ankle brachial index (ABI) is a noninvasive way to evaluate for peripheral arterial disease. An **ABI** is calculated by dividing the systolic pressure measured in the limb (usually by Doppler at the dorsalis pedis or posterior tibialis artery) by the brachial artery pressure. For example, if systolic pressure is below 60 mmHg at the ankle and 120 mmHg at the arm, the ABI would be 0.50. When ABIs are below normal, the probability of healing an ulcer or surgical wound is decreased. ABI may be interpreted as follows:
- **>1.30:** Indicates a noncompressible artery
- **0.91–1.30:** Normal
- **0.41–0.90:** Mild-to-moderate peripheral arterial disease
- **0.00–0.40:** Severe arterial disease

13. **What are the levels of amputation for the lower extremities?**
In 1974, the Task Force on Standardization of Prosthetic-Orthotic Terminology developed an international classification system to define amputation level (Table 33-4).

14. **Describe the major criteria in determining amputation level in the dysvascular limb.**
1. Palpable pulses at the next more-proximal joint have clinical significance only when present, and their presence is a very positive indication of the likelihood of healing at any given level.
2. Skin temperature is a representative measure of collateral circulation. Skin temperature should always be compared to the opposite limb and evaluated throughout the diseased limb.
3. Dependent rubor indicates marginal viability of the skin. Incision through rubrous tissue may not heal.
4. Degree of sensory loss is of significance in the diabetic patient whose ischemic process is frequently accompanied by peripheral neuropathy.
5. Bleeding of the skin edges at the time of surgical incision is probably the best clinical sign available to predict healing at the intended level.
6. Consideration of functional goals of the patient includes evaluation of premorbid mobility.

15. **What are the limb-salvage decision-making variables in trauma patients?**
Patient variables
- Age (usually unfavorable result after age 50)
- Occupational considerations
- Patient and family desires
- Underlying chronic disease (e.g., diabetes)

TABLE 33-4.   LEVELS OF AMPUTATION IN THE LOWER EXTREMITIES

Level of Amputation	Comments
Partial toe	Excision of any part of one or more toes
Toe disarticulation	Disarticulation at the MTP joint
Partial foot/ray resection	Resection of the 3rd, 4th, 5th, metatarsals, and digits
Transmetatarsal	Amputation through the mid section of all metatarsals
Syme's	Ankle disarticulation with attachment of heel pad to distal end of tibia; may include removal of all malleoli and distal tibial/fibular flares
Long below-knee (transtibial)	50% of tibial length
Below-knee (transtibial)	20–50% of tibial length
Short below-knee (transtibial)	<20% of femoral length
Knee disarticulation	Amputation through the knee joint, femur intact
Long above-knee (transfemoral)	>60% of femoral length
Above-knee (transfemoral)	35–60% of femoral length
Short above-knee (transfemoral)	<35% of femoral length
Hip disarticulation	Amputation through hip joint, pelvis intact
Hemipelvectomy	Resection of lower half of the pelvis
Hemicorpectomy	Amputation of both lower limbs and pelvis below L4, L5 level

MTP = metatarsophalangeal.

Extremity variables
- Mechanism of injury (soft tissue injury kinetics; massive crush or high-energy soft tissue injuries have poor prognosis)
- Arterial/venous injury location (e.g., poor prognosis with infrapopliteal arterial injury)
- Neurologic (anatomic) status
- Injury status of ipsilateral limb
- Intercalary ischemic zone after revascularization

Associated variables
- Magnitude of associated injury
- Severity and duration of shock
- Warm ischemia time (unfavorable prognosis if warm ischemia time is >6 hours)

Lange R: Limb reconstruction versus amputation: Decision making in massive lower-extremity trauma. Clin Orthop Relat Res 243:92–99,1989.

16. **Why is preoperative amputee assessment an important part of the rehabilitation program?**

Rehabilitation consultation should be requested before amputation to assess nutrition, weight, diabetes control, strength, flexibility, and ideal level of amputation for prosthetic fitting. Patient education with exposure to actual prostheses and other amputee peers reduces fear, shortens recovery time, and maximizes the fullest effort in rehabilitation.

Amputees at various levels have distinctive problems of anatomic and functional loss, fitting and alignment of the prosthesis, gait abnormalities, and medical issues that require continued care for the remainder of their lives. A neglected part of total patient management is the preamputation stage. When amputation is anticipated or planned, rehabilitation clinicians have the opportunity to help prepare the patient physically and psychologically.

Questions can be answered and instructions given to alleviate anxieties of the unknown. Patients want to know what a prosthesis looks like, what it is made of, and how much it costs. The patient should be shown what type of exercise program is expected and how ambulation is performed with crutches or a walker on flat surfaces and stairs. Addressing these issues *before amputation* not only shortens the recovery time but also gives the patient a psychological edge.

17. **What is the segmental weight of the limbs and its percentage of total body weight?**
In a typical rehab setting, knowing the approximate segmental weight of each limb at different levels can be helpful in managing various clinical situations, including nutritional assessment of an amputee. Table 33-5 shows segmental weights of the limbs and percentage of the total body weight for a 150-lb man.

TABLE 33-5. SEGMENTAL WEIGHT OF THE LIMBS AND PERCENTAGE OF BODY WEIGHT

	Weight (lb)	Percentage of Total Body Weight for 150-lb Man
Lower Limb		
Entire length	23.4	15.6
Thigh	14.5	9.7
Leg	6.8	4.5
Foot	2.1	1.4
Upper Limb		
Entire length	7.3	4.9
Arm	4.0	2.7
Forearm	2.4	1.6
Hand	0.9	0.6

18. **What is the difference between myoplasty and myodesis?**
In **myoplasty,** opposing muscle groups are joined to each other by sutures through myofascia and investing fascia over the end of the bone. In a severely dysvascular residual limb with marginal muscle viability, myoplasty is probably the preferable method, but it should be done with little closure tension.

The most structurally stable residual limbs are achieved with **myodesis,** in which the surrounding muscles and their fasciae are sutured directly to the bone through drill holes. In the case of transfemoral amputation, the additional advantages of myodesis are stabilization of the femur in adduction by the adductor magnus, enhanced hip flexion by the rectus femoris, and enhanced hip extension by the biceps femoris, all three being muscles that cross the hip joint.

19. **What are the postoperative dressing options in lower-extremity amputation?**
   - **Immediate postoperative fitting prosthesis** (IPOP) or **rigid dressing:** IPOP is done more easily in below-knee amputation than at the above-knee level, because the use of rigid spica, particularly in elderly people, causes physical difficulties and hygienic problems. IPOPs and rigid dressings also prevent knee flexion contractures, control edema, and can prevent trauma to the residual limb from inadvertent falls. Rigid dressing is preferred over an

IPOP in dysvascular patients because of the risk of wound dehiscence with premature weight bearing, resulting in poor wound healing. Some report psychological benefit associated with use of an IPOP.

- **Semirigid postoperative dressing:** A variety of semirigid dressings have been used to provide wound support and pressure. The **Unna paste dressing,** a compound of zinc oxide, gelatin, glycerin, and calamine, may be used as a wrapping over conventional soft dressings. It allows limited joint movement.
- **Soft dressing:** The oldest method of postoperative residual limb management and includes two forms: elastic shrinker and elastic bandages. Soft dressings are inexpensive and lightweight, and they can be reapplied several times daily. Their disadvantages include poor control of edema, and they require a skilled individual to wrap the residual limb properly. The preferred technique is a figure-eight method, which uses a diagonal wrapping technique. Soft dressings are not recommended for below-knee amputations, as they do not prevent contracture and do not protect from trauma.

20. **To what degree does malnutrition affect the healing of lower-extremity amputations?**
Diabetics with dysvascular limbs often have open wounds and systemic sepsis, causing increased metabolic demands and an increased energy requirement 30–55% above basal values. Despite the technical expertise that yields an 86% success rate for healing of well-nourished patients after amputations, one study showed an 85% failure rate in malnourished amputees, defined as serum albumin of <3.4 gm/dL and total lymphocyte counts <1,500 cells/mm^3. Surgical procedures on these patients should be delayed until their nutritional status is improved.

Dickhaut SC, DeLee JC, Page CP: Nutritional status: importance in predicting wound-healing after amputation. J Bone Joint Surg Am 66A:71–75, 1984.

Pederson NW, Pederson D: Nutrition as a prognostic indicator in amputations. A prospective study of 47 cases. Acta Orthop Scand 63(6):675–678, 1992.

21. **What are the primary goals of treatment during the preprosthetic phase (POD 1—until the prosthetic is fitted) after amputation in the dysvascular patient?**
- Promote wound healing
- Prevent injury to surgical site
- Achieve sufficient mobility and activities of daily living function and to safely return home if possible
- Provide psychological support
- Assess depression risk
- Adjust to changes in body image
- Control pain adequately
- Prepare for eventual prosthetic fitting
- Range of motion: Prevent knee and hip contractures
- Strengthening
  - □ Lower extremity (LE): Exercise both side intact and amputated side
  - □ Upper extremity (UE): Important for both transfer and gait activities
- Aerobic conditioning
- Balance training

22. **Explain the difference between phantom limb pain and stump pain.**
Phantom pain can be defined as pain referred to a surgically removed limb or portion of the limb. **Residual limb (stump) pain** is a different entity and should be distinguished from phantom pain The three most commonly described painful sensations include postural type of cramping or squeezing sensation; burning pain; and sharp, shooting pain. Many patients may complain of a mixed type of pain, but often the major sensation falls into one of the above three categories. Other unpleasant sensory occurrences, such as paresthesia, hypothesia, and dysesthesia, should be excluded from the definition (they may coexist with phantom pain).

23. **What is phantom sensation?**

    This term is usually reserved for individuals who have an awareness of the missing portion of their limb in which the only subjective sensation is **mild tingling**. It is rarely unpleasant or painful. The incidence of phantom sensation is 80–100% in amputees immediately after amputation. Only 10% develop it after 1 month. Phantom sensation may appear in children with congenitally missing limbs and those who had amputations in early childhood.

    Most of the available data indicate that nonpainful phantom sensation seems to be the normal experience of the body, encoded (neurosignature) over a precise brain region (neuromatrix) from birth. Phantom sensation experience is produced by networks in the brain that are normally triggered by the continuous incoming modulated flow from the periphery. As soon as this flow ceases, nonpainful phantom sensation replaces the lost organ. To most patients, the limb feels perfectly normal or somewhat shortened; this is known as the telescoping phenomenon. Patients can "move" this phantom limb normally into various positions. This can be used therapeutically to prevent or treat phantom pain and transition to functional use of a prosthesis.

24. **How common is phantom pain in the lower extremity?**

    Recent studies show that 72% of all lower extremity amputees report phantom limb pain, and 74% report residual limb pain. Of those, 14% report phantom limb pain that is severely limiting. In a survey of 5,000 veteran amputees, phantom pain prevented 18% from working and interfered with the work of 33.5% who were employed; 36% found it hard to concentrate because of pain, 82% had sleep disturbances, and 45% could not carry out social activity.

    Ehde DM, Czerniecki JM, Smith DG, et al: Chronic phantom sensations, phantom pain, residual limb pain, and other regional pain after lower limb amputation. Arch Phys Med Rehabil 81:1039–1044, 2000.

25. **Is phantom pain more common with war injuries?**

    No. The incidence of phantom pain is the same in civilian and war-related amputations. Pain may occur immediately after the amputations, and 50–75% of patients have pain within 1 week postoperatively. Pain may be delayed weeks, months, or years after the amputation.

26. **Is there any treatment for phantom pain?**

    Therapeutic regimens have had <30% long-term efficacy. Although at least 68 methods of treatment have been identified, most report varying success. Initial treatment methods include transcutaneous electrical nerve stimulation (TENS), tricyclic antidepressants, anticonvulsants, beta blockers, chlorpromazine, chemical sympathectomy, neurosurgical procedures, analgesics, anesthetic procedures, and sedative/hypnotic medications. Interventional treatments such as chemical sympathectomy, anesthetic procedures, or other neurosurgical procedures are reserved for refractory cases. Usually, treatments reducing stump problems (e.g., neuroma, infection) also decrease phantom pain.

    Treatment measures that create increased peripheral control input may provide at least temporary relief of the phantom pain. One of the more effective adjuncts is extensive use of the prosthesis. Other treatments include gentle manipulation of the stump by massage, a vibrator, stump wrapping, baths, ultrasound, and application of hot packs if sensation is intact. No single drug has been proved effective in long-term control of phantom pain (narcotics should be avoided). Trigger point injection on or near the stump may be useful (aqueous steroid and local anesthetic agents). The treatment plan for each patient needs to have an interdisciplinary approach that involves physical, pharmacologic, and psychological support.

    Czerniecki JM, Ehde DM: Chronic pain after lower extremity amputation. Crit Rev Phys Med Rehabil 15:3–4, 2003.

27. **What are the common skin problems of amputees?**

    Amputation at any level is accompanied by distinct problems of functional loss, prosthetic fitting and alignment problems, and medical conditions such as skin disorders. Skin lesions, however minute they may appear, are nevertheless of great importance because they can be the beginning of an extensive skin disorder that may be physically, mentally, socially, and economically disastrous (Table 33-6).

TABLE 33-6. SKIN PROBLEMS IN AMPUTEE STUMPS AND THEIR TREATMENT

Problem	Cause	Treatment
Excessive sweating	Lack of evaporation	Antiperspirants, wicking garments
Nonspecific eczema	Associated with chronic edema and congestion of distal part of stump, characterized by weeping and itching	Modification of prosthesis, topical steroids
Fungal infection	Secondary to increased moisture	Fungistatic creams, keep dry
Skin adherence	Constant rubbing of scar tissue on prosthesis may cause skin breakdown and ulceration.	Massage to soften scar tissue, modification of prosthetic socket
Folliculitis, cysts, furuncles	Hair follicle and sweat gland occlusion with staphylococcal infection	Clean often with antibacterial soap. Remove pressure, lance to drain as needed.
Open ulcer	Pressure, shear	Discontinue wearing prosthesis until ulcer is healed, modification of socket, wound care
Epidermoid cysts	Follicular keratin plugs, very sensitive (at socketrim)	Surgical incision and drainage, systematic antibiotics, discontinue wearing prosthesis until stump is healed
Painful neuromas and hypersensitivity	A natural repair phenomenon that occurs in any transection of a peripheral nerve	Desensitize by tapping, local injection, surgical excision
Choked stump syndrome, painful verrucous hyperplasia with cracking and weeping of stump	Insecure suspension and lack of total contact distally stretching the skin over the end of the bone with each step. Underlying vascular disorder usually present.	Refitting with new total contact socket usually solves the problem, and skin gradually changes to normal. Proximal pressure must be avoided.

28. **Does energy expenditure differ between dysvascular and traumatic amputees during ambulation?**

Older dysvascular amputees use more energy during walking than their younger, usually traumatic counterparts. A comparison of the two etiologies of amputation at the below-knee (BK) and above-knee (AK) levels reveals that comfortable walking speed is slower and the O_2 consumption higher for the dysvascular BK amputee than for the traumatic BK amputee (45 m/min and 0.20 mL/kg/m versus 71 m/min and 0.16 mL/kg/m, respectively). The same differences were observed at the AK level between dysvascular and traumatic amputees (36 m/min and 0.28 mL/kg/m versus 52 m/min and 0.20 mL/kg/m). Many older patients who have AK or higher amputations for vascular disease are not successful prosthetic community ambulators; many will require an assistive device. If able to walk, they have a very slow walking speed and an elevated heart rate if crutch assistance is required (Table 33-7).

TABLE 33-7.   ENERGY EXPENDITURE IN TRAUMATIC VERSUS VASCULAR AMPUTATION

Amputation Level and Etiology	Increased Metabolic Costs
Traumatic BK	15%
Vascular BK	40%
Traumatic AK	40%
Vascular AK	>100%

BK = below knee, AK = above knee.

29. **How does energy expenditure differ between crutch and prosthetic ambulation?**
    Direct comparison of walking in unilateral traumatic and dysvascular amputees at the Syme's, BK, and AK levels using a prosthesis or a swing-through crutch-assisted gait without a prosthesis reveals that almost all amputees have a lower rate of energy expenditure, heart rate, and O_2 cost when using a prosthesis. This difference is insignificant in dysvascular AK patients and is related to the fact that, even with a prosthesis, most of these patients require crutches for some support, thereby increasing the O_2 rate and heart rate. It can be concluded that a well-fitted prosthesis that results in a satisfactory gait not requiring crutches significantly reduces the physiologic energy demand. Because crutch-walking requires more exertion than walking with a prosthesis, crutch-walking without a prosthesis should not be considered an absolute requirement for prosthetic prescription and training.

    Waters RK, Mulroy S: The energy expenditure of normal and pathological gait. Gait Posture 9:207–231, 1999.

30. **What is the goal in rehabilitation of the geriatric bilateral amputee?**
    The great majority of bilateral lower-limb amputees today are elderly who lose their limbs secondary to diabetes and peripheral vascular disease. In general, dismissing these patients as poor prosthetic candidates is a grave mistake, and it compromises their rehabilitation potential when immediate postsurgical treatment is delayed. Lack of exercise and mobility will encourage joint contractures, weaken the patient, cause loss of independence, bring on depression, and maybe even become life-threatening. Unfortunately, the challenge of rehabilitating these patients is frequently complicated by the presence of other illnesses, such as diabetes, chronic infection, kidney disease, cardiovascular disease, respiratory disease, arthritis, impaired vision, delayed wound healing, and neuropathy. These coexisting diseases warrant additional consideration and precautions, but chronologic age *alone* should not determine whether an amputee is a prosthetic candidate. Each patient should receive a thorough functional evaluation to determine suitability for prosthetic ambulation. Some key components to this evaluation are determination of upper and lower extremity strength, presence of contractures, cardiovascular function, cognitive ability, as well as clear determination of realistic patient goals. Also note the importance of using a wheelchair with a posteriorly placed axle to prevent rear tipping of the chair in this population.

WEBSITES

1. www.amputee-coalition.org
2. http://ndep.nih.gov/diabetes/diabetes.htm

CHAPTER 34

UPPER LIMB ORTHOSES: SUPPORT, ALIGNMENT PROTECTION, AND FUNCTION

John B. Redford, MD, Abna A. Ogle, MD, and Richard C. Robinson, MD

A complex system that works is invariably found to have evolved from a simple system that works.

—John Gaule

1. **What is an orthosis?**

   An orthosis is an external apparatus worn to restrict or assist movement. An orthosis can be used to transfer load from one area to another. The terms *brace* and *splint* are used interchangeably with orthosis.

   McKee P, Morgan L: Orthotics in Rehabilitation: Splinting the Hand and Body. Philadelphia, F.A. Davis, 1998, pp 1–17.

2. **State three general reasons why orthotics are prescribed.**

   The mnemonic **SAP** highlights the three broad cardinal indications for the orthotic prescription:

   - **S** = **S**upport
   - **A** = **A**lignment
   - **P** = **P**rotection

   By supporting, aligning, and protecting body parts, orthotics can enhance the function of movable body regions and prevent or correct deformities. Orthotics can be used to enhance functionality.

   Braddom RL: Physical Medicine and Rehabilitation, 3rd ed. Philadelphia, W.B. Saunders, 2007, pp 325–342.

3. **State four functions of upper limb movement that must be considered in the orthotic prescription.**

   - **Reach:** Primarily accomplished by shoulder and elbow positioning and function; severe loss of shoulder function is devastating to reach and difficult, yet hard to treat with orthoses
   - **Carry:** The action of transporting a load; orthotic substitutions are of little consequence
   - **Prehension pattern:** All the functional aspects of holding objects in the hand; this aspect is very important in orthotic prescription and follow-up
   - **Release:** Active digital extension accompanied by relaxation of digital flexors; this is an essential reverse action in all prehensile function, and it may need special orthotic attention

   Fess EE: Hand and Upper Extremity Splinting: Principles and Methods, 3rd ed. St. Louis, Mosby, 2004, pp 37–41.

4. **It is said that monkeys cannot use their hands like humans. What does that mean?**

   Hook prehension (such as carrying a suitcase) or **cylindrical grasp** (such as grabbing a rail) are tasks monkeys can do as easily as humans. However, because only humans have an **opposable thumb,** monkeys cannot perform fine motions such as **fingertip pinch, lateral pinch** (holding a key), and **palmar prehension** (three jaw-chuck prehension or opposition between the thumb and second and third digits). Monkeys cannot be baseball pitchers because they lack the **spherical grasp** that is needed to hold the ball well. These observations imply that for any hand orthosis to work—in conjunction with hand therapy—it must restore these unique human functions as closely to normal as possible.

Fess EE: Hand and Upper Extremity Splinting: Principles and Methods, 3rd ed. St. Louis, Mosby, 2004, pp 37–41.

5. **Why are upper limb splints used?**
   - **To rest the body part** so that the patient does not hurt inflamed joints or further injure muscles, ligaments, or fractured bones.
   - **To prevent contractures**—that is, to prevent patients from losing adjoining joint motion as the result of untreated burns, injury to nerves, or spasticity.
   - **To correct deformity,** in conjunction with surgery and occupational or physical therapy—a splint will be formed to keep the treated parts on a stretch.
   - **To promote exercise** for recovery of weak muscles or to correct muscle imbalances—splints are worn to strengthen certain key muscles.
   - **To substitute for lost function**—if the patient has lost a certain muscle action, it may be partly restored or retrained with an orthosis.

   Redford JB: Orthotics: Clinical Practice and Rehabilitation Technology. New York, Churchill Livingstone, 1995, pp 103–119.

6. **How do static and dynamic orthoses differ?**
   - **Static orthoses** keep underlying segments from moving. They are often used to rest body parts during healing, to reduce tone in spastic muscles, or to decrease or prevent deformity. In some cases, they can substitute for lost joint function (e.g., an orthotic thumb post makes the thumb rigid to oppose the fingers).
   - **Dynamic orthoses** move. They have external or internal power sources and encourage restoration and control of joint movements. External power means providing motion primarily by elastics, springs, or, rarely, pneumatic or electrical systems; internal power means providing motion through action of another body part, such as using wrist extension or a shoulder motion via harness and cable to operate finger grasp and release. The prescription should always indicate which motion a dynamic orthosis is to assist. For example, the phrase *finger flexion assist* would be part of the prescription for an orthosis to restore prehension.

   Shurr DG: Prosthetics and Orthotics, 2nd ed. Upper Saddle River, NJ, Prentice Hall, 2001, pp 173–181.

7. **How long should patients expect to wear an orthosis?**
   Generally no more than a month or two. Most upper limb orthoses are to be worn only during postoperative recovery or until the useful effects of medication, physical modality, or exercise to improve mobility and strength evidently have overcome the acute problem. At first, orthoses are applied 2–3 hours once or twice a day. Gradually, patients may wear them longer, depending on the condition. Some are worn mainly at night.

8. **When are upper limb orthoses, most likely to be used?**
   Indications include:
   - Trauma and surgery
   - Tendon repair
   - Post reconstructive surgery (Dupuytren's contracture release)
   - Joint injuries
   - Nerve injuries
   - Painful disorders (rheumatoid arthritis, carpal tunnel syndrome)
   - Improve function after disease (poststroke, neuromuscular disease, peripheral nerve disorders)

   Irani KD: Wrist and hand orthoses. Phys Med Rehabil State Art Rev 6:137–160, 1993.

9. **What are static shoulder orthoses?**

Because we rely heavily on free, unrestricted motion for shoulder function, orthoses that immobilize fractures of the upper arm can be used only for short periods. Effective immobilization is difficult to achieve unless the orthosis applies most of the force through the longitudinal axis of the upper arm and combines this with a force in the frontal plane to hold the humerus into the glenoid cavity.

Most varieties of static or partly dynamic shoulder slings do not really perform well biomechanically. Many orthoses tried for the subluxed paralyzed shoulder—a frequent sequela of stroke—help to relieve pain but do little to promote function. An **airplane splint** holds the arm out like a wing (Fig. 34-1). It is designed to promote healing of fractures or to immobilize the shoulder in abduction after reconstructive surgery or injury. However, it is an example of a good mechanical or orthotic idea, but a bad human interactive idea, because patients often tolerate them so poorly. Nevertheless, an airplane splint may be the only useful device to prevent an axillary burn from causing a contracture or to ensure healing of a shoulder fusion.

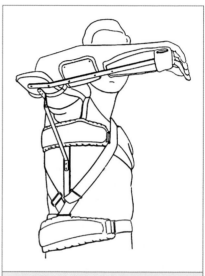

Figure 34-1. Airplane splint: a static shoulder orthosis.

Redford JB: Orthotics: Clinical Practice and Rehabilitation Technology. New York, Churchill Livingstone, 1995, pp 103–110.

Redford JB: Orthotics, Etcetera, 3rd ed. Baltimore, Williams & Wilkins, 1986, pp 198–227.

10. **Is a ballbearing feeder used to feed patients ball bearings?**

No! A ballbearing feeder is an old name for the dynamic shoulder orthosis called a **balanced forearm orthosis** (BFO). This device attaches to the upright of a wheelchair and supports the forearm with a freely moving rod located beneath the forearm trough. The BFO works to modify the effects of gravity so that persons confined to a wheelchair and with slight use of the shoulder or elbow (grade 2 at least in area muscles) may be more functional in their wheelchair. A BFO is not useful unless some hand function remains and the patient really wants to feed himself or herself or perform other activities that require reach. An occupational therapist must make the necessary adjustments before conducting training. The patient should have a trial of a dynamic overhead sling suspension orthosis before applying the BFO because the sling is much easier to set up and use for evaluation.

Redford JB: Orthotics: Clinical Practice and Rehabilitation Technology. New York, Churchill Livingstone, 1995, pp 103–110.

11. **What are some purposes for elbow orthoses?**

Elbow orthoses are used most commonly to **reduce flexion contractures** by employing a static type with hinged bars attached by Velcro to the upper arm and forearm cuffs. Single-axis elbow joints can be sequentially adjusted to extend the elbow farther. A tension spring to extend the elbow joint dynamically, or a turnbuckle applied between the upper arm and the lower forearm cuffs, can provide steady stretch to reduce the contracture. Less commonly, a static or dynamic orthosis is used to **reduce an extension contracture.** Dynamic elbow orthoses are rarely used to substitute for muscle loss, such as lost elbow flexion, because they lack cosmetic appeal and are just not very effective.

McKee P, Morgan L: Orthotics in Rehabilitation: Splinting the Hand and Body. Philadelphia, F.A. Davis, 1998, pp 1–17.

12. **What special problems must be considered when splinting the wrist or hand?**
Any surgery or injury to the hand will cause swelling. Unless this **edema** is properly approached, joints may become stiff as a result of the subsequent overactivity of fibroblasts. It has been said that "Hand therapy is behavior modification of fibroblasts during the healing response." As part of this hand therapy, you do not want hand splints applied incorrectly during recovery. Orthoses may aggravate edema. Their use must be carefully monitored, especially in patients with limited cognition or inappropriate emotional reactions to using splints.

The hand has great **sensibility,** and any sensory loss results in significant effects on function. Unfortunately, sensory loss is very common. Its extent must be mapped carefully, and orthotic pressure over insensate areas should be kept to a minimum. Because the hand is the organ of touch, the orthosis must be designed to avoid blocking sensation to critical areas, such as the fingertips. The hand is so sensitive that fitting must be exact; any discomfort will result in rejection of the orthosis.

There is a multiplicity of joints in the hand. It may be necessary to make an orthosis that immobilizes one or more joints to allow movement in others. Deciding how to do this requires good judgment and wide experience with the various materials needed for fabrication. A good example is the metacarpophalangeal (MCP) block orthosis: The MCP joints are held in flexion to block the action of the long finger extensors and allow the proximal interphalangeal (PIP) and distal interphalangeal (DIP) joints to extend.

Fess EE: Hand and Upper Extremity Splinting: Principles and Methods, 3rd ed. St. Louis, Mosby, 2004, pp 37–41.

13. **What is a SEWHO?**
Upper limb orthoses are named for the parts that they incorporate, and these are then usually abbreviated. Some examples include:
- Shoulder-elbow-wrist-hand orthosis: SEWHO
- Hand orthosis: HO
- Wrist-hand orthosis: WHO
- Finger orthosis: FO

Redford JB: Orthotics: Clinical Practice and Rehabilitation Technology. New York, Churchill Livingstone, 1995, pp 103–110.

KEY POINTS: UPPER LIMB ORTHOSES

1. Orthoses support, align, and protect body parts.

2. They also restrict or assist movement.

3. Static splints stabilize; dynamic splints promote movement.

4. Orthoses are named with the series of capital letter representing the first letter of the joint they cross over (e.g., WHO stands for wrist-hand orthosis).

14. **Hand therapists, like all specialists, have their own language. Define some of the more common terms.**
   - **Assist:** Any dynamic component designed to provide a certain motion
   - **Block or stop:** Any part of an orthosis designed to block a given motion as in the MCP block orthosis; the block is sometimes in the form of a lock (e.g., an elbow lock)
   - **C-bar:** A C-shaped strip of plastic or metal applied in the thumb/index finger webspace to prevent thumb adduction against the palm
   - **Dorsal wrist-hand orthosis:** An orthosis applied to the superior surface of the hand and wrist; it contrasts with the more common palmar or volar WHO
   - **Finger deviation splint:** A hand orthosis with components to prevent abduction or adduction of the fingers, as incorporated in splints for the rheumatoid arthritic hand to prevent ulnar drift; whether they really help prevent drift is controversial
   - **Opponens bar:** A component for positioning the thumb, such as a bar outside the thumb to prevent it from extending
   - **Opponens splint:** An orthosis that holds the thumb in opposition to the fingers; sometimes described as "short" (below the wrist) or "long" (incorporating the wrist and hand)
   - **Outrigger:** A component applied above or below an orthosis to provide a platform from which various dynamic components can pull against the digits with elastics and cuffs or springs

   Fess EE: Hand and Upper Extremity Splinting: Principles and Method, 3rd ed. St. Louis, Mosby, 2004, pp 37–41.

15. **How should you order and classify orthoses for the wrist and hand?**
   The easiest way to describe a hand orthosis is to state whether it is static or dynamic and locate the main area it encompasses or immobilizes. In any orthosis the prescriber should also say if it is to mobilize, assist, or apply traction to a certain joint or movement. The authors of the American Society of Hand Therapists Splint/Orthotic Classification System recommend further distinction between static and dynamic orthoses by clarifying the purpose of an orthosis as immobilizing, mobilizing, restricting, or a combination of several of these terms (Table 34-1).

   Redford JB: Orthotics: Clinical Practice and Rehabilitation Technology. New York, Churchill Livingstone, 1995, pp 103–110.

TABLE 34-1. COMMON KINDS OF HAND ORTHOSES

Type	Description
Wrist orthosis	Ends in the palm
Wrist-hand orthosis	Ends over digits
Wrist-thumb orthosis	Extends into webspace of thumb
Wrist-MCP orthosis	Extends just distal to PIP crease
Forearm-wrist-finger orthosis	Many variations, but must end on fingers
Hand orthosis	Starts below the wrist
Thumb orthosis	Incorporates the thumb in some way
Finger orthosis	One finger only
Tenodesis orthosis	A special class of orthosis prescribed mainly in tetraplegic patients, employing the natural tendency of the fingers to close when the wrist is extended and open when it is flexed

MCP = metacarpophalangeal, PIP = proximal interphalangeal.

16. **What are some design categories of upper limb splints?**
   - **Nonarticular** splints provide support for a body part without crossing any joints (e.g., the humeral fracture splint with circumferential support to the upper arm).
   - **Static motor blocking** splints permit motion in one direction by blocking motion in another (e.g., a swan-neck finger orthosis that allows flexion in a PIP joint but blocks hyperextension of that same joint).
   - **Serial static** splints are periodically changed to alter joint angle and generally used to regain motion.
   - **Static progressive** splints help to regain motion using a static line of pull that is tightened periodically to regain tissue length. One such splint (available commercially) has a MERIT component that resembles a tuning screw on a guitar; tension increases on the static line length as the MERIT is turned, thus increasing the motion into flexion of a digit.

   Braddom RL: Physical Medicine and Rehabilitation, 3rd ed. Philadelphia, W.B. Saunders, 2007, pp 325–342.

17. **Making splints is expensive. Why not just buy off-the-shelf orthoses?**
   Many static splints and a few dynamic ones can be prefabricated and kept in stock. A common WHO, for example, is the Futuro line of products. However, like army clothing that is designed to fit everyone but really fits no one, prefabricated orthoses may produce unexpected problems if poorly fitted. Custom-made orthoses used to be more expensive when they were made from metal or polyester resins, but now almost all are made from low-temperature thermoplastic and take much less time to make than the older ones. Because hands differ dramatically in size, shape, and even innervation, only custom-made orthoses can be used in many situations.

18. **What are the main considerations in prescribing upper limb orthoses?**
   - **Patient cooperation:** The patient must understand the purpose of the splint, and the therapist must judge the likelihood of patient use.
   - **Comfort and cosmesis:** The splint must be comfortable to the wearer and as light as possible. In addition, the patient should be able to choose the color and suggest cosmetic considerations to satisfy concerns about appearance.
   - **Wearing schedule:** This requires discussion of the time the splint must be worn in order to meet the goals of the patient and therapist. Most splints are used only temporarily and are only part of any treatment plan.
   - **Design:** The splint must be biomechanically suited to reach optimum goals, and prescriber follow-up is needed to make design alterations as condition improves or changes.

   Irani KD: Wrist and hand orthoses. Phys Med Rehabil State Art Rev 6:137–160. 1993.
   Braddom RL: Physical Medicine and Rehabilitation, 2nd ed. Philadelphia, W.B. Saunders, 1996, pp 321–322.

WEBSITE

Upper limb orthotics (search publications: Journal of Orthotics and Prosthetics)
www.oandp.com

BIBLIOGRAPHY

1. Butner PA: A comparison of static and dynamic wrist splints using electromyography in individuals with rheumatoid arthritis. J Hand Ther 16:320–325, 2003.
2. Collier S: Range of motion at the wrist: A comparison of four wrist extension orthoses and the free hand. Am J Occup Ther 56:180–184, 2002.
3. King S: The immediate and short-term effects of a wrist extension orthosis on upper-extremity kinematics and range of shoulder motion. Am J Occup Ther 57:517–524, 2003.

CHAPTER 35

UPPER LIMB PROSTHESES: CABLE AND MYOELECTRIC CONTROL

Atul T. Patel, MD, and Subhadra Lakshmi Nori, MD

Do not let what you cannot do interfere with what you can do.

–John Wooden (1910–)

1. **What is the most common congenital upper-extremity limb deficiency?**
   The most common deficiency is a unilateral short, below-elbow deficiency, with absence of the forearm, wrist, and hand (terminal transverse radial limb deficiency).

2. **What is the most common cause of upper limb amputations in the United States?**
   In adults, upper limb amputations are most frequently caused by work-related civilian trauma. In an epidemiologic study in Maryland, the leading causes of trauma-related amputations (upper and lower limb) were injuries involving machinery (40%), powered tools and appliances (28%), firearms (8.5%), and motor vehicle accidents (8%). Congenital limb deficiency is the most common cause of upper limb amputations in children and second most common cause overall for upper limb amputations. The third most common cause of an upper limb amputation is cancer.

   Atkins DJ, Heard DCY, Donovan WH: Epidemiologic overview of individuals with upper-limb loss and their reported research priorities. J Prosth Orthot 8:2–11, 1996.
   Dillingham TR, Pezzin LE, MacKenzie EJ: Incidence, acute care length of stay, and discharge to rehabilitation of traumatic amputee patients: An epidemiologic study. Arch Phys Med Rehabil 79:279–287, 1998.
   National Limb Loss Information Center: Fact sheet. Amputation Statistics by Cause, 2004: www.amputee-coalition.org/fact_sheets/amp_stat_cause.pdf

KEY POINTS: COMMON CHARACTERISTICS OF AN UPPER LIMB AMPUTEE IN THE UNITED STATES

1. Young worker (20–50 years old)

2. Amputation caused by a work-related injury

3. Dominant upper limb is the one that is involved

4. More likely to be an amputation below the elbow

3. **What is the prevalence of upper limb amputations among all amputees in the United States?**
   Approximately 10% of all amputations involve the upper limb, most frequently below the elbow. The ratio of lower- to upper-extremity amputations is approximately 5:1.

4. **How are congenital upper limb deficiencies classified?**
   The International Terminology for the Classification of Congenital Limb Deficiencies defines limb deficiencies as either terminal or intercalary.
   - **Terminal** is used to define a deficiency in which a limb has developed normally to a certain level, beyond which no further skeletal elements exist (e.g., terminal transverse radial limb deficiency).
   - **Intercalary** refers to deficiencies in the long axis, where normal skeletal elements may be present distal to the affected segment (e.g., partial reduction of the ulna with normal radius and hand elements).

5. **At what age should an infant with a congenital limb deficiency be fitted with an upper-extremity prosthesis?**
   From 3 to 6 months of age, when the child begins to sit and needs the arms for prop support. At first, a passive-type prosthesis is provided; active components are added as motor landmarks are reached and approached.

6. **How are upper-extremity amputations classified?**
   For **below-elbow amputations**, the length of the stump remaining below the elbow is measured from the medial epicondyle of the humerus to the end of the longer residual bone (the radius or ulna). For **above-elbow amputations**, the length of the stump remaining above the elbow is measured from the tip of the acromion to the end of the residual humerus. This length is expressed as a percentage of the distance from the acromion to the lateral humeral epicondyle of the sound limb (Fig. 35-1).

7. **Why is it so important to preserve as much of the limb as possible during surgical amputation?**
   A longer residual limb provides more stump-to-prosthesis contact, more proprioceptive sensation, and a longer lever arm to power the prosthesis.

8. **In child amputees, the disarticulation level of amputation is preferred. Why?**
   The goal is to preserve the epiphyses, to allow maximum limb growth, and to avoid bony overgrowth that can occur in amputations performed through the shaft of a long bone.

9. **What are the goals of upper-extremity stump care?**
   To control pain and swelling, maintain strength and range of motion (ROM), and to promote wound healing and residual limb maturation. In the upper limb it is also important to manage the skin carefully to preserve sensation, because, in essence, the amputation site becomes the hand.

10. **What is the primary goal of the preprosthetic training period?**
    The primary goal is to help the patient achieve functional independence in activities of daily living (ADLs) by using the remaining normal arm. This promotes self-esteem and encourages the patient to realize that he or she can accomplish more than he or she thought possible.

11. **What are the essential goals of prosthetic training?**
    During early prosthetic training the patient wears the prosthesis for short periods, usually not longer than 15 minutes. Skin integrity is carefully monitored. The amputee progresses from learning to put on (don) and take off (doff) the prosthesis to executing and controlling ROM of the prosthetic joints and developing basic essential prehension movements. The final step is learning terminal-device dexterity in various elbow and shoulder positions. Bilateral amputees need one functional prosthesis as soon as possible; ideally, this should be provided to the dominant limb.

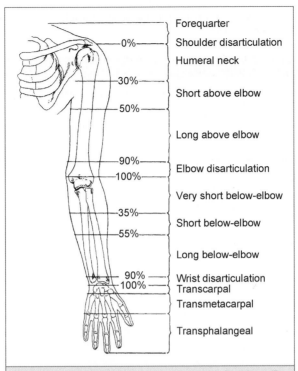

Figure 35-1. Upper limb amputation levels. (From Kottke EJ, Lehman JF [eds]: Krusen's Handbook of Physical Medicine and Rehabilitation, 4th ed. Philadelphia, W.B. Saunders, 1990.)

12. **What requirements must an amputee meet before he or she can be fitted with a permanent upper-extremity prosthesis?**
    - The stump must be free of edema and skin breakdown for comfortable fitting.
    - The patient must have adequate active ROM and motor strength to operate the prosthetic control system.
    - The patient must demonstrate adequate cognitive ability and perseverance to successfully participate successfully in prosthetic training.

13. **Name the most important things to keep in mind when developing the prescription for an upper-extremity prosthesis.**
    Function and comfort, rather than cosmesis, are most important. The patient's avocational and vocational habits must be evaluated to determine the combination of components that will best meet his or her needs—for example, the requirements of a farmer who operates heavy equipment will differ substantially from those of a secretary. It is also important that the patient receive appropriate training to increase the chance of prosthetic acceptance and long-term functional use.

    Lake C: Effects of prosthetic training on upper-extremity prosthesis use. J Prosth Orthot 9:3–11, 1997.

14. **How soon should a person with an upper limb amputation be fitted with a prosthesis?**
    There is a 3–6 month window of opportunity to fit an amputee with a prosthesis to significantly increase the likelihood of long-term prosthetic use. Once a person achieves independence in

performing ADLs with the preserved upper limb, the chance of fully incorporating the prosthesis in routine activities is reduced.

KEY POINTS: UPPER LIMB AMPUTEE REHABILITATION

1. Early rehabilitation management after upper limb amputation improves acceptance of prosthetic use.

2. A comprehensive life goal and vocationally focused rehabilitation program maximizes functional outcomes.

3. A carefully designed and crafted upper limb prosthetic prescription promotes continued use.

4. Quality of training determines how well individuals use the prosthesis for the rest of their lives.

15. **After successful fitting of the definitive prosthesis, is further medical follow-up needed?**
    Yes—usually within 4–6 weeks. But this depends on several factors, including how well the patient functions at home and whether medical problems develop, such as phantom limb pain, neuroma, diminished joint mobility, bony overgrowth, and—the most common problem— skin complications such as blisters, ulcers, infections, or stasis eczema.

16. **What are the essential components of every prescription for a functional upper limb prosthesis?**
    Suspension system (cuffs and harness), socket, **control system** (cables for a body-powered prosthesis, batteries for an externally powered prosthesis), **elbow hinge, wrist component**, and **terminal device** (hook or hand). A nonfunctional or cosmetic prosthesis is usually indicated when the patient is unable to operate a functional prosthesis for his or her level of amputation.

17. **A 30-year-old right-hand-dominant man has a right below-elbow amputation secondary to a farm accident. His forearm stump is approximately 50% in length, and his wounds are well healed with sensation loss limited to the scar. Name the most commonly prescribed components of a below-elbow prosthesis for this type of patient.**
    Figure-eight harness with a triceps pad/cuff; plastic laminate double-walled socket; Bowden single-control cable system; flexible elbow hinges; friction wrist unit; and voluntary opening (VO) split hook (Fig. 35-2). He would be expected to be able operate farm equipment, handle simple farm tools, and be independent with basic ADLs.

18. **A 60-year-old left-hand-dominant man has an above-elbow amputation secondary to burns. The wounds over the entire distal stump are healed, with a significant amount of scarring and decreased sensation. The stump is approximately 50% in length. Name the most commonly prescribed components of an above-elbow prosthesis for this type of patient.**
    Figure-eight harness; double-walled plastic laminant socket; internal locking elbow; dual-control cable system; friction wrist unit; and VO split hook (Fig. 35-3).

19. **What is the purpose of the terminal device?**

    To provide **prehension** (the ability to grasp objects). The human hand is capable of **six types of prehension:** lateral, palmar, tip, cylindrical grasp, spherical grasp, and hook or snap. The terminal device replaces the types of prehension that allow the amputee to perform ADL skills using one or two devices.

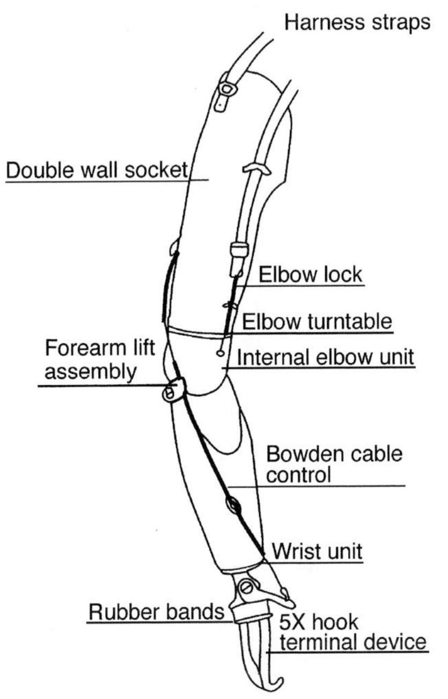

20. **What are the advantages of a hook terminal device compared to a prosthetic hand?**

    Normal **lateral prehension** (or pinch) is grasping an object between the pad of the thumb and the lateral surface of the index finger. The **hook** provides this function and is better suited for tasks requiring manual dexterity than a prosthetic hand. It is lighter in weight and easier to maintain, and its simple design allows for maximal visualization of objects manipulated to compensate for touch sensation loss.

    Normal **palmar prehension** (three-jaw chuck pinch) is grasping an object between the pad of the thumb and the pads of the index and middle fingers. The **prosthetic hand** provides this function and can be used to grasp larger objects as well as rounded ones. It also provides better cosmesis. The selection of a hook or a prosthetic hand is determined by the needs and preferences of the amputee.

Figure 35-2. Body-powered transradial prosthesis with components identified. (From Esquenazi A: Upper limb amputee rehabilitation and prosthetic restoration. In Braddom RL [ed]: Physical Medicine and Rehabilitation, 2nd ed. Philadelphia, W.B. Saunders, 2000, pp 263–278.)

21. **What is the most commonly used terminal device?**

    The **Dorrance voluntary opening (VO) split hook**. This device was patented in 1912 by D.W. Dorrance, who was a bilateral upper-extremity amputee. Before the invention of the "split" hook, terminal devices were actually hooks and provided no prehension at all.

22. **What functions do wrist units provide?**

    Both the friction and locking types of wrist units serve as the attachment point for the terminal device. They do not function as true wrist joints, but they provide passive pronation and supination, which the patient controls by using the normal hand to rotate the wrist.

23. **Explain the advantages of the epicondyle suspension prosthesis (Muenster-type below-elbow prosthesis).**

    Used with very short below-elbow amputations, the socket of this prosthesis is set at 30 degrees of elbow flexion. Because this shortens the lever arm during flexion movements, it requires much less effort to operate. Because the socket is securely fitted above the humeral

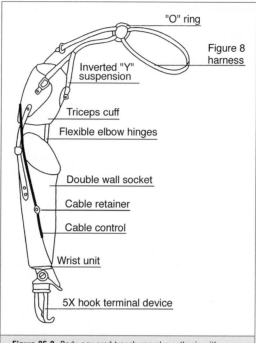

Figure 35-3. Body-powered transhumeral prosthesis with components identified. (From Esquenazi A: Upper limb amputee rehabilitation and prosthetic restoration. In Braddom RL [ed]: Physical Medicine and Rehabilitation, 2nd ed. Philadelphia, W.B. Saunders, 2000, pp 263–278.)

epicondyles, and the hook is fitted behind the olecranon process, a high degree of retention is attained without the use of suspension devices, such as elbow hinges, cuffs, or pads.

24. **What type of suction of suspension system can be used to support an upper limb prostheses?**
Silicon suction suspension. This type of system has been found to be useful in patients with delicate or sensitive skin, such as burn patients or those with degloving-type injuries. It has also worked well in patients who play sports and are very active.

25. **Name the three basic types of below-elbow hinges. What are their indications?**
Flexible, rigid, and **step-up hinge.** The selection of the type of hinge depends on the level of amputation and on the functional status of the residual limb. A long below-elbow amputee will use the **flexible hinge** (allows for some use of residual forearm rotation); the short below-elbow amputee requires more stability and needs the **rigid hinge** (protects residual limb against torque loads). When the below-elbow stump is very short and flexion is severely limited, the gear arrangement of the **step-up hinge** (used to enhance elbow flexion by using a split socket) permits the socket to flex through a greater range than the residual elbow joint would otherwise allow. Keep in mind that with short below-elbow stumps, the supracondylar suspension prosthesis is often a good alternative to hinges.

26. **How does the amputee operate the body-powered upper-extremity prosthesis?**
An amputee is trained to protract the shoulders, which transmits tension along a cable system that slides inside one or more flexible housings. The stainless-steel cable is attached proximally to the harness and distally to the terminal device. With an above-elbow prosthesis, the cable is also attached to the elbow unit.
   - An amputee with a **below-elbow prosthesis** uses a single-control system (Bowden control system) to operate the terminal device through coordinated elbow flexion, shoulder abduction, and protraction.
   - An amputee with an **above-elbow** or **very short below-elbow prosthesis** needs a dual-control system (fair-lead system) in which arm flexion operates the terminal device and controls forearm flexion, and arm extension operates the elbow lock. When the elbow is locked between 90 and 135 degrees, the terminal device is operated by biscapular abduction (shoulder protraction).

27. **Why is the figure-eight harness the most commonly used? What are some other types?**
It provides the widest range of everyday activities with the least restrictions of the body. Other harness types meet more specific requirements of an amputee. The **figure-nine harness**, for example, affords more freedom of movement of the prosthetic limb and is used with the supracondylar socket. The **triple-control system harness**, which separates terminal-device operation from forearm flexion and replaces the dual-control system, is useful for people with above-elbow amputations. The **modified shoulder saddle harness** provides a larger weight-bearing area and permits the amputee to lift heavy objects without transmitting excessive pressure to the sound axilla.

28. **How much weight can typically be lifted with the upper limb fitted with a prosthesis?**
A person with a transradial amputation can typically lift 20–30 lb, whereas a person with a transhumeral amputation can be expected to lift 10–15 lb.

29. **How does the myoelectric-type prosthesis work?**
When this type of prosthesis is worn by a patient with an upper-extremity amputation, surface electrodes housed in the socket are brought into contact with muscles that have been trained to contract, and generate a minimum signal of 10 μV. This voltage, which is amplified 20,000–40,000 times, activates a rechargeable nickel-cadmium battery that then operates the small reversible electric motors in the terminal device and prosthetic joints.

30. **What is the value of the myometric evaluation?**
This evaluation uses a myotester to measure the action potentials of the amputee's stump muscles and to determine whether the muscles are capable of activating the surface electrodes of the prosthesis that operate the terminal device.

31. **Which type of prosthesis requires more time for training—externally powered or body powered?**
Generally, the control training for an externally powered prosthesis is more complex; and it requires more time to learn the appropriate muscle motions and contractions needed to operate the device precisely.

32. **What particular difficulties does a patient with a shoulder disarticulation or forequarter amputation face?**
These patients have no residual stumps and therefore cannot easily mobilize their shoulder girdle strength to operate the control systems. In the forequarter amputation (interthoracoscapular amputation), the problem is even more difficult, because there is no

residual shoulder girdle. Thus an amputee must expend great effort and be highly motivated to operate a body-powered shoulder disarticulation prosthesis.

33. **What are the essential components of the body-powered shoulder disarticulation prosthesis?**
This appliance, also called the active prehensile arm, consists of the shoulder component, arm section, elbow unit, forearm section, wrist unit, and terminal device. All these are operated by shoulder girdle movements.

34. **What is the Krukenberg procedure?**
It is a procedure that reshapes the forearm of the transradial amputee into radial and ulnar rays. These rays then function as muscle-powered pincers or forceps. The procedure was introduced in 1916 by the German army surgeon Hermann Krukenberg.

Poonekar PD: The Krukenberg procedure. In Smith DG, Michael JW, Bowker JH (eds): Atlas of Amputation and Limb Deficiencies. Surgical, Prosthetic, and Rehabilitation Principles, 3rd ed. AAOS, 2004, pp 231–237.

WEBSITES

1. www.amputee-coalition.org

2. www.ispo.ca/default.asp

3. www.oandp.com

4. www.oandp.org

5. www.orthopaedic.ed.ac.uk/amputations/

BIBLIOGRAPHY

1. Atkins DJ, Meier RH III: Comprehensive Management of the Upper-Limb Amputee. New York, Springer-Verlag, 1989.

2. Esquenazi A: Upper limb amputee rehabilitation and prosthetic restoration. In Braddom RL (ed): Physical Medicine and Rehabilitation, 2nd ed. Philadelphia, W.B. Saunders, 2000, pp 263–278.

3. Meier RH III, Atkins DJ (eds): Functional Restoration of Adults and Children with Upper Extremity Amputation. New York, Demos Medical, 2004.

4. Nader EHM (ed): Otto Bock Prosthetic Compendium—Upper-Extremity Prostheses. Berlin, Schliele & Schon, 1990.

5. Smith DG, Michael JW, Bowker JH (eds): Atlas of amputations and limb deficiencies: Surgical, prosthetic and rehabilitation principles, 3rd ed. Rosemont, IL, American Academy of Orthopaedic Surgeons, 2004, pp 101–343.

LOWER LIMB ORTHOSES: STABILIZATION, AMBULATION, AND ENERGY CONSERVATION

Kristjan T. Ragnarsson, MD, and Richard A. Frieden, MD

CHAPTER 36

Some great men owe most of their greatness to the ability of detecting in those they destine for their tools the exact quality of strength that matters for their work.
—Joseph Conrad (1857–1924)

1. How are shoes modified to correct leg-length discrepancy?
Minor leg-length discrepancies of up to ½ inch may be left uncompensated or are corrected by placing ¼-inch heel pads inside the heel only of the shoe. Any lift >½ inch should be added externally to both the heel and sole of the shoe. The outer sole elevation should be approximately half of the heel elevation and taper forward from the ball of the shoe to the toe.

Ragnarsson KT: Lower extremity orthotics, shoes, and gait aids. In DeLisa JA, Gans BM (eds): Rehabilitation Medicine: Principles and Practice, 4th ed. Philadelphia, Lippincott Williams & Wilkins, 2005, pp 1377–1391.

2. How can shoes be modified to control knee, foot, and ankle motions throughout the gait cycle?
Shaving the heel of a shoe can bring the ground reaction force closer to the axis of knee rotation, thus stabilizing the knee at heel strike. A cushioned heel can reduce the knee flexion moment by permitting faster ankle plantar flexion. A medial wedge can limit pronation caused by a weak tibialis posterior muscle. A lateral wedge can limit supination caused by a weak peroneus longus muscle. A rigid sole and a rocker bar can take pressure off the metatarsal heads and reduce hyperextension of the metatarsophalangeal joints.

www.podiatrytoday.com/podtd/displayArticleaa.cfm?articleID=article2961

3. What is the impact of footwear on orthoses?
For an orthosis to transmit and modify applied forces in the desired manner, the shoe must hold the footplate of the orthosis in the correct position. If the upper (of the shoe) is too soft or the counter is too flexible, the patient will ride over or roll over the shoe during the stance phase of gait. This may decrease the efficacy of the ankle-foot orthosis (AFO), especially to control mediolateral stability. A shock-absorbing material built into the soles of the shoes may reduce the forces imparted to the legs during ambulation with **knee-ankle-foot orthoses** (KAFOs).

Biering-Sorensen F, Ryde H, Bojscn-Moller F, Lyquist E: Shock absorbing material on the shoes of long leg braces for paraplegic walking. Prosthet Orthot Int 14:27–32, 1990.

4. Explain the role of orthoses in preventing diabetic foot ulcers.
Foot orthoses can provide relief for bony prominences, support bony structures, reduce heat buildup, reduce shear forces, and absorb perspiration.

5. What is "Charcot foot"? How can it be treated?
Jean-Martin Charcot (1825–1893) was a French physician who some have called the founder of modern neurology. In addition to work on hysteria, he was also the first to describe the

degeneration of ligaments and joint surfaces caused by lack of use or control, now called Charcot's joint. More specifically, a Charcot's joint develops from repeated trauma to an anesthetic joint. This can result in widening and deformity of the joints, and the potential loss of bony architecture. A foot with Charcot (neuropathic) joints can develop bony prominences and plantar surface ulcerations. This can lead to infection, osteomyelitis, and increased risk for amputation.

An off-loading or anterior-tibial weight-bearing AFO, usually with anterior and posterior shells to take pressure off the bones of the ankle and foot, will help protect against further deterioration of the joints. It may actually permit healing of ulcers and allow "solidification" of the bony structures.

Pinzur M. Surgical versus accommodative treatment for Charcot arthropathy of the midfoot. Foot Ankle Int 25(8):545–549, 2004.

6. List the indications for using an AFO to improve a patient's gait.

- Mediolateral instability at the ankle
- "Foot-drop," that is, passive plantar flexion during swing phase
- "Foot-slap" at heel strike as a result of weak ankle dorsiflexors
- Weak pushoff at late stance phase
  For more information, visit www.oandp.org/jpo/library/1990_01_014.asp.

7. What requirements must the patient meet in order to use an AFO effectively?

- Knee extension strength > 3/5
- Stable limb size without fluctuating edema for use of a plastic AFO
- Skin pressure tolerance and patient compliance with skin checks

Lehmann JF: Biomechanics of ankle-foot orthosis: Prescription and design. Arch Phys Med Rehabil 60:200–207, 1979.

8. What are anterior and posterior stops on an AFO?

Anterior and posterior stops are used to control ankle dorsiflexion and plantar flexion on a jointed AFO. A posterior stop limits plantar flexion during swing phase; an anterior stop limits dorsiflexion following midstance. Limiting dorsiflexion at the ankle allows less knee flexion moment during stance and stabilizes it. Energy efficiency and speed of gait are enhanced with limitation of dorsiflexion at late stance, which replaces pushoff and passively raises the center of gravity. The posterior stop prevents plantar flexion during swing phase, preventing sole friction and maximizing step length. A posterior stop is also helpful when moderate spasticity is present to control plantar flexion spasms and to prevent equinus deformity from developing.

9. How do AFO stops differ from AFO assists?

An anterior stop limits dorsiflexion. An anterior assist (spring) aids in plantar flexion, substituting for a weak gastrocsoleus muscle. A posterior stop limits plantar flexion. A posterior assist (spring) aids in dorsiflexion, substituting for a weak tibialis anterior muscle.

10. How can an AFO be altered to stabilize the knee?

An AFO can be adjusted to alter the forces that are transmitted from ground reaction through the closed kinetic chain of the limb to the knee. When the AFO is set into plantar flexion, the knee is provided with a stabilizing extension moment during stance in foot-flat and pushoff. The opposite result can occur if the AFO is set in dorsiflexion, causing a destabilizing knee flexion moment at heel strike (Fig. 36-1).

11. Which type of AFO is used when clonus is present at the ankle?

Spring action may perpetuate ankle clonus. Therefore the ankle joint should usually be locked by using a solid AFO.

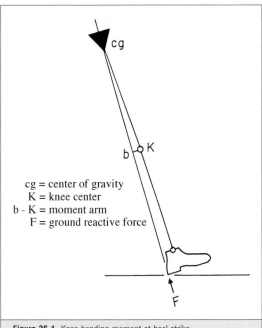

cg = center of gravity
K = knee center
b - K = moment arm
F = ground reactive force

Figure 36-1. Knee-bending moment at heel strike.

12. **What is a floor-reaction orthosis?**
The floor-reaction orthosis is an AFO with the footplate set in slight plantar flexion. The extension moment created by plantar-flexing the orthosis is transferred to the patellar tendon by a band of material on the top of the orthosis. The extension moment helps to stabilize the knee. Floor-reaction orthoses are prescribed to help with knee extension in patients who have less than fair (3/5) quadriceps motor strength, or for children with crouched gait.
    For more information, visit www.oandp.org/jpo/library.

13. **Why do we use "old-fashioned" metal bracing to support limbs weakened by poliomyelitis?**
    1. If the patient is an experienced user of metal AFOs or KAFOs, then the rate of acceptance of plastic orthoses is low.
    2. Metal uprights can accommodate a deformity well by adding extra padded straps, thus avoiding excessive pressure on bony prominences.
    3. The open nature of metal uprights means better accommodation to fluctuating edema than that provided by the intimate fit of plastic orthoses.
    4. Hybrids of metal and plastic are becoming more popular, as technology improves.
    For more information, visit www.post-polio.org/ipn/pph21-1b.html and www.disabilitymuseum. org/lib/subject/medicine/rehabilitation.

14. **What should be checked when a patient receives a new AFO?**
If the orthosis is jointed, the anatomic ankle joint that runs through the malleoli should be in the same axis as the orthotic joint. In stance, the knee should be fully extended and the sole of the shoe should be flat on the floor. In swing, there should be adequate toe clearance. The knee should flex slightly immediately following heel strike. There should be a 1-inch or

2-inch clearance from the upper brim of the orthosis to the fibular head in order to prevent pressure on the peroneal nerve.

15. Does prophylactic knee bracing prevent knee injuries in football?
There is some controversy on this issue. A study of college football players at West Point found a statistically significant decline in medial collateral injuries in defensive players who used prophylactic knee braces. A larger study on NCAA collegiate football players actually showed more knee injuries in those using prophylactic knee orthoses. Currently, it appears that there is no compelling evidence to recommend prophylactic knee bracing to football players.

Deppen RJ, Landfried MJ: Efficacy of prophylactic knee bracing in high school football players. J Orthop Sports Phys Ther 20(5):243–246, 1994.
Hardin GT, Farr J, Stiene HA: Prophylactic knee braces for football: Do they work? Indiana Med 86(4):308–311, 1993.

KEY POINTS: LOWER LIMB ORTHOSES

1. Attempt to direct the forces acting on the lower extremity from below as much as possible, using the least extensive device.

2. There is an inverse correlation between support and comfort, and between restriction of unwanted joint movement and freedom of forward motion.

3. An orthosis is most effective when it is held in a stable position by the footwear.

4. It is important to periodically monitor the fit of an orthosis because of the effects of wear and tear on the device, as well as the effects of fluctuations in body weight, foot dimensions, and muscle strength.

5. To assess the ability of an orthosis to reduce gait deviations, it is important to analyze gait patterns before and after applying the device.

16. Which type of orthosis is used in Legg-Calvé-Perthes disease?
Legg-Calvé-Perthes disease is a childhood disorder with avascular necrosis of the capital femoral epiphysis. The goal of bracing in this disorder is to maintain the femoral head completely within the acetabulum in order to maintain its sphericity. This is achieved by using plaster casts or orthoses of different designs to place the hip in hyperabduction and external rotation.

17. What type of orthosis is used for persons with spina bifida who are community ambulators?
Persons with spina bifida who can ambulate successfully in the community generally must have intact neurologic function to include at least the L3 neurologic level and thus have at least fair (3/5) quadriceps strength. Such a person should be provided with bilateral solid AFO. It is unwise to extend the orthoses to the knee, because the person may not be able to advance the limb with the knee locked in extension. An assistive device for balance is often needed.

18. Should you prescribe KAFOs for a patient with thoracic paraplegia?
Few persons with thoracic paraplegia use KAFOs (long leg braces) for functional ambulation, due in part to the high energy expenditure and the slow speed of such gait. There are, however, significant psychological and functional benefits for persons who achieve the ability to stand erect and perform some ADLs upright. There may also be considerable physiologic benefits

from regularly assuming the standing position and performing the physical exercise associated with KAFOs (swing-to or swing-through) ambulation. Therefore, KAFOs should not be denied to a person based only on the spinal cord injury (SCI) level and the poor prospects for functional ambulation. However, the person with paraplegia must be advised that KAFOs are only an adjunct to, and not a replacement for, the wheelchair as primary means of locomotion.

Stauffer ES, Hussey RW: Spinal cord injury: Requirements for ambulation. Arch Phys Med Rehabil 54:544–547, 1973.

19. **Why is ambulation with bilateral KAFOs and crutches so much more energy consuming than wheelchair propulsion?**
Ambulation requires moving the center of gravity up and down as well as side to side, and along with it the whole weight of the body. Bilateral KAFO ambulation requires lifting the limbs with shoulder depressors and swinging them forward while on crutches. This tripod or swing-through gait is energy consuming. A wheelchair translates the center of gravity horizontally and in a straight line without the energy cost associated with moving the center of gravity vertically or laterally. Recent design improvements, such as the stance-control knee joint, may reduce energy expended during ambulation with KAFOs by reducing the vertical displacement of the center of gravity.

Hebert JS, Liggins AB: Gait evaluation of an automatic stance-control knee orthosis in a patient with postpoliomyelitis. Arch Phys Med Rehabil 86(8):1676–1680, 2005.

Merkel KD: Energy expenditure in patients with low, mid, or high thoracic paraplegia using Scott-Craig knee-ankle-foot orthoses. Mayo Clin Proc 60:165–168, 1985.

20. **What is the difference between the reciprocating gait orthosis (RGO) and other types of hip-knee-ankle-foot orthoses (HKAFOs)?**
The RGO is designed to include a custom-molded pelvic girdle with a thoracic extension (as required by the patient for balance) that is attached with ballbearing hip joints to bilateral KAFO components. The unique characteristic mechanism consists of two cables with conduits that translate hip extension movement on one side into hip flexion on the other. The RGO is usually used with a walker and infrequently with crutches. The unloaded limb is thereby advanced forward with forces transmitted from the loaded side, thus providing a "reciprocating" gait. Experimental work continues to focus on enhancement of ambulation efficiency, that is, reduction of both energy expenditure over distance and energy cost over time, by using the RGO in combination with functional electrical stimulation (see Chapter 85).

www.ifess.org/cdrom_target/ifess04/control%20techniques/oral/toc.pdf

Merati G, Sarchi P, Ferrarin M, et al: Paraplegic adaptation to assisted-walking: Energy expenditure during wheelchair versus orthosis use. Spinal Cord 38(1):37–44, 2000.

WEBSITES

1. www.emedicine.com/pmr/topic172.htm

2. www.ifess.org/cdrom_target/ifess04/control%20techniques/oral/toc.pdf

3. www.ifess.org/Services/Consumer_Ed/References/Walking-references.htm

CHAPTER 37

LOWER LIMB PROSTHESES AND GAIT: PRESCRIPTION AND EVALUATION

Joan E. Edelstein, MA, PT

Of all exercises, walking is the best.

–Thomas Jefferson (1743–1826)

1. **What is the most common prosthesis for a patient with transtibial (below-knee) amputation?**

   Medicare regulations specify reimbursement levels for unilateral transtibial or transfemoral prostheses as follows:

   - **Level 0:** Unable, or no potential, to ambulate or transfer with or without assistance; prosthesis does not enhance mobility
   - **Level 1:** Ability or potential to use prosthesis for transfers, ambulate on level surface, fixed cadence; household ambulatory
   - **Level 2:** Ability or potential to ambulate curbs, stairs, uneven surfaces; limited community ambulatory
   - **Level 3:** Ability or potential to ambulate with variable cadence, traverse environmental barriers
   - **Level 4:** Ability or potential for ambulation that exceeds basic skills, exhibits high-impact stress or energy levels

   Thus, for levels 1 and 2, a prosthesis with a **SACH (solid ankle cushion heel)** foot-ankle assembly, endoskeletal shank with foam cover, plastic total contact socket with polyethylene foam liner, and cuff suspension is appropriate. The traditional socket is **patellar tendon–bearing;** however, all portions of the amputation limb support some weight. Newer sockets, such as **total surface bearing** and **hydrostatic,** place less stress on the patellar ligament. The foam liner accommodates changes in limb volume and distributes forces through the gait cycle. The endoskeletal shank can be adjusted in length and alignment; the cover contributes to the look and feel of the prosthesis. The cuff is readily adjustable. The SACH foot is least expensive; the cushion heel absorbs shock at heel strike.

   Davies B, Datta D: Mobility outcome following unilateral lower limb amputation. Prosthet Orthot Int 27:186–190, 2003.

   Johannesson A, Larsson GU, Oberg T: From major amputation to prosthetic outcome: A prospective study of 190 patients in a defined population. Prosthet Orthot Int 28:9–21, 2004.

2. **When should the transtibial prosthetic prescription differ from the basic prescription?**

   Individuals at levels 3 and 4 are able to walk rapidly and engage in sports. They will benefit from an energy-storing foot, such as the Flex-Foot, Seattle Foot, or Springlite Foot, as well as a shock-absorbing endoskeletal shank and distal pin suspension. Someone who does heavy labor may need an exoskeletal shank; this shank is less expensive and more durable than the endoskeletal one. Alternative liners include those made with silicone or those that have oil-filled chambers to distribute pressure hydraulically. The person with a very short amputation limb may require supracondylar/suprapatellar suspension. Supracondylar suspension eliminates the need to buckle a strap and thus is more streamlined, particularly when the wearer sits. Corset suspension is heavier and should be reserved for the patient who has knee instability.

Beil TL, Street GM: Comparison of interface pressures with pin and suction suspension systems. J Rehabil Res Dev 41: 821–828, 2004.

Coleman KL, Boone DA, Laing LS, et al: Quantification of prosthetic outcomes: Elastomeric gel liner with locking pin suspension versus polyethylene foam liner with neoprene sleeve suspension. J Rehabil Res Dev 41:591–602, 2004.

Gard SA, Konz RJ. The effect of a shock-absorbing pylon on the gait of persons with unilateral transtibial amputation. J Rehabil Res Dev 40:109–124, 2003.

Sanders JE, Nicholson BS, Zachariah SG, et al: Testing of elastomeric liners used in limb prosthetics: Classification of 15 products by mechanical performance. J Rehabil Res Dev 41:175–186, 2004.

Selles RW, Janssens PJ, Jongenengel CD, Bussman JB: A randomized controlled trial comparing functional outcome and cost efficiency of a total surface-bearing socket versus a conventional patellar tendon-bearing socket in transtibial amputees. Arch Phys Med Rehabil 86:154–161, 2005.

3. **What is the most common prosthesis for a patient with transfemoral (above-knee) amputation?**
    Patients in Medicare level 1 or 2 benefit from a prosthesis that has a SACH foot-ankle assembly, endoskeletal shank, single-axis knee unit with constant sliding friction and an extension aid, plastic total contact socket, and partial suction suspension with Silesian belt as auxiliary suspension. The endoskeletal shank is appreciably lighter than the exoskeletal one for transfemoral prostheses. Socket contour may be **quadrilateral** (high anterior and lateral walls, relatively narrow anteroposteriorly) or **ischial containment** (high posterior and medial walls, relatively narrow mediolaterally).

    Schoppen T, Boonstra A, Groothoff JW, et al: Physical, mental, and social predictors of functional outcome in unilateral lower-limb amputees. Arch Phys Med Rehabil 84:803–811, 2003.

    van der Linde H, Hofstad CJ, Geurts ACH, et al: A systematic literature review of the effect of different prosthetic components on human functioning with a lower-limb prosthesis. J Rehabil Res Dev 555–570, 2004.

4. **When should the transfemoral prosthetic prescription differ from the basic prescription?**
    People at level 3 or 4 should ambulate rapidly and are candidates for fluid friction in the knee joint, either pneumatic or hydraulic; microprocessor-controlled knee units, such as the C-Leg, are designed for active patients who walk on ramps, stairs, and similar terrain. Those at level 1 or 2 may need a knee unit that has a friction weight-bearing brake or a manual lock. The individual with stable limb volume can manage with total suction suspension, eliminating the Silesian belt. A pelvic band provides maximum hip stabilization.

    HCFA Common Procedure Coding System, Chapter 5.3. Washington, DC, U.S. Government Printing Office, 2001.

    Johansson JL, Sherrill DM, Riley PO, et al: A clinical comparison of variable-damping and mechanically passive prosthetic knee devices. Am J Phys Med Rehabil 84:563–575, 2005.

    Swanson E, Stube J, Edman P: Function and body image levels in individuals with transfemoral amputations using the C-Leg®. J Prosthet Orthot 17:80–84, 2005.

    van der Linde H, Hofstad CJ, Geurts ACH, et al: A systematic literature review of the effect of different prosthetic components on human functioning with a lower-limb prosthesis. J Rehabil Res Dev 555–570, 2004.

5. **How do energy-storing feet work? What effect do they have on gait?**
    Energy-storing feet, such as Springlite, Flex-Foot, Carbon-Copy, or Seattle Foot, have a flexible keel made of carbon fiber or nylon. The **keel** is the longitudinal structural support of the foot. Depending on the design, during stance on the prosthesis, the load applied by the patient bends the keel, thereby storing energy. Just before swing phase, the keel recoils, producing a ground reaction force from below and behind and propelling the patient up and forward. Prosthetic foot action imitates the propulsive force normally provided by gastrocnemius-soleus contraction. If the patient is too feeble to apply substantial force to the foot, the energy-storing effect is minimal.

Casillas JM, Dulieu V, Cohen M, et al: Bioenergetic comparison of a new energy-storing foot and SACH foot in traumatic and vascular below-knee amputations. Arch Phys Med Rehabil 76:39–44, 1995.

Torburn L, Powers CM, Gutierrez R, et al: Energy expenditure during ambulation in dysvascular and traumatic below-knee amputees: A comparison of five prosthetic feet. J Rehabil Res Dev 32:111–119, 1995.

6. **What factors influence energy consumption during walking?**
Residual limb length and etiology of the amputation are the principal factors. Individuals with transtibial amputations consume less energy per distance walked than those with transfemoral amputation. Those with longer residual limbs are more energy-efficient. Disease that affects cardiovascular, pulmonary, nervous, or muscle function reduces the safety, quality, and efficiency of gait.

Gonzalez EG, Edelstein JE: Energy expenditure during ambulation. In Gonzalez EG, Myers SJ, Edelstein JE, et al (eds): Downey and Darling's Physiological Basis of Rehabilitation Medicine, 3rd ed. Boston, Butterworth Heinemann, 2001, pp 417–447.

7. **Which patients are not candidates for a prosthesis?**
Level 0 designates individuals with moderate or severe cognitive impairment and those with exercise-limiting cardiopulmonary disease who will not benefit from prosthetic rehabilitation. Severe arthritis, obesity, and neurologic disease do not contraindicate fitting, but patients with such disorders may experience difficulty ambulating.

Bussman JB, Grootscholten EA, Stam HJ: Daily physical activity and heart rate response in people with a unilateral transtibial amputation for vascular disease. Arch Phys Med Rehabil 85:240–244, 2004.

Dillingham TR, Pezzin LE, Shore AD: Reamputation, mortality, and health care costs among persons with dysvascular lower-limb amputations. Arch Phys Med Rehabil 86:480–485, 2005.

HCFA Common Procedure Coding System, Chapter 5.3. Washington, DC, U.S. Government Printing Office, 2001.

8. **What anatomic factors interfere with the gait of patients with amputation?**
Hip and knee contractures compromise stability, even when the prosthesis is aligned to compensate for the deformity. A short residual limb limits the surface for prosthetic contact and presents a short lever arm for force transmission.

Rabuffetti M, Recalcati M, Ferrarin M: Trans-femoral amputee gait: Socket-pelvis constraints and compensation strategies. Prosthet Orthot Int 29:183–192, 2005.

9. **How do you evaluate the gait of a patient with amputation?**
Ask the patient to walk at a comfortable pace (80 m/min) along an unobstructed walkway at least 4 meters (12 ft) long. Stand behind the patient to observe the width of the walking base and movements in the frontal and transverse planes. Stand on the side of the prosthesis to observe sagittal movements. From each observation position, systematically note the action of the foot, knee, hip, and trunk in comparison with joint action in the gait of able-bodied people. Other clinical means of assessing gait include recording step length, cadence (steps per minute), and velocity.

Edelstein J: Prosthetic assessment and management. In O'Sullivan SB, Schmitz TJ (eds): Physical Rehabilitation: Evaluation and Treatment Procedures, 5th ed. Philadelphia: F.A. Davis, 2006 pp 1251–1286.

10. **When watching the knee joint from the side, what specifically should be evaluated?**
When an able-bodied adult walks at a comfortable speed (approximately 80 m/min), the knee flexes about 15 degrees between heel strike and foot-flat. At the slower walking speed of the person with unilateral transtibial amputation, the knee flexes less following heel strike. The observer must note whether knee flexion on the amputated side is significantly more or less than the expected 10 degrees.

Detrembleur C, Vanmarsenille J-M, De Cuyper F, Dierick F: Relationship between energy cost, gait speed, vertical displacement of centre of body mass and efficiency of pendulum-like mechanism in unilateral amputee gait. Gait Posture 21:333–340, 2005.

Edelstein J: Prosthetic assessment and management. In O'Sullivan SB, Schmitz TJ (eds): Physical Rehabilitation: Evaluation and Treatment Procedures, 5th ed. Philadelphia: F.A. Davis, 2006, pp 1251–1286.

Isakov E, Keren O, Benjuya N: Transtibial amputee gait: Time-distance parameters and EMG activity. Prosthet Orthot Int 24:216–220, 2000.

Nolan L, Wit A, Dudzinski K, et al: Adjustments in gait symmetry with walking speed in transfemoral and transtibial amputees. Gait Posture 17:142–151, 2003.

11. **Excessive knee flexion in early stance is termed** *buckling*. **What might cause this deviation?**

Any factor that places the floor reaction behind the knee will cause excessive knee flexion.

- **Shoe heel too high:** The floor reaction passes behind the knee, causing knee flexion. To determine whether the shoe is the source of buckling, have the patient change to a shoe with a lower heel.
- **Heel cushion or plantar bumper too stiff:** Normally, as a result of ankle plantar flexion and knee flexion, the forefoot descends to the floor quickly after heel contact. If plantar flexion is restricted by a stiff prosthetic heel, the knee will flex excessively (>10 degrees) after heel contact. The forefoot slaps the floor rapidly. An overly stiff heel will not absorb the impact shock as the prosthetic foot strikes the floor.
- **Foot in dorsiflexion:** If the foot is attached to the shank in excessive dorsiflexion, when the forefoot contacts the floor, the shank is inclined forward and the knee is markedly flexed.
- **Socket too far forward over the foot:** The force transmitted through the socket (force A in Fig. 37-1) and the reaction force from the floor (force B in Fig. 37-1) constitute a force couple that tends to rotate the prosthesis in the clockwise direction around the heel. This rotation is seen as excessive knee flexion immediately after heel strike. The quadriceps, which is active in early stance, must contract more forcefully to resist the increased flexion moment. As the quadriceps contracts to control the flexing knee, compression and shear between the socket and residual limb increase dramatically, particularly at the anterior-distal tibia.
- **Knee flexion contracture, uncompensated:** Contracture places the socket of an uncompensated prosthesis considerably ahead of the foot. An exaggerated knee flexion

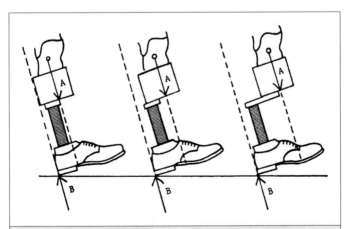

Figure 37-1. Force transmitted through the socket (force A) and the reaction force (force B) from the floor constitute a force couple that tends to rotate the prosthesis clockwise around the heel as a fulcrum.

moment increases anterior-distal tibial pressure. If the residual limb is short and the contracture is not great, the prosthetist can move the foot forward under the socket.

Rabuffetti M, Recalcati M, Ferrarin M: Trans-femoral amputee gait: Socket-pelvis constraints and compensation strategies. Prosthet Orthot Int 29:183–192, 2005.

12. **What happens during late-stance phase?**
    At heel-off, the body's center of gravity passes over the portion of the prosthetic foot corresponding to the metatarsophalangeal (MTP) joints. The knee, which had been extending, begins to flex. If body weight passes over the forefoot too soon, the premature loss of anterior support would allow the knee to flex too soon, and the torso would drop abruptly (**"drop off"**) until arrested by contralateral heel contact. Many factors that cause knee buckling also cause drop off, such as foot in dorsiflexion, anterior displacement of the socket, and knee flexion contracture.

    Edelstein J: Prosthetic assessment and management. In O'Sullivan SB, Schmitz TJ (eds): Physical Rehabilitation: Evaluation and Treatment Procedures, 5th ed. Philadelphia: F.A. Davis, 2006, pp 1251–1286.

13. **What causes insufficient knee flexion?**
    Any factor that places the floor reaction in front of the knee will cause insufficient knee flexion.
    - **Heel cushion or plantar bumper too soft.** The soft heel absorbs shock so quickly that the floor reaction passes in front of, rather than behind, the knee. The anterior floor reaction resists knee flexion.
    - **Prosthetic foot in excessive plantarflexion.** The forefoot reaches the floor too quickly after heel strike.
    - **Socket too far posterior over the foot.** The clockwise rotation of the prosthesis (flexion moment) produced by the force couple is reduced as the socket force moves closer to the floor reaction.
    - **Quadriceps weakness.** Supporting body weight over a flexed knee is possible only if the quadriceps can prevent the knee from buckling. The individual with weak knee extensors avoids collapse by walking over a stiffly extended knee, with the gluteus maximus largely responsible for maintaining knee extension. Leaning the trunk forward enhances knee extension.
    - **Anterior-distal tibial discomfort.** Increased pressure between the anterodistal tibia and the socket stems primarily from exaggerated quadriceps activity controlling the rate and extent of knee flexion after heel contact. To alleviate discomfort, the patient may hold the knee in full extension. The gait may mimic that with weak quadriceps, even though quadriceps strength is normal. Differentiating between these two causes requires muscle testing, residuum and socket inspection for evidence of high-pressure injury, and questioning of the patient who may fear allowing the knee to flex.

    Schmalz T, Blumentritt S, Jarasch R: Energy expenditure and biomechanical characteristics of lower limb amputee gait: The influence of prosthetic alignment and different prosthetic components. Gait Posture 16:255–263, 2002.

14. **What is "climbing the hill"?**
    A patient with transtibial amputation may complain of "**climbing the hill**" during late stance if the prosthesis is excessively stable. A foot malaligned too far anteriorly or plantar flexed, a socket set too far posteriorly or insufficiently flexed, or a suspension cuff or thigh corset attached too far anteriorly contributes to this effect. Quadriceps weakness may be compensated by keeping the knee extended; this maneuver may produce or aggravate pain at the anterodistal aspect of the amputation limb. Hyperactive quadriceps, as occurs in extensor synergy after stroke, also prevent knee flexion and produce the sensation of climbing the hill.

    Edelstein J: Prosthetic assessment and management. In O'Sullivan SB, Schmitz TJ (eds): Physical Rehabilitation: Evaluation and Treatment Procedures, 5th ed. Philadelphia: F.A. Davis, 2006, pp 1251–1286.

15. **What is "lateral thrust"? How is it observed?**
Midstance on the prosthesis is the period of single support. Because the socket surrounds soft tissue, some shifting (thrusting) of the proximal portion of the socket relative to the amputation limb occurs. The transtibial prosthesis is aligned to maximize load on pressure-tolerant tissue, namely the proximomedial aspect over the pes anserinus, and to minimize pressure on the proximolateral aspect over the fibular head and peroneal nerve. A properly aligned prosthesis thrusts laterally at midstance, that is, exhibits slight varus movement. Excessive lateral thrust, produced by aligning the prosthetic foot too far medial, is undesirable because high pressure is felt at the distolateral portion of the amputation limb.

Edelstein J: Prosthetic assessment and management. In O'Sullivan SB, Schmitz TJ (eds): Physical Rehabilitation: Evaluation and Treatment Procedures, 5th ed. Philadelphia: F.A. Davis, 2006, pp 1251–1286.

16. **Describe the gait of the patient with transfemoral (above-knee) amputation.**
As compared to the transtibial gait, the patient with transfemoral amputation walks more slowly, expends more energy, is more likely to use a cane or other support, and exhibits more deviation from the able-bodied pattern. These are the consequences of loss of the anatomic knee.

Ordinarily, without quadriceps, the prosthetic knee must be fully extended through early and midstance to avoid buckling. Maintaining extension requires gluteus maximus contraction, prosthetic alignment that brings the floor reaction anterior to the knee, a relatively soft prosthetic heel to absorb heel contact impact and thereby limit the knee flexion moment, and sometimes a knee friction unit that inhibits or prevents flexion during early stance. Microprocessor-controlled knee units enable the patient to pass through early stance with a slightly flexed knee.

During swing phase, the quadriceps normally function to limit knee flexion immediately after toe-off, while the hamstrings act to decelerate the lower leg before heel strike. In the absence of these muscular controls, the speed and arc of the swinging shank must be regulated by the knee unit. Fluid-controlled knee units, with or without microprocessor control, automatically accommodate to changes in walking velocity, enabling the prosthetic shank and the sound leg to swing approximately the same extent, regardless of walking speed.

Jaeger SM, Arendzen JH, de Jongh JH: Prosthetic gait of unilateral transfemoral amputees: A kinematic study. Arch Phys Med Rehabil 76:736–743, 1995.

Nolan L, Wit A, Dudzinski K, et al: Adjustments in gait symmetry with walking speed in transfemoral and transtibial amputees. Gait Posture 17:142–151, 2003.

KEY POINTS: LOWER LIMB PROSTHESES

1. Medicare regulations specify four levels of reimbursement based on the patient's functional potential.

2. The transtibial prosthesis for level 1, household ambulation, includes a SACH (**s**olid **a**nkle **c**ushion **h**eel) foot-ankle assembly, endoskeletal shank with foam cover, total contact socket with liner, and cuff suspension.

3. The transfemoral prosthesis for level 1 includes a SACH foot-ankle assembly, endoskeletal shank with cover, single-axis knee unit, total contact socket, and partial suction suspension with Silesian belt.

4. Energy consumption during walking is influenced primarily by residual limb length and amputation etiology.

5. Excessive knee flexion in early stance on a transtibial prosthesis ("buckling") is caused by any factor that places the floor reaction behind the knee.

17. **Describe the causes of lateral trunk bending.**
   As soon as the sound limb lifts off the floor to begin its swing phase, the pelvis tends to drop on the unsupported (sound) side. The hip abductors on the prosthetic, stance-phase side contract strongly to limit the pelvic drop. In the absence of hip abductor control, the trunk must lean toward the prosthetic side to counteract the instability toward the swing-phase side. Conditions that interfere with pelvic control by the hip abductors, and thus are causes of lateral trunk bending, include the following:
   - **Weak hip abductors:** Insufficient abductor force fails to counteract pelvic drop.
   - **Hip abduction contracture or abducted socket:** The shortened abductors are ineffective.
   - **Poor fit of the lateral socket wall:** Gluteus medius contraction causes the femoral remnant to exert force at both its origin and its insertion, that is, on the pelvis and femur. For it to stabilize the pelvis, the femur must be prevented from moving. This is the primary function of the lateral socket wall, which must fit snugly to limit femoral abduction.
   - **Laterodistal femoral discomfort:** If thigh abduction against the lateral wall results in discomfort, the patient may bend laterally to reduce pressure.
   - **Short amputation limb:** Insufficient bony leverage prevents the patient from achieving frontal plane stability.
   - **Lack of distal stabilization of the femur:** This problem is eliminated by osseous integration of the prosthesis with the femur, so that the patient has a stable connection between the hip on the amputated side to the prosthesis and thus to the floor.

   Schmid M, Beltrami G, Zambarbieri D, Verni G: Centre of pressure displacements in trans-femoral amputees during gait. Gait Posture 21:255–262, 2005.

18. **What causes abducted gait (wide walking base)?**
   A wide walking base is >10 cm between heel centers. The prosthetic foot is held away from the midline throughout the gait cycle and is associated with lateral trunk bending. Major causes include:
   - Perineal discomfort. When the patient experiences crotch pain, widening the base moves the medial socket brim away from the sensitive area.
   - Excessively long prosthesis. Although few prostheses have a thigh or shank that is too long, apparent lengthening occurs with failure to lodge the thigh properly in the socket.
   - Abduction contracture, uncompensated
   - Poor balance
   - Hip arthritis
   - Hip dislocation
   - Inguinal hernia

   A cane, preferably held in the contralateral hand, minimizes both lateral bending and wide base.

   Edelstein J: Prosthetic assessment and management. In O'Sullivan SB, Schmitz TJ (eds): Physical Rehabilitation: Evaluation and Treatment Procedures, 5th ed. Philadelphia: F.A. Davis, 2006, pp 1251–1286.

19. **What causes the knee on a transfemoral prosthesis to swing through an excessively large range, also known as high heel rise?**
   Swing-phase biomechanics depend on the wearer's walking speed and the adjustment of the knee unit. At a given walking speed, the patient will exhibit **high heel rise** (excessively acute knee flexion) during early swing phase if the friction mechanism, the extension aid, or both components are relatively loose. During late-swing phase, a loose friction mechanism or a tight extension aid will cause rapid, abrupt extension, known as **terminal impact**. Some patients like the sound at impact because it indicates that the knee is extended and will be stable during early-stance phase. A person who walks rapidly while wearing a prosthesis that has a sliding friction knee unit will experience high heel rise and terminal impact. A fluid-controlled knee unit adjusts automatically to changes in walking speed, thus minimizing high heel rise and terminal impact.

   Edelstein J: Prosthetic assessment and management. In O'Sullivan SB, Schmitz TJ (eds): Physical Rehabilitation: Evaluation and Treatment Procedures, 5th ed. Philadelphia: F.A. Davis, 2006, pp 1251–1286.

20. **How do you determine the cause of circumduction?**
This swing-phase deviation is characterized by a laterally curved line of progression—that is, the prosthesis swings to the side then brought back to the midline for the next heel contact. Patients who fear stubbing the prosthetic toe adopt this maneuver to ensure that the prosthetic foot clears the floor. Examine the patient for conditions that create a "functionally long" prosthesis:
- Foot in plantarflexion: Toe tends to scuff the floor
- Socket so small that the amputation limb cannot enter fully
- Inadequate suspension causes the socket to slip during swing phase
- Insufficient or no knee flexion during swing because the knee unit includes a manual lock, has excessive friction, or has a tight extension aid
- Patient is reluctant to flex the knee during swing because of poor balance or fear

Edelstein J: Prosthetic assessment and management. In O'Sullivan SB, Schmitz TJ (eds): Physical Rehabilitation: Evaluation and Treatment Procedures, 5th ed. Philadelphia: F.A. Davis, 2006, pp 1251–1286.

21. **What are whips? Why do they occur?**
A whip is a sudden abrupt rotation of the prosthesis that occurs at the end of stance phase as the knee flexes to begin swing. If the prosthetic heel moves medially, a **medial whip** is noted, while lateral rotation of the heel denotes a **lateral whip**.
Mechanically, flexion and extension of the prosthetic knee (i.e., motion of the shank and foot) occurs in a plane perpendicular to the knee axis. Thus for the shank to swing along a sagittal line, the knee axis must be perpendicular to that line. If the knee axis were externally or internally rotated, the shank swings diagonally. Major causes of whips are as follows:
- **Improper alignment of the knee axis:** An externally rotated axis produces a medial whip, because at initial flexion of the knee the prosthesis rotates to a position perpendicular to the axis. An internally rotated axis causes a lateral whip.
- **Flabby musculature that rotates freely around the femur:** The prosthesis rotates with the soft tissue unless a suspension component, such as a Silesian belt, controls rotation.

Edelstein J: Prosthetic assessment and management. In O'Sullivan SB, Schmitz TJ (eds): Physical Rehabilitation: Evaluation and Treatment Procedures, 5th ed. Philadelphia: F.A. Davis, 2006, pp 1251–1286.

22. **What is vaulting? What are its causes, and who is most apt to vault?**
Vaulting refers to exaggerated plantar flexion on the contralateral intact leg during swing phase of the prosthesis. Vaulting increases the distance between the prosthetic foot and the floor, thus reducing the likelihood of tripping on the prosthesis. Because this deviation is arduous, it is primarily seen in children and young adults. Older adults who formed the habit years earlier may persistently vault.

Edelstein J: Prosthetic assessment and management. In O'Sullivan SB, Schmitz TJ (eds): Physical Rehabilitation: Evaluation and Treatment Procedures, 5th ed. Philadelphia: F.A. Davis, 2006, pp 1251–1286.

23. **What causes a long step on the prosthetic side?**
- **Hip flexion contracture:** In order for the sound limb to take a normal-length step, the hip on the prosthetic side must hyperextend. A hip flexion contracture on the amputated side prevents hyperextension, causing asymmetrical step lengths.
- **Insufficient socket flexion:** Aligning the transfemoral socket in flexion enables the prosthesis to reach a position of hyperextension. Whether this can be accomplished depends on the degree of contracture and the length of the amputation limb; the shorter the thigh, the more compensatory socket flexion that can be introduced.
- **Pain, insecurity, fear:** Discomfort from an ill-fitting socket or fear of balancing on an insensate stilt will cause the patient, whether having transfemoral or transtibial amputation,

to minimize time in prosthetic-stance phase. Body weight is shifted quickly back to the sound side, which has taken a rapid, short step to prepare to accept weight.

Edelstein J: Prosthetic assessment and management. In O'Sullivan SB, Schmitz TJ (eds): Physical Rehabilitation: Evaluation and Treatment Procedures, 5th ed. Philadelphia: F.A. Davis, 2006, pp 1251–1286.

24. **Describe the mechanics of uneven heel rise.**
Normally, the quadriceps is responsible for limiting knee flexion in early swing. Without a quadriceps, the patient with transfemoral amputation must depend on resistance to motion provided by the prosthetic knee unit through a friction mechanism, whether sliding, pneumatic, or hydraulic, or an extension aid. If these produce too little resistance to motion, the prosthetic knee will flex excessively in early swing, and will be obvious as high heel rise. Conversely, too much resistance to knee motion causes insufficient heel rise as the knee flexes too little.

Edelstein J: Prosthetic assessment and management. In O'Sullivan SB, Schmitz TJ (eds): Physical Rehabilitation: Evaluation and Treatment Procedures, 5th ed. Philadelphia: F.A. Davis, 2006, pp 1251–1286.

25. **How do you recognize terminal impact?**
Noisy extension at the end of swing phase on the prosthetic side indicates **terminal impact.** Toward the end of swing phase, the hamstrings normally decelerate the shank—that is, control the rate of knee extension. Without intact hamstrings, the patient with transfemoral amputation must depend on the knee unit to resist shank motion. Too little resistance from the friction mechanism allows inertia to swing the shank forward so rapidly that it produces a forceful impact into full extension. Alternatively, a taut extension aid will accelerate the shank forward.

A small amount of terminal impact is often beneficial because the impact provides auditory and vibratory feedback, signaling that the prosthetic knee is fully extended and that it is safe to contact the floor with the prosthetic foot.

Edelstein J: Prosthetic assessment and management. In O'Sullivan SB, Schmitz TJ (eds): Physical Rehabilitation: Evaluation and Treatment Procedures, 5th ed. Philadelphia: F.A. Davis, 2006, pp 1251–1286.

26. **What effect does the shoe have on the gait of patients who wear prostheses?**
The shoe is an integral part of the prosthesis. A loose shoe will slip from the prosthetic foot during late stance. A tight shoe will interfere with forefoot action during late stance. An excessively high heel reduces knee stability, both in the anatomic knee of the person wearing a transtibial prosthesis and the knee unit in a transfemoral prosthesis. Too low a heel or an excessively compressible heel makes the knee on the prosthetic side overly stable. A stiff boot restrains dorsiflexion and plantar flexion.

Edelstein J: Prosthetic assessment and management. In O'Sullivan SB, Schmitz TJ (eds): Physical Rehabilitation: Evaluation and Treatment Procedures, 5th ed. Philadelphia: F.A. Davis, 2006, pp 1251–1286.

BIBLIOGRAPHY

1. Carroll K, Edelstein JE (eds): Prosthetics and Patient Management: A Comprehensive Clinical Approach. Thorofare, NJ, Slack, 2006.
2. Smith DG, Michael JW, Bowker JH (eds): Atlas of Amputations and Limb Deficiencies, 3rd ed. Chicago, American Academy of Orthopaedic Surgeons, 2004.

CHAPTER 38

SPINAL ORTHOSES: PRINCIPLES, DESIGNS, INDICATIONS, AND LIMITATIONS

Abna A. Ogle, MD, and John B. Redford, MD

...and the crooked shall be made straight...

—Isaiah 40:4

1. What is a spinal orthosis?

The word *orthosis* is derived from the Greek word meaning "making straight." Spinal orthoses or braces are appliances used in an attempt to correct and support the spine. The application of neck braces was described during the fifth Egyptian dynasty, and thoracic bandages were used in the mid-18th century to correct scoliosis. The use of the halo vest in the 1960s helped revolutionize spinal cord injury rehabilitation.

Smith GE: The most ancient splints. BMJ 1:732–734, 1908.
www.biomech.com
www.oandp.com

2. Why are spinal orthoses used in clinical care?

- Stabilization and maintenance of spinal alignment
- Prevention and correction of spinal deformities
- Relief of pain by limiting motion or weight-bearing
- Reduction of axial loading of the spine
- Improvement of spinal function
- Provision of effects such as heat, massage, and kinesthetic feedback

Lusskin R, Berger N: Prescription principles. In American Academy of Orthopedic Surgeons (ed): Atlas of Orthotics: Biomechanical Principles and Applications. St. Louis, Mosby, 1975, pp 105–129.
Redford JS, Patel AT: Orthotic devices in the management of spinal disorders. Phys Med Rehabil State Art Rev 9:709–724, 1995.

3. List the three principal functions of the vertebral column.

- Protect the spinal cord and its nerve roots
- Absorb axial compressive forces
- Provide a base for mobility of the human skeleton

4. How do spinal orthoses work?

Spinal orthoses, when applied to the body, exert forces on the spine. This is accomplished in one or more of the following ways:

- **Three-point pressure system:** See Figure 38-1.
- **Fluid compression:** When the brace encompasses the trunk, it forms a semirigid cylinder surrounding the vertebral column. This results in an increase in intraabdominal pressure, which measurably decreases intervertebral disc pressure and shearing forces across the lowest functional units.
- **Irritant:** The brace is constructed so that the wearer is forced into the desired posture to avoid discomfort (kinesthetic feedback) or is reminded to voluntarily restrict motion.

- **Skeletal fixation:** The scientific basis for orthotic use is well delineated in the correction of certain progressive spine deformities. However, as orthopedic surgery has advanced, the use of external corrective devices has declined. Braces are commonly used in nonsurgical musculoskeletal complaints, such as back or neck strains. It is in this arena that empirical evidence is incomplete. However, clinical experience and patient reports provide justification for their continued use.

  Sypert GW: External spinal orthotics. Neurosurgery 20(4):642–649, 1987.

5. **What are the potential complications of spinal orthoses?**
   - Loss of skin integrity because of compressive forces
   - Weakening of axial muscles
   - Soft-tissue contractures
   - Increased movement at the ends of immobilized segments
   - Physical and psychological dependence
   - Osteopenia (through misuse/overuse)

   Eisinger DB, Kumar R, Woodrow R: Effect of lumbar orthotics on trunk muscle strength. Am J Phys Med Rehabil 75(3):194–197, 1996.

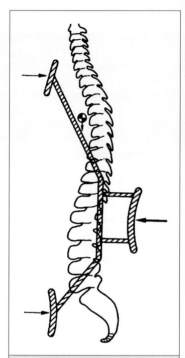

Figure 38-1. Three-point pressure as applied in a hyperextension thoracolumbosacral orthosis.

6. **There are so many different orthoses. How can I remember their names?**
   There is a bewildering variety, several even sporting the name or hometown of the creator. To avoid confusion and aid in classification of braces, the American Academy of Orthopaedic Surgeons and the American Academy of Prosthetists and Orthotists together have devised a uniform naming system (Table 38-1).

   Harris EE: A new orthotics terminology. Ortho Prosthet 27:6–10, 1973.

TABLE 38-1.   COMMONLY USED SPINAL ORTHOSES

Orthoses	Uniform Naming System
Cervical orthosis	CO
Cervicothoracic orthosis	CTO
Cervicothoracolumbosacral orthosis	CTLSO
Thoracolumbosacral orthosis	TLSO
Lumbosacral orthosis	LSO
Sacroiliac orthosis	SIO

7. **How is an orthosis prescription developed?**
   The spinal segments have very different characteristics. The specific complaint, anatomic pathology, and unique properties of the spinal segment must be considered when

recommending an orthosis. Once a specific diagnosis is made, objectives for treatment are prioritized: stability, deformity corrections, pain relief, comfort, and function. A brace is then selected based on its particular capabilities.

KEY POINTS: SPINAL ORTHOSES

1. The cervical spine has the greatest range of motion of all segments of the vertebral column. It is capable of motion in three planes: flexion/extension, lateral rotation, and side bending.

2. Nearly half (~45%) of all cervical rotation occurs at the atlantoaxial joint (C1–C2).

3. The greatest amount of cervical flexion occurs between C5 and C6.

4. Between 80% and 90% of available motion in the lumbar spine occurs at L4–L5 and L5–S1, making these joints more susceptible to degenerative change.

5. The thoracic spine is the least mobile and most stable segment of the spine. It owes its rigidity to its attachment to the ribs and sternum.

8. **Your patient has an acute but uncomplicated cervical strain. What orthosis do you prescribe?**
The **soft collar** is probably the most commonly used orthosis. It is made of a firm foam covered with cotton and fastened posteriorly with Velcro. It is usually prescribed for cervical muscle strain. It provides little restriction of cervical movement. Flexion and extension are reduced only by approximately one fourth, and virtually no reduction of lateral bending or rotation is present. However, the collar allows soft tissues to rest, provides warmth to strained muscles, and reminds the patient to avoid extremes of neck movement.

Sandler AJ, Dvorak J, Humke T, et al: The effectiveness of various cervical orthoses. An in vivo comparison of the mechanical stability provided by several widely used models. Spine 21(14):1624–1629, 1996.

9. **When is a Philadelphia collar used?**
This type of cervical orthosis provides more restriction of movement than does the soft collar, but less than a halo vest or custom-made plastic cervicothoracic orthosis (CTO). The Philadelphia collar is made of a foam reinforced by firm thermoplastic material. It has an anterior and posterior portion that conform to the chin and occiput.

A Philadelphia collar is frequently prescribed after cervical surgery, when very strict neck immobilization is not necessary. It may also be used in cases with cervical ligament rupture and in some relatively stable cervical spine fractures. It provides more limitation in flexion/extension and side-bending than a soft collar, but it does not significantly limit rotation. Patients frequently complain of feeling hot and sweaty under this type of collar, but it is generally well tolerated.

10. **What is a halo vest orthosis?**
This CTO consists of two parts. The halo portion is a circular band of steel attached to the skull via threaded pins. Adjustable rods connect the halo to a vest that encircles the trunk. This device provides the most rigid fixation of the cervical spine and is the orthosis most widely used after cervical fractures. This brace makes possible early mobilization and rehabilitation of the patient after spinal surgery, while maintaining a stable spine.

Botte MJ, Byrne TP, Abrams RA, Garfin SR: The halo skeletal fixator: Current concepts of application and maintenance. Orthopedics 18(5):463–471, 1995.

11. **How do you choose a cervical orthosis?**
    See Table 38-2.

TABLE 38-2. CHOOSING A CERVICAL ORTHOSIS

Main Goals	Type of Collar
Kinesthetic feedback, comfort/warmth	Soft cervical collar
Limit cervical flexion and lateral bending	Philadelphia collar
	Aspen collar
	Miami collar
Limit cervical flexion, lateral bending, and most rotation	Halovest
	SOMI
	Minerva

SOMI = sterno-occipital-mandibular immobilizer.

12. **What braces are used for thoracic deformities?**
    The best demonstrable results are for low thoracic scoliosis with the Milwaukee and Boston braces. For middle and high thoracic scoliosis, the efficacy of corrective orthoses remains debatable. Idiopathic or paralytic scolioses are amenable to surgery (Table 38-3).
    - **Milwaukee bracing** for progressive spinal curvature consists of two posterior and one anterior upright attached to a ring around the neck and pelvic girdle. Straps with pressure pads are mounted on the brace to improve spinal alignment.
    - The **Taylor brace** is prescribed for countering kyphosis. It has high thoracic uprights and shoulder straps. These straps must be tightened (often to the discomfort of the patient) to provide adequate antideformity force. This brace is uncomfortable with generally poor patient compliance. Molded plastic jackets are more acceptable to patients who need extensive spinal immobilization.
    - The **CASH** (cruciform anterior spinal hyperextension) orthosis is also used to decrease kyphosis. It has an anterior cross-bar with pads at the four ends of the cross. This orthosis adjusts posteriorly with straps held closed with Velcro. It is lightweight and easy to put on but may require frequent repositioning.
    - The **Jewett** (hyperextension thoracolumbosacral [TLSO]) orthosis uses the three-point system to facilitate thoracic hyperextension. The two anterior pads are positioned over the sternum and pubic symphysis, while the third opposing posterior pad lies over the thoracolumbar junction. It does not limit spine rotation but is fairly comfortable to wear and more easily adjusted than the CASH orthosis. The Jewett orthosis is prescribed to prevent spinal flexion after a middle or lower level thoracic vertebral compression fracture.

    McLain RF, Karol L: Conservative treatment of the scoliotic and kyphotic patient. Arch Pediatr Adolescent Med 148:646–665, 1994.

13. **How is a painful nondisplaced thoracic compression fracture treated?**
    Clinical experience indicates that orthoses can alleviate acute pain, but no scientific evidence exists as to how this may occur. Short-term use of a corset is acceptable in the first 7–10 days following a fracture (in the authors' experience).

14. **How are unstable thoracic fractures treated?**

Generally, after acute decompression of the spinal cord and spinal fusion at thoracic (and sometimes lumbar) level are accomplished, a custom bivalve TLSO is prescribed for up to 3 months. The patient is usually instructed to wear this at all times, removing it only for purposes of hygiene.

Benzel EC, Larson SJ: Postoperatiave stabilization of the post traumatic thoracic and lumbar spine: A review of concepts and orthotic techniques. J Spinal Disord 2(1):47–51, 1989.

15. **When are lumbosacral orthoses used?**

They are frequently prescribed for uncomplicated low back pain but are primarily used for support and immobilization of the spine after trauma or surgery. Application of these orthoses for low back pain is controversial. Some clinicians cite the lack of consistent scientific evidence to support their use, especially in chronic low back pain. Others would agree with their limited use during high-impact activities, along with patient education and an exercise program.

Hodgson EA: Occupational back belt use: A literature review. AOHN J 44(9):438–443, 1996.

16. **There are so many LSOs on the market. How can I choose appropriately?**

One way to keep straight the ever-increasing multitude of LSOs is to consider them in order from the least to the most immobilizing:

- **Corsets** provide the least restriction in spinal movement. These can be made of canvas or elasticized material and can be reinforced with metal or plastic stays or even a thermomolded plastic plate. Corsets are more comfortable than rigid metal orthoses, such as the chair-back brace, and achieve lumbar support by increasing intra-abdominal pressure. They also provide some warmth to extensor muscles of the spine and can remind the wearer to avoid extremes of movement.
- **Spinal braces,** reinforced with rigid metal bars and rigid plastic jackets, are more restrictive than corsets and vary in length: the greater the length, the more immobilizing the effect. An example is the short flexion jacket **(Rainey orthosis)** that has been advocated by some for preventing extension in the lumbar spine; it is used in low back pain, particularly that caused by spondylolisthesis. This orthosis is made of thermomolded plastic anterior and posterior parts and fastened with Velcro. The anterior portion presses into the abdomen, causing increased intra-abdominal pressure. The forced flexion of the lumbar spine may also alleviate pressure in the posterior elements of the vertebral column.
- **Lumbosacral spicas** provide the most effective way of immobilizing the lower lumbar spine. They are made of thermomolded plastic extending from 2 cm below the inferior angle of the scapulae to the sacrum. A unilateral side piece is extended distally, usually immobilizing the hip in 15 to 20 degrees of flexion. Investigation of lumbosacral movements has demonstrated that the lower lumbar vertebrae are best immobilized when there is fixation of the pelvis (via the extended thigh piece). This orthosis is useful for postoperative immobilization and unstable lower spine fractures.

See Table 38-3 for specific guidelines.

van Poppel MN, de Loose MP, Koes BW, et al: Mechanisms of action of lumbar supports: A systematic review. Spine 25(16):2103–2113, 2000.

17. **What about sacroiliac orthoses?**

These belts or bands of fabric fit between the iliac crests and the greater trochanter of the femur. They are prescribed for sacroiliac dysfunction. It is important to note that the underlying pathomechanics and efficacy of these devices remain controversial. Generally speaking, it is recommended that these orthoses are used in combination with an appropriate strengthening, stretching, and posture education program.

Don Tigny RL: Function and pathomechanics of the sacroiliac joint. A review. Phys Ther 65(1):35–44, 1985.

TABLE 38-3. CHOOSING A TLSO, LSO, OR SIO

Application	Orthotic Device
Limits bending and reduces pain with nondisplaced spinal fracture	Thoracolumbar corset
To decrease thoracic kyphosis with or without compression fracture in a stable spine	Taylor brace
	CASH
	Molded plastic TLSO
Unstable fracture in thoracolumbar spine	Jewett brace
	CASH
	Molded plastic TLSO
Low back pain with or without history of trauma	Off-the-shelf LSO with rigid frame
	Corset with LS pad, custom-molded over SI area with Velcro closure
Nontraumatic sacroiliac pain	SIO (wide belt)
Low back pain during pregnancy	

CASH = cruciform anterior spinal hyperextension, LS = lumbosacral, LSO = lumbosacral orthosis, SI = sacroiliac, SIO = sacroiliac orthosis, TLSO = thoracolumbosacral orthosis.

BIBLIOGRAPHY

1. Redford J, Basmajian JB, Trautman P (eds): Orthotics, Clinical Practice and Rehabilitation Technology. New York, Churchill Livingstone, 1995.
2. Orthotics and Prosthetics: Physicians Pocket Guide. New York, Rehabilitation Designs of America, 1999.
3. Tan T (ed): Practical Manual of PM&R. St. Louis, Mosby, 1998.

CHAPTER 39

WHEELCHAIRS: MANUAL AND POWER

R. Lee Kirby, MD, Rory A. Cooper, PhD, and Michael L. Boninger, MD

Freedom and constraint are two aspects of the same necessity, which is to be what one is and no other.

—Antoine de Saint-Exupery (1900–1944)

Among the therapeutic tools in rehabilitation, the wheelchair is where the rubber really meets the road!

1. **Discuss the importance and prevalence of wheelchair use.**

   The wheelchair acts as an interface between the person and the environment, establishing mobility and enhancing independence. It is arguably the most important therapeutic tool in rehabilitation. In 2000, there were 2.2 million wheelchair users in the United States, approximately 75% of whom used manually propelled wheelchairs. This figure has been increasing at a rate of approximately 5% per year for 30 years. The prevalence is about fivefold greater among the elderly than the general population. The mechanical efficiencies of wheeling and walking are comparable, varying from 8% to 20%, depending on the population and technology evaluated.

   LaPlante MP: Demographics of wheeled mobility device users. Conference on Space Requirements for Wheeled Mobility, an International Workshop, October 9–11, 2003. Center for Inclusive Design and Environmental Access, University at Buffalo, State University of New York, Buffalo, New York: www.ap. buffalo.edu/idea/space%20workshop/papers/mitchell%20laplante/demographics%20of%20wheeled%20mobility%20-%20mitchell%20p%20laplante.htm

2. **How safe are wheelchairs?**

   The long-term use of wheelchairs can adversely affect the health of users as a result of chronic or repetitive stresses—for instance, by affecting shoulders, peripheral nerves, and skin. In the United States, there are more than 50 wheelchair-related deaths per year and more than 100,000 wheelchair-related injuries per year that are serious enough to require attention at a hospital's emergency department. The majority (approximately 75%) of these injuries are caused when the wheelchair users tip over and/or fall from their chairs. The best means for preventing these problems is through selecting the proper wheelchair to fit the user, to recommend only high-quality wheelchairs that have undergone rigorous testing, and to provide training in safe and effective use.

   Boninger ML, Koontz AM, Sisto SA, et al: Pushrim biomechanics and injury prevention in spinal cord injury: Recommendations based on CULP-SCI investigations. J Rehab Res Dev 42(Suppl 1):9–19, 2005.

   Calder CJ, Kirby RL: Fatal wheelchair-related accidents in the United States. Am J Phys Med Rehabil 69:184–190, 1990.

   Xiang H, Chany AM, Smith GA: Wheelchair-related injuries treated in US emergency departments. Injury Prevention 12:8–11, 2006.

3. **Compare the rides of folding- and rigid-frame manual wheelchairs.**

   The flexibility of the folding frame leads to a more comfortable ride and makes it more likely that all four wheels will remain in contact with uneven terrain. Rigidity provides a responsive feel to wheelchair propulsion and turning, because the applied forces are not dampened by the chair flexing. A rigid frame also allows more precise wheel alignment, which reduces the forces required for mobility.

4. **Review the considerations in prescription of a wheelchair for an experienced person with spinal cord injury at T9.**
An individual with T9 spinal cord injury is typically a candidate for a manual wheelchair; however, the case history and secondary conditions of the user need to be considered. The key factors to consider are user experience with wheelchairs, the user's current wheelchair, the anthropometry of the user, user strength and range of motion, user functional mobility and transfer skills, and home and transportation settings. Most active users should initially use a lightweight wheelchair with adjustability to permit adapting the wheelchair to changes in their bodies and skills. Experienced wheelchair users may be better served by a wheelchair made to exacting specifications.

> Cooper R: Wheelchair selection and configuration. New York, Demos Medical Publishing, 1998.
> Preserving upper limb function in spinal cord injury: A clinical practice guideline for health-care professionals. Spinal Cord Medicine, Clinical Practice Guideline. Washington, DC, Consortium for Spinal Cord Medicine, 2005.

5. **Compare the performance of front-, rear-, and center-wheel drive powered wheelchairs.**
Rear-wheel drive electric-powered wheelchairs provide greater directional stability (i.e., less tendency to wander to the left or right) and control over uneven terrain. Front-wheel drive provides enhanced obstacle climbing (e.g., curbs) but at the expense of directional stability. They are susceptible to turning unexpectedly and to difficulty in controlling turns. Center-wheel drive minimizes the turning radius and makes it easier to maneuver the wheelchair, especially indoors.

6. **What are the types of powered wheelchair controls?**
Analog devices (e.g., joysticks) allow the user to generate a continuous control command for the wheelchair. Continuous input signals allow smoother and more precise control over the wheelchair. Switched devices (e.g., sip and puff) provide discrete commands to the wheelchair, typically forward, backward, left, and right.

> Dan D, Cooper RA: Review of control technology and algorithms for electric powered wheelchairs. IEEE Controls Systems Magazine 25:22–34, 2005.

7. **How and why might you change the seat height?**
To lower the seat height for manual wheelchairs, one can use drop hooks to lower a rigid seat surface below the level of the side rails (to allow foot propulsion), adjust tip back of the seat-plane angle (also known as seat "dump"), select a higher axle position for the rear wheel, or use a rear wheel with a smaller diameter. Note that the latter two actions will tilt the seat backward unless the casters are also modified. For electric-powered wheelchairs, one can use a power base of a different height. Alternatively, in some chairs, power-seating functions control the seat height. Seat height affects a number of functions, such as foot propulsion (of manual wheelchairs), transfers, eating, and reaching (e.g., floor, medicine cabinet, or light switches).

8. **What are the pros and cons of increasing the seat-plane angle?**
The seat-plane angle (the angle of the seat-plane relative to the horizontal) is typically 3–5 degrees upward at the front. The advantages of increasing the seat-plane angle are to reduce spasticity, to reduce the tendency for the user to slide forward on the seat, to help bring the pelvis firmly against the back of the seat, and to reduce lumbar lordosis. However, the accentuated angle makes transfers more difficult and may put more weight on the ischial tuberosities.

9. **What should the backrest angle be for the active user?**
The backrest is commonly tilted back about 8 degrees from vertical (i.e., approximately 95 degrees from the seat-plane). Users of lightweight wheelchairs may prefer to increase the

seat-plane angle and reduce the backrest-to-seat-plane angle ("squeeze") to help apply force to the wheels by preventing the trunk from being pushed backward with each arm thrust.

10. **What is the major problem with wheelchair "recline"?**
Despite its numerous benefits, changing to and from the reclined position can result in shear forces between the chair and user, because the mechanical axis of a backrest with variable recline is usually below and behind the anatomic axis of the user's hip joints. This can produce skin ulcers.

11. **What is "tilt"? Why is it used?**
Tilt is a change in the seat's position or attitude rather than a change in the posture (relative position of body parts). Tilt obviates the shear problem of recliners and is less likely to trigger spasms. It also reduces the pressure on the ischial tuberosities, in proportion to the extent of the tilt.

12. **What are the pros and cons of elevating footrests?**
Elevating the footrests may reduce edema and knee-flexion contractures but decreases forward stability, both because the center of gravity is altered and because footrests serve as forward antitip devices. This latter effect can lead to a violent yawing tip when only a single footrest is elevated. Also, there can be relative movement (and shear) between the elevating footrest and the user if the axes of the mechanical and anatomic joints are not colinear. Some elevating footrests prevent or compensate for shear by using a gooseneck attachment (to raise the mechanical axis) or a telescoping mechanism that lengthens the footrest as it is elevated. Elevating footrests also add weight, a consideration in manual wheelchairs, and are more prone to failure when hitting a structure.

Kirby RL, Atkinson SM, MacKay EA: Static and dynamic forward stability of occupied wheelchairs: Influence of elevating footrests and forward stabilizers. Arch Phys Med Rehabil 70:681–686, 1989.

13. **What are the pros and cons of positioning the knees in >90 degrees of flexion?**
Although the usual "hanger angle" is 80–90 degrees (0 degrees being full knee extension) for manual wheelchairs, some wheelchairs position the knees in >90 degrees of flexion. This has several benefits: closer access to objects, protection of the feet, ease of wheelchair transport, inhibition of spasticity, tighter turns, and better traction. In addition, by bringing the limb segments closer to the yaw axis, turns can be faster because of reduced moment of inertia (analogous to a spinning skater who speeds up when bringing the arms closer to the body). However, users with long legs may be difficult to accommodate, a small caster diameter and caster trail may be needed to avoid having the caster swivel into the footrests/heels when changing direction, and the footrests are less effective as forward antitip devices.

MacPhee A, Kirby RL, Bell AC, MacLeod DA: The effect of knee-flexion angle on wheelchair turning. Medical Engineering and Physics 23:275–283, 2001.

14. **How does rear-axle position affect the manual wheelchair?**
Raising the rear axles (i.e., closer to the seat-plane) lowers the seat height, tilts the wheelchair backward, lowers rear stability, raises forward stability, and causes a cambered wheel to toe out. Lowering the rear axles has the converse effects. Moving the axle back raises rear stability, interferes with the user's ability to grasp as much of the push-rim (i.e., reduces the propulsive arc), decreases the ease of doing wheelies, limits the ability of a caregiver to lift the front wheels, reduces traction, lengthens the wheelbase, raises rolling resistance, and raises downhill-turning tendency. Moving the rear axle forward has the converse effects.

Kirby RL: Wheelchair stability: Important, measurable and modifiable. Technol Disabil 5:75–80, 1996.

15. **What is camber? How does it affect the manual wheelchair?**
Camber, usually 3–9 degrees, is present when the distance between the tops of the rear wheels is less than the distance between the bottoms. Camber provides a natural angle for the arms to address the wheels during propulsion, protects the user's hands from doorways or from other players in sports, reduces downhill-turning tendency on side slopes, increases the ease of turning, and increases lateral stability. However, increasing the camber angle induces many mechanical effects that may require lengthening of the wheelbase, tilting the wheelchair backward, toe out, and altering the caster-stem angle and the caster-trail distance. Camber causes more wear on wheel bearings and more rolling resistance and creates a wider track (causing more difficulty in tight spaces). A cambered wheel, even if perfectly aligned when all four wheels are on the ground, will toe out during a wheelie, in proportion to the wheelie angle. Unless compensations are made, camber increases forward and reduces rear stability as well, as a result of some of the aforementioned effects that are coupled to camber angle. These mechanical effects may need to be considered or compensated for to optimize wheelchair safety and performance.

Trudel G, Kirby RL, Bell AC: Mechanical effects of rear-wheel camber on wheelchairs. Assist Technol 7:79–86, 1995.

KEY POINTS: WHEELCHAIR SAFETY AND PERFORMANCE

1. The wheelchair is arguably the most important therapeutic tool in rehabilitation.

2. The long-term use of manual wheelchairs can cause chronic overuse problems of the upper extremities, and injuries caused by tip over are common.

3. Many wheelchair users do not achieve as much community mobility and participation as they could.

4. Proper wheelchair prescription, setup, and training have the potential to prevent overuse injury, to enhance wheelchair safety and performance, and to reduce pain.

5. Wheelchair science is a complex and rapidly evolving rehabilitation subspecialty. To optimize activity and participation outcomes, rehabilitation professionals should make every effort to formalize the wheelchair-provision process.

16. **What is "toeing error"? What are its adverse effects?**
The rear wheels are "toed in" when the fronts of the rear wheels are closer to each other than the backs; the opposite is "toe out." Symmetrical toeing error increases the rolling resistance quite dramatically, even for a malalignment of as little as 2 degrees by generating shear at the tire–floor interface. Asymmetrical toeing can cause the wheelchair to persistently deviate to one side.

17. **What is a "wheelie"? Why is it useful?**
A rear wheelie for a manual wheelchair occurs when the front wheels, ordinarily in contact with the support surface, are intentionally caused, by means of a transient or sustainable rear pitch, to lift from the surface while the rear wheels remain on the surface. The wheelie position is useful to reduce the loads on the ischial tuberosities, to decrease neck discomfort when talking to a standing person, to help turn in tight spaces, and to negotiate such obstacles as rough ground, inclines (Fig. 39-1), and curbs.

Seaman R, Macleod DA, Parker K: The manual wheelchair wheelie: A review of our current understanding of an important motor skill. Disabil Rehabil 1:119–127, 2006.

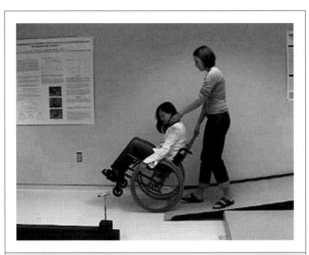

Figure 39-1. The wheelie position can be used to descend steep inclines. Note the spotter holding a spotter strap with one hand, while the other hand is ready in the event of a forward pitch.

18. **What are the limitations of fixed rear antitip devices?**

    Most fixed rear antitip devices have a limited range of adjustability and, when adjusted in a way that makes them effective in preventing full rear tips, they interfere with maneuverability (e.g., by "grounding out" during incline transitions (Fig. 39-2) or by preventing the wheelchair from being tipped back sufficiently to get the casters up a curb or to get into the wheelie position). Emerging designs may be able to circumvent these problems.

    Kirby RL, Lugar J, Breckenridge C: New wheelie aid for wheelchairs: Controlled trial of safety and efficacy. Arch Phys Med Rehabil 82:380–390, 2001.

    Kirby RL, Thoren F, Ashton B, Ackroyd-Stolarz SA: Effect of the position of rear antitippers on safety and maneuverability. Arch Phys Med Rehabil 75: 525–534, 1994.

19. **What is the role of wheelchair-skills training for wheelchair users and caregivers?**

    Wheelchair-skills training is an important component of the wheelchair provision process. For instance, manual wheelchair users should be taught proper propulsion technique—wheelchair users should use a long, smooth stroke that uses as much of the push-rim as possible, letting the hand drift below the rim in the recovery phase. Wheelchair users and caregivers should also be taught to negotiate curbs (Fig. 39-3), ramps, and small obstacles, and maneuvering in compact spaces. Electric-powered wheelchair users need to be taught how to tune the user adjustable controls and the effects of these changes. There is emerging evidence that a formal approach to such training is considerably more efficacious than ad hoc approaches.

    Wheelchair Skills Program: www.wheelchairskillsprogram.ca

20. **How much input should the wheelchair user have in the prescription process?**

    The prescription process should fully involve the user (and, if appropriate, the family or other caregivers). For their first wheelchairs, the limited experience of users will mean that they will need to rely heavily on the clinical team. However, as users develop more experience, they are able to participate more fully in the process. All the users' activity capabilities (transfers,

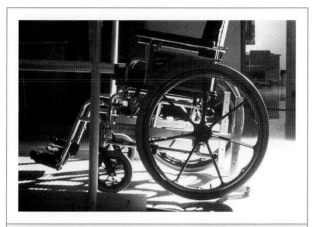

Figure 39-2. Low rear antitip devices can cause rear-wheel "float" at incline transitions.

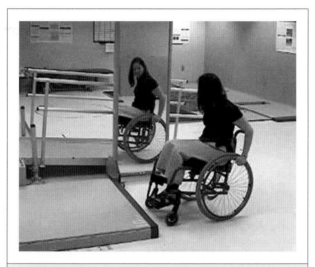

Figure 39-3. A mirror provides feedback while practicing popping the casters onto a 10-cm curb.

wheelchair skills) need to be considered as well as all areas of the environment where the wheelchair will be used (car/van access, home door widths, bathroom access).

21. **How do you decide when to use a power wheelchair rather than rely on exclusive use of a manual wheelchair?**
The patient's weight, strength, life demands, living environment, and transportation are all considered. Prevention of upper extremity overuse can be achieved with power assist wheels.

Some patients may benefit from use of a power wheelchair when at work, in the community, or in traveling the natural environment. Many users can utilize a manual wheelchair for much of the day and transfer to a power wheelchair when needed. Careful attention to problems of upper extremity overuse improves mobility and prevents further damage before transfer performance is significantly affected.

NECK PAIN: ANATOMY, PATHOPHYSIOLOGY, AND DIAGNOSIS

Rene Cailliet, MD, Dheera Ananthakrishnan, MD, MSE, and Stephen P. Burns, MD

Having critics praise you is like having the hangman say you've got a pretty neck.
—Eli Wallach (1915–)

1. **What functional anatomy of the cervical spine must be understood to evaluate pain in and from the neck?**
   The cervical spine is composed of two segments. The upper segment consists of the occiput, atlas (C1), and axis (C2). The lower segment includes the functional units C3–C7. The movements of the occiput on C1 allows flexion-extension, the movement of C1 on C2 allows rotation, and the movements of C3–C7 contribute to movement in all planes of motion.

2. **Describe a functional unit.**
   A functional unit is two adjacent vertebrae separated by an intervertebral disc and posteriorly two laminae, two pedicles, and zygapophyseal joints, termed *facets*.

3. **A "pain in the neck" is a common complaint. Where in the cervical spine does pain originate?**
   Nearly two thirds of the population will experience neck pain at some point in their lives, and at any one time about 5% of the population has sufficient neck pain to cause disability. The majority of neck pain is muscular in origin; however, there are pain generators within the vertebral column itself. The tissue sites where nociception occurs are the posterior longitudinal ligaments, nerve roots and their dural sheaths, the facet capsules, and the neck muscles. Nociception results from injury, irritation, inflammation, or infection of these sites.

4. **"Disc pain" is a common complaint. Is there such a thing?**
   Yes, but it is difficult to differentiate with certainty the etiology of disc pain and pain from the surrounding structures. The intervertebral disc consists of annular fibers within a mucopolysaccharide matrix with no blood supply and no nerve endings other than minimal unmyelinated nerve endings in the outer peripheral annulus fibrosus. Consequently, only damage to the outer annular fibers can conceivably cause pain. With disc herniation, the nociceptors in other structures, such as nerve roots, may become activated by compression or inflammation.

5. **In evaluating pain originating from the cervical spine, what should be emphasized in the physical examination? What are the anatomic correlates?**
   Range of motion should be evaluated first, followed by a thorough neurologic evaluation. The nerve roots emerge from the cervical spine through the foramina, which contain the dorsal root ganglion and their dural sheath (both sites of nociception). Flexion opens the foramina, and extension closes them. Rotation and lateral flexion of the neck close the foramina on the concave side and open those on the convex side. Passive and active neck movements trigger pain by nerve compression.

6. **In obtaining a history, what are the major factors to be determined?**
Every chief complaint can be elucidated using the mnemonic **PQRST**:
- **P** = **P**alliative—determine the precise position or alleviating and exacerbating factors
- **Q** = **Q**uality of symptoms
- **R** = **R**adiation of symptoms
- **S** = **S**everity as experienced throughout the day and with various activities
- **T** = **T**emporal factors—onset, duration, time the pain is worst, any movement(s) that cause or aggravate the pain

7. **What is the Spurling test?**
The test defined by Spurling is reproduction of radicular pain by extending the neck, rotating it to one side, and pressing down on the head toward the side of complaint. A positive test reproduces the radicular pain. The site of referred pain indicates which nerve root has been compressed: arm/forearm, C5; thumb, C6; middle finger, C7; fifth finger, C8.

8. **Is it radicular pain or radiculous pain?**
Radicular pain indicates that a radicle (nerve root) has been compressed; for example, C5–C6 intervertebral disk protrusion will encroach on the C6 spinal nerve emerging through the C5–C6 intervertebral foramen (Fig. 40-1), causing a radiating pain from the neck to the thumb. Radiculous pain is pain without anatomic basis, pathophysiologic pattern, or consistent findings.

9. **Do cervical spine x-ray studies have precise diagnostic value?**
Plain radiographs are an important first step in a cervical spine evaluation following trauma but have less value in patients with chronic neck pain. Information about alignment, canal size, disc degeneration, and foraminal compromise can be gleaned from cervical spine x-rays. In addition, the behavior of the cervical spine in an upright position can be great value. However, x-rays often show "pathology" that is irrelevant to the complaints. X-rays are only of value if they confirm the presence and indicate the site of pathology that can explain the symptoms and physical signs.

10. **What are the most common causes of neck pain or pain from the neck?**
Acute or chronic trauma. The trauma can result from an accident (often vehicular), postural position (e.g., poor ergonomics such as prolonged computer usage), or emotional tension. The most common site of neck pain is muscular. Trauma can cause ecchymosis of the muscles, resulting in obliteration of the muscle planes and fibrosis. Abnormal motion and stiffness can then occur. Repetitive stress injuries can cause muscle tension, resulting in neck pain and headaches.

11. **Is posture an important factor in causing neck pain?**
Yes. An exaggerated dorsal kyphosis (round back) places the head ahead of the center of gravity, increasing the cervical lordosis. The weight of the head in this position is borne by the zygapophyseal joints (facets) and causes pain.

12. **Is there one particular tissue site in the cervical spine that is considered the prevalent site of neck pain?**
There is no one tissue site that can be considered the prevalent site of neck pain. The majority of neck pain is of a muscular etiology. The discs, facet joints, and nerve roots can all be pain generators. The zygapophyseal joints (facets) have been singled out as a specific post-traumatic cause by some investigators, because injection of an irritating substance in them reproduces the pain and injecting an analgesic relieves the pain.

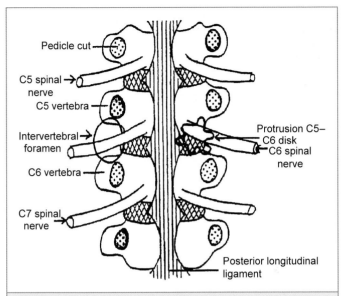

Figure 40-1. Example of a C5–C6 intervertebral disk protrusion. (From Schneck CD: Functional and clinical anatomy of the spine. In Young MA, Lavin RA [eds]: Conservative Care and Spinal Rehabilitation. Spine: State of the Art Reviews. Philadelphia, Hanley & Belfus, 1998, pp 525–558.)

13. **What is a whiplash injury?**

In a rear-end motor vehicle accident, the impact acutely forces the entire body forward, but the head does not move at the same time and undergoes translation forces with initial extension then reflex flexion. Normal flexion-extension does not occur, but translatory forces can cause disc annular fiber damage and facet capsule excessive stress. In addition, the intermuscular planes can be obliterated by bleeding and fibrosis, which can cause persistent long-term neck pain.

14. **Should soft cervical collars be prescribed after whiplash injury?**

If there is possible spinal instability, use of an orthosis that restricts range of motion to a much greater degree than a soft collar would be required. For most patients, there is no concern about cervical instability. Although optimal treatment for whiplash injuries has not been determined, it is clear from prospective randomized trials that use of soft cervical collars and activity restriction are associated with a *worse* outcome than if usual activity is maintained.

15. **What is a stinger?**

A stinger results from sudden forceful stretch in the nerve roots and brachial plexus as they emerge from the cervical spine. Typically, in a fall onto the turf, the shoulder is forced down and the neck is bent forcefully to the side in the opposite direction.

Acute cervical injury in athletes may result in a transient paresis (paraplegia/quadriplegia) caused by stretching of the cervical roots and/or the brachial plexus. The symptoms are usually not in a radicular distribution. The symptoms usually last for a short period, but they may persist for weeks. If they do persist, evaluation with magnetic resonance imaging of the cervical spine is indicated. Athletes with persistent symptoms should not be playing while evaluations are ongoing.

16. **Degenerative disc disease of the cervical spine is considered a cause of neck pain as well as arm pain from the neck. Is this a valid assumption? What are the causative factors?**

Neck pain and arm pain are two distinct problems, and every attempt should be made to distinguish between the two. Arm pain of cervical etiology is usually caused by compression of neural elements, by either enlarged facet joints and/or bulging degenerated discs that narrow the available space for these elements. Neck pain, as has already been discussed, is of a multifactorial etiology. Degenerative disc disease occurs from age 30 on as a result of the aging process but is aggravated and accentuated by trauma. The disc dehydrates and narrows with age, allowing the longitudinal ligaments to be separated from the vertebral bodies. The blood that seeps in between the ligament and the body gradually ossifies and forms osteophytes (spurs). These spurs narrow the foramen and can entrap the nerve roots.

17. **Can headaches be caused by injury to the cervical spine?**

A condition termed **cervicogenic headache** occurs after an injury and responds favorably to neck therapy. Its pathoanatomic basis is not clear, but it is generally thought to be muscular in nature.

18. **What is a "computer headache"?**

Although not yet an official disorder, computer headache occurs in people who spend much time at the computer, especially if they wear bifocal glasses. The dorsal kyphotic posture with head forward and up increases the cervical lordosis. Also, emotional tension from intensity of work can cause neck and head pain.

KEY POINTS: NECK PAIN

1. To perform the Spurling test: Close the neural foramina by actively extending the neck and side, bending the neck toward the affected side.

2. A positive Spurling test produces radiating pain in a radicular dermatomal distribution.

3. Apply cervical traction 30 degrees forward from the vertical baseline for 30 minutes, up to three times per day.

19. **What is thoracic outlet syndrome?**

The thoracic outlet is the space between the first rib, the clavicle, and the two scalene muscles. The nerves of the brachial plexus and the subclavian blood vessels pass through this space. Acute contraction or chronic contraction of the scalene muscles can compress the nerves and blood vessels, causing paresthesia of the arm and hand. Diagnosis is made by the **Adson sign**—diminished radial pulse produced by having the patient take a deep breath with his or her head turned all the way to the affected side.

20. **What causes the headache from greater superior occipital neuralgia?**

The greater superior occipital nerve contains roots from C1 and C2 and a branch from C3. It emerges through the extensor capitis muscles and supplies the dermatomes of C1, C2, and C3 of the posterior occiput. When entrapped or traumatized, it causes a vertex occipital headache. An injection of an anesthetic agent around the nerve at the occiput confirms the diagnosis and relieves the headache.

21. **Is cervical traction a viable therapeutic modality?**
    Properly applied cervical traction has great value in cervical problems. It must comfortably pull the head upward and forward at a 30-degree angle forward from vertical and be applied twice daily and for periods of 30 minutes.

WEBSITES

1. BC Whiplash Initiative
   www.health-disciplines.ubc.ca/whiplash.bc/

2. Clinical Evidence Concise: Neck Pain
   www.aafp.org/afp/20050101/bmj.html

3. The enigma of whiplash injury: Current management strategies and controversies
   www.postgradmed.com/issues/2001/03_01/young.htm

4. What a Pain in the Neck! Good Habits to Remember to Prevent Neck Pain
   www.aapmr.org/condtreat/pain/necktips.htm

BIBLIOGRAPHY

1. Cailliet R: Neck and Arm Pain, 3rd ed. Philadelphia, F.A. Davis, 1991.

2. Malanga GA (ed): Cervical Flexion-Extension/Whiplash Injuries. Spine: State of the Art Reviews. Vol 12, No. 2. Philadelphia, Hanley & Belfus, 1998.

CHAPTER 41

LOW BACK PAIN: PERSPECTIVES ON MANAGEMENT

Maury R. Ellenberg, MD, and Joseph C. Honet, MD, MS

The art of medicine consists of amusing the patient while nature cures the disease.
—Voltaire (1694–1778)

1. **Is low back pain (LBP) a common problem?**
   Yes. Epidemiologic studies show that by the age of 20, 50% of the population has experienced LBP. By age 60, the cumulative incidence is more than 80%. It is present in all societies and cultures. LBP is second only to the common cold when it comes to symptoms prompting a physician visit.

2. **What causes LBP?**
   A number of structures can potentially cause LBP. Anatomic studies have identified structures that have free nerve endings that transmit pain sensations. Irritating material can be injected into structures to determine the source and reproducibility of pain. Newer techniques attempt to distinguish some of the structures leading to LBP in a particular patient by differential injection, specifically into the facet and sacroiliac joints or by performing a discogram. These techniques remain controversial and are ideally suited for reliable patients free of psychological, legal, or monetary reinforcer.

3. **Can the cause of back pain be determined by imaging?**
   Definitely not! Although many abnormalities can be visualized on imaging studies, there is no conclusive evidence that these abnormalities are, in fact, responsible for the patient's complaints. Results of numerous studies since the 1950s have shown a poor correlation between spinal x-ray abnormalities and LBP. More recent studies using computed tomography (CT) and magnetic resonance imaging (MRI) show a natural progression of abnormalities of the disc. These anatomic changes are part of aging and are considered the gray hair or wrinkles of the spine. There has been limited evidence to suggest that these changes correlate with LBP. Discogram continues to be a very controversial procedure; therefore, decisions about major procedures such as spine surgery or other invasive interventions should not be based on discography alone.

4. **What are the most common diagnoses in a patient with LBP?**
   In a number of studies the most common diagnoses are "nondiagnoses," such as nonspecific LBP musculoskeletal or degenerative "disease." More specific diagnoses include compression fracture (4%), spondylolisthesis (3%), malignancy (0.7%), ankylosing spondylitis (3%), and infection (0.01%). Approximately 2% of patients with LBP are diagnosed with "radiculopathy" or incorrectly misdiagnosed with "sciatica." At least 85% or more are not diagnosed and fall into the category of "nonspecific LBP."

5. **Once LBP is present, does it ever go away?**
   LBP is usually self-limited. Because the incidence is more than 50%, and with point prevalence in the 10–20% range, it is obvious that most individuals are able to deal with their pain until resolution. However, in certain populations, the pain, complaints, and subsequent disability

become significant and difficult to resolve. Furthermore, the natural history of LBP is often marked by unpredictable recurrence over time.

6. Are recurrences preventable?
There are ways to try to prevent recurrence, but few have proved effective. Education about proper back care and proper exercises is helpful. Exercises should include abdominal and back stabilizer muscle strengthening as well as stretches for the back and hamstrings. Patients should be educated to respond to an acute episode with nonsteroidal anti-inflammatory drugs (NSAIDs), ice or heat, maintenance of activities, and expected resolution over 3–7 days.

7. What is the most important tool to assess patients with LBP?
The history (Hx) and physical examination (PEx) remain the mainstays in evaluation of LBP, despite new, expensive technology.

8. What factors of the history are most important?
The history should separate innocuous LBP from serious causes of LBP. The red flags, if present, indicate a need for further imaging or laboratory testing. Issues of work injury, litigation, and other general factors may point to other issues that are contributing to complaints, despite negative examination, testing, and poor response to usual treatments (Table 41-1).

9. Which areas should be examined in a patient with LBP, and how is the examination performed?
The physical examination requires precision and a great deal of practice. Stereotype your examination and examine the back in all patients, even if they come in for a neck problem. This will give you a good basis for what "normal" is. Keep in mind the following factors:
1. **Back motion,** for asymmetric movement, recreation of pain, and areas of mechanically limited or guarded motion (so-called spasm).
2. **Tenderness,** especially percussion tenderness over bony areas in the back and pelvis or palpation tenderness over the sacroiliac joint or greater trochanter.
3. **Gait and balance,** including heel and toe walking, squat and raise, and ascending and descending a stool and chair. Evaluate for Trendelenburg gait.
4. **Range of motion (ROM)** of the lower limbs and quadriceps and muscle tightness, especially in the hamstrings. Pay particular attention to hip ROM, which is best examined in the prone position. *Note:* LBP and hip pain with limited hip range may indicate osteoarthritis or other hip abnormality.
5. **Full peripheral neurologic examination:** Test reflexes, strength, and sensation.
6. If pain is accompanied by **other symptoms** such as abdominal pain, nausea, vomiting, or groin pain, examine the abdomen. Look for pancreatic, renal, or vascular (abdominal aortic aneurysm) causes of the pain.
    Remember that few physical exam techniques have been proven to identify the specific structure or disorder that is the cause of pain and that no one's back is completely symmetric.

10. Even though laboratory and imaging studies are not always accurate for diagnosing low back problems, should any tests be performed?
Imaging studies can be used to diagnose major disease. They are indicated only if "red flags" are present or if there is no improvement after several weeks of treatment. The initial study may be a plain x-ray. Other tests include bone scan, cross-sectional imaging (e.g., CT and MRI), and special tests, such as single photon emission computed tomography (SPECT) scanning and discography. Remember that "abnormal" findings are expected on cross-sectional imaging. If leg pain is present, electromyography, which is more specific than imaging, can be performed.

TABLE 41-1. HISTORY OF LOW BACK PAIN

General Characteristics	Characteristics (of Pain)	Characteristics of Associated Symptoms	History of Tests and Treatment	Red Flags
Onset	Intensity	Extremity pain	Imaging studies	Fever
Duration	Location	Numbness or tingling	Electromyography	Significant
Reason it occurred	Character (aching, burning, sharp, etc.)	Bowel or bladder dysfunction	Medications taken and benefit	Trauma
Relation to work, accident, or injury	Relation to position, time of day, or activity		Therapy, type and duration	Cancer history
Litigation present	Relieving or exacerbating factors		Injection procedures	Unexplained weight loss
Financial remuneration			Surgical interventions	Failure to improve with treatment
				Age > 50
				Alcohol or drug abuse

11. **Is disability from LBP common?**

Patients with disability from LBP present a very different picture from those with acute, acute recurrent, or even chronic LBP who are still functioning. Despite improvement in diagnostic and treatment techniques, disability from LBP has risen astronomically in the past few decades (as much as 2500%). Explanations beyond the purely physical account for this increase. Patients with disability from LBP that occurred either spontaneously or, more commonly, from an injury must also be assessed from psychoemotional, social, and vocational viewpoints.

12. **What are signs to look for in identifying the "disability syndrome"?**

The most common associations that indicate disability from an injury are *not* physical ones. Table 41-2 outlines some of the factors that allow diagnosis of this syndrome. The importance of diagnosis of the syndrome cannot be overemphasized. Treatment of this syndrome as a purely organic problem leads to unnecessary tests and procedures rather than appropriate therapy.

13. **How do you treat the patient with acute LBP?**

When the offending structure is not known, the natural history is to improve regardless of (or despite) treatment. Few treatments have been proven to be beneficial, but several strategies may hasten the healing process.

1. Reassurance is vitally important. Advise the patient that the process is "benign," will not lead to long-term impairment, and is unlikely to require major intervention.
2. NSAIDs can give the double benefit of pain relief and decreased inflammation (assuming inflammation is part of the pain generator), but be aware of ulcer history or anticoagulants. Data also indicate the possibility of adverse cardiac events (particularly related to coronary artery disease) with COX2 inhibitors and a number if NSAIDs.
3. Educate the patient about proper back care and exercises. Other treatments for acute LBP are usually not necessary. Several studies suggest that manipulation during the first 3 weeks decreases painful episodes; however, this is controversial.

There is a lack of research support for lumbar supports, traction, transcutaneous electrical nerve stimulation (TENS), and intradiscal electrothermal therapy (IDET), although anecdotal studies suggest that some of these may prove helpful. Possibly effective treatments include manipulation and tricyclic antidepressants. A good principle is that if side effects are minor, a method can be can tried, even without definite proven effectiveness. Avoid major invasive procedures unless very well proven by randomized controlled trials.

14. **Is bed rest helpful?**

Bed rest was once the mainstay of treatment. However, a number of studies show that the patient is better off carrying out as many normal activities as possible. It seems to shorten the course of disability and allow an earlier return to work. It is recommended that the patient be upright as much as is tolerable and avoid anything that results in significant pain increase.

15. **What should be done if the pain persists for several weeks after the initial treatment?**

If the pain still does not resolve after a number of months and the individual is not disabled but distressed, repeat reassurances, because patients may fear severe illness. If not already performed, imaging studies are appropriate. Bone scan and MRI should be interpreted cautiously and correlated clinically. Next, determine severity of pain perception and how it interferes physically, psychosocially, and psychoemotionally with function. Treatment options include medications such as NSAIDS, tricyclic antidepressants, acetaminophen; injections (including sacroiliac joint, facet joint, and local myofascial trigger points); and alternative medicine techniques such as acupuncture.

16. **How should the patient who is disabled by the pain be treated?**

Other factors contributing to the pain must be identified. There has been a large movement toward treating "benign" or "nonmalignant" pain problems with opioid medications, various

TABLE 41-2. INDICATORS OF THE DISABILITY SYNDROME AND NONORGANIC FACTORS CONTRIBUTING TO PAIN COMPLAINTS

History	Physical Exam	Testing	Special Signs (Waddel and Others)
■ Prior back pain with work loss	■ Appears comfortable despite high pain ratings	■ MMPI high scale 3	■ Neck extension or rotation without back motion causing LBP
■ Fault finding	■ Grimacing, demonstrative during exam	■ High work APGAR	■ General overreactions to examination
■ Numerous tests	■ Bizarre gait	■ Imaging that doesn't correlate with Hx and PEx	■ Superficial tenderness
■ Many health care providers	■ Break weakness on muscle testing		■ Regional weakness or sensory loss not following anatomic pattern
■ Many ineffective treatments and medications	■ Unusual body positioning		■ Distracted SLR
■ Surgical procedures	■ Pain with minor movement		
■ Extremely high pain ratings (8–10)			
■ Abuse history			

Hx = history, LBP = low back pain, MMPI = Minnesota Multiphasic Personality Inventory, PEX = physical examination, SLR = straight leg raising.

injections, disc dissolution techniques, device insertion (spinal stimulatOR, morphine pumps), and surgery. However, these methods are unproved and invasive, may have a high complication rate, and are unlikely to treat the entire problem or restore functional loss. When etiology is not clearly defined and multiple inorganic signs are present, treat the functional loss and disability. It is our view that this type of patient is best served by an interdisciplinary (not multidisciplinary) team approach, such as a functional restoration program. At this point, acceptance of pain and restoration of function are paramount; chasing the pain with diagnostic or treatment measures becomes counterproductive.

KEY POINTS: THE TRUTH ABOUT LOW BACK PAIN

1. LBP is ubiquitous in the human race and not a disease.

2. Degenerative discs and some of the anatomic sequelae of facet arthropathy and spurring are usual consequences of aging.

3. The natural history of LBP is to improve with or without treatment, but certain treatments can hasten the process and are worthwhile.

4. There is little or no correlation between anatomic abnormalities as seen on imaging and the patient's clinical symptoms or signs.

5. It is our job to discover serious problems presenting as LBP by identifying the red flags as outlined in the Agency for Health Care Policy & Research guideline number 14 (*see* Bibliography). This guideline is worth requesting. (Remember the guideline only applies to acute LBP.)

6. Treatment consists of reassurance, NSAIDs, and staying out of bed and being active.

7. Disability from LBP is a different disorder than acute LBP, and a host of factors contribute to it. It must be evaluated and treated differently from acute LBP.

8. Special injection techniques are occasionally indicated in patients with LBP.

17. **Is LBP usually remediable without surgery?**
    Yes, in 99% of cases. The reasons for the marked increase in spinal fusion (more than the increase in hip and knee replacement) are multifactorial. As more imaging abnormalities become visible, surgery has been recommended to remove the architecturally observable, but nonoffending, discs. Even today, degenerative discs are blamed for LBP. Spinal fusion, IDET (heat dissolution of discs), and a variety of other procedures are being performed to "fix" the problem. Any major procedure such as these should be performed only when shown effective. Such procedures, when performed without adequate indication, can be counterproductive and potentially harmful.

18. **Who should treat patients with LBP?**
    A variety of clinicians can initiate treatment of LBP, and it is appropriate for a primary care physician to start the process. Unfortunately, by the time the patient comes to a specialist, he or she may already have undergone an MRI and been told the pain is caused by disc problems or been given other misinformation. It is then difficult to "unteach" the patient, especially because the general population places such credence in MRI. Physiatrists (physical medicine and rehabilitation physicians) are the best next line of treatment. Ideally, a physiatrist would be the best primary physician as well.

19. **When should a neurosurgeon or orthopedic surgeon be consulted?**
The physiatrist should be consulted first in all patients with back or back and limb pain. In the rare circumstance when there is a neurosurgical emergency, such as cauda equina syndrome (bladder or bowel incontinence or retention), the patient should go to an emergency department where he or she can receive immediate care, including surgical treatment if needed.

WEBSITES

1. www.nlm.nih.gov/medlineplus/ency/article/003108.htm

2. http://orthoinfo.aaos.org/brochure/thr_report.cfm?Thread_ID=10&topcategory=Spine

BIBLIOGRAPHY

1. Agency for Health Care Policy & Research Clinical Practice Guideline #14. Acute Low Back Problems in Adults. Rockville, MD, U.S. Department of Health & Human Services, Public Health Service, 1994.

2. Carragee EJ: Persistent low back pain. N Engl J Med 352:1891–1898, 2005.

3. Carragee EJ, Tanner CM, Khurana S, et al: The rates of false-positive lumbar discography in select patients without low back symptoms. Spine 25:1373–1381, 2000.

4. Cutler R, Fishbain D, Rosomoff H, et al: Does nonsurgical pain center treatment of chronic pain return patients to work?. Spine 19:643–652, 1996.

5. Deyo RA, Rainville J, Kent D: What can the history and physical examination tell us about low back pain? JAMA 268:760–765, 1992.

6. Deyo RA, Nachemson A, Mirza SK: Spinal-fusion surgery: The case for restraint. N Engl J Med 350:7, 2004.

7. Dreyfuss P, Michaelsen M, Pauza K, et al: The value of medical history and physical examination in diagnosing sacroiliac joint pain. Spine 21:2594–2602, 1996.

8. Frymoyer J, Ducker T, Hadler N, et al (eds): The Adult Spine: Principles and Practice, Vol. 1. New York, Raven Press, 1991.

9. Haldeman S: Diagnostic tests for the evaluation of back and neck pain. Neurol Clin 14:103–117, 1996.

10. Jensen M, Brant-Zawadzki M, Obuchowski N, et al: Magnetic resonance imaging of the lumbar spine in people without back pain. N Engl J Med 331:69–73, 1994.

11. Leboeuf-Yde C, Kyvik K: At what age does low back pain become a common problem: A study of 29,424 individuals aged 12–41 years. Spine 23:228–234, 1998.

12. Malmivaara A, Hakkinen U, Aro T, et al: The treatment of acute back pain—bedrest, exercise, or ordinary activity. N Engl J Med 332:351–355, 1995.

13. van Tudler M, Ostelo R, Vlaeyen J, et al: Behavioral treatment for chronic low back pain. A systematic review within the framework of the Cochrane Back Review Group. Spine 26:270–281, 2000.

CHAPTER 42

LOW BACK PAIN: THE BASICS

James W. Leonard, DO, PT, and Bryan J. O'Young, MD

The best lightning rod for your protection is your own spine.

—Ralph Waldo Emerson (1803–1882)

EPIDEMIOLOGY

1. **What are the more common causes of lumbar pain by age group?**
   - **Teenager:** Spondylolysis, especially in the athletic population
   - **Ages 20–60:** Disc abnormalities
   - **Age > 60:** Stenosis or compression fractures

2. **What are the most common diagnoses seen in a spine clinic?**
   Only approximately 15% of patients presenting with acute low back pain (LBP) can be given a specific diagnosis. It is important for the reader to be aware of the most common diagnoses that enter a spine center. If the provider understands the diagnosis, pathophysiology, indicated studies, and natural course of these common disorders, then more expedient care can be provided. The 10 most common diagnoses include:
   - Strain/sprain
   - Myofascial pain/fibromyalgia
   - Disc herniation
   - Facet syndrome
   - Stenosis
   - Spondylolysis/spondylolisthesis
   - Spondyloarthropathy
   - Fracture
   - Infection
   - Tumor

PATHOPHYSIOLOGY

3. **What are the four forces that act on the spine?**
   - Compression
   - Tension
   - Torque
   - Shear
   Injury is a result of the combination of one or more of these forces.

   Gratovesky S: The Spinal Engine. Springer-Verlag, New York, 1988.

4. **What is the most significant difference between degenerative and isthmic spondylolisthesis?**
   - **Degenerative:** No pars interarticularis fracture occurs, so when there is slippage, stenosis of the central canal usually develops. This is most frequently noted at L4–L5.

- **Isthmic:** Because of the pars interarticularis fracture (spondylolysis), stenosis does not develop with the slippage (spondylolisthesis). This is most frequently noted at L5–S1.

5. **What are the differences among spondylitis, spondylosis, spondylolysis, and spondylolisthesis?**
   - **Spondylitis:** An inflammatory condition of the spine.
   - **Spondylosis:** A degenerative condition (osteoarthritis) of the spine.
   - **Spondylolysis:** A defect of the pars interarticularis; may be congenital or a result of repetitive traumatic stress. The L5 vertebra is most commonly involved, followed by L4.
   - **Spondylolisthesis:** Subluxation of vertebra on one another. It is a forward slippage of the superior on the inferior vertebra (e.g., L5 spondylolisthesis is an anterior slippage of L5 on the S1 vertebra). Spondylolisthesis most commonly occurs at the L5–S1 junction.

6. **What is lumbar stenosis?**
   When the lower limit of normal for the anterior-posterior diameter of the lumbar spinal canal is <11 mm, it is considered to be stenotic. Although we are familiar with central stenosis, it can also occur in the lateral recess (bordered by the vertebral body, pedicle, and superior facet) and in the neuroforamina.

   Cole A, Herring S: Low Back Pain Handbook, 2nd ed. Hanley & Belfus, 2003, p 110.

7. **Outline the natural history of idiopathic LBP.**
   - **Phase 1 (dysfunction):** Minor pathology results in abnormal function of the posterior joints and disc.
   - **Phase 2 (instability):** Repetitive trauma results in laxity of the posterior joint capsule and annulus.
   - **Phase 3 (stabilization):** Fibrosis of the posterior joints and capsule, loss of disc material, and formation of osteophytes render the segment stable because motion is reduced.

   Kirkaldy Willis WH: Managing Low Back Pain, 2nd ed. New York, Churchill-Livingstone, 1988.

HISTORY AND PHYSICAL EXAMINATION

See Chapter 41 for coverage of basic history and physical examination.

8. **What are the top 10 key points in the history of a patient with LBP?**
   - Numbness
   - Radiating pain
   - What increases/decreases pain
   - Inciting events
   - Course of pain over 24 hours
   - Current activity level
   - Past medical history
   - Medications/allergies
   - Bowel/bladder involvement
   - Weakness

9. **During the evaluation and treatment process, when is the physician's input most critical?**
   The physician's input is most critical during the following time periods:
   - Initial evaluation and establishment of a treatment plan
   - Confirmation in a follow-up visit to assess if the treatment plan is appropriate
   - Exacerbation episodes
   - At the time of return to work and/or increased activity level
   - At the time of case closure and transition to long-term treatment plan

10. **What should the physical exam include?**
    - Gait
    - Posture
    - Range of motion (spine and extremities)
    - Palpatory findings
    - Neurologic tests
    - Special tests (e.g., straight leg raise)

11. **What are Waddell's tests?**
    If three out of the following five tests are positive, then a nonorganic psychological cause is likely:
    - Tenderness, superficial or nonanatomic
    - Pain on simulated stressing tests
    - Inconsistent findings when testing the patient while he or she is distracted
    - Nonanatomic regional disturbance
    - Overreaction

    Waddell G: Non-organic physical signs in low back pain. Spine 5:117–125, 1980.

12. **Describe the straight leg raise test.**
    The straight leg raise test is usually done with the patient supine, the hip in a neutral position, and the knee extended. One leg at a time is passively raised, and the angle at which the patient has pain is noted. True stretch on the nerve occurs between 30 and 60 degrees of hip flexion. When recording the result of the test, note at what degree of flexion the patient had pain and where the pain was located. Also, note whether the crossed straight leg raise is positive. This occurs when the straight leg raise brings pain on the opposite side.

    Konin T, Wiksten D, Isear J, Brader H: Special Tests for the Orthopedic Examination, 2nd ed. Thorofare, NJ, Slack, 2002.

13. **Is there a specific test for sacroiliac joint (SIJ) pain? What role does the SIJ dysfunction play in low back pain and how is it best diagnosed and treated?**
    No. While there is not a single physical diagnostic test or maneuver that can definitively confirm the presence of SIJ abnormality, three commonly used clinical tests (which lack absolute sensitivity and specificity) include Gaenslen's test, Patrick's test, and the FABER maneuver (Flexion, Abduction, External Rotation of the proximal lower extremity). Since SIJ dysfunction has been shown to be present in as many as 30% of low back pain sufferers, it is essential that clinicians routinely screen for dysfunction of the SIJ.

    As the largest axial joint in the body, the SIJ is bolstered by a complex network of articulating muscles and ligaments that support and deliver muscular forces to the pelvic bones. The SIJ provides stability to the spine above and functions to transmit and dissipate of truncal loads to the lower extremities as well as restrict axial rotation. A retrospective study by Kirkaldy-Willis demonstrated a 22.5% prevalence rate in 1293 patients with low back pain. Although frequently the SIJ is the primary pain generator accounting for low back pain, SIJ pain frequently co-exists with other sources of pain. Since SIJ dysfunction is not easily detectable with standard radiological methods, intrarticular injection of the SIJ with anesthetic and/or steroid has been shown to be both diagnostic and therapeutic. Intrarticular SIJ injections are best performed in a "radiologically guided" fashion, using either fluoroscopy or ultrasonic visualization. Although fluoroscopic guidance has been customarily used, the recent availability of musculoskeletal ultrasound has enabled a more cost effective, non-ionizing radiation and functionally pertinent form of localization according to recent studies.

    SIJ injections performed under ultrasound offer several distinct advantages, including non-ionizing radiation mode of imaging, portability within the clinic setting, capacity for "dynamic" (motion) assessment of the joint, greater cost-effectiveness, and convenience.

    Bernard TN, Kirkaldy-Willis WH: Recognizing specific characteristics of nonspecific low back pain. Clin Orthop 217:266–280, 1987.

Cohen, SP: Sacroiliac joint pain: A comprehensive review of anatomy, diagnosis, and treatment. Anesth Analg 101:1440–1453, 2005.

Pekkafal MZ, Kralp MZ, et al. Sacroiliac joint injections performed with sonographic guidance. J Ultrasound Med 22:553–559, 2003.

14. **How does one measure leg length?**
Measure from the most prominent portion of the anterior superior iliac spine to the medial malleolus in supine and standing positions. Inequalities > 1 cm may benefit from a lift device.

Maigne R: Diagnosis and Treatment of Pain of Vertebral Origin. Baltimore, Williams & Wilkins, 1996, p 98.

15. **How does one clinically differentiate between neurogenic and vascular claudication?**
See Table 42-1.

LABORATORY TESTS

16. **What are the guiding principles for ordering laboratory tests for a patient with LBP?**
   - Guided by the clinical examination
   - May include complete blood count, erythrocyte sedimentation rate, and other specific tests when **chronic inflammatory disease, infection,** or **malignancy** is considered
   - Potentially useful, nonspecific lab tests include alkaline phosphatase (osteomalacia, Paget's disease), amylase (pancreatitis), rheumatoid factor/antinuclear antibody (connective tissue disease), serum protein electrophoresis (multiple myeloma), and urinalysis (prostatitis, renal stones, urinary tract infection)

DIAGNOSTIC IMAGING

17. **What radiologic studies should be done in the lumbar spine?**
The minimum views include the anterior-posterior and lateral views. To evaluate for a pars interarticularis fracture (spondylolysis), oblique views should be obtained.

18. **What are the essential anatomic points to observe in a lumbar spine film?**
It is essential to look for 10 points and to define them on the different views. The 10 points are divided into three soft tissue spaces and seven bony structures:
Three soft tissue spaces
   - Intervertebral disc
   - Spinal canal
   - Intervertebral foramen

TABLE 42-1. NEUROGENIC VERSUS VASCULAR CLAUDICATION		
Characteristic	**Neurogenic Claudication**	**Vascular Claudication**
Pain increased with	Spine extension, walking downhill, ambulation	Exercise
Pain decreased with	Spine flexion, walking uphill	Rest
Leg/foot pulses	Normal	Decreased or absent
Skin/trophic changes	Absent	Present
Pain pattern	Progresses from proximal to distal	Progresses from distal to proximal

Seven bony structures
- Vertebral body
- Superior facet pedicle
- Inferior facet
- Transverse process
- Lamina
- Spinous process

Kricun ME: Imaging Modalities in Spinal Disorders. Philadelphia, W.B. Saunders, 1988.
Spine Universe: www.spineuniverse.com

19. **Should magnetic resonance imaging (MRI) or a computed tomographic (CT) scan be ordered as a definitive diagnostic test?**
    - **CT:** Superior in imaging bony abnormalities (such as fractures or spondylolysis)
    - **MRI:** Superior in evaluating discs for hydration (on T2- or water-weighted images) and in imaging the conus medullaris portion of the spinal cord; also superior in detecting soft tissue abnormalities, such as facet cysts, hematomas, and inflammation of soft tissues.

      In this age of cost-effective medicine, it is important to define the goal and usefulness of the MRI of CT scan before ordering it.

20. **How are disc abnormalities graded on MRIs?**
    The North American Spine Society (NASS) has advocated the following set of terms to describe disc changes:
    - **Disc bulge:** A circumferential extension of the annulus 3 mm or more beyond the end plate. The circumferential character distinguishes the bulging disc from a protruded or extruded disc.
    - **Disc degeneration:** Seen on T2-weighted images of MRI scans. The more the disc is degenerated, the darker the signal of the nucleus.
    - **Annular fissure:** Fluid may be evident in the annulus, described as a "high intensity zone." (There appears to be a cyst in the annulus.)
    - **Disc protrusion:** A focal, asymmetric condition in which a segment of the disc contour extends beyond the margin of the adjacent vertebra into the spinal canal. Some of the outermost annular fibers are noted to be intact.
    - **Disc extrusion:** The nucleus extends beyond the annulus and posterior longitudinal ligament into the epidural space. It may migrate up or down the spinal canal.
    - **Disc sequestration:** A free fragment of disc that is detached from the remaining portion of the disc.

      The term *disc herniation* is not considered as specific as the aforementioned terms are, and it should be used cautiously when referring to specific findings on MRI or CT scan. See also Chapter 31 (Spine: Interventional Physiatric Care) for additional discussion of disc changes.

Mink J, Deutsh AL, Goldstein TB, et al: Spinal imaging and intervention. Phys Med Rehabil Clin N Am 9:343–360, 1998.

21. **What other imaging studies may be helpful? When?**
    Bone scans, particularly SPECT (single photon emission computed tomography) scans, are very helpful in defining subtle abnormalities, such as acute spondylolysis or evidence of bone trauma, that may not be evident on other studies. Myelograms and discograms, while useful, are not commonly required for the planning and implementation of nonoperative approaches.

22. **How is a lumbar fracture determined to be stable or unstable?**
    Follow the criteria developed by Denis. Divide a vertebra into three columns (anterior, middle, and posterior), with each including:
    Anterior
    - Anterior portion of disc and vertebra
    - Anterior longitudinal ligament

Middle
- Posterior portion of vertebra and disc
- Posterior longitudinal ligament

Posterior
- Pedicle, facets, lamina, spinous process
- Supraspinous and intraspinous ligaments

A fracture involving two of the three columns is considered unstable.

Denis F: The three column spine and its significance in the classification of acute thoracolumbar spinal injuries. Spine 8:817–831, 1983.

MANAGEMENT

23. **What are the main approaches in treating LBP**
    There are many approaches in the treatment of LBP. The proper sequencing of the modalities can be as important as which one is chosen (Table 42-2).

    Spitzer WO, LeBlanc F, Dupuis M, et al: Scientific approach to the assessment and management of activity-related spinal disorders. A monograph for physicians. Report of the Quebec Task Force on Spinal Disorders. Spine 12:S1–S59, 1987.

24. **What is the proper sequencing of a rehabilitation program?**
    - Control of inflammation
    - Control of pain
    - Restore spine and extremity range of motion
    - Improve muscular strength

TABLE 42-2. TREATMENT APPROACHES TO LOW BACK PAIN	
Treatment Approach	**Example(s)/Comment(s)**
Rest/activity modification	Avoid trunk extension in patient with lumbar spondylolisthesis
Thermal	Heat/cold/ultrasound
Electrical	Electrical stimulation, transcutaneous electrical nerve stimulation (TENS), spinal cord stimulation
Mechanical	Bracing/traction/canes
Injection	Joint/trigger point/epidural/nerve root block
Exercise (aerobic)	Walking
Exercise (specific for spine and extremity)	Lumbar stabilization
Medications	Analgesics/anti-inflammatories/antispasmodics
Hydrotherapy	Whirlpool/warm water pool/regular pool
Psychological	Cognitive therapy/biofeedback
Manual medicine	Mobilization/manipulation
Integrative medicine	Acupuncture/massage/yoga
Vocational	Retraining
Ergonomics	Job site evaluation/modification
Surgery	Discectomy/fusion/artificial disc placement
Case closure	Finalizing opinions on work/personal injuries

- Improve muscular endurance
- Improve neuromuscular coordination

Saal J: Rehabilitation of the injured athlete. In Delisa J (ed): Rehabilitation Medicine, Principles and Practice, 2nd ed. Philadelphia, J.P. Lippincott, 1988, p 847.

25. **What general exercise approaches should be recommended?**
Aerobic exercises are best for general conditioning. For the majority of patients this would include walking an acceptable distance at a relaxed pace with the goal of not increasing pain by overdoing it. Many patients with stenosis fare better in a flexed posture on a recumbent exercise bicycle. If a patient enjoys water exercise, this is superior in relieving stress on the spine while working the major muscle groups. In addition, mild strengthening exercises of the major muscle groups of the upper and lower extremities can be done as long as pain is not noticeably increased.

26. **When are lumbar flexion, extension, or stabilization approaches indicated?**
If there is a mechanical basis to the pain, with a flexion or extension bias (i.e., the patient feels better moving into one or the other of these two positions), pursue exercises accordingly. For example, lumbar stenosis is usually better with flexion approaches, whereas extension exercises are usually preferred initially for discogenic pain. Stabilization approaches are preferred for patients with LBP that is easily flared. However, this approach can be used in conjunction with the other two (e.g., physioball exercises). See Table 42-3.

Twomey L, Taylor J: Physical therapy of the low back. In Twomey L, Taylor J (eds): Clinics in Physical Therapy. New York, Churchill-Livingstone, 1994, pp 379–408.

27. **How do I define restrictions for a patient?**
Talk to the patient and base any restrictions on the limits the patient has self-imposed on activities of daily living. Also, have the patient perform a Functional Capacities Test and compare the results with the "essential functions" of his or her job description to see if there is a match. The key components of defining restrictions include the following:

- Posture (sit/stand/walk time limits at one time and during an 8-hour day)
- Force (lift limits)
- Repetition (e.g., climbing, bending)
- Number of hours able to work per day and total hours during the week
- Frequency of required breaks

TABLE 42-3. EXERCISE APPROACHES AND GENERAL INDICATIONS FOR THEIR USE

Diagnosis	Aerobics	Flexion	Extension	Stabilization
Myofascial pain	+	+	+	+
Herniated disc (not a free fragment)	+	±	±	+
Spondylolysis	+	+	Not acutely	+
Fracture (stable)	+	Not acutely	Not acutely	+
Facet syndrome	+	+	−	+
Spinal stenosis	+	+	−	+
Fibromyalgia	+	+	+	+
Infection	Mild	±	±	±
Spondyloarthropathy	+	±	±	+
Tumor	Varies	±	±	±

28. **When is surgery indicated?**
    - **Absolute indications:** Cauda equina syndrome, progressive neurologic deficit
    - **Relative indications:** Intolerable pain, persistent pain that markedly compromises a patient's functional abilities

29. **When can an athlete return to competition after a lumbar pain episode?**
    Although most of the literature addresses this topic in relation to cervical spine injuries, certain principles can be extrapolated to the lumbar region.
    - Full range of motion
    - No neurologic deficit
    - Little or no pain
    - Athlete can practice without symptoms
    - Proper protective equipment is available
    - Participation will not place the athlete at risk for further injury
    - Athlete has confidence that he or she can play without further injury

    Eck J: Return to play after lumbar spine conditions and surgery. Clin Sports Med 23:367–379, 2004.
    Maorganti C: Recommendations for return to sports following cervical spine injuries. Sports Med 33(8):563–573, 2003.

30. **What are the alternative decisions when a patient is not progressing?**
    Inability to improve with a lumbar pain episode causes emotional stress in a patient and may instill a lack of confidence in the practitioner. The physician needs to step back from the situation and readdress the thought process that was followed in arriving at a diagnosis and treatment plan. Altering one of the following five parameters of decision alternatives may allow the patient to get beyond an impasse and progress to a more realistic outcome level. The five parameters include:
    - Diagnosis
    - Treatment process
    - Time frame of treatment
    - Expected outcome
    - "Rules" of treatment

    Brandenburger A, Nalebuff B: Co-opetition. New York, Currency-Doubleday, 1996.

31. **What are some common "red flags" that identify the 10–20% of cases less likely to improve well?**
    - Poor educational level (less than a high school degree)
    - Tobacco/alcohol use
    - Presence of significant emotional stressors
    - Pending medical–legal issues

KEY POINTS: LOW BACK PAIN

1. Lumbar stenosis is associated with degenerative, not isthmic, spondylolisthesis.
2. Lumbar stenosis is defined as an anterior-posterior diameter of the central spinal canal of <11 mm.
3. Patients with neurogenic claudication feel better walking uphill (spinal flexion).
4. Divide the spinal column into three parts when evaluating for stability with fractures.
5. Posture, force, repetitions, and endurance are key components of defining restrictions.
6. In a degenerative process leading to increased stiffness from fibrosis, there should be gradually less pain at the involved lumbar segment, as long as there is no neurovascular compromise from scarring and osteophytes.

32. **How should end of healing and maximal medical improvement issues in workers' compensation injury and personal injury cases be approached?**
Workers' compensation injuries
- Diagnosis
- Restrictions (if any)
- Date of end of healing
- Impairment or disability rating
- Future diagnostic and treatment needs

Personal injury
- Diagnosis
- Date of end of healing
- Causation of pain (if applicable)
- Prognosis
- Future diagnostic and treatment needs
- Restrictions (if applicable)
- Impairment rating (if applicable)

33. **How can patient encounters be efficient, yet still effective?**
Just as an airplane pilot has to develop "situational awareness," so does a physician by using the following strategies:
1. Look for patterns of symptoms, exam findings, and injuries commonly seen in specific occupations and age brackets.
2. With an injury, there is inflammation, followed by repair. Attempt to determine where the patient is in this process.
3. Know the culture and background of the patient. This affects how patients react to pain.
4. If the case is complicated, do not try to do everything in one visit. Set the expectations for the encounter early in the evaluation.
5. Always follow up on your recommendations and impressions. Only fools believe that they are always right the first time. Pain is a dynamic process; expect it to change.

34. **How is the physician's role defined in the treatment of patients with spinal pain?**
There are several options, which include either one or a combination of the following:
- A consultant, who sees the patient for only a few visits and then forwards recommendations to the primary physician.
- A specialist, who takes over management of a complex case of spinal pain until the episode subsides or stabilizes. In the "court of last resort" the specialist takes over long-term management of complex spine pain cases.
- An interventionalist, who performs specific procedures but does not manage cases of spine pain.
- A primary care musculoskeletal physician, who follows the total spectrum of spine pain patients.
- An urgent care musculoskeletal physician, who sees the patient for a brief encounter.
- An independent medical examiner, who evaluates the patient one time only for a medical–legal opinion.

35. **What are the keys to successful treatment?**
- Identifying proper diagnosis
- Defining the problem for the patient
- Having a motivated patient
- Correctly structuring the treatment program
- Knowing the patient and his or her problem well enough to set realistic expectations for final outcome in an appropriate time frame

36. **What are the most important points to impress on a patient?**
    - A severe medical or surgical condition has either been addressed or ruled out.
    - Back pain is usually a lifestyle issue, and unless there is an alteration of risk factors, there is a high rate of recurrence.

Note: On subjects relating to bone metastasis to the spine, see Chapter 67 (Cancer Rehabilitation: General Principles). For lumbar radiculopathy, see Chapter 17 (Radiculopathies: Symptoms, Differential Diagnosis, and Treatment).

WEBSITES

1. American Academy of Physical Medicine and Rehabilitation (AAPMR)
   www.aapmr.org

2. American Society of Interventional Pain Physicians (ASIPP)
   www.asipp.org

3. International Spinal Injection Society (ISIS)
   www.spinalinjection.com

4. Physiatric Association of Spine, Sports, and Occupational Rehabilitation (PASSOR)
   www.aapmr.org/passor.htm

5. Spine Universe
   www.spineuniverse.com

BIBLIOGRAPHY

1. Cole A, Herring S: The Low Back Pain Handbook, 2nd ed. Hanley & Belfus, 2003.
2. Kirkaldy-Willis WH: Low Back Pain, 2nd ed. New York, Churchill-Livingstone, 1988.
3. Konin J, Wiksten D, Isear J, Brader H: Special Tests for the Orthopedic Examination, 2nd ed. Thorofare, NJ, Slack, 2002.
4. McKenzie R: The Lumbar Spine: Mechanical Diagnosis and Therapy. Upper Hut, New Zealand, Spine Publications, 1981.
5. Spitzer WO, LeBlanc F, Dupuis M, et al: Scientific approach to the assessment and management of activity-related spinal disorders. A monograph for clinicians. Report of the Quebec Task Force on Spinal Disorders. Spine 12(Suppl 7):S1–S59, 1987.
6. White AA, Panjabi MM: Clinical Biomechanics of the Spine, 2nd ed. Philadelphia, J.B. Lippincott, 1990.
7. Young MA, Lavin R: Conservative Care and Spinal Rehabilitation. Spine: State of the Art Review. Philadelphia, Hanley & Belfus, 1995.

CHAPTER 43

THE SHOULDER: ANATOMY, PATHOLOGY, AND DIAGNOSIS

Mark Harrast, MD, Rene Cailliet, MD, Edward McFarland, MD, Tsai Chao, MD, and Atsushi Tasaki, MD

A dwarf standing on the shoulders of a giant may see farther than the giant.
—Robert Burton (1577–1640)

ANATOMY AND BIOMECHANICS

1. **Name all of the joints involved in the shoulder girdle complex.**
   - Glenohumeral joint
   - Acromioclavicular joint
   - Costovertebral joint
   - Sternoclavicular joint
   - Sternocostal joint
   - Scapulocostal joint
   These many joints indicate why the term *shoulder girdle complex* is better than *shoulder joint*.

2. **Which muscles control the primary movements about the glenohumeral (GH) joint and scapulothoracic interface?**
   Primary movers at GH joint
   - Flexion: Pectoralis major, anterior deltoid
   - Extension: Latissimus dorsi, posterior deltoid
   - Internal rotation: Pectoralis major, latissimus dorsi, teres major, subscapularis
   - External rotation: Infraspinatus, teres minor, posterior deltoid
   - Abduction: Deltoid, supraspinatus
   - Adduction: Pectoralis major, latissimus dorsi, teres major, subscapularis
   Primary movers at scapulothoracic interface
   - Elevation: Upper trapezius, rhomboids, levator scapulae
   - Depression: Latissimus dorsi, pectoralis major, lower trapezius
   - Protraction: Serratus anterior, pectoralis major
   - Retraction: Trapezius, rhomboids
   - Upward rotation: Trapezius, serratus anterior
   - Downward rotation: Rhomboids, levator scapulae, pectoralis major

3. **What muscles comprise the rotator cuff?**
   One way of remembering the rotator cuff muscles is by using the mnemonic **SITS**: **s**upraspinatus, **i**nfraspinatus, **t**eres minor, and **s**ubscapularis. At rest, their function is glenohumeral stabilization. All contract isometrically in the dependent arm to prevent subluxation. Dynamically, all contract to abduct and forward flex the arm. All but the subscapularis contract in external rotation of the arm.

4. **What muscles are considered the primary scapular stabilizers? List exercises that are used to train and strengthen them.**
   - **Teres major:** Pull-downs
   - **Rhomboids:** Standard rows, low rows, prone arm lifts

- **Serratus anterior:** Push-ups with a plus, punches
- **Trapezius:** Train/target complete scapular rotation
- **Levator scapulae:** Shoulder shrugs, seated press-ups

5. **Describe the importance of the scapula in shoulder function and rehabilitation.**
   The scapula is the platform for glenohumeral articulation and motion. Very commonly after shoulder injury, the serratus anterior and lower trapezius (prime scapular stabilizers) are reflexively inhibited, thus "destabilizing" the platform. This produces a retracted and downwardly rotated scapula, which can exacerbate the primary shoulder pathology (e.g., impingement or rotator cuff disease). Neuromuscular reeducation of the serratus anterior and lower trapezius, and then strengthening, are the initial rehabilitation steps for many shoulder disorders.

   Kibler WB: The role of the scapula in athletic shoulder function. Am J Sports Med 26:325–327, 1998.

6. **What are the components of scapulohumeral rhythm?**
   This term indicates the movement of the humerus within the glenoid fossa and the scapula upon the rib cage when the arm abducts or forward flexes. At rest they are vertical, but as the humerus abducts/flexes, the scapula initially remains static then rotates to permit overhead elevation. The rhythm implies that for every degree of scapular rotation on the rib cage, there are 2 degrees of glenohumeral abduction movement. The ratio 2:1 is not totally accurate for the entire 180 degrees.

   Cailliet R: Shoulder Pain, 3rd ed. Philadelphia, F.A. Davis, 1991.

7. **An injury to which sets of nerves and muscles can result in scapular winging?**
   See Table 43-1.

TABLE 43-1. MUSCLE/NERVE INJURIES RESULTING IN SCAPULAR WINGING	
Muscle/Nerve	**Resulting Scapula Position**
Rhomboids/dorsal scapular	Protracted and upwardly rotated
Serratus anterior/long thoracic	Retracted and downwardly rotated
Trapezius/spinal accessory	Protracted and downwardly rotated

8. **Is posture a factor in evaluating shoulder pain?**
   Yes. An exaggerated thoracic kyphosis causes the scapula to rotate downward. This changes the alignment of the glenoid fossa and the proximity of the acromium, making impingement more possible.

9. **Is there a difference between subdeltoid bursitis and supraspinatus tendinitis?**
   The synovial linings of both the subdeltoid bursa and the glenohumeral capsule are contiguous with the supraspinatus tendon. Inflammation of the sheath inflames both.

10. **Name the three most common anatomic structures of the shoulder involved in shoulder impingement syndrome.**
    1. Subacromial bursa
    2. Supraspinatus
    3. Biceps tendon

11. **What are the work-related factors in the development of subacromial shoulder impingement?**
    - Arm position required
    - Weight-lifting requirements
    - Number of repetitions

    Isernhagen SJ: Principles of prevention of cumulative trauma. Occup Med 7:147–153, 1992.

CLINICAL PRESENTATION

12. **What clinical tests suggest the diagnosis of a complete torn rotator cuff tear? How can the diagnosis be confirmed?**
    No test on physical examination confirms the diagnosis of a complete tear. Clinically, a complete tear is indicated by inability to abduct the arm from dependency, inability to externally rotate the arm, and a positive **drop arm test**. Magnetic resonance imaging (MRI) studies are useful in confirming tears and evaluating the extent of tendon damage.

13. **What is the mechanism of the "drop arm test"?**
    The arm cannot abduct, but once abducted to horizontal, it can be briefly held there by the deltoid muscle. Because the supraspinatus muscle is not seating the humeral head into the glenoid fossa, the arm gradually, or with minimal weight, "drops."

14. **Aside from faulty shoulder abduction, is there another test to determine the presence of a complete rotator cuff tear?**
    Yes. Because a portion of the rotator cuff is represented by the tendinous insertion into the tuberosity from the supraspinatus and infraspinatus muscles, in a complete tear, active external rotation of the arm is not possible.

15. **Describe the standard radiographic views to evaluate a patient with glenohumeral arthritis.**
    - **True anteroposterior (AP) view** of the glenohumeral joint with the humerus in 35 degrees of external rotation and 45 degrees of abduction. This view places the humeral neck in maximum profile and centers the humerus in the glenoid fossa; thus showing the thickness of the cartilage space, the degree of deformity of the humeral articular surface, and superior humeral migration (especially if a complete rotator cuff tear is present).
    - **Axillary lateral view** allows assessment of glenoid erosion, abnormal glenoid version, and humeral subluxation.

    Matsen FA, Rockwood CA, Wirth MA, Lippitt SB: Glenohumeral arthritis and its management: In Rockwood CA, Matsen FA (eds): The Shoulder, Vol. 2. Philadelphia, W.B. Saunders, 1998, pp 840–964.

16. **What findings of MRI are associated with shoulder impingement and rotator cuff disease?**
    - Subacromial fluid
    - Anterior acromial enthesophytes
    - Signal abnormalities of the rotator cuff
    - Acromioclavicular arthropathy with downward-projecting osteophytes

    Iannotti JP, Zlatkin MB, Esterhai JL, et al: Magnetic resonance imaging of the shoulder: Sensitivity, specificity and predictive value. J Bone Joint Surg 73A:17–29, 1991.

17. **Describe common radiographic findings after a traumatic anterior shoulder dislocation.**

    Traumatic shoulder dislocation most frequently occurs in the anterior direction. Such dislocations involve injury to the anterior-inferior glenohumeral joint capsule (middle glenohumeral ligament or anterior band of the inferior glenohumeral ligament) or a Bankart lesion, which is the detachment of the anterior-inferior glenoid labrum from the glenoid rim. If a fracture of the anterior-inferior glenoid rim is involved, it is referred to as a *bony* **Bankart** lesion. A **Hill-Sachs defect** refers to a compression fracture of the posterolateral aspect of the humeral head.

DIFFERENTIAL DIAGNOSIS

18. **Is it possible to differentiate a rotator cuff tendon partial tear from tendinitis by clinical means?**

    No. A partial tear of the rotator cuff tendon causes segmental swelling that becomes entrapped under the coracoacromial ligament, similar to tendinitis.

19. **Describe the stages of adhesive capsulitis.**

    Adhesive capsulitis, also known as frozen shoulder, is classically divided into three stages (Table 43-2), which are not discreetly defined entities but, rather, represent a continuum of the disease process.

    Rizk TE, Pinals RS: Frozen shoulder. Semin Arthr Rheum 11:440–452, 1982.

20. **What is bicipital tendinitis?**

TABLE 43-2. STAGES OF ADHESIVE CAPSULITIS	
Stage I: "The painful phase"	Spontaneous shoulder pain with ensuing stiffness; lasts 2.5–9 months
Stage II: "The stiff phase"	Continued shoulder stiffness but improved pain; lasts 4–12 months
Stage III: "The resolution phase"	Gradual functional recovery with a progressive increase in shoulder range of motion due to capsular remodeling from the use of the arm and shoulder; lasts 5–26 months

The biceps tendon acts passively (mechanically) on the humerus during abduction and forward flexion as the bicipital fossa passes over the tendon. Inappropriate glenohumeral friction that occurs over the tendon, which is contiguous to the subdeltoid bursa and glenohumeral capsule, results in tendinitis.

21. **Describe the two types of shoulder impingement.**

    - **Primary outlet impingement** implies extrinsic compression of the rotator cuff and/or biceps tendon by the acromion or coracoacromial ligament, which can be exacerbated by a subacromial osteophyte, hooked acromion, exaggerated thoracic kyphosis, and/or protracted and downwardly rotated scapula. It is more common in patients age >40 years.
    - **Secondary (internal or glenoid) impingement** implies irritation of the articular (glenoid) side of the rotator cuff tendons typically seen in young overhead-throwing athletes. It may be related to subtle instability.

    Karzel RP, Pizzo WD: Rotator cuff impingement in athletes. In Pettrone FA (ed): Athletic injuries of the shoulder. New York, McGraw-Hill, 1995, pp 143–153.

22. **How is acromioclavicular (AC) pain manifested?**
Usually, there is a history of trauma, with pain and tenderness located at the AC joint. Crepitation is elicited by circumduction of the shoulder. Cross-body adduction creates a compressive force across the AC joint and thus is considered a provocative diagnostic maneuver. Diagnosis and possible relief are gained by intra-articular local anesthetic injection. AC separation can be evaluated with plain radiographs to determine the severity.

Rockwood CA, Williams GR, Young DC: Disorders of the acromioclavicular joint. In Rockwood CA, Matsen FA (eds): The Shoulder, 2nd ed. Philadelphia, W.B. Saunders, 1998, pp 483–553.

23. **Classify the types of AC joint separation and their treatment.**
The Rockwood Classification is summarized in Table 43-3.

TABLE 43-3. ROCKWOOD CLASSIFICATION OF AC JOINT SEPARATION	
Type	**Treatment**
I. AC ligament sprain	Nonoperative
II: Torn AC and sprained CC ligaments	Nonoperative
III: Torn AC and CC ligaments; CC space is 25–100% widened	Controversial (tending toward nonoperative)
IV: Type III with clavicle displaced posteriorly	Operative
V: Type III with CC space widened > 100% and deltoid and trapezius are detached from distal clavicle	Operative
VI: Type III with clavicle displaced inferiorly through or behind the biceps tendon	Operative

AC = acromioclavicular, CC = coracoclavicular.

24. **What are the mechanism, diagnosis, and management of shoulder subluxation?**
Subluxation is partial glenohumeral dislocation that results from direct trauma, but it also occurs after acute stroke. Stability is maintained by the glenohumeral capsule and the rotator cuff muscles. In acute stroke the supraspinatus muscle becomes frail. Management entails positioning the patient to avoid downward traction, or increasing supraspinatus muscle contraction, mechanically or electrically.

25. **Besides rotator cuff disease, what other differential diagnostic possibilities must be considered in evaluating shoulder pain?**
See Table 43-4.

TABLE 43-4. DIFFERENTIAL DIAGNOSIS OF SHOULDER PAIN	
Suprascapular nerve entrapment	Cervical radiculitis
Shoulder instability	Cervical facet syndrome
Acromioclavicular degenerative joint disease	Cardiac ischemia
Bicipital tendinopathy	Diaphragmatic irritation
Gallbladder disease	Upper lobe/pleural irritation

TREATMENT

26. What are the six phases of general shoulder rehabilitation?
1. Control of pain and inflammation
2. Restoration of motion
3. Neuromuscular retraining and strengthening
   a. Scapular stabilizers are generally first line of focus
   b. Rotator cuff muscles
   c. Prime movers—initially start with isolated strengthening; then progress to more functional exercises in multiple planes and in conjunction with lower limb activities and engaging core musculature
4. Proprioceptive training
5. Endurance training
6. Return to task-specific or sport-specific activities

27. What is the treatment for rotator cuff tendinitis?
Treatment of rotator cuff tendinitis begins with frequent applications of ice, NSAIDs for 4–6 weeks, avoidance of painful motions, and physical therapy. Exercises should be performed in a pain-free range. Focus on stretching to avoid loss of motion followed by activation and strengthening the scapular stabilizers and later, if necessary, the rotator cuff. Persistent pain warrants subacromial corticosteroid injection. An MRI or arthrogram may confirm a rotator cuff tear. Arthroscopic evaluation with acromioplasty is sometimes necessary.

28. What is the optimum treatment of a frozen shoulder?
- Prevention by early mobilization with pendulum exercises
- Avoidance of splinting
- Minimization of pain and inflammation
  Once there is adhesion, active and passive mobilization exercises are effective, particularly stretching in the plane that has lost motion. Stretching exercises should be recommended at least 2–3 times daily. Oral pain medicine and oral steroids can be helpful with controlling pain.

KEY POINTS: TREATMENT OF A STIFF SHOULDER

1. Aggressive passive (then active-assisted) range of motion

2. Medications for pain relief (especially before stretching):
   a. Nonsteroidal anti-inflammatory drugs (NSAIDs) and/or nonnarcotic and narcotic analgesics orally
   b. Intra-articular (with or without subacromial) steroids or oral steroids

3. Manipulation under anesthesia

4. Arthroscopic or open surgical evaluation and release of adhesions, followed by aggressive physical therapy

5. Hospitalization with an indwelling interscalene catheter and aggressive physical therapy

29. How do you treat patients with severe arthritis of the shoulder?
Treatment of arthritis of the shoulder is aimed at maintaining range of motion (ROM), through stretching at home and with use of ice, heat, and NSAIDS. Impingement or rotator cuff tendonitis is addressed. When nonoperative treatment fails, joint replacement is the best

surgical option. Either the humeral head (hemiarthroplasty) or the humeral head and socket/glenoid (total shoulder replacement) can be replaced. Severe arthritis with rotator cuff tears can be treated with a reverse prosthesis. A one- or two-night hospital stay is typical. Rehabilitation begins the day after surgery (*see* Table 43-5).

TABLE 43-5. REHABILITATION AFTER TOTAL SHOULDER REPLACEMENT		
Duration	**Treatment**	**Precautions**
Phase 1		
0–3 weeks	Gentle passive and active ROM to full flexion as tolerated, abduction to 90 degrees, internal rotation and external rotation as dictated by surgeon	No weight-bearing Sling worn at all times, except with exercise Avoid active abduction, extension >0 degrees, external rotation as dictated by surgeon
	Pendulum exercises	
	Isometric strengthening as tolerated by pain in flexion, extension, and internal and external rotation	
	One-handed ADLs	
3–6 weeks	Vigorous isometrics as tolerated	Continue sling at night and non–weight-bearing
	Active-assisted progressing to active ROM	
	"Wall-walking" with hand used as stabilizer	May begin active abduction
Phase 2		
6–12 weeks	Vigorous isometrics	May lift up to 2 lb
	Progressive isotonics (e.g., elastic-tubing exercises)	Discontinue sling
	Active-assisted ROM and active ROM past 90 degrees	Discontinue ROM precautions in external rotation
	Two-handed ADLs encouraged	Can begin to work on external rotation
Phase 3		
>12 weeks	Active ROM exercises, progressive resistance, strengthening	Discontinue ROM precautions
	Stretching in flexion, abduction, and rotation	

ADLs = activities of daily living, ROM = range of motion.

30. **What is the treatment for shoulder instability?**
   In some cases, shoulder instability can be controlled with muscle strengthening and careful positioning. Rehabilitation is particularly effective in patients with signs of instability but no

history of trauma. Patients with a traumatic dislocation, younger patients (<25 years old), and athletic individuals have a greater chance of recurrence.

Surgery for instability involves repair of the torn labrum to the glenoid rim (Bankart repair) and shortening of the ligaments (capsular shift). Both can be performed with an open incision or arthroscopically. Arthroscopic capsule tightening and Bankart repair has effectiveness similar to open techniques. Shifting has been described but is used currently only in select cases. The arm is put in a sling for 3 weeks while the ligaments become tight, then rehabilitation is similar to the open procedure (Table 43-6).

Kirkley A, Griffin S, Richards C, et al: Prospective, randomized clinical trial comparing the effectiveness of immediate arthroscopic stabilization versus immobilization and rehabilitation in first traumatic anterior dislocations of the shoulder. Arthroscopy 15:507–514, 1999.

TABLE 43-6. REHABILITATION AFTER BANKART AND CAPSULAR SHIFT (OPEN), BANKART AND SHIFT (ARTHROSCOPIC), AND THERMAL CAPSULORRAPHY*

Duration	Treatment	Precautions
Phase 1		
0–3 weeks	Passive ROM in abduction in scapular plane	No weight-bearing
	Passive ROM in ER to operative limit	No active external rotation
	Pendulum exercises	Wear immobilizer to sleep and for most of the day for 2 weeks, then just to sleep
	Begin scapular retraction and depression exercises	
	Active flexion as tolerated	
	After 1 week, add active-assisted ROM for ER to operative limit	
	Gradually progress to isometric flexion and ER without weight below shoulder level	
Phase 2		
3–6 weeks	Progressive isotonic exercises (e.g., elastic-tubing exercises) as tolerated	May lift objects up to 2 lb
	Full ROM forward flexion, abduction	
	Progressive external rotation as tolerated after 4–6 weeks	
6–9 weeks	Progressive isotonic exercises as tolerated	Discontinue night bracing
	Emphasis on gently regaining ER	May lift objects up to 5 lb
Phase 3		
9–12 weeks	Begin isokinetic IR/ER/FF, abduction	
	Active ROM exercises, progressive resistance, strengthening	Discontinue all ROM precautions
	Stretching in flexion, abduction, and rotation	

ER = external rotation, FF = forward flexion, IR = internal rotation, ROM = range of motion.
*In thermal shift, motion of the shoulder is not begun for 3 weeks.

31. **How do fractures of the shoulder affect rehabilitation?**
    Shoulder fractures requiring incision and fixation with pins, plates, or screws can begin motion of the fingers, wrist, and elbow in a few days. When the fracture can withstand stress and is cleared for active ROM, pendulum exercises should be started, followed by active-assisted motion and active motion. Pain, loss of motion, and poor function should be evaluated with radiographs to check for hardware failure, avascular necrosis of the humeral head, and proper location of the humeral head in the socket. Sometimes the bones heal in a position that will not allow full motion. Re-evaluation by the surgeon may be necessary.

32. **List the types of potential therapeutic and/or diagnostic shoulder girdle complex injections and their anatomic sites.**
    See Table 43-7.

TABLE 43-7. TYPES AND ANATOMIC SITES OF THERAPEUTIC AND DIAGNOSTIC SHOULDER GIRDLE COMPLEX INJECTIONS	
Injection Location	**Anatomic Structure**
Anterior	Acromioclavicular joint
	Glenohumeral joint
	Sternoclavicular joint
	Biceps tendon sheath
Lateral/posterolateral	Subacromial bursa
Posterior	Glenohumeral joint

33. **Suggest a convenient way of initiating active-passive shoulder movement.**
    Pendulum (Codman's) exercises are a simple way of instituting active-passive motion of the glenohumeral joint. This is best achieved with the patient bent forward, with the arm in the dependent (pendular) position and the body "actively" moving to "passively" move the pendular arm.

34. **What does rehabilitation after acromioplasty entail?**
    Lifting anything heavier than a coffee cup is prohibited for 2–3 weeks. If the deltoid muscle was removed and reattached, active motion above table level is not allowed for 4–6 weeks. Otherwise, full motion is gradually attained with physical therapy as pain permits. The goal is full motion in 2–3 months.

35. **What does rehabilitation after rotator cuff repair entail?**
    See Table 43-8.

36. **Discuss rehabilitation after shoulder replacement.**
    External rotation should be avoided for 6–8 weeks. Interestingly, elevation in front of the body does not stress the subscapularis in most cases and can be instituted soon after surgery. Strengthening is important. The most serious complication is infection. Drainage from the

TABLE 43-8. REHABILITATION AFTER ROTATOR CUFF REPAIR

Duration	Treatment	Precautions
Phase 1		
0–3 weeks	Elbow, wrist, finger ROM	No weight-bearing
	Passive ROM in abduction in scapular plane	No active ROM above table level
	Passive ROM in forward flexion	Sling or immobilizer at all times except exercise
	Pendulum exercises	Avoid arm adduction across body and internal rotation; avoid shoulder extension and external rotation as dictated by surgeon
	Begin scapular retraction and depression exercises	
Phase 2		
4–6 weeks	Start active-assisted ROM in flexion and abduction	Start active ROM
	Active ROM of flexion less than 90 degrees	No lifting of objects causing axial distraction
6–8 weeks	Continue active-assisted ROM	Patient allowed to use arms in front of body, below shoulder level
	Isometric strengthening as tolerated by pain in flexion, extension, and internal and external rotation	
8–10 weeks	Progressively more vigorous isometrics	
	Progressive isotonic exercises	
Phase 3		
10–12 weeks	Active ROM exercises, progressive	
	Discontinue ROM precautions, resistance, strengthening	
	Stretching in flexion, abduction, and rotation	

ROM = range of motion.

wound after 4–5 days is abnormal. If the subscapularis tendon repair fails, dislocation of the prosthesis can occur. Stiffness is common, and most patients do not entirely regain normal motion.

37. **What are the indications for shoulder arthroscopy?**
The most common shoulder arthroscopy indication is for diagnostic purposes; however, the following disease entities can be assessed and treated arthroscopically: rotator cuff disease, impingement, shoulder instability, GH and AC joint arthritis, adhesive capsulitis, biceps tendon and labral pathology, and loose bodies.

Rao AG, Yokota A, McFarland EG: Shoulder arthroscopy: Principles and practice. In Harrast MA, Paynter KS, Barr KP (eds): Shoulder Rehabilitation. Philadelphia, Elsevier, 2004, pp 627–642.

WEBSITES

1. http://hopkinsmedicine.org/orthopedocsurgery/sportsguide.html

2. Nicholas Institute of Sports Medicine and Athletic Trauma: This site is particularly useful for the basics of physical exam.
www.nismat.org/orthocor/exam/shoulder.html

3. UW Medicine Orthopaedics and Sports Medicine: Great website for shoulder disorders in general, but particularly helpful for shoulder arthritis, instability, and rotator cuff disease.
www.orthop.washington.edu

4. A service of the United Kingdom Association of Doctors in Sports: This site is particularly helpful for patient education material on a wide range of shoulder disorders.
www.shoulderdoc.co.uk

CHAPTER 44

THE ELBOW: ANATOMY, PATHOLOGY, AND DIAGNOSIS

Richard A. Rogachefsky, MD, Michael E. Frey, MD, Vivencio Salcedo, MD, and Francisco H. Santiago, MD

A problem well stated is a problem half solved.
—Charles F. Kettering (1876–1958)

She was a woman who, between courses, could be graceful with her elbows on the table.
—Henry James (1843–1916)

1. **Name the major muscles of the elbow, the movements performed, and their nerve supply.**
   See Table 44-1.

   ### TABLE 44-1.   MUSCLES OF THE ELBOW

Muscle	Movement	Nerve Supply
Biceps	Flexion, supination	Musculocutaneous (C5, C6)
Brachioradialis	Flexion	Radial (C5, C6)
Brachialis	Flexion	Musculocutaneous (C5, C6)
Triceps	Extension	Radial (C5–C8)
Anconeus	Extension (weak) Stabilizes elbow joint	Radial (C7, C8)
Supinator	Supination	Radial (C5, C6)
Pronator quadratus	Pronation	Median (anterior interosseous) (C8, T1)
Pronator teres	Pronation Least effective as a pronator with elbow in full flexion	Median (C6, C7)

2. **Is there anything unique about the brachioradialis muscle?**
   It is the only muscle that attaches from the distal end of one bone to the distal end of another bone and the only muscle producing flexion of the elbow that is supplied by the radial nerve instead of the musculocutaneous nerve. Depending on the position, it may also act as a pronator or supinator.

3. **What is the most powerful supinator in the arm?**
   Biceps brachii.

4. **Specify the articulations of the elbow and where movement occurs.**
   - The humeroulnar joint, between the trochlear notch of the ulna and the humerus
   - The humeroradial joint, between the radial head and capitulum of the humerus
   - The radioulnar joint

Flexion and extension occur at the axis of the trochlear and capitulum. Supination–pronation occurs through the longitudinal axis of rotation at the radial head and the radial ulnar notch of the ulna (Fig. 44-1).

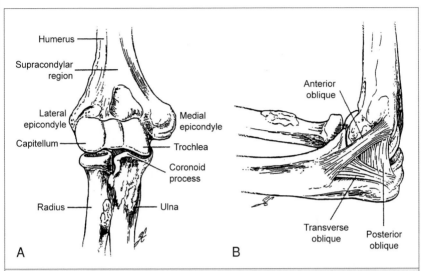

Figure 44-1. *A,* Anterior view of the elbow. *B,* The three components of the ulnar collateral ligament. (From Nicholas JA, Hershman EB: The Upper Extremity in Sports Medicine. St. Louis, Mosby, 1990.)

5. **What is elbow angulation? What is carrying angle?**
The normal anatomic valgus angulation, or carrying angle, is the angle between the upper arm and forearm when the elbow is fully extended. The normal angle for males is 5–10 degrees and for females is 10–15 degrees. Greater than 20 degrees is considered abnormal.

KEY POINTS: CAUSES OF ELBOW INJURY

1. Fall on an outstretched arm

2. Fall on a bent elbow

3. Overuse of elbow motion (e.g., repetitious movements in sports)

4. Carrying angle (greater in women than in men, posing a heightened injury risk in sporting competition)

6. **What is olecranon bursitis? How is it treated?**
Olecranon bursitis is inflammation of the olecranon bursa, sometimes referred to as draftsman's elbow or student's elbow. It causes pain and swelling at the posterior elbow and may be associated with trauma or systemic conditions such as gout, rheumatoid arthritis, pseudogout, tuberculosis, chondrocalcinosis, xanthomatosis, or infection. A septic bursa is ruled out by Gram stain and culture. Radiographs rule out osteomyelitis and bone spurs. Treatment of nonseptic olecranon bursitis includes protective padding, nonsteroidal anti-inflammatory drugs

(NSAIDs), maintenance of functional range of motion (ROM), a trial of aspiration (often unsuccessful), or local cortisone injection. Surgical intervention is rarely required.

7. **What is medial epicondylitis (golfer's elbow)?**
This repetitive strain injury usually affects the flexor pronator musculature, such as pronator teres, flexor carpi radialis, flexor carpi ulnaris, and, rarely, the flexor digitorum superficialis. Pain is present with resisted wrist flexion or pronation with the elbow extended. Causes include an improper serve in tennis, throwing a baseball, a golf swing, or use of hand tools.

8. **What is lateral epicondylitis (tennis elbow)?**
Tennis elbow is an overuse syndrome caused by repetitive microtrauma to the musculotendinous unit along the radial extensors of the wrist in the lateral epicondyle region. It causes inflammation and degenerative tissue damage and presents as pain in the lateral elbow that can radiate down the forearm to the wrist. Pain worsens with grasping or wrist extension. Less than 5% of patients get tennis elbow by playing tennis. The four sites of occurrence from proximal to distal are supracondylar, tenoperiosteal, tendinous, and muscular. A point of tenderness is usually palpated in one of the four locations. Diagnosis should not be confused with radioulnar or radiohumeral bursitis, annular or collateral ligament sprains, osteoarthritis of the radioulnar joint, or radial nerve entrapment at the supinator or arcade of Frohse.

Tennis elbow (lateral epicondylitis): http://Orthoinfo.aaos.org

9. **What is pushed or pulled elbow in a child? How is it treated?**
In a **pulled elbow** the head of the radius is dislocated from the annular ligament, usually caused by a forceful pull on a child's extended arm. Supination is limited. If the pull cannot be reduced by flexion and supination, the following manual maneuver can be used to correct it. The child stands against the wall with the upper arm abducted and the elbow flexed at 90 degrees. The examiner grasps the lower forearm with the ipsilateral hand, pushes the radius upward toward the humerus by pressing the elbow against the wall, and rapidly rotates the forearm in both directions. Usually, on full supination, the radial head will click back into place.

A **pushed elbow** describes subluxation of the radial head in a proximal direction, often seen when a person falls on an outstretched hand. The radial head impinges on the capitulum. It is occasionally associated with the Colles' fracture. Treatment consists of traction and repetitive stretching.

10. **What is a little leaguer's elbow?**
This injury in children and adolescents is caused by repetitive valgus stress in which the medial epicondyle is inflamed. Partial separation of the apophysis can occur. A common symptom is pain when throwing. Radiographs are important in diagnoses and may show widening of the apophyseal line or an avulsion fracture, which needs surgical correction.

Throwing injuries in the elbow: http://Orthoinfo.aaos.org

11. **Describe pronator syndrome.**
This entrapment neuropathy affects the median nerve distal to the antecubital fossa. In most cases the nerve pierces the two heads of the pronator teres muscle, where hypertrophy or an anomalous band may injure the nerve. Presentation includes pain in the anterior elbow that increases with resisted pronation, numbness in the hand, and weakness of the wrist and finger flexors. Compression over the median nerve at the pronator teres often reproduces symptoms within 30 seconds. Other sites of compression can be at the lacertus fibrosis or in the flexor digitorum superficialis muscle. Median nerve compression proximal to the pronator teres can occur at the ligament of Struthers at the medial epicondyle.

12. What is cubital tunnel syndrome?

Cubital tunnel syndrome is entrapment of the ulnar nerve along the cubital tunnel at the medial aspect of the elbow. It is associated with Tinel's sign. Paresthesia and numbness can occur in the fourth and fifth fingers. Over time there may be weakness in grasp and pinch and loss of dexterity. The three zones of compression are:

- Zone I: Proximal to the medial epicondyle
- Zone II: At the level of the medial epicondyle
- Zone III: Distal to the medial epicondyle (cubital tunnel)

Overuse injuries can cause entrapment with a tight flexor carpi ulnaris muscle in zone III. Treatment is with NSAIDs, elbow pad to protect the nerve, avoidance of aggravating activities, and exercises in the pain-free range. Surgical release or transposition may be required.

Grana W: Medial epicondylitis and cubital tunnel syndrome in the throwing athlete. Clin Sports Med 20:541–548, 2001.

13. What is posterior interosseous nerve syndrome?

It is an entrapment neuropathy of the posterior interosseous nerve branch of the radial nerve at the fibrous arch of the supinator or within the muscle belly. Symptoms may include pain with resisted pronation or supination, Tinel's sign over the nerve, resisted pronation or supination, and weakness in wrist or finger extension. There is no associated numbness. Diagnosis is made with electromyography (EMG). Muscles involved can be the extensor carpi ulnaris, extensor digitorum communis, extensor indicis, abductor pollicis longus, and extensor pollicis longus and brevis. The extensor carpi radialis longus and brevis muscles are spared.

Markiewitz AD, Merryman J: Radial nerve compression in the upper extremity. J Am Soc Surg Hand 5:87–99, 2005.

14. Describe Panner disease.

Panner disease is osteochondrosis of the capitulum. The etiology is unclear, but it is seen most often in young boys. Patients present with tenderness and swelling over the lateral aspect of the elbow with limited extension. Radiographs show patchy areas of sclerosis and lucency, which may appear fragmented. Treatment includes immobilization with a long arm cast, followed by protected motion.

15. Describe a Galeazzi's fracture.

It is a fracture of the distal radial shaft with a dislocation or subluxation of the inferior radioulnar joint.

Forearm fractures in children: http://Orthoinfo.aaos.org

16. What is Monteggia's fracture?

It is a fracture of the upper third of the ulna and dislocation of the head of the radius. It is classified based on location and displacement of the radius.

Forearm fractures in children: http://Orthoinfo.aaos.org

17. What is boxer's elbow? What causes it?

Also known as **hyperextension overload syndrome** or **olecranon impingement syndrome**, boxer's elbow is caused by repetitive valgus extension of the elbow in the boxer's jab or in sports that involve throwing.

18. **What is the terrible triad? Describe surgical treatment and postoperative rehabilitation.**

    The terrible triad is an elbow fracture dislocation that includes radial head fracture, coronoid fracture of the olecranon, and tearing of the medial and/or lateral collateral ligaments. The elbow is extremely unstable and poor results are common. Surgical intervention is the treatment indicated. The surgery involves repair of the torn ligaments and open reduction and internal fixation of the radial head and coronoid fracture, most commonly with plates or screws. If the radial head is not able to be repaired, then a radial head metallic prosthesis is placed. Postoperative rehabilitation includes splinting for 1 day and then active and active-assisted ROM exercises. Forearm pronation and supination are done with the elbow in a flexed position. The last 30 degrees of elbow extension is avoided for 1 month. Then full unrestricted elbow flexion and extension is instituted.

    McKee MD, Pugh DMW, Wild LM, et al: Standard surgical protocol to treat elbow dislocations with radial head and coronoid fractures: Surgical technique. J Bone Joint Surg 87A:22–32, 2005.

19. **What is posterolateral rotatory elbow instability? What is the main structure involved?**

    Posterolateral rotatory instability is the subluxation of the radial head posteriorly and rotatory subluxation of the ulna on the humeral articulation. The stress maneuver to confirm the diagnosis on physical examination is with the elbow flexed 40 degrees and the forearm supinated; valgus stress and compressive load are placed on the elbow. As the radius subluxes out of the joint, a dimpling of the skin may be seen at the lateral elbow region. The lateral ulnar collateral ligament of the elbow is the main stabilizer to the lateral aspect of the elbow, and disruption of this ligament leads to posterolateral rotatory instability.

    Chen FS, Diaz VA, Loenberg M, Rosen J: Shoulder and elbow injuries in the skeletally immature athlete. J Am Acad Orthop Surg 13:172–185, 2005.

20. **What is osteochondritis desiccans of the elbow?**

    This idiopathic condition affects the capitulum of the humerus, with ensuing avascular necrosis. It is usually seen in the dominant arm of teenage boys involved in throwing sports. It is characterized by poorly localized elbow pain. The radial head is sometimes involved. Treatment includes immobilization followed by gentle ROM exercises.

    Cain EL Jr., Dugas JR, Wolf RS, Andrews JR: Elbow injuries in throwing athletes: A current concept review. Am J Sports Med 32:621–635, 2003.

    Peterson RK, Savoie FH III, Field LD: Osteochondritis dissecans of the elbow. Instr Course Lect 48:393–398, 1999.

21. **Describe myositis ossification.**

    It occurs after injury to muscle fibers, connective tissue, and blood vessels underlying the periosteum and presents with a triad of symptoms: pain, palpable mass, and flexion contracture. It is most common in the brachioradialis of the elbow and in males 15–30 years of age.

22. **What is heterotopic ossification of the elbow?**

    Heterotopic ossification of the elbow is an abnormal growth of bone across the elbow joint and results in restricted motion. The causes include trauma to the elbow such as fractures and dislocations, burns, head trauma, etc. More information about heterotopic ossification is available elsewhere in this text.

    Hotchkiss RN: Elbow contracture. In Green DP, Hotchkiss JW, Pederson WC (eds): Green's Operative Hand Surgery, 4th ed. New York, Churchill Livingstone, 1999, pp 667–682.

WEBSITES

1. http://anatomy.med.umich.edu/limbs/forearm_tables.html

2. www.emedicine.com/SPORTS/fulltopic/topic87.htm

3. http://Orthoinfo.aaos.org

4. www.rad.washington.edu/atlas/

5. www.upstate.edu/cdb/grossanat/limbs4.shtml#Anchor-Chart-49575

6. www.wheelessonline.com/ortho/elbow_joint_menu

CHAPTER 45

THE WRIST AND HAND: ANATOMY, ASSESSMENT, AND TREATMENT

Jaywant J.P. Patil, MBBS, and Richard A. Rogachefsky, MD

The movement of the thumb underlies all the skilled procedures of which the hand is capable.
—John Napier (1550–1617)

1. **Name the carpal bones.**
   A "handy" mnemonic is **S**cared **L**overs **T**ry **P**ositions **T**hat **T**hey **C**annot **H**andle:

S = **S**caphoid (1)	**T** = **T**rapezium (5)
L = **L**unate (2)	**T** = **T**rapezoid (6)
T = **T**riquetrum (3)	**C** = **C**apitate (7)
P = **P**isiform (4)	**H** = **H**amate (8)

   Numbers in parentheses refer to Fig. 45-1.

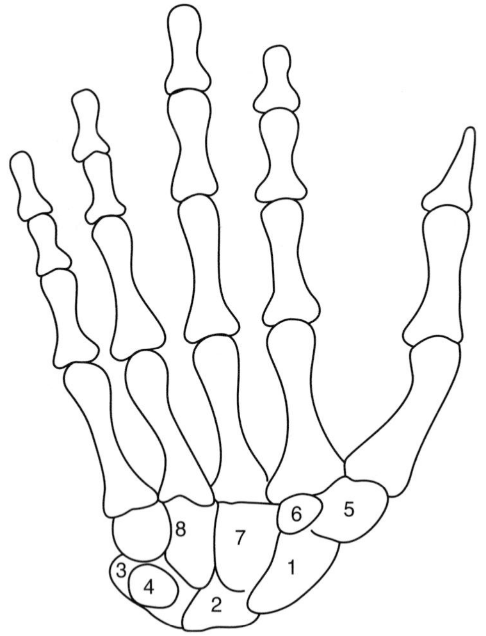

Figure 45-1. Bones of hand and wrist.

2. **What structures are found in the dorsum of the hand?**
    The **extensor tendons** of the hand are divided into six dorsal compartments. From radial to ulnar, they are as follows:
    1. Abductor pollicis longus, extensor pollicis brevis
    2. Extensor carpi radialis longus, extensor carpi radialis brevis
    3. Extensor pollicis longus
    4. Extensor digitorum communis, extensor indices proprius
    5. Extensor digiti minimi
    6. Extensor carpi ulnaris

3. **Describe the key actions of the interossei muscles.**
    Remember **dab** and **pad**:
    ■ **dab** = **d**orsal interossei—**ab**duct and assist in metacarpophalangeal (MCP) flexion
    ■ **pad** = **p**almar interossei—**ad**duct and assist in MCP flexion

4. **What are the borders of the anatomic snuff box?**
    ■ Floor: **S**caphoid bone
    ■ Radial border: **A**bductor pollicis longus and extensor pollicis brevis
    ■ Ulnar border: **E**xtensor pollicis longus.

    Cailliet R: Functional anatomy. In Cailliet R (ed): Hand Pain and Impairment, 4th ed. Philadelphia, F.A Davis, 1994.

5. **Where is "no man's land" in the hand?**
    This is the area of the hand where the flexor tendons (i.e., the flexor profundus and sublimis) are tightly enclosed within the tenosynovium. It is located in the palm between the distal palmar crease and the crease of the proximal interphalangeal (PIP) joints in the palm. Generally, primary repair of the tendons in this region is contraindicated.

    Cailliet R: Common tendonitis problems of the hand and forearm. In Cailliet R (ed): Hand Pain and Impairment, 4th ed. Philadelphia, F.A Davis, 1994.

6. **Explain how lumbrical muscle function is related to its anatomy.**
    Because the lumbrical muscles originate from the tendons of the flexor digitorum profundus and insert into the extensor hood tendons, their main action is flexion of the MCP joints and extension at the interphalangeal (IP) joints.

    Conolly B, Prossor R: Functional anatomy and assessment. In Prossor R, Conolly B (eds): Rehabilitation of Hand and Upper Limb. New York, Butterworth-Heinemann, 2003.

KEY POINTS: FUNCTION OF THE INTRINSIC MUSCLES OF THE HAND

1. Lumbricals flex the metacarpophalangeal joint but extend the interphalangeal joints.

2. Palmar interossei adduct the fingers.

3. Dorsal interossei abduct the fingers.

---

7. **How do you test the integrity of the flexor digitorum superficialis tendon?**
    Perform the superficialis test to assess the tendon's integrity. (Keep in mind that the flexor digitorum superficialis flexes the PIP joint.) While the examiner holds the adjacent fingers in full

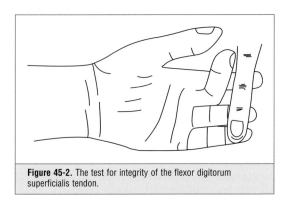

Figure 45-2. The test for integrity of the flexor digitorum superficialis tendon.

extension, the patient flexes the problematic finger (Fig. 45-2). If there is no injury or tear in the flexor digitorum superficialis tendon, the patient is able to flex the PIP joint, while the distal interphalangeal (DIP) joint remains in extension or neutral.

Hoppenfeld S: Physical Exam of the Spine and Extremities. Norwalk, CT, Appleton & Lange, 1999.

8. **How can you test the integrity of the flexor digitorum profundus tendon to one particular finger?**
In this test, the MCP and PIP joints are held in extension by the examiner while the patient flexes the DIP joints. If the patient is able to flex, then the long flexor (or the profundus tendon) to that finger is intact.

Hoppenfeld S: Physical Exam of the Spine and Extremities. Norwalk, CT, Appleton & Lange, 1999.

9. **What type of deformity results from edema in the hand due to burns, and how does one prevent this from occurring?**
Edema is one of the main causes of a typical claw-hand deformity, which includes hyperextension of the MCP joints, flexion of the proximal and DIP joints, and the thumb experiencing adduction and external rotation deformity. Antideformity splints that hold the wrist in slight extension can be helpful. Edema can be treated by elevating the arm and performing active exercises.

Helm PA, Fisher S: Rehabilitation of patients with burns. In Delisa J (ed): Rehabilitation Medicine: Principles and Practice, 2nd ed. Philadelphia, J.B Lippincott, 1988.

10. **How is the Finkelstein test performed?**
The patient flexes the thumb into the palm of the hand and folds the fingers over the thumb. The examiner then twists the wrist inward (ulnar deviation). This maneuver maximizes tension on the abductor pollicis longus and extensor pollicis brevis tendon (Fig. 45-3). In deQuervain's disease (stenosing tenosynovitis), pain is reproduced over the radial wrist. This condition is commonly seen in women aged 30–50 years.

Cailliet R: Common tendonitis problems of the hand and forearm. In Cailliet R (ed): Hand Pain and Impairment, 4th ed. Philadelphia, F.A Davis, 1994.

11. **What is Froment's sign?**
Although the adductor pollicis is paralyzed in ulnar nerve lesions, the movements of palmar and ulnar adduction can still be performed. Grasping an object such as a piece of paper between the thumb and the edge of the palm is accomplished by flexing the thumb at the IP joint by

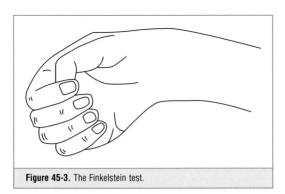

Figure 45-3. The Finkelstein test.

means of the flexor pollicis longus, which is supplied by the median nerve. This is described as a positive Froment's sign.

Cailliet R: Nerve control of the hand: In Cailliet R (ed): Hand Pain and Impairment, 4th ed. Philadelphia, F.A Davis, 1994.

12. **Name the two different types of grips in the hand.**
   - **Prehension,** which includes pinch, tip, and lateral grip
   - **Power,** which includes hook, grasp, and palmar grip

13. **Describe the Bunnell-Littler test.**
   This test evaluates the tightness of the intrinsic muscles of the hand (lumbricals and the interossei). To assess the tightness of the intrinsic muscles, hold the MCP joint in a few degrees of extension and try to move the PIP joint into flexion. If the PIP can be flexed in this position, the intrinsics are not tight. If the PIP joint cannot be flexed, either the intrinsics are tight or there are joint capsule contractures.

   Hoppenfeld S: Physical Exam of the Spine and Extremities. Norwalk, CT, Appleton & Lange, 1999.

14. **Briefly describe the autonomic innervation of the hand.**
   The sympathetic nerves arise from the stellate ganglion in the neck and control all the autonomic function of the hand and the upper limb. There are no parasympathetic fibers in the hand. Sympathetic nerves arise from the stellate ganglion in the neck. The post-ganglionic fibers travel mainly in the upper trunk of the brachial plexus, but some fibers also travel along blood vessels (the periarterial sympathetic plexus).

   Conolly B, Prossor R: Functional anatomy and assessment. In Prossor R, Conolly B (eds): Rehabilitation of Hand and Upper Limb. New York, Butterworth-Heinemann, 2003.

15. **What is a trigger finger?**
   Trigger finger occurs secondary to tenosynovitis involving the flexor tendon sheaths. The usual presentation is a fusiform swelling around the area of the flexor sublimis tendon in the vicinity of the metacarpal head. A constriction of the tendon sheath results in locking or obstruction of finger flexion.

   Finger locking often occurs in the morning. At times, a popping sensation may be perceived when the fingers go from the flexed to the extended position. This type of trigger finger could be associated with trauma, osteoarthritis, or inflammatory arthritis, such as rheumatoid arthritis.

   Cailliet R: Common tendonitis problems. In Cailliet R (ed): Hand Pain and Impairment, 4th ed. Philadelphia, F.A Davis, 1994.

16. **Name the two common deformities associated with rheumatoid arthritis in the hands, excluding ulnar deviation of the fingers. Describe the mechanism of the deformities.**
    - **Boutonnière deformity.** This includes hyperextension at the MCP joint, flexion at the PIP joint, and extension at the DIP joint (Fig. 45-4). Often in the rheumatoid process, there is weakness and tearing of the terminal portion of the extensor's hood, which tends to hold the lateral band in place. In this deformity the lateral bands tend to slip down, flex the PIP joint, and exert tension to hyperextend the DIP joint.
    - **Swan-neck deformity.** This often occurs as a result of contractures and shortening of the intrinsic muscles, which causes flexion at the MCP joint, hyperextension at the PIP joint, and flexion at the DIP joint (*see* Fig. 45-4). Contractures and spasms of the intrinsic muscles cause dorsal subluxation of the tendons that results in hyperextension of the PIP joint. Synovitis further aggravates hyperextension by causing laxity of that joint. Flexion and tension on the long flexor cause flexion of the DIP joint.

    Conolly B, Prossor R: Rheumatoid arthritis. In Prossor R, Conolly B (eds): Rehabilitation of Hand and Upper Limb. New York, Butterworth-Heinemann, 2003.

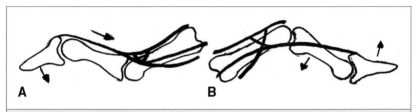

Figure 45-4. Swan-neck **(A)** and Boutonnière **(B)** deformities.

17. **Describe the mechanism of ulnar deviation of the fingers in rheumatoid arthritis.**
    This deformity is often associated with ulnar deviation of the wrist. Basically, the flexor tendons enter the tunnel of the flexor pulley. In rheumatoid arthritis the mouth of the tunnel becomes more relaxed, which causes the flexor tendons to deviate more toward the ulnar side.

    Conolly B, Prossor R: Rheumatoid arthritis. In Prossor R, Conolly B (eds): Rehabilitation of Hand and Upper Limb. New York, Butterworth-Heinemann, 2003.

18. **Where are Heberden's nodes usually found?**
    These discrete but palpable bony nodules are found on the dorsal and lateral surfaces of the DIP joint and may be features of osteoarthritis. The nodules found in the PIP joint are called Bouchard's nodes.

    Hoppenfeld S: Physical Exam of the Spine and Extremities. Norwalk, CT, Appleton & Lange, 1999.

19. **Describe briefly the pathology in Dupuytren's contracture and indications for surgery.**
    Dupuytren's disease is a form of proliferative fibroplasias of the palmar fascial bands, which displaces the neurovascular bundles. This displacement then results in soft tissue and joint contractures in genetically susceptible individuals. Indications for surgery are mainly to restore hand function and/or to reduce disability. Surgery does not involve radical excision.

    Conolly B, Prossor R: Dupuytren's contracture. In Prossor R, Conolly B (eds): Rehabilitation of the Hand and Upper Limb. New York, Butterworth-Heinemann, 2003.

20. **What is a boxer's fracture?**
    This injury is more appropriately considered a street fighter's fracture because it results from an unskillful blow with a clenched fist. The blow fractures the neck of the fifth metacarpal bone.

    Conolly B, Prossor R: Hand and wrist injuries. In Prossor R, Conolly B (eds): Rehabilitation of Hand and Upper Limb. New York, Butterworth-Heinemann, 2003.

21. **Describe a Bennett's fracture.**
    In adults, a longitudinal force along the axis of the first metacarpal in the flexed thumb may produce a serious intra-articular fracture or dislocation of the carpometacarpal joint. A small triangular-shaped fragment at the base of the metacarpal remains in proper relationship to the trapezium, but the remainder of the metacarpal, which carries with it the majority portion of the joint surface, is dislocated and assumes a position of flexion.

    Conolly B, Prossor R: Hand and wrist injuries. In Prossor R, Conolly B (eds): Rehabilitation of Hand and Upper Limb. New York, Butterworth-Heinemann, 2003.

22. **Who usually gets a scaphoid fracture?**
    Fracture of the carpal scaphoid is relatively common in young adults, particularly males. The injury responsible for the fracture is usually a fall on the open hand, with the wrist dorsiflexed and radially deviated. This fracture is frequently overlooked at the time of injury and is usually dismissed as a sprain. Scaphoid fracture can be associated with serious complications, including avascular necrosis, delayed union, nonunion, and post-traumatic degenerative joint disease.

    Conolly B, Prossor R: Hand and wrist injuries. In Prossor R, Conolly B (eds): Rehabilitation of Hand and Upper Limb. New York, Butterworth-Heinemann, 2003.

23. **Who gets Kienböck's disease?**
    Osteochondrosis or avascular necrosis of the lunate occurs most frequently in young adults and may be secondary to trauma. The disease often affects workers such as carpenters and riveters.

    Prossor R, Herbert T: Carpal fractures. In Prossor R, Conolly B (eds): Rehabilitation of Hand and Upper Limb. New York, Butterworth-Heinemann, 2003.

24. **How could a gamekeeper and a skier possibly develop the same sort of thumb injury?**
    Both gamekeeper's thumb and skier's thumb are caused by forcible abduction of the thumb associated with injury to the ulnar collateral ligament of the first MCP. Gamekeeper's thumb earned its name from British gamekeepers who sustained this injury when shooting rabbits. A skier who falls is at risk for an injury through a similar mechanism.

    Scougall P, Prossor R: Metacarpal and phalangeal fractures. In Prossor R, Conolly B (eds): Rehabilitation of Hand and Upper Limb. New York, Butterworth-Heinemann, 2003.

25. **What does the absence of "okay" sign mean?**
    The inability to make an "okay" sign demonstrates the absence of flexion of the IP joint of the thumb and the DIP joint of the index finger, and therefore the inability to make an "okay" sign may signal a deficit in the anterior interosseus nerve innervated muscles.

26. **How is deQuervain's tenosynovitis treated?**
    Conservative management includes a thumb spica splint, corticosteroid injection, nonsteroidal inflammatory drugs, activity modification, therapeutic modalities (Coban wrap for edema, ice massage over the radial styloid, phonophoresis with 10% hydrocortisone), and gentle passive and active range of motion. If surgical decompression is required, IP joint motion starts immediately after surgery. The presurgical spica splint may be worn for 2 weeks and may be needed for postoperative hypersensitivity.

27. **What type of tendon transfers are commonly done to restore finger flexion in a tetraplegic patient?**
Patients with tetraplegia lack finger and thumb flexion. To restore finger flexation, the extensor carpi radialis longus tendon that performs wrist extension is transferred to the flexor digitorum profundus tendons of the index, long, ring, and small fingers. The brachioradialis is transferred to the flexor of the thumb to restore thumb flexion.

28. **What is the postoperative protocol after tendon transfers are done to restore finger flexion in a tetraplegic patient?**
The arm is immobilized in a long arm cast for 4 weeks with the wrist slightly flexed, the finger flexed to 70 degrees at the MCP joint, the PIP joints in extension, and the thumb in abduction for 4 weeks. After that, the patient is started on active and passive motion and is placed in a wrist-control Polyform splint. Strengthening exercises are started at 3 months postoperatively.

Ejeskar A, Dahlgrin A, Friden J: Clinical and radiographic evaluation of surgical reconstruction of finger flexion in tetraplegia. J Hand Surg 30A:842–849, 2005.

29. **What is a mallet finger? What is the nonsurgical treatment protocol?**
A mallet finger is a rupture of the insertion of the extensor tendon's form at the base of the distal phalanx. The patient is unable to extend the DIP joint, which sits in a flexed position. Treatment for mallet finger is 6 weeks in a volar static splint with the DIP joint in 10 degrees of hyperextension. Afterward, the patient starts on active and passive range of motion at the DIP joint. The patient continues to wear the volar static splint at night for 2 more weeks.

Bendre A, Harrigan B, Kalainov D: Mallet finger. J Am Acad Orthop Surg 13:336–344, 2005.

30. **Describe the treatment for first carpometacarpal arthritis and the postsurgical rehabilitation protocol.**
When the degenerative arthritis is mild, treatment is a short opponens thumb splint to restrict the motion of the carpometacarpal joint and thereby relieve pain. In cases of severe arthritis, operative intervention is recommended and includes excision of the trapezium, reconstruction of the volar ligament with the flexor carpi radialis (FCR) tendon to stabilize the base of the first metacarpal, and placement of the rest of the FCR tendon in the trapezial space as a spacer cushion. Postoperatively, the hand is kept in a thumb spica cast for approximately 5–6 weeks. When the cast is removed, active and passive range-of-motion exercises are performed to increase thumb motion. Strengthening exercises are started approximately 8 weeks later.

Young SD, Mikola EA: Thumb carpometacarpal arthrosis. J Am Soc Surg Hand 4:73–93, 2004.

WEBSITES

1. www.apta.org/AM/Template.cfm?Section=Home&CONTENTID=24768&TEMPLATE=/CM/MLDisplay.cfm

2. www.assh.org/Content/NavigationMenu/PatientsPublic/HandConditions/Default798.htm

3. www.nlm.nih.gov/medlineplus/handinjuriesanddisorders.html

4. http://orthoinfo.aaos.org/category.cfm?topcategory=Hand

THE HIP: ANATOMY, PATHOLOGY, DIAGNOSIS, TREATMENT, AND REHABILITATION

Michael A. Mont, MD, German A. Marulanda, MD, Ronald E. Delanois, MD, Thorsten M. Seyler, MD, and Alan Friedman, MD

Live long enough, and you will win a measure of this ailment which has, more than any other, come to be synonymous with the decay of aging. That it is most apparent in the spine and hips is no more than the wages we are made to pay for the sins of our forefathers.
  –Richard Selzer, describing osteoarthritis in *Mortal Lessons: Notes on the Art of Surgery*

1. **Why is the hip joint so stable?**
   The hip joint is a multiaxial ball-and-socket joint comprising a femoral and acetabular component. The femoral head forms approximately two thirds of a sphere and inserts deeply into the acetabulum, which is approximately half a sphere. The fibrocartilaginous labrum of the acetabulum contributes to the depth of the "socket." A tough joint capsule surrounds the articulating surfaces and provides further stability. Muscles play less of a role in providing joint stability at the hip than they do at other joints.

2. **What is the price of this joint stability?**
   The hip joint has a high degree of stability at the expense of some movement. In contrast, the glenohumeral joint has greater freedom of movement but less stability.

3. **What are the named ligaments of the capsule of the hip joint?**
   There are three named ligaments (or thickenings) of the capsule:
   - **Iliofemoral** ligament (Y ligament of Bigelow), which is considered the strongest ligament in the body
   - **Ischiofemoral** ligament
   - **Pubofemoral** ligament

4. **In which direction is the hip most likely to dislocate?**
   Posterior. The patient typically presents in severe pain with a hip fixed in adduction, flexion, and internal rotation. It is associated with sciatic nerve injury in 8–20% of cases. Evaluation should include testing of toe and ankle movement and sensory exam of the foot.

5. **How do anterior dislocations present?**
   Anterior dislocations present as painful hips that are fixed in abduction, flexion, and external rotation. There may be an associated femoral nerve injury.

6. **What are the innervation and blood supply to the hip joint? Why is this information clinically important?**
   The hip joint is supplied by multiple nerves, including the femoral nerve, obturator nerve, superior gluteal nerve, and the nerve to the quadratus femoris. Pain in the true hip joint frequently refers to the groin and other sensory distributions of these nerves. Blood supply to

the head of the femur comes from the branch of the obturator artery that passes through the ligament of the head of the femur, as well as from multiple branches that pierce the capsule, originating from the femoral circumflex arteries, superior gluteal artery, and obturator artery. These arteries are often damaged during fracture, making healing difficult.

7. **What is the most common site of osteonecrosis?**
The femoral head. However, the humeral head and distal femur are involved in 10–15% of osteonecrosis cases.

8. **What is hip dysplasia?**
Hip dysplasia is a comprehensive term that has been used to include a spectrum of related developmental hip problems in infants and children, often present at birth. Other frequently used terms include the following:
- Congenital hip dislocation: The hip is frankly dislocated at birth.
- Congenital dislocatable hip: The hip is in place at birth but dislocates fully when stressed.
- Congenital subluxable hip: The hip is in place but dislocates partially when stressed.
- Acetabular dysplasia: The hip socket is shallow and remains shallow, so that the hip is unstable.
- Developmental dysplasia (or dislocation) of the hip: This is a more widely accepted and recent term, reflecting the fact that some patients have apparently normal hips at birth but develop the problem in the first year of life.

9. **What is Legg-Calvé-Perthes disease?**
Legg-Calvé-Perthes disease is avascular necrosis of the femoral head. It usually occurs in children aged 5–12 years and may result from interruption of the vascular supply of the hip, leading to ischemic necrosis.

10. **What are common causes of a "snapping hip"?**
Snapping in and around the hip (coxa saltans) is sometimes felt when ligamentous structures about the hip travel over bony prominences during movement of the joint. The most common cause is a tight iliotibial band or gluteus maximus tendon riding over the greater tuberosity of the femur. This may happen during hip flexion or extension and is worsened if the hip is held in internal rotation or in the setting of trochanteric bursitis. Other sources of coxa saltans include the iliofemoral ligament riding over the femoral head and the iliopsoas tendon snapping over the pectineal eminence of the pelvis, over an osseus ridge of the lesser trochanter, or over the anterior acetabulum. Snapping hips also can be associated with intra-articular pathology, including acetabular labral tears or loose bodies. With intra-articular pathology, pain is localized to the groin and anterior thigh when pivoting movements occur. Clicking is felt and heard in hip extension and adduction with lateral rotation.

11. **What is SCFE or "hip slip"?**
A **s**lipped **c**apital **f**emoral **e**piphysis is typically seen in overweight adolescents, more commonly in males. Hormonal effects on epiphyseal plate development have been suggested as an etiologic factor. Onset is often insidious. There may be some initial hip stiffness, which is followed by a limp and then hip pain. The affected leg may become externally rotated. A true leg-length discrepancy may be noted. In later stages, blood supply to the head of the femur may be compromised, and avascular necrosis may result. Anteroposterior (AP) and lateral "frog leg" x-rays may show widening of the epiphyseal line or displacement of the femoral head. Orthopedic consultation is critical because SCFE is typically progressive, and surgical correction is often warranted.

12. **Name the most common cause of a painful hip in children younger than 10 years of age.**
Acute transient synovitis, which is usually nonspecific and self-limited.

13. **What is an intertrochanteric fracture?**
An intertrochanteric fracture occurs between the greater and lesser trochanters along the intertrochanteric line and outside the hip joint capsule. The treatment of choice is a sliding hip screw.

14. **What is meralgia paresthetica? How does it present? What are some causes?**
Pathology of the lateral femoral cutaneous nerve is commonly called meralgia paresthetica. Patients complain of pain, burning, or hypoesthesia over the anterolateral thigh. Common causes include entrapment under the inguinal ligament, surgical injury, acute blunt injury, and external pressure from belts or clothing. Pregnancy may worsen symptoms by changing the angle between the nerve and the inguinal ligament. Less common causes include hematomas and tumors.

15. **What causes of osteoarthritis in the hip may lead to a total hip arthroplasty (THA)?**
   - Idiopathic primary osteoarthritis
   - Slipped capital femoral epiphysis
   - History of trauma leading to joint incongruity
   - Rheumatoid arthritis
   - Developmental dysplasia of the hip
   - Osteonecrosis (avascular necrosis [AVN])
   - Other inflammatory arthritides

16. **Where are the most frequent sites of hip fracture in the elderly?**
Femoral neck and the intertrochanteric and subtrochanteric areas.

17. **What are the most common associated factors of avascular necrosis of the hip in adults?**
Steroid use and alcohol use account for approximately 90% of known associated factors of avascular necrosis in the patient population younger than age 45. Other conditions associated with osteonecrosis include myeloproliferative disorders, Gaucher disease, trauma, chronic pancreatitis, Caisson disease, sickle cell and other anemias, and radiation.

18. **What is the incidence of bilaterality for osteonecrosis?**
Literature shows an 80% risk of bilateral involvement. One side may be entirely asymptomatic.

19. **What are the different methods of evaluating osteonecrosis of the femoral head?**
Adequate AP and lateral radiographs are the first step in osteonecrosis evaluation. Magnetic resonance imaging (MRI) is the most sensitive and specific modality. Computed tomographic (CT) scan can be used to assess femoral head collapse. Invasive modalities include direct pressure measurements, venography, and biopsy.
   Note: Technetium scans have recently been shown to be less sensitive and less specific.

20. **Why and how is the Thomas test performed?**
The Thomas test is performed to assess flexion contracture of the hip. The patient lies supine on the examining table. To test the right hip, instruct the patient to maximally flex the left hip and knee. A positive result (flexion contracture) is present if the right thigh elevates above the table passively. If the right thigh is pushed down to the table and excessive passive lordosis of the spine occurs, this is also positive.

21. **What is the FABER test?**
    FABER stands for **fl**exion, **ab**duction, **e**xternal **r**otation. This nonspecific test (also known as the Patrick test) helps detect pathology in the hip and sacroiliac (SI) joint. The patient is in the supine position, and the foot of the tested side is placed on the knee of the opposite side. The tested hip is then lowered to a flexed, abducted, and externally rotated position (the "frog leg" position). Inguinal pain is suggestive of hip pathology. Increased pain elicited by increasing the range of motion (ROM) by placing pressure on the opposite anterior superior iliac spine suggests SI joint pathology.

22. **Why and how is the Ober test performed?**
    The Ober test is used to evaluate contracture of the tensor fasciae latae (TFL) and iliotibial band. The patient lies on his or her side with the lower leg flexed at the hip and knee for stability. The examiner flexes and abducts, then extends the patient's upper leg with the knee flexed to 90 degrees. The examiner then releases the upper leg. If a contracture is present, the upper leg will remain abducted and will not fall to the table.

23. **What changes in the physical exam are noted in hip osteoarthritis?**
    The typical first sign of osteoarthritis is loss of internal rotation, followed by loss of flexion and extension, and eventually contracture. An antalgic gait and abductor lurch (swaying of the trunk over the side of the affected hip) also may be noted.

24. **What is the Garden classification of fractures?**
    See Table 46-1.

TABLE 46-1. GARDEN CLASSIFICATION OF FEMORAL NECK FRACTURES	
Grade	**Description**
I	Incomplete or impacted fractureTrabeculae of the inferior neck still intact
II	Complete fracture without displacementFracture lines across entire femoral neckSlight varus deformityDisplacement will occur unless internally fixed
III	Complete fracture with partial displacementNeeds reductionShortening and external rotation of distal fragment often occursIncomplete displacement between femoral fragments
IV	Complete fractured with total displacementNo continuity between proximal and distal fragmentsAcetabulum and the femoral head are aligned

25. **Why should a patient with unilateral hip osteoarthritis carry a cane on the unaffected side?**
    It decreases pelvic drop on the side of the cane. This decreases the load on the affected hip and the amount of work the gluteus medius-minimus complex has to accomplish. (A cane on the ipsilateral side does not effectively reduce either of these.) This is consistent with a normal physiologic gait because the upper limb will be moving in concert with the opposite and advancing lower limb.

26. **Discuss the symptoms and treatment of trochanteric bursitis.**
    Classic symptoms of trochanteric bursitis include gradual onset pain in the bursa region, pain on arising in the morning, aggravation of pain during ambulation, and an antalgic gait. Pain can

radiate down the lateral aspect of the leg and into the buttock. Thus the syndrome is sometimes confused with sciatica. Physical exam will reveal point tenderness over the greater trochanter, which can be exacerbated by external rotation and abduction of the hip. Conservative treatment includes anti-inflammatories and an iliotibial band–stretching program. Injection of local anesthetic and corticosteroids into the bursa may relieve symptoms.

27. **What are treatment options for femoral neck fractures?**
For patients younger than 65, femoral neck fractures that are impacted, nondisplaced, or adequately reduced should be fixed internally with screws or pins. For patients older than 65, a fixed unipolar or bipolar endoprosthesis may be used when satisfactory reduction and fixation cannot be achieved. Endoprosthesis is favored if rheumatoid, degenerative, or malignant disease has caused preexisting articular damage.

28. **What are some significant complications after total hip replacement, and how often do they occur?**
The most common hip replacement complication is usually thromboembolic disease, including deep venous thrombosis (DVT) and pulmonary embolism (PE). PEs are the leading cause of death after hip replacement. Aside from death, the most significant long-term complication is aseptic loosening of the prosthesis (either the femoral or acetabular component). Heterotopic ossification can occur in up to 50% of cases, but only a small percentage will experience loss of motion.

29. **How does loosening of the hip prosthesis present? How is it usually detected?**
Loosening at the cement-bone or cement-prosthesis interface presents with new onset of thigh or groin pain that worsens during transfers and early ambulation. Plain x-rays may pick up a bone cement lucency >2 mm wide.

30. **For a patient requiring ipsilateral hip and knee replacements, in which order should the surgeon proceed?**
The hip should be replaced first because (1) it may rule out a source of referred knee pain from the hip, (2) it is easier to rehabilitate a hip arthroplasty with a diseased knee than the other way around, and (3) some orthopedists believe there is less chance of damage to a prosthetic hip when replacing a knee than to a prosthetic knee when replacing a hip.

31. **What is an osteotomy?**
A hip osteotomy is a surgical procedure in which the bones of the hip joint are cut, reoriented, and fixed in a new position. Healthy cartilage is placed in the weight-bearing area of the joint, followed by reconstruction of the joint in a more normal position.

32. **How does an intertrochanteric osteotomy affect the leg length?**
Open valgus osteotomy generally lengthens the limb; varus osteotomy usually shortens the limb.

33. **Who is the ideal patient for hip arthrodesis?**
Young adults or older adolescents with end-stage arthritis who are engaged in heavy labor types of work are the ideal type of patients for a hip arthrodesis.

34. **What are the indications for hip arthroscopy?**
- Removal of loose bodies
- Repair of torn labrum
- Synovitis (the synovial lining of the hip joint is inflamed, causing disabling pain that may be relieved by a synovectomy)
- Palliative treatment to buy time for a future hip arthroplasty

35. **What is the difference between THA and hemiarthroplasty?**
A THA resurfaces the femoral head and neck and acetabulum. A hemiarthroplasty replaces the femoral head and neck only.

36. **What are the indications for total hip arthroplasty?**
The goal of hip arthroplasty is to relieve pain, correct deformity, and restore ROM and function. Indications include severe degenerative changes and failure of nonoperative treatment for 3–6 months. Occasionally, THA is chosen when a fracture of the femoral head or neck cannot be repaired or repair has little chance for clinical success (e.g., an 80-year-old with a severely displaced femoral neck fracture).

37. **What is metal-on-metal hip resurfacing?**
Hip resurfacing is a surgical alternative to conventional hip arthroplasty. The femoral head is reshaped to accept a metal cap with a small guide stem. The head size is approximately 50 mm in diameter and a metal cup is set into the acetabulum.

38. **What are the advantages to the use of metal on resurfacing devices?**
   - Femoral head is preserved.
   - Femoral canal is preserved and there is no associated femoral bone loss with future revision.
   - Larger size of implant "ball" reduces the risk of dislocation significantly.
   - Stress is transferred in a natural way along the femoral canal and through the head and neck of the femur. With the standard total hip replacement, some patients experience thigh pain because the bone has to respond and reform to less natural stress loading.
   - Use of metal rather than plastic may reduce osteolysis and associated early loosening risk.

39. **What are the disadvantages to the use of metal devices?**
   - Lack of long-term follow-up: Current device has only been used for approximately 7 years.
   - Despite known low wear rate, longevity and long-term effects of wear debris are unknown.
   - For some surgeons, the procedure has a longer surgical time.
   - The procedure requires somewhat more skill of surgeon (learning curve).

40. **What are the different bearing surfaces available for THAs?**
   - Metal-on-metal (cobalt-chrome alloy)
   - Ceramic-on-ceramic
   - Ceramic-on-polyethylene
   - Metal-on-polyethylene

41. **What are the recently publicized concerns with ceramic-on-ceramic fractures?**
Recent use of ceramic-on-ceramic resurfacing devices has led to very low fracture rates where the reported risk is 0.015%, which should not be a concern. Ninety percent of fractures occur within 3 years of implantation.

42. **What are the recently publicized concerns about metal ion toxicity?**
Metal ion concentrations have been found to be increased in patients with metal-on-metal prostheses, but these increases have been maintained over 6–7 year follow-up and have not caused problems. There have been no reports of adverse toxic effects of these metal-on-metal devices, so this still should be known, but it only represents a minor concern.

43. **Are there any advantages to the use of so-called large femoral heads?**
Large femoral heads may have advantages of reducing dislocation rates and wear and improving range of motion. Various companies have developed these large femoral heads, mostly with

metal-on-metal devices, although various other metal-on-plastic or ceramic-on-ceramic units have larger heads that have been previously used.

44. **What are minimally invasive approaches to the hip?**
Minimally invasive approaches to the hip involve less tissue disruption through smaller skin incisions. There are two incision approaches—small posterolateral and small anterolateral. Most studies have shown no difference in outcome, and some studies have shown increased complication rates. Minimally invasive approaches are still being studied, and certainly the field has led to smaller incisions. At this point, small incision may have no advantage except for a cosmetic one.

45. **Define weight-bearing.**
Body weight supported through the affected limb is measured by placing the limb on a weight scale and applying force (*see* Table 46-2).

TABLE 46-2. DEFINITION OF WEIGHT-BEARING STATUS	
Weight-Bearing	**Percentage of Body Weight**
None	0
Toe-touch weight-bearing	Up to 20
Partial weight-bearing	20–50
Weight-bearing as tolerated	50–100
Full weight-bearing	100

46. **How does mode of fixation affect rehabilitation?**
Patients with cemented prostheses are capable of bearing full weight immediately after surgery because the cement reaches 90% of its strength 10–15 minutes after mixing. Patients with a porous ingrowth prosthesis should be on protected weight-bearing up to 12 weeks.

47. **Why should physiatrists be aware of the surgical approach used in a hip arthroplasty?**
Because muscle groups should be targeted according to approach. The lateral approach involves splitting the hip abductors (gluteus medius and minimus) with repair back to the greater trochanter or trochanteric osteotomy with repair of the osteotomy. The hip abductors should be a target of strengthening. The posterior approach involves splitting the gluteus maximus and releasing the short external rotators, which are repaired. The hip extenders and the short external rotators are targeted.

48. **How long will patients have significant pain after hip surgery?**
Arthritis pain is typically eliminated immediately. Surgical pain can last 2–3 weeks. Pain may be elicited by activities and ambulation for several months depending on various factors, such as preoperative deformity and degree of muscle atrophy. It may take months to rebuild muscle mass and strength to reduce activity-related pain.

49. **Can patients return to playing sports after hip replacement surgery?**
Most patients can return to low-impact sports (e.g., golf, doubles tennis, bowling, walking, and using exercise machines). High-impact exercises (running, singles tennis, basketball, volleyball, and football) should be avoided because they may lead to excessive wear of the prosthesis.

50. **When will the patient receive full benefit after hip arthroplasty?**
Typically by 3 months, the patient will have regained most of his or her strength across the joint and ROM. By 1 year, the patient usually will have achieved full benefit from the operation.

51. **Describe a general management approach in a patient with total hip arthroplasty.**
See Table 46-3.

TABLE 46-3. SCHEDULED REHABILITATION MANAGEMENT OF THA

Schedule	Management
Day of surgery	Deep breathing exercises, incentive spirometry, active ankle ROM exercises
Postoperative day 1	Quadriceps isometric exercises, gluteus muscle isometrics (depending on surgical approach), maintain hips in abduction, active-assisted and knee flexion exercises as tolerated
Postoperatives day 2–6 Cemented THA Bony ingrowth THA Trochanteric osteotomy	Begin ambulation with a walker or crutches, progressive gait trainingBegin reconditioning exercises to unaffected limbs; transfers to the unaffected sideToe-touch weight-bearing for 6 weeks; advance to weight-bearing as tolerated (WBAT)If secure reattachment, start WBAT; if tenuous, partial weight-bearingInstruct on hip precautions, energy conservation, and work simplification techniquesActive-assisted exercise; progress to active ROM motion and strengthening exercisesTeach adaptive ADLs
Weeks 1–12	Add light resistance exercises; hip flexor stretches; emphasize transfers—begin on affected sideProgressive strengthening and ranging of the trunk, hip, and kneeClosed kinetic chain exercisesImprove endurance and gait patternEliminate the use of assistive devicesPool therapy, bicycling, long-distance walking, progressive stair climbing, and isotonic exercises with weights are encouraged
Postoperative month 3	Follow-up visitFocus on level and location of pain, daily walking distance, sitting or standing duration, use of assistive devices, stair climbing method, analgesics, and community reintegration

ADLs = activities of daily living, ROM = range of motion, THA = total hip arthroplasty.

52. **How long should a patient maintain total hip precautions?**
From 10–12 weeks. This allows for a pseudocapsule to form and soft tissue to heal. Incidence of dislocation is reduced by greater than 95% after 12 weeks. The use of an anterior approach to the hip may further reduce the incidence of dislocation.

KEY POINTS: REHABILITATION AFTER HIP REPLACEMENT

1. Hold cane on the opposite side of the affected hip.

2. Hip precautions and weight-bearing status are crucial to initial postoperative rehabilitation.

3. Monitor for neuropathy.

4. Maintain total hip precautions for 10–12 weeks.

---

53. **How should a patient negotiate stairs after hip surgery?**
"Up with the good and down with the bad." When going up stairs, the patient should lead with the nonoperative extremity and follow with crutches and operative extremity. When descending, he or she should lead with crutches and the operative extremity and follow with the nonoperative extremity.

54. **What are the most common causes of falls after hip surgery?**
Decreased visual acuity and balance sensation in the elderly population are the most common causes of falls. Accident prevention tips should be stressed. An in-home visit for safety should be considered. Throw rugs, thick carpets, and poor lighting may cause stumbling and should be avoided. All rooms must be well-lit. The path from the bed to the bathroom is especially important, because many falls occur when trying to get to the bathroom at night.

55. **Do patients need prophylaxis for deep venous thrombosis after hip replacement?**
The incidence of DVT after hip surgery is greater than 50% in most reports. It is standard to give some form of prophylaxis, which can include mechanical adjuncts such as support hose and pneumatic compression devices, and should be continued throughout hospitalization. Pharmacologic prophylaxis includes warfarin, heparin, and aspirin.

56. **Why should abduction pillows be utilized? When? For how long?**
An abduction pillow prevents dislocation of the hip prosthesis (adduction, internal rotation) while the patient is sleeping or resting in bed. It is used for the first 6–12 weeks.

57. **What is the sequence of ambulatory aids usually given to patients after THA?**
Parallel bars (days 1–2), crutches or a walker (first 6 weeks), and one crutch or cane (next 6 weeks). Greater than 70% of patients are ambulatory without an assistive device at the end of 3 months.

58. **Give four goals of occupational therapy after THA.**
   - Reestablish basic activities of daily living (ADLs) with modifications that keep the patient's ROM within the restricted limits
   - Teach joint protection
   - Review fall risks
   - Provide equipment with training

59. **Are resisted concentric exercises important after hip or knee surgery?**
For the first 6–8 weeks the patient can perform isometrics and active ROM exercises against gravity. Concentric exercises against resistance should be avoided. After 6–8 weeks, resisted open kinetic chain strengthening with 1–10 lb can begin. Heavier weights cause undue wear on the prosthetic components.

60. **How do you assess flexion contracture of the hip?**
The Thomas test. The patient tries to lower the extremity flat on the examination table while holding the opposite thigh against the abdomen. The test is positive if the hip does not extend fully.

61. **What are the surgical indications and rehabilitations for the various hip fracture types?**
See Table 46-4.

TABLE 46-4. SURGICAL PROCEDURES AND REHABILITATION WEIGHT-BEARING STATUS FOR HIP FRACTURES

Fractures and Type	Surgical Procedure	Weight-bearing Status
Femoral neck		
Displaced fracture (Garden III and IV)	Hemiarthroplasty; ORIF (in younger patients)	WBAT
Undisplaced and impacted fractures (Gardens I and II)	ORIF	Depends on the stability of surgical fixation
Intertrochanteric		
Undisplaced, displaced two-part fractures, or unstable three-part fractures	Treated operatively with multiple pins or screws and side-plate devices	Depends on degree of fracture stabilization, bone stock, patient's frailty, and risks of immobilityMost patients are WBAT
Subtrochanteric		
Simple, fragmented, or comminuted	ORIF with a blade plate and screws or an intramedullary nail	Delayed until fracture demonstrates evidence of healing

ORIF = open reduction and internal fixation, WBAT = weight-bearing as tolerated.

62. **What are the negative predictors of ambulation after hip fracture?**
Negative predictors of ambulation after hip fracture include lack of social support, lower-limb contractures, age older than 85, and poor prefracture functional status. Generally, a patient will lose one level of function after a hip fracture. Inability to transfer or ambulate, incontinence, dementia, fewer hours of physical therapy, and lack of family involvement may require institutionalization.

63. **What are the major postoperative complications after THA that the physiatrist must be aware of during a rehabilitation program?**
Complications after THA include DVT (and PE), deep infection, and dislocation. The risk of all of these increases with a surgical revision compared to primary THA. Other complications include gastrointestinal (GI) (paralytic ileus), urinary retention, and neuropathy.

64. **What nerves may be damaged during THA surgery?**
The sciatic nerve is most often involved. The peroneal fibers tend to be more affected because of their relative outer location within the nerve. Femoral neuropathies can also occur.

65. **When can patients begin to drive?**
Patients who underwent a right THA and who use their right foot while driving in a vehicle with automatic transmission can usually begin to drive after 4–6 weeks. After a THA of the left side, 1 week is usually enough. However, total hip precautions must be maintained.

WEBSITES

1. http://orthopedics.about.com/cs/hipsurgery/a/hippain.htm

2. http://jointpaininfo.com

BIBLIOGRAPHY

1. Allen WC: Coxa saltans: The snapping hip revisited. J Am Acad Orthop Surg 3:303–308, 1995.

2. Bitar AA, Kaplan RJ, Stitik TP, et al: Rehabilitation of orthopedic and rheumatologic disorders. Total hip arthroplasty rehabilitation. Arch Phys Med Rehabil 86(3 Suppl 1):S56–S60, 2005.

3. Callaghan JJ, Dennis DA, Paprosky WG, Rosenberg AG (eds): Orthopedic Knowledge Update: Hip and Knee Reconstruction. Rosemont, IL, American Academy of Orthopaedic Surgeons, 1995.

4. Evarts CM (ed): Surgery of the Musculoskeletal System, 2nd ed, Vol. 3. New York, Churchill Livingstone, 1998.

5. Ganz SB, Levin AZ, Peterson MG, Ranawat CS: Improvement in driving reaction time after total hip arthroplasty. Clin Orthop 413:192–200, 2003.

6. Hoppenfeld S: Physical Examination of the Spine and Extremities. Norwalk, CT, Appleton & Lange, 1976.

7. Hoppenfeld S: Treatment and Rehabilitation of Fractures. Philadelphia, Lippincott Williams & Wilkins, 2000.

8. Kasser J (ed): Orthopedic Knowledge Update 5. Rosemont, IL, American Academy of Orthopaedic Surgeons, 1996.

9. Magee D: Orthopedic Physical Assessment. Philadelphia, W.B. Saunders, 1997.

10. Mont MA, Hungerford DS: Non-traumatic avascular necrosis of the femoral head. J Bone Joint Surg 77A:459–474, 1995.

CHAPTER 47

THE KNEE: ANATOMY, PATHOLOGY, DIAGNOSIS, TREATMENT, AND REHABILITATION

Michael E. Frey, MD, Bryan J. O'Young, MD, German A. Marulanda, MD, Michael A. Mont, MD, and Thorsten M. Seyler, MD

In matters of style, swim with the current; in matters of principle, stand like a rock.
—Thomas Jefferson (1743–1826)

1. **How does one view the knee from a musculoskeletal viewpoint?**
   The knee is the most complicated joint in the whole body. Its function is related to its gross bony anatomy, integrated muscular activity, and precise restrictive ligamentous structures. Despite its complex structure, one method of assessing the knee is by anatomically dividing it into anterior and posterior components, the ligamentous structures supporting the knee, and the meniscus in between (Fig. 47-1).

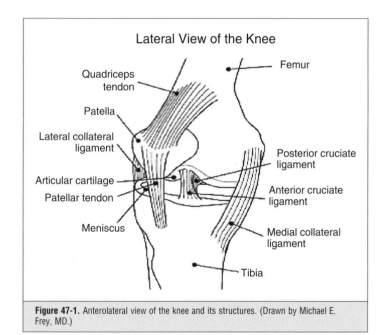

Figure 47-1. Anterolateral view of the knee and its structures. (Drawn by Michael E. Frey, MD.)

2. **What are the two primary joints of the knee?**
   - **Tibiofemoral:** Largest joint in the body; provides great range of motion (ROM) in flexion and extension, limited rotation, and minimal adduction and abduction

- **Patellofemoral:** Protects the anterior knee; provides a mechanical advantage for the quadriceps unit

3. **What anatomic structures may cause referred pain to the knee?**
   Lumbar spine, hip joint, sacroiliac joint, ankle joint, and/or foot

ANTERIOR KNEE

4. **What are some common conditions, other than meniscal and ligament injury, that can cause anterior knee pain?**
   See Table 47-1.

5. **Describe the typical signs and symptoms of patellofemoral pain.**
   - Anterior knee pain with gradual onset that worsens with repetitive knee flexion
   - Pain with prolonged sitting or on arising after sitting (positive theater sign)
   - Pain with squatting or with descending stairs

6. **What are treatment strategies for patellofemoral pain?**
   - Treatment should be directed at quadriceps (especially the vastus medialis obliques [VMO]) strengthening and flexibility stretching exercises, including the stretching of the quadriceps, hamstrings, iliotibial band (ITB), and gastrocsoleus muscles.
   - Initially, full-arc quadriceps exercises (0–90 degrees) should be avoided, and closed kinetic chain exercises with short-arc activities (0–45 degrees) emphasized.
   - Patella femoral taping is helpful.
   - Once quadriceps strength and flexibility are achieved, increased ROM exercise, such as bicycling, can be initiated.
   - It is important to assess excessive pronation or supination of the foot and determine if orthotics are necessary.
   - Surgery is rarely indicated and is considered in the case of persistent patellar instability.

7. **Identify two key abnormal positions of the patella.**
   - **Patella alta:** A high-riding patella (in a proximal direction to the joint level) or in relation to the femur. Patella alta is also seen in patellar tendon rupture. It can lead to pain, weakness, or inability to extend the knee.
   - **Patella baja:** Abnormally low patella that most often results from soft tissue contracture (scarring) and hypotonia of the quadriceps muscle (abnormal weak function) after surgery or trauma to the knee. Patella baja typically leads to a stiff and less functional knee.

8. **How does ITB "syndrome" present? How is it treated?**
   Clinical presentation
   - Lateral knee pain after excessive running, bicycling, or hiking. This may also occur as a lateral snapping hip.
   - Runners who present with symptoms typically state that faster running and sprinting do not cause this pain. The reason is that they spend more time with their knee at angles greater than 30 degrees.
   - Physical exam reveals tenderness at the lateral epicondyle of the femur, approximately 3 cm proximal to the joint line. Soft tissue swelling may be present, but there is no joint effusion.

   Treatment
   - Includes activity modification; protection, relative rest, ice, compression, elevation (PRICE) method; and possible corticosteroid injection.

TABLE 47-1. CONDITIONS OTHER THAN MENISCAL AND LIGAMENT INJURY THAT CAN CAUSE ANTERIOR KNEE PAIN

Diagnosis	Distinguishing Symptoms	Physical Findings/Comments	Treatment/Comments
Patellar tendinopathy	Squats (especially rapid) may exacerbate pain Patellar tendon pain	Tenderness along the inferior margin of the patella and pain on resisted quadriceps during contraction or squatting	Taping should have minimal to no effect Modify activities to reduce the load on the tendon Nonsteroidal anti-inflammatory drugs (NSAIDs) Low-resistance bicycling
Patellofemoral syndrome	Squats and/or stairs may aggravate patellofemoral joint (PFJ) Taping should decrease pain (see question 5)	Vague/nonspecific; may be medial, lateral, or infrapatellar (see question 5)	Orthotic bracing to correct pes planus or foot pronation Brace with patella opening Patella taping Closed kinetic chain quadriceps strengthening exercise Stretching of the quadriceps, hamstrings, iliotibial band (ITB) and gastrocsoleus muscles Surgery rarely indicated (see question 6)
Fat-pad impingement	Often, sudden onset anterior knee pain with hyperextension injury Does not respond well to stretching	Tenderness in fat-pad region behind the inferior pole of patella and deep to patellar tendon	Taping a "V" below the fat pad, with the point at the tibial tubercle, coming wide to the medial and lateral joint lines Tape is pulled toward the joint line and the skin is lifted toward the patella Muscle retraining to improve mechanics

Recurrent patellar subluxation	Subjective feeling of the patella slipping or moving laterally Knee buckling	Retinacular tenderness Patella alta Increased Q angle Patellar hypermobility Effusion Muscle atrophy	Quadriceps strengthening Specialized brace to control motion If conservative management fails, consider arthroscopic surgery
Synovial plica (see question 14)	Variable sharp pain located anteriorly (front), medially (inside edge), or posteriorly (at the back) of the patella or kneecap Pain may be sharp when squatting	Intermittent anterior knee pain Painful clicking with activity Buckling Palpable tender plica Definitive diagnosis of the condition is possible primarily through arthroscopy	Closed chain quadriceps kinetic exercise Hamstring stretching Knee stabilization brace If conservative management fails, consider arthroscopic surgery
Stress fracture of the patella	History of chronic anterior knee pain with tenderness over the patella	Patellar pain and difficulty in extending the knee Gold standard for diagnosis of a stress fracture is the bone scan	Non–weight-bearing exercise, such as swimming Bone stimulation, especially in poor healers (smokers, diabetic persons) If conservative management fails, consider surgery
Quadriceps tendinopathy	Tenderness along the superior margin of the patella and pain on resisted quadriceps contraction	Tenderness and swelling over the tubercle	Modify activities to reduce the load on the tendon NSAIDs Low-resistance bicycling Swimming

Continued

TABLE 47-1. CONDITIONS OTHER THAN MENISCAL AND LIGAMENT INJURY THAT CAN CAUSE ANTERIOR KNEE PAIN—CONT'D			
Diagnosis	Distinguishing Symptoms	Physical Findings/Comments	Treatment/Comments
Degenerative joint disease (see question 36)	Pain increases with loading; morning stiffness	Crepitus Limited range of motion Change in structural alignment Hallmark x-ray findings include asymmetric joint narrowing, sclerosis, cysts, and osteophytes	NSAIDs Medial or lateral unloading brace Cortisone injections Viscous supplementation Surgery, if conservative management fails
Common peroneal nerve entrapment	Tenderness over area of entrapment Pain may increase with exertion	Local tenderness over area of entrapment Positive nerve conduction test	Rest Elimination of triggering factors, such as leg crossing If associated with acute compartment syndrome, surgery may be warranted
ITB syndrome	Lateral knee pain after running (see question 8)	Tenderness at the lateral epicondyle of the femur, approximately 3 cm proximal to the joint line (see question 8)	Activity modification NSAIDs Rest, ice, compression, elevation (RICE) Friction massage Cortisone injection (see question 8)
Pes anserinus bursitis	Anterior medial knee pain (see question 9)	Tenderness at the superior medial tibia (see question 9)	NSAIDs RICE principle Cortisone injection

- Rehabilitation consists of ultrasound; electrical stimulation; increasing flexibility of the ITB, iliopsoas, gluteus maximus, quadriceps, and gastrocsoleus muscles; and correction of foot pronation.
- Final stages of rehabilitation include joint mobilization, strengthening weaker muscles, and videotaping to find biomechanical deficits.

9. What is pes anserinus syndrome?

Pes anserinus syndrome causes anterior medial knee pain because of friction of the sartorius, gracilis, and semitendinosus tendons on the medial aspect of proximal tibia, medial to the tuberosity of the tibia. Treatment includes applying the RICE principle and stretching of the medial hamstrings. Cortisone injections, which are often effective, may be indicated with failed conservative treatment.

10. What is osteochondritis dissecans (OCD)?

OCD is a fragmentation of the articular cartilage with subchondral bone, most commonly affecting the medial femoral condyle or patella. It can be a result of trauma but is often of unknown (idiopathic) etiology. It predominantly occurs in adolescent males. The usual presentation is stiffness and aching with an effusion. Sometimes it can be treated nonsurgically, but it may need to be treated operatively to prevent further joint collapse.

11. What is jumper's knee, and where is the most common location?

Jumper's knee is insertional tendinopathy (inflammation where the muscle joins the bone) of the quadriceps or the patellar tendons. The site of involvement is most commonly the inferior pole of the patella in 20- to 40-year-old patients. In patients older than 40, the quadriceps tendon is affected more frequently.

12. How do you treat jumper's knee?

- Nonoperative measures (RICE)
- NSAIDs such as aspirin or ibuprofen
- Ice massage after activity (control the swelling and inflammation)
- Strengthening the quadriceps (to balance the forces across the patella)
- Hamstring stretching (take pressure off the anterior structures of the knee)
- Neoprene sleeves or braces (similar to the ones used for tennis elbow)
- Surgery reserved for patients who experience pain for 6–12 months despite close adherence to treatment and for those who have suffered a complete tendon rupture

13. What is Osgood-Schlatter disease?

Apophysitis (abnormality) at the insertion of the patellar tendon into the tibial tubercle. Osgood-Schlatter disease is probably the most frequent cause of knee pain in children. It is always characterized by activity-related pain that occurs at the tibial tubercle. It usually responds to rest and gradual resumption of activities and does not require surgery.

14. What is plica?

Plica is the extra synovium ("remnant") present in the knee joint. During fetal development the knee is divided into three separate compartments. As the fetus develops, these compartments develop into one large cavity (synovial membrane). The majority of people have remnants of these three cavities, referred to as a plica. Most often the plica is on the medial (inside) of the knee at the level of the medial femoral condyle. Most individuals are not adversely affected by the presence of plicas. The plica only becomes a problem when there is an inflammation (thickening) in the synovial sack, causing it to catch on the femur as the knee moves (plica syndrome).

15. **What is the Q angle? How can it be reduced?**

The **quadriceps angle (Q angle)** or **patellofemoral angle** is the angle formed between a line drawn from the anterior superior iliac spine (ASIS) to the midpoint of the patella and a line drawn from the tibial tubercle to the midpoint of the patella with the hip and foot in neutral position. A normal angle is 13–18 degrees (although if the quadriceps is contracted, the normal angle is 8–10 degrees). The angle in men tends to be lower than in women. A higher end of the normal range indicates a tendency for added biomechanical stress during strenuous or repetitive activities using the knee. These problems are dependent on a number of factors, including habitual forces on the knee and other alignment abnormalities.

The most effective way **to decrease a high Q angle** and lower the biomechanical stresses on the knee joint is to prevent excessive pronation with orthotics. Stretching of tight muscles and strengthening of weak areas should be included in the therapeutic program. Muscles commonly found to be tight include the quadriceps, hamstrings, ITB, and gastrocnemius. The vastus medialis obliquus is usually weaker than the opposing vastus lateralis muscle. Strengthening may require special focus on the timing of muscle contractions. Closed-chain exercises (such as wall squats), performed only to 30 degrees of flexion, are currently recommended.

POSTERIOR KNEE

16. **What are some common conditions that can cause posterior knee pain?**

See Table 47-2.

17. **If kneeling in prayer causes vicar's knee and housework causes housemaid's knee, what causes a Baker's cyst?**

Housemaid's knee is a prepatellar bursitis related to excessive kneeling. Vicar's knee is a superficial infrapatellar bursitis. In children, Baker's cyst is usually congenital. In adults, it is usually secondary to an underlying articular pathology or trauma. By definition, it is a herniation of synovial tissue through a weakening posterior capsular wall that causes swelling in the popliteal fossa (popliteal cyst). The general population is susceptible. It is a response to events happening in the anterior aspect of the knee. It is not a "true" cyst.

18. **How does hamstring tendinitis present? How is it treated?**

Hamstring tendinitis is inflammation of the hamstring tendon as it attaches to the ischial tuberosity. It can follow a tear of a poorly treated hamstring tendon or, more often, is an overuse injury. Pain can occur anywhere within the muscular unit. The patient typically presents with pain and tenderness at the ischial tuberosity, pain when stretching the hamstring, pain when flexing the knee against resistance, or a gradual onset of pain after a sprinting session. Treatment consists of cold therapy, NSAIDs, and deep tissue sports massage techniques to decrease the incidence of fibrosis formation once the acute stage has passed.

LIGAMENT

19. **List the ligaments of the knee and their function.**
- **Anterior cruciate ligament (ACL):** Prevents anterior displacement of the tibia over the femur and provides rotational (torsional) stability
- **Posterior cruciate ligament (PCL):** Prevents the femur from sliding forward on the tibia (or the tibia from sliding backward on the femur)
- **Medial collateral ligament (MCL):** Connects the femur to the tibia and stabilizes the medial side of the knee
- **Lateral collateral ligament (LCL):** Connects the femur to the fibula and stabilizes the lateral side of the knee

TABLE 47-2. CONDITIONS THAT CAN CAUSE POSTERIOR KNEE PAIN

Diagnosis	Distinguishing Symptoms	Physical Findings/Comments	Treatment/Comments
Baker's cyst	Feeling of fullness in the popliteal fossa	Crescent sign May simulate venous thrombosis	NSAIDs RICE principle Surgery rarely indicated
Soft-tissue or bone tumor	Palpable mass Pain without weight-bearing	Limited knee flexion	Surgery or radiation, depending on type of tumor
Meniscal tear (see questions 33 and 34)	Increasing pain with deep knee flexion	Point joint-line tenderness Positive McMurray's test Possible joint effusion	Depending on the location and degree of tear: Bracing RICE principle NSAIDs Cortisone Consider surgery with persistent mechanical symptoms, including buckling, locking, or swelling with pain, if conservative management fails (see questions 34 and 35)
Hamstring injury (see question 18)	Posterior knee pain with sudden acceleration or deceleration	Tenderness at distal biceps femoris tendon Pain with knee flexion	NSAIDs RICE principle Running backward Swimming Most heal without surgery
Popliteus tendon injury	Pain with running downhill	Pain during knee flexion with internal rotation of the tibia in the prone position	NSAIDs RICE principle Running upward Ultrasound
Gastrocnemius tendinitis	Posterior knee pain with knee extension and dorsiflexion	Point tenderness in the proximal gastrocnemius tendon insertion	NSAIDs RICE principle Ultrasound Consider surgery if conservative management fails

Continued

TABLE 47-2. CONDITIONS THAT CAN CAUSE POSTERIOR KNEE PAIN—CONT'D

Diagnosis	Distinguishing Symptoms	Physical Findings/Comments	Treatment/Comments
Posterolateral corner injury	Varus thrust in stance or with ambulation, hyperextension, or external rotation (peroneal nerve could be injured)	Corner comprised of popliteus muscle, lateral collateral ligament, the posterolateral capsule, and the popliteofibular ligament Varus thrust Positive external recurvatum test (see question 25)	Depending on the degree of injury: Bracing RICE principle NSAIDs Cortisone Consider surgery if conservative management fails
Popliteal artery entrapment syndrome	Hypertrophy of calf muscles; claudication Paresthesias below the knee	Distal pulses may disappear with hyperextension and active plantar flexion or passive dorsiflexion Trophic changes below the knee Pulsatile mass	Vascular surgery, especially if aneurysm
Tibial nerve entrapment	Tenderness over area of entrapment Pain may increase with exertion	Local tenderness over area of entrapment Positive nerve conduction test	Unload pressure-sensitive area Consider surgery if causing weakness and significant pain
Degenerative joint disease (see question 36)	Pain increases with loading Morning stiffness	Crepitus; limited range of motion Change in structural alignment	NSAIDs Medial or lateral unloading brace Cortisone injections Viscous supplementation Consider surgery if conservative management fails
Postsurgical arthrofibrosis	Limited range of motion Stiffness	Limited knee extension	NSAIDs RICE principle PT to increase ROM Arthroscopic surgery

NSAIDs = nonsteroidal anti-inflammatory drugs; PT = physical therapy; RICE = rest, ice, compression, elevation; ROM = range of motion.
Adapted from Muché JA, Lento PH: Posterior knee pain and its causes. A clinician's guide to expediting diagnosis. Physician Sports Med 32(3):22–30, 2004.

20. **How should one approach the patient with an ACL injury?**
Patients typically develop a rapidly developing effusion (hemarthrosis) and "pop" sign, usually during a pivot motion. The most common tests are the Lachman, anterior drawer sign, and pivot shift test (*see* next question). In an acute injury, depending on the size of effusion, ACL injury may be difficult to assess. The gold standard imaging study is MRI (magnetic resonance imaging) of the knee. To prevent anterior subluxation of the tibia, rehabilitation should focus on the strengthening of the hamstrings and proprioceptive training. To prevent patellofemoral pain, a frequent occurrence after ACL injury, quadriceps should be strengthened through terminal-range squats. ACL reconstruction is considered depending on the patient's age, level of activity, expectations, degree of instability, and associated injuries.

KEY POINTS: GENERAL REHABILITATION PRINCIPLES FOR OSTEOARTHRITIS OF THE KNEE

1. Non–weight-bearing strengthening exercises should be emphasized, particularly on the quadriceps muscle group.

2. Hydrotherapy provides the appropriate environment in which knee osteoarthritic patients can exercise at intensities that improve strength and mobility.

3. Exercise load should increase each week and maintenance of cardiovascular conditioning is a must, even before a total joint replacement.

4. Evaluation of activities of daily living is essential and should include evaluation for assistive devices to maximize independence and ensure safety in the home environment.

21. **Name and describe three common tests for an ACL injury.**
    - **Lachman test:** Patient lies supine. Knee is flexed approximately 20 degrees and the proximal tibia is pulled forward to assess excessive translation (more than 5 mm).
    - **Anterior drawer test:** Patient lies supine. Knee is flexed at 90 degrees and the hip is flexed at 45 degrees. The proximal tibia is pulled anteriorly to assess excessive translation (more than 5 mm).
    - **Pivot shift test:** Patient lies supine. Knee is placed in extension. The examiner supports the leg by the upper tibia and flexes the knee while applying a slight valgus stress to the knee (pushing the knee toward the midline) and internal rotation stress about the femur. In a knee with an ACL injury, the femur sags backward on the tibia (or conversely, the tibia moves forward on the femur), creating a subluxation of the lateral tibiofemoral compartment. At approximately 30 degrees of flexion, the subluxed tibia suddenly reduces and externally rotates about the femur. The subluxation and the sudden reduction of the knee joint during flexion are termed the *pivot shift*.

22. **Does a positive Lachman test always mean ACL injury?**
No. Laxity may also be present in the other knee. Knee clinical examination requires comparing both knees.

23. **Identify the cause and acute signs of PCL injury. Discuss a treatment approach.**
The most common mechanism of injury of the PCL is the so-called dashboard injury (while the knee is bent, an object forces the tibia backward). Another mechanism of injury is hyperflexion of the knee, with the foot held pointing downward. The acute signs include swelling in the popliteal space with bruising present during the first 36–48 hours, and no effusion as a result of the extra-articular nature of the PCL. Pain and instability are also common.

Rehabilitation should concentrate on regaining ROM and substituting the lost function of the PCL by strengthening the quadriceps. If conservative therapy fails, then surgical reconstruction is considered.

24. **Name and describe common tests for PCL injury.**
   - **Posterior drawer test:** Patient lies supine. Knee is flexed at 90 degrees and the hip is flexed at 45 degrees. The proximal tibia is pushed posteriorly to assess excessive translation (more than 5 mm).
   - **Posterior sag test:** Patient lies supine and flexes both hips to 45 degrees and both knees to 90 degrees with examiner supporting both heels. The tibia will "drop back" or sag if there is a PCL tear.
   - **Reversed pivot shift test:** Patient lies supine. Knee is placed in flexion at 90 degrees. The examiner supports the leg by the upper tibia and extends the knee while applying a slight valgus stress to the knee (pushing the knee toward the midline) and external rotation stress about the femur. In a knee with a PCL injury, the femur moves forward on the tibia (or conversely, the tibia moves backward on the femur). The subluxed tibia will shift into anterior reduction at 20–30 degrees.

25. **Name and describe two common tests for a posterolateral corner injury (PLC).**
   - **External rotation recurvatum test:** While the patient is supine, with slight downward pressure to the femur, the great toe is lifted and the amount of recurvatum is assessed. Compare to the contralateral knee.
   - **Varus stress test:** While the patient is supine, the leg is placed over the examining table with one hand over the lateral joint line and the other holding the ankle with the knee flexed to 30 degrees. Varus stress is applied to the knee to assess the integrity of the fibular collateral ligament and other PLC structures. Compare to the contralateral knee.

26. **Describe the MCL and LCL stress test.**
   The patient is supine, and the knee is examined at neutral and at 30 degrees. Valgus and varus stress is applied at both degrees. Valgus stress examines the MCL and varus stress examines the LCL. The posterior capsule is relaxed at approximately 30 degrees of knee flexion. The maneuver can also be completed by rotating internally and externally the tibia while palpating the joint space.

27. **What are the degrees of MCL strains?**
   - **Grade 1 (first degree):** Valgus stress results in medial pain but no increased laxity; laxity = 0–5 mm
   - **Grade 2 (second degree):** Valgus stress demonstrates increased laxity and an endpoint is appreciated; laxity = 6–10 mm
   - **Grade 3 (third degree):** Valgus stress demonstrates increased laxity with no appreciable endpoint, indicating rupture of the ligament and the surrounding capsular structures; laxity = 11–15 mm

28. **When can an athlete return to competitive sports after an MCL grade 1 strain?**
   When the patient's strength is near normal (90%) and the valgus instability is reduced to a point that a brace is no longer required. The patient should be able to perform one-legged hopping, jumping rope, and climbing stairs before returning to the playing field.

29. **What is an "extensor lag"?**
   Extensor lag refers to the inability to fully extend the knee actively, although passively full extension is possible. This results from lengthening of the extensor mechanism or weakening of the quadriceps. Component malposition may also produce this problem.

MENISCUS

30. What is the purpose of the knee meniscus?
The meniscus is a half moon–shaped piece of cartilage that lies between the weight-bearing joint surfaces of the femur and the tibia. It is triangular in cross-section and is attached to the lining of the knee joint along its periphery. There are two menisci in a normal knee; the outer one is called the lateral meniscus and the inner one the medial meniscus. Their purposes include lubrication, nutrition, shock absorption, and prevention of cartilage wear. The menisci are primarily avascular, especially the inner two thirds.

31. What is O'Donoghue's triad?
O'Donoghue's triad is a complex of meniscoligamentous lesions entailing injuries to the medial meniscus, MCL, and ACL, caused by a valgus force to a flexed, externally rotated knee. This injury is second only to an isolated ACL tear as the most common injury.

32. Describe McMurray's test.
McMurray's test is useful for diagnosing meniscal injury. The test is performed with the patient lying supine with the knee and hip maximally flexed. The examiner stabilizes the thigh and rotates the tibia either medially or laterally. With medial rotation the presence of a loose fragment in the lateral meniscus can cause a snap or click that is often accompanied by pain. With lateral rotation the presence of a loose fragment in the medial meniscus can be similarly detected. By repeatedly adjusting the amount of flexion, the examiner can test the entire posterior aspect of the meniscus from the posterior horn to the medial component. The anterior half of the meniscus is not as easily examined because the pressure exerted on the meniscus is not as great.

33. Describe the Apley maneuver.
The Apley maneuver is another commonly used test for diagnosing meniscal injury. The patient lies prone with the knee flexed 90 degrees. While the examiner stabilizes the thigh, the tibia is rotated medially and laterally, with downward pressure. Joint-line tenderness with this movement is considered positive.

34. Can meniscal injuries be treated without surgery?
Yes. Initially, the **PRICE** regimen is prescribed. One could change the pneumonic to **CRISP** (**S** for **s**teroid intra-articular injection) if conservative care is failing. In fact, most meniscal tears can be treated without the need for surgical intervention.

35. When is surgical treatment indicated for a meniscal tear?
- Locking or inability to fully extend the knee because of mechanical blockage
- Motion restricted despite a trial of physical therapy
- Instability, which may predispose to further intra-articular damage
- Persistent Baker's cyst, resulting from a meniscal tear
- Pain not improving with physical therapy and symptomatic treatment

OSTEOARTHRITIS

36. What are the signs and symptoms of knee osteoarthritis?
Knee osteoarthritis is characterized by joint pain, tenderness, and decreased ROM. Patients can have swelling, joint effusion, and pain with weight-bearing activity. Physiatric

treatment consists of using a cane in the opposite hand, NSAIDs, intra-articular joint injections, knee brace, and physical therapy.

37. **What are the general principles of rehabilitation of arthritis of the knee?**
    - Non–weight-bearing strengthening exercises should be emphasized, particularly with emphasis on the quadriceps.
    - Hydrotherapy provides the appropriate environment in which osteoarthritic patients can exercise at intensities that improve strength and mobility.
    - Exercise load should increase each week, and maintenance of cardiovascular conditioning is a must—even before a total joint replacement.
    - Activities of daily living and transfer/ambulatory evaluation are essential and should include evaluation for assistive devices, including raised toilet seats, shower grab bars, reachers, and ambulatory aids to maximize independence and ensure safety in the home environment.

38. **How should knee ROM be measured and recorded?**
    ROM should be measured from the lateral side of the patient's leg with a goniometer. Full extension, an angle between the femur and tibia of 0 degrees, should be recorded as 0 degrees. Full flexion is recorded as a positive number, somewhere between 0 and 135 degrees. If the patient's leg cannot be fully extended, the number of degrees possible short of full extension is recorded as a positive number. For example, the patient who lacks 10 degrees of full extension but is able to flex to 100 degrees should be recorded as having a ROM +10–110 degrees. If the patient's knee comes to hyperextension, the amount past 0 degrees should be recorded as a negative number. For example, if the patient hyperextends approximately 5 degrees and flexes to 100 degrees, the ROM is recorded as +5–100 degrees.

39. **What are the types and indications for the use of a knee brace?**
    According to the American Academy of Orthopaedic Surgeons, knee braces can be classified as:
    - **Prophylactic braces:** Intended to prevent or reduce the severity of knee injuries in contact sports; these braces are often not recommended because of excessive preloading of the MCL, limited speed and athleticism, false sense of security for previously injured knee, and brace-related contact injuries to other players
    - **Functional braces:** Designed to provide stability for unstable knees
    - **Rehabilitative braces:** Designed to allow protected and controlled motion during the rehabilitation of injured knees
    - **Patellofemoral braces:** Designed to improve patellar tracking and relieve anterior knee pain

40. **What is the rationale for the use of knee injections?**
    There are two types of injections used to treat symptoms of knee osteoarthritis:
    - **Viscosupplementation therapy** involves injecting a gel-like substance directly into the knee joint. These injections help to restore the lubrication lost by damaged cartilage and may have anabolic (beneficial) effects on articular cartilage. Usually people who respond to this form of treatment will experience some improvement for 6–12 months, but it sometimes takes longer.
    - **Cortisone injections** are reserved for people suffering from a severely inflamed knee with uncontrolled pain. Cortisone injections can provide rapid relief from a tender, swollen osteoarthritic knee that has failed to respond to other forms of treatment. The benefit of an injection may last from a few days to more than 6 months. Cortisone injections can be repeated safely every few months.

41. **What is the role of pulsed electrical fields in the treatment of osteoarthritis of the knee?**
The limited capacity of articular cartilage to heal has stimulated a number of approaches to try to effect cartilage repair. Animal and clinical studies have suggested that pulsed electrical stimulation may have beneficial effects on articular cartilage healing. One company markets a product (Bionicare, Bionicare Medical Technologies, Sparks, MD) that appears to be a safe and effective method for avoiding total knee arthroplasty and relieving clinical signs and symptoms of osteoarthritis of the knee in some patients.

42. **What are the surgical options for osteoarthritis of the knee?**
   - Arthroscopic débridement: Includes irrigation and removal of loose bodies from the knee.
   - Cartilage transplantation: For small isolated areas, portions of autologous articular cartilage can be grafted into the defect.
   - Osteotomies of the distal femur or proximal tibia are used for isolated lateral or medial compartment arthritis.
   - Unicompartmental knee arthroplasty can be performed for isolated lateral or medial compartment arthritis.
   - Patellofemoral replacement replaces just the patellofemoral joint (anterior part of the knee).
   - Total knee arthroplasty is used to treat severe arthritis.

43. **What are the indications for total knee arthroplasty?**
The primary indication is to relieve pain caused by arthritis. Secondary goals are to restore functions and correct deformity. Candidates should show degenerative changes on radiographs and have failed other nonoperative methods (and occasionally other types of operative care). Nonoperative modalities may include anti-inflammatory medications, assistive devices, weight loss, behavioral modification, oral and intra-articular chondroprotective agents, and intra-articular corticosteroid injections. In select cases, surgical options before total knee arthroplasty include arthroscopy and osteotomies.

44. **Identify one condition in which a patient is at great risk for peroneal nerve palsy after a total knee arthroplasty.**
The patient with a valgus knee with a fixed flexion contracture is at high risk of peroneal nerve palsy. The peroneal nerve is at risk when a retractor is placed on the lateral side of the knee during surgery. However, injury from this is not a common occurrence. Neurapraxias more often result from stretching of the nerve with correction of the limb deformity. If a patient presents with a foot drop, then all dressings should be removed and the knee should be flexed to relieve tension across the peroneal nerve. If there is no resolution of the palsy, surgical exploration and decompression should be considered.

45. **What is the weight-bearing status immediately after total knee arthroplasty?**
There are different protocols, and it is important to discuss this with the operating physician. In the most common situation, when cement is used to fix both the femoral and tibial components, the patient is routinely allowed to bear weight as tolerated. Rarely, fixation requires bony ingrowth; then partial weight-bearing may be utilized.

46. **Outline a rehabilitation program for the patient with a total knee replacement.**
   - **Day of surgery:** Deep breathing exercises, active ankle ROM
   - **Postoperative day 1:** Lower-limb isometric exercises (quadriceps, hamstrings, and gluteal sets), passive and active ROM exercises
   - **Postoperative day 2:** Active-assisted ROM
   - **Postoperative day 3:** Progressive isotonic and isometric knee and hip muscle strengthening. (Concentrate on terminal knee extension through active knee extension exercises.)

47. **What muscles should be targeted after total knee arthroplasty?**
The quadriceps muscles are significantly weaker after total knee arthroplasty. This is, in part, related to the exposure required. Tourniquet and ischemic time also may play a part in muscular weakness. The quadriceps are important for stability during the stance phase of gait. Isometric strengthening and active ROM should begin immediately after surgery and continued for the first 6 weeks. Resisted isokinetic or isotonic strengthening should be added. Other muscles that should be strengthened after total knee arthroplasties include the hamstrings, gastrocsoleus, and ankle dorsiflexors.

48. **List the usual sequence of ambulatory aids after a total knee replacement.**
    - Parallel bars in inpatient physical therapy
    - Crutches or a walker, depending on patient stability and comfort
    - One crutch or cane
    - Most patients do not require assistive devices by 6–12 weeks postoperatively

49. **What rehabilitation approach should be used to treat a stiff knee post knee arthroplasty?**
The authors recommend a multimodality approach, which combines revising the joint, performing an arthrolysis, and excising any adhesions present with a strict rehabilitation protocol. A customized device may also be used to gain extension or flexion when physical therapy alone (e.g., moderate-intensity isometric sets of gluteal, quadriceps, and ankle pumps, active-assistive flexion and passive extension exercises, and active exercise of the hamstring muscles to relax the quadriceps mechanism by reciprocal inhibition) fails.

OTHER

50. **Name three types of knee effusions.**
Synovial, hemarthrosis, and purulent

51. **What should be done when evaluating an edematous knee?**
If the patient has a history of an acute, hot edematous knee, it is important to obtain Gram stain and culture before injecting it with steroids.

52. **Identify three key deformities of the knee.**
    - **Genu recurvatum:** Hyperextension or excessive backward knee joint mobility; often resulting from individuals with generally lax ligaments
    - **Genu varum:** Bowleg or excessive outward (lateral) deviation of the leg at the knee joint level
    - **Genu valgum:** Knock-knee or excessive medial deviation of the leg (at the knee joint level)

WEBSITES

1. www.emedicinehealth.com/articles/9051–1.asp

2. www.kneepaininfo.com

3. www.kneeguru.co.uk

4. http://orthopedics.about.com

BIBLIOGRAPHY

1. Calliet R: Knee Pain and Disability, 3rd ed. Philadelphia, F.A. Davis, 1983.

2. Eisle MA: A precise approach to anterior knee pain. Phys Sports Med 19:315–327, 1991.

3. Ellen MI, Young JL, Sarni JL: Musculoskeletal rehabilitation and sports medicine. III. Knee and lower extremity injuries. Arch Phys Med Rehabil 80:S59–S67, 1999.

4. Foley A, Halbert J, Hewitt T, et al: Does hydrotherapy improve strength and physical function in patients with osteoarthritis—a randomised controlled trial comparing a gym based and a hydrotherapy based strengthening programme. Ann Rheum Dis 62:1162–1167, 2003.

5. Magee DJ: The knee. In Quillen W (ed): Orthopedic Physical Assessment, 2nd ed. Philadelphia, W.B. Saunders, 1992, pp 372–447.

6. Mont MA, Alexander N, Krackow KA, Hungerford DS: Total knee arthroplasty after failed high tibial osteotomy. Orthop Clin North Am 23:515–525, 1994.

7. Mont MA, Mathur SK, Krackow KA, et al: Cementless total knee arthroplasty in obese patients: A comparison to matched control group. J Arthroplast 11:153–156, 1996.

8. Sheon RP, Moskowitz RW, Goldberg VM: Soft Tissue Rheumatic Pain: Recognition, Management, and Prevention, 3rd ed. Baltimore, Williams & Wilkins, 1996.

9. Snyder R: Essentials of Musculoskeletal Care. Rosemont, IL, American Academy of Orthopedic Surgeons, American Academy of Pediatrics, 1997.

CHAPTER 48

THE FOOT AND ANKLE: CLINICAL PRESENTATION, DIAGNOSIS, AND TREATMENT

Karen Barr, MD, Marta Imamura, MD, PhD, and Barry Rosenblum, DPM

A slip of the foot you may soon recover but a slip of the tongue you may never get over.
—Benjamin Franklin (1706–1790)

1. **For clinical discussions, how are the regions of the foot divided? What structures are in each region?**
   The foot is generally divided into three regions: the **hindfoot,** which consists of the calcaneus, talus, and related soft tissues; the **midfoot,** which consists of the cuneiform, navicular, cuboids, and related soft tissues; and the **forefoot,** which consists of the metatarsals and phalanges (Fig. 48-1). For further anatomic details, see also www.rad.washington.edu/anatomy/index.html.

2. **Describe common diagnoses seen by rehabilitation physicians for each region of the foot.**
   Some common causes of hindfoot pain include plantar fasciitis, fat pad contusions, and S1 radiculopathy. Causes of midfoot pain include tendinopathies (such as posterior tibialis or peroneal tendon) and navicular stress fractures. Forefoot pain may be caused by metatarsal stress fractures, metatarsalgia, interdigital neuromas, extensor and flexor tendinitis, and first metatarsal phalangeal conditions such as hallux valgus and rigidus.

3. **How do most patients with plantar fasciitis present?**
   The most common complaint of patients with plantar fasciitis (PF) is pain (sharp or bruising) in the plantar (the medial inner heel) associated with taking the first few steps in the morning, weight-bearing near the end of the day, and arising from a seated position.

4. **What are some risk factors for PF that can be addressed by rehabilitation?**
   Increased body mass index is a risk factor. In studies of runners, older age and heavier weight (i.e., bigger runners, not just fatter ones) were found to increase the risk of PF. Another study found that limited foot dorsiflexion caused an exponential increase in the risk of having PF. Those with limited dorsiflexion (6–10 degrees) had an odds ratio of 2.9:1 compared to age-matched controls with normal dorsiflexion (greater than 10 degrees). Those with 0 degrees or less of dorsiflexion had an odds ratio of more than 23! The literature is unclear as to whether those who overpronate or oversupinate are at increased risk of getting PF.

   Riddle DL, Pulisic M, Pidcoe P, et al: Risk factors for plantar fasciitis: A matched case control study. J Bone Joint Surg 85A(5):872–877, 2003.
   Taunten JE, Ryan MB, Lement DB, et al: A retrospective case control analysis of 2002 running injuries. Br J Sports Med 6(2):95–101, 2002.

5. **What is the main cause of acquired flatfoot in the adult?**
   Posterior tibial tendon (PTT) insufficiency occurs more in females and in persons over 40 years old. It has an insidious onset and is characterized by pain along the posterior tibial tendon, usually posterior to the medial malleolus. There is progressive flatfoot deformity and difficulty in walking long distances, especially over uneven surfaces. Physical examination

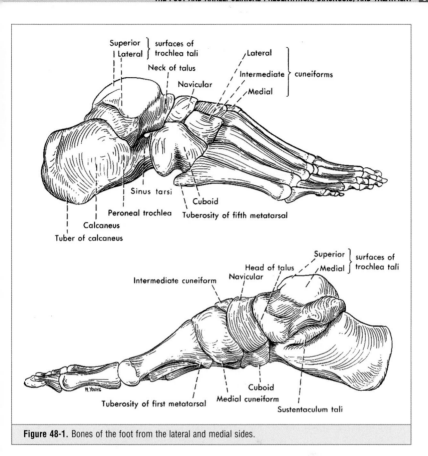

Figure 48-1. Bones of the foot from the lateral and medial sides.

shows decreased height of the longitudinal arch, external rotation deviation of the foot axis, and a pronated and abducted foot. A positive sign is "too many toes"; this can be observed when the person is standing and the hindfoot is viewed posteriorly. More toes are seen laterally on the affected side. Swelling is seen posterior to the medial malleolus. There is decreased heel motion into varus position during heel lift, as well as pain on palpation of the tibialis posterior tendon with active resisted inversion of the foot.

6. **What is the aggressive conservative treatment of PTT insufficiency?**
    Conservative treatment of PTT insufficiency or rupture has been considered ineffective, and surgical intervention is widely recommended. Recently, experts reported successful outcome with early aggressive conservative treatment addressing the biomechanics, using the University of California Biomechanics Lab (UCBL) orthosis or ankle-foot orthoses instead of simple foot orthoses. UCBL and ankle-foot orthoses align the subtalar joint (STJ) by direct control of the calcaneus, allowing PTT to heal. In patients with excessive obesity, fixed deformity of the STJ, and tight heel cord, the UCBL orthosis is not effective.

7. **What is tarsal coalition?**
    Tarsal coalition is the congenital connection of two or more tarsal bones. Coalitions can be fibrous, cartilaginous, or bony. Clinical findings are foot pain during adolescence, stiff hindfoot,

decreased range of motion at the STJ, and flatfoot caused by peroneal hyperactivity. Most common coalitions are calcaneus/navicular (13–16 years old) seen at the anteroposterior/lateral and with oblique x-rays. Talus/calcaneus (9–13 years old) is often seen only with a computed tomographic scan. Operative coalition resection is the main treatment when symptoms are present.

8. **Describe tarsal tunnel syndrome and its treatment.**
   Tarsal tunnel syndrome is the entrapment of the tibial nerve under the flexor retinaculum by tenosynovitis of the tibialis posterior tendon, flexor digitorum longus, flexor hallucis longus, and posterior tibial artery and vein. Increased pressure at the tunnel can also be caused by exostosis due to fractures, synovial sheath cysts, tumors, venous stasis, accessory soleus muscle, talocalcaneal coalition, and severe hindfoot planovalgus deformity. Systemic diseases such as gout, systemic lupus erythematosus, rheumatoid arthritis, diabetes mellitus, and hypothyroidism should also be ruled out. Pain, tingling, and burning on the sole can be worse during activity or even at rest. Positive Tinel's sign is detected by occurrence of tingling or paresthesia from tapping the tibialis nerve located posterior to the medial malleolus. Plain x-rays are normal, electromyography confirms the diagnosis, and magnetic resonance imaging (MRI) can help find a mass lesion. Treatments include nonsteroidal anti-inflammatory drugs (NSAIDs), steroid injections, and surgical release.

9. **What are the main pathologic changes found in the talipes equinovarus congenital clubfoot deformity? How do they correlate to treatment?**
   In **plantar-flexed ankle (equinus), inverted hindfoot (varus), adducted forefoot**, and **cavus midfoot,** soft tissue presents with tightness of tibionavicular ligament and flexor digitorum longus, tibialis anterior, flexor hallucis longus, and tibialis posterior tendons. Manipulation of tight soft tissue followed by casting can be performed while the child is non–weight-bearing. The cavus is corrected first by supinating the forefoot and dorsiflexing the first metatarsal. To correct the varus and adduction, the foot is abducted while counterpressure is applied against the head of the talus. Surgical correction by release of soft tissue and lengthening should be followed by postoperative casting.

10. **How useful are x-rays in diagnosing metatarsal stress fractures?**
    Imaging devices have varying levels of usefulness. Plain films may remain normal for 3–6 weeks after stress fracture. The first sign usually seen is subperiosteal bone formation. Bone scans will be positive in 20–40% of cases in which clinical suspicion is high, but plain films are normal. MRIs are very sensitive in showing stress fractures; some clinicians would say they are too sensitive because they sometimes show bony reaction in asymptomatic athletes. Grading scales have been developed to correlate MRI changes with prognosis.

    Arendt E, Agel J, Heikes C, et al: Stress injuries to bone in college athletes: A retrospective review of experience at a single institution. Am J Sports Med 31(6):959–968, 2003.

11. **What is a Jones fracture? What can cause it? If not significantly displaced, how can it be treated?**
    A Jones fracture is located at the **metaphyseal–diaphyseal junction of the fifth metatarsal** (within 1.5 cm distal to the tuberosity of the fifth metatarsal) and often results in delayed healing if untreated. This injury is usually caused by stress placed across the bone when the heel is off the ground and the forefoot is planted. Treatment of an acute Jones fracture that is not significantly displaced consists of a non–weight-bearing cast for 6–8 weeks and progressive ambulation after removal of the cast. Fractures about the base of the fifth metatarsal are termed *avulsion type* fractures and will usually heal with a stiff-soled shoe.

    American Academy of Family Physicians: Fractures of the Proximal Fifth Metatarsal. May 1, 1999: www.aafp.org/afp/990501ap/2516.html

12. **Define bunion and bunionette deformities.**
    A **bunion,** or **hallux valgus deformity,** develops when the great toe deviates laterally and the first metatarsal head develops a medial prominence. Conversely, a **bunionette,** or tailor's bunion, arises when a similar process develops laterally over the fifth metatarsal head.

13. **What are some of the most common etiologies of bunion deformities?**
    Congenital bunions often occur in family lines. Certain foot types, such as flatfeet, are prone to pathologic changes by causing an imbalance of the tendons that control the great toe, which results in abnormal motion about the metatarsophalangeal joint (MTPJ). Shoes with a narrow toe box may also create similar tendon imbalances, which may contribute to a bunion deformity over time. Other causes include inflammatory arthritides and trauma.

14. **What joint is the most common location for a gout attack?**
    The first MTPJ. This is called "podagra."

15. **What is an interdigital neuroma?**
    Often misunderstood as a tumor, this pathology is actually a benign enlargement of the fibrotic layer surrounding one of the common plantar digital nerves. This enlargement is typically the result of inflammation and irritation caused by shearing forces between the metatarsal heads or entrapment from a tight or enlarged deep transverse intermetatarsal ligament.

16. **What is the most common location for an interdigital neuroma, otherwise known as a Morton's neuroma, to occur?**
    The third interspace.

17. **Describe the first-line management of Morton's interdigital neuritis.**
    Because tight shoes are the main culprit of interdigital neuritis, wearing roomy footwear is the first step. Often this is enough to resolve symptoms. Other treatment options (metatarsal pads, neuroma pads, injection, or surgery) are adjunctive.

KEY POINTS: ANKLE AND FOOT DISORDERS

1. Eccentric calf strengthening has been found to be helpful to treat both the pain and the tendon abnormality of Achilles tendinosis.

2. Risk factors for plantar fasciitis include obesity, age, and limited ankle dorsiflexion.

3. The anterior talofibular ligament is the most commonly injured ligament in an ankle sprain.

4. Morton's neuroma is a benign enlargement of the fibrotic layer around the digital nerve in the third interspace that is irritated by tight footwear.

18. **How do plantar callus and warts differ?**
    See Table 48-1.

19. **What is the impact of weight-bearing on the motion of the STJ?**
    - **Open-chain kinetics** occurs with non–weight-bearing status; during this time, motion of the foot occurs about a stable talus at the STJ.
    - **Closed-chain kinetics** restricts the motion of the calcaneus and requires motion of the talus to allow function of the STJ.

TABLE 48-1. CALLUSES VERSUS PLANTAR WARTS

Characteristics	Calluses	Plantar Warts
Localization	High shear/friction area	Any location
Skin lines	Cross through the lesion	Pass around the lesion
Satellite lesion (mother–daughter)	No satellite lesions	Multiple daughter lesions
Local tenderness/pain	Pain on direct compression	Pain on side-to-side squeeze
Punctuate hemorrhages	Central core with punctuate on shaving	Hemorrhages around the base
Age	Common in elderly	Rare in elderly

20. **What is flexor stabilization?**
    Excessive STJ pronation causes the midtarsal joint to unlock, resulting in hypermobility of the forefoot structures. The flexors attempt to steady the forefoot by contracting earlier and longer, which overpowers the intrinsic musculature and can result in digital pathology.

21. **What is the biomechanical effect of pronation or supination?**
    See Table 48-2.

TABLE 48-2. BIOMECHANICAL EFFECT OF PRONATION OR SUPINATION

Body Part	Pronation Response	Supination Response
Hindfoot (coronal)	Eversion	Inversion
Forefoot/midfoot (sagittal)	Dorsiflexion	Plantar flexion
Forefoot (transverse)	Abduction	Adduction
Ankle	Dorsiflexion	Plantar flexion
Tibia	Internal rotation	External rotation
Knee	Flexion, valgus	Extension, varus
Femur	Internal rotation	External rotation
Hip	Flexion	Extension
Leg length	Shortened	Lengthened
Effect during gait	Absorbs impact, adapts to uneven	Provides solid leverage for terrain pushoff

Adapted from Wernick J, Volpe RG: Lower extremity function and normal mechanics. In Valmassy R (ed): Clinical Biomechanics of the Lower Extremities. St. Louis, Mosby, 1996, pp 2–57.

22. **How are hallux rigidus (HR) and hallux limitus (HL) treated?**
    First, determine if the condition is primary or secondary. Secondary HL is caused by the following:

- Dorsiflexed first ray in excessive pronation, collapsed medial longitudinal arch from neuroarthropathy, foot orthosis with excessively high medial arch support, or surgery.
- Tethering the flexor hallucis longus (FHL) after an ankle fracture, deep posterior compartment syndrome of the leg, or diabetes mellitus Charcot joint.
Treat underlying causes (e.g., lengthening exercise of gastrocsoleus muscle, lowering the arch of foot orthosis). Footwear modifications (rocker sole with steel shank, toe-spring, or Springlite carbon plate) are often helpful.

23. **What kind of physical therapy has been found to help treat Achilles tendinosis?**
Eccentric calf-strengthening exercises have been found in multiple studies to treat the pain of Achilles tendinosis and to normalize tendon structure on ultrasound. The mechanism is believed to involve strengthening and hypertrophy of the gastrocnemius muscles, lengthening of the muscle tendon unit, increased tendon tensile strength, and decreased tendon neovascularity. The important component to this exercise program appears to be the intense, eccentric nature of the exercises and that they are done at an intense level, despite producing pain.

    Ohberg L, Lorentzon R, Alfredson H: Eccentric training in patients with chronic Achilles tendinosis: Normalized tendon structure and decreased thickness at follow up. Br J Sports Med 38(1):8–11, 2004.

24. **What ligaments are involved in the common ankle sprain?**
Ankle sprains typically involve an inversion moment of the ankle that, most commonly, injures the **anterior talofibular ligament (ATFL)**, followed by involvement of the **calcaneofibular ligament (CFL)**, and, least commonly, the **posterior talofibular ligament (PTFL),** which causes severe instability of the ankle. Together, these ligaments form the **lateral ligament complex** of the ankle (Fig. 48-2).

25. **Name and describe the two tests used to detect injury and instability of the lateral ankle ligament complex.**
    - The **anterior drawer test** evaluates the ATFL and is performed by applying a forward stress to the ankle while stabilizing the tibia, with the ankle in slight plantar flexion.
    - The **talar tilt test** evaluates the CFL and is performed by applying an inversion stress to the ankle while stabilizing the tibia, with the ankle in neutral flexion. The quality of the endpoint and the amount of translation are noted.

26. **How are ankle sprains commonly graded?**
Ankle sprains are most commonly graded by the amount of ligament damage.
    - **Grade I:** Ligament sprain or strain and no increase in translation on stress testing
    - **Grade II:** Partial ligament tearing and minimal increase in translation on stress testing
    - **Grade III:** Complete tearing of one or both of the lateral ligaments and no endpoint noted on stress testing

27. **How are ankle sprains usually treated?**
In the acute phase, **RICE** measures (**r**est, **i**ce, **c**ompression, and **e**levation) and NSAIDs are commonly indicated. **Immobilization** with a plaster cast or splint should be performed for 4 weeks in grade III injuries. Functional treatment includes an early ankle-mobilization program associated with use of an external support, such as a semirigid or lace-up ankle brace, elastic bandages, and ankle taping. **Ankle-strengthening exercises** should be followed by ankle proprioceptive and coordination retraining. **Operative ligament repair or reconstruction** is indicated in the case of severe injury and in the presence of an associated lesion, such as syndesmosis rupture or osteochondral lesion of the talar dome.

    Pijnenburg ACM, Van Dijk CN, Bossuyt PMM, et al: Treatment of ruptures of the lateral ankle ligaments: A meta-analysis. J Bone Joint Surg 82A(6):761–773, 2000.

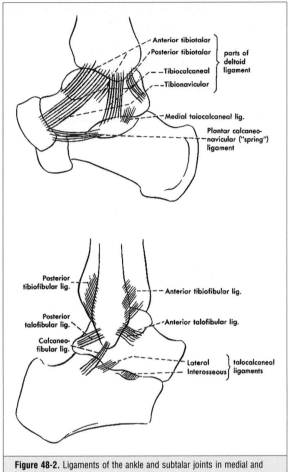

Figure 48-2. Ligaments of the ankle and subtalar joints in medial and lateral views.

28. **What are some outcome measures that can be used to evaluate recovery from an ankle sprain?**

Outcome measures include **subjective measures,** such as pain or subjective instability ("give-way"); **objective measures,** such as swelling, objective instability (anterior drawer and talar tilt test), or ankle range of motion; and **functional measures,** such as return to the previous performed sport at the same level or work (time to achieve). Assessments can be performed within 6 weeks of treatment (to identify early significant complications, short-term results), at 6 weeks to 1 year follow-up (to identify intermediate-term results), and at 1–2 years after treatment (long-term results).

29. **Who has a higher risk of recurrent ankle sprains? How can ankle sprains be prevented?**

Athletes who engage in high-risk sports (basketball players with a history of ankle injury are nearly five times more likely to sustain an ankle injury) and those who have suffered a previous injury to the ankle ligament complex have a higher risk of recurrent ankle sprains. Prophylactic interventions include the application of an external ankle support in the form of a semirigid orthosis, an air-cast brace, or high-top shoes during high-risk sporting activities (e.g., soccer, basketball, volleyball); ankle-disc training aimed at enhancing coordination and retraining proprioception; ankle taping; muscle stretching; and the use of modified footwear and associated supports.

Handoll HHG, Rowe BH, Quinn KM, et al: Interventions for preventing ankle ligament injuries. In The Cochrane Library, Issue 2. Oxford, Update Software, 2005.

McKay GD, Goldie PA, Payne WR, et al: Ankle injuries in basketball: Injury rate and risk factors. Br J Sports Med 35(2):103–108, 2001.

30. **List possible complications after an ankle fracture.**
Post-traumatic osteoarthritis and pain, decreased motion or stiffness, muscle atrophy, ankle instability, delayed union, nonunion, malunion, and complex regional pain syndrome.

31. **How many degrees of dorsiflexion at the ankle joint are required for normal gait?**
A minimum of 10 degrees of dorsiflexion is required for normal gait.

32. **What are the two more common theories regarding the development of Charcot neuroarthropathy in the diabetic foot?**
The neurotraumatic (German) and neurovascular (French) theories.

33. **What are the grades of diabetic ulcers according to Wagner?**
- Grade 1: Superficial
- Grade 2: Deep ulcer to tendon, bone, or joint
- Grade 3: Deep ulcer with abscess or osteomyelitis
- Grade 4: Gangrene of the forefoot
- Grade 5: Gangrene of the entire foot

34. **Describe the primary aspects of good local wound care in the diabetic foot.**
- Ensure adequate perfusion
- Débridement of devitalized tissue
- Antibiotic therapy if infected
- Offloading areas of increased pressure

35. **Name a surgical technique that has been shown to reduce plantar pressures in the neuropathic foot.**
Achilles tendon lengthening.

WEBSITES

1. American Orthopaedic Foot and Ankle Society
   www.aofas.org

2. University of Washington Anatomy Modules
   www.rad.washington.edu/anatomy/index.html

BIBLIOGRAPHY

1. Magee DJ: Orthopedic Physical Assessment Enhanced Edition, 4th ed. Philadelphia, W.B. Saunders, 2005.
2. Snider R (ed): Essentials of Musculoskeletal Care. Rosemont, IL, American Academy of Orthopaedic Surgeons, 1997.

CHAPTER 49

FRACTURE REHABILITATION: GENERAL PRINCIPLES

Arun J. Mehta, MB, and Tarek S. Shafshak, MD

A broken bone can heal, but the wound a word opens can fester forever.
—Jessamyn West (1902–1984)

1. **How common are musculoskeletal injuries?**
   Fractures are the fifth leading diagnosis in hospital discharges in the United States. It is estimated that in 1999, 28.6 million Americans sustained a musculoskeletal injury. Sprains, dislocations, and fractures account for nearly 65% of all injuries. More than 320,000 Americans are hospitalized for a hip fracture every year. About 200,000 osteoporotic fractures occur in Britain each year and 1.5 million in the United States. Common sites for osteoporotic fractures are the spine, hip, and wrist.

2. **Describe the mechanisms of injury that lead to fracture.**
   - **Direct injury:** Direct blow fractures the bone at site of impact
   - **Indirect injury:** Force applied at one point, fracture occurs at a remote site
   - **Transverse or oblique fracture:** Force bends a long bone
   - **Spiral fracture:** Result of a twisting force
   - **Compression fracture:** Compressive forces crush soft spongy bone (e.g., vertebral body)

3. **Name the factors that predispose a patient to fractures.**
   - **Age:** As we age, the risk of fracture increases because of increased prevalence of osteoporosis and falls. Approximately 40% of people over 65 years of age and 50% of those over 80 fall in a year. Children usually break bones because they are more active and take more risks. Vision, sense of balance, and muscle strength also decline as we age.
   - **Sex:** Women lose bone density at a faster rate and earlier in life than men do. However, men are not immune to developing osteoporosis.
   - **Heredity:** Caucasians and Asians have a higher risk for developing osteoporosis. Genetic factors influence bone size, bone mass, and bone density. A light-weight, small-boned, slender person is at an increased risk for osteoporosis.
   - **Osteoporosis:** In the United States, osteoporosis causes more than 1.5 million fractures every year—most of them in the spine, hip, or wrist. It is estimated that there are 28 million people with osteoporosis in the United States. It is seen 10–15 years earlier in women than in men. Prevalence of osteoporosis is 3–6% in males and 13–18% in females over the age of 50 years. One of every two women and one of every eight men older than age 50 will have an osteoporosis-related fracture in their lifetime. Although it is often thought of as a woman's disease, osteoporosis affects many men as well.
   - **Falls:** The elderly are more likely to fall and break a bone because of neurologic disorders, such as peripheral neuropathy, cerebrovascular accidents, visual impairment, Parkinson's disease, dementia, or cardiac factors (orthostatic hypotension, arrhythmias, or syncope). These medical problems may lead to impaired proprioception, reduced muscle strength, poor coordination, or postural sway. Medications for insomnia and other medical conditions may affect judgment and balance. A patient who falls more than once in a year, sustains an injury as a result of a fall, or has unstable gait deserves a detailed investigation for a correct diagnosis and management.

- **Poor nutrition:** Lack of calcium and vitamin D in diet, anorexia nervosa, and bulimia may lead to osteoporosis.
- **Tobacco and alcohol use:** Smoking and excessive consumption of alcohol are also associated with osteoporosis.
- **Medications:** Long-term use of corticosteroids, anticonvulsants, thyroid medications, and certain diuretics and blood thinners may lower bone mass. Other medications (e.g., sedatives, tranquilizers, antidepressants, cold and allergy medications, pain relievers, sleep and blood pressure medications) affect balance, cause dizziness, and lead to falls.
- **Environmental hazards:** Loose rugs, poor lighting, exposed electrical cords, and stairs with no handrails may increase the risk of falling.

  Falls and osteoporosis are two independent and additive risk factors for fractures around the hip.

Morris CD, Einhorn TA: Bisphosphonates in orthopedic surgery. J Bone Joint Surg 87A:1609–1618, 2005.
Papapoulos SE, Quandt SA, Liberman UA, et al: Meta-analysis of the efficacy of alendronate for the prevention of hip fractures in postmenopausal women. Osteoporosis Int 16:468–474, 2005.

4. **Is there a role for vitamin D supplement in the treatment of patients with osteoporosis?**
Approximately 60–70% of patients with osteoporotic fracture of the neck or femur have low blood levels of 25 hydroxyvitamin D. Those who sustain a fracture of the neck of the femur and survive are five to ten times more likely to have another one. Treatment of osteoporosis with bisphosphonates, calcium, and vitamin D supplements has been suggested. Vitamin D helps by increasing the bone mass and muscle function.

Harwood RH, Sahota O, Gaynor K, et al: A randomised, controlled comparison of different calcium and vitamin D supplementation regimes in elderly women after hip fracture: The Nottingham Neck of Femur (NoNOF) Study. Age Aging 33:45–51, 2004.

5. **What more can be done to prevent fractures in the elderly population?**
- Exercises to strengthen paraspinal muscles can reduce the risk of vertebral fractures in postmenopausal women. Progressive resistive exercises and functional activity training can improve muscle strength, balance, and performance of motor functions. These exercises need to be continued to maintain the gains. Tai chi exercises and walking also reduce the incidence of falls.
- The living facility—home or nursing home—can be made safe by removing loose rugs and other obstacles to walking.
- Proper evaluation, diagnosis, and treatment of medical conditions can help patients predisposed to falls.

6. **What systemic complications can occur after a fracture?**
- Urinary tract infections (indwelling catheter)
- Fat embolism
- Constipation (secondary to opioid analgesics)
- Deep venous thrombosis
- Pressure ulcers (pressure of the cast or bedrest)
- Pneumonia
- Anemia (injury-related or perioperative blood loss)

7. **How does a fracture heal?**
When blood vessels are injured, blood accumulates in tissues and forms a hematoma, which is replaced by new blood vessels and fibroblasts. Later, osteoblasts from the periosteum and endosteum proliferate and form the intercellular matrix, in which calcium salts are deposited to form a callus. Mechanical loading generates electrical potentials, known as the

piezoelectric property of the bone. These electrical potentials are recognized by osteoblasts and guide new bone formation. Increasing compression force or stress at the fracture site signals formation and orientation of collagen fibers, deposition of minerals, and strengthening of callus.

8. **How would you describe a fracture on plain x-rays?**
   - Fracture location
   - Involvement of diaphysis, metaphysis, epiphysis, or articular surface
   - Fracture line—transverse, oblique, or spiral
   - Deformity—alignment, angulation, and rotation
   - Number and location of bony fragments, displacement, direction, and distance from normal location, distance between fragments
   - Dislocation or effusion of adjacent joints
   - Swelling or blood loss

9. **When should you suspect pathologic fracture?**
   A pathologic fracture occurs after a minor trauma that would not ordinarily break a bone. The patient may have had pain before the fracture, especially at night. If a patient has a malignant tumor and later develops a fracture, it may be due to metastatic disease. Pathologic fractures can also occur with hormonal deficiency states (e.g., estrogen and testosterone deficiency).

10. **Which malignant tumors commonly metastasize to bone?**
    Malignant tumors of the breast, lung, prostate, colon, rectum, kidney, thyroid, and bladder

11. **Is magnetic resonance imaging (MRI) useful in the diagnosis and management of fractures?**
    Yes. MRI is useful for early diagnosis of infection, tumor, early diagnosis of stress fracture, bone and muscle hematomas, partial and complete tears of ligaments, hematomas within ligaments, and avascular necrosis. It is also useful in skull, spinal, and pelvic fractures with suspected soft tissue injury.

    Spitz DJ, Newberg AH: Imaging of stress fractures in the athlete. Radiol Clin North Am 40:313–331, 2002.

12. **What are some local complications of a fracture?**
    - **Nerve and blood vessels** (are) may be damaged during injury, manipulation, or orthopedic procedures.
    - **Compartment syndrome** is suspected when the patient complains of very severe pain, numbness of toes or fingers, inability to move toes or fingers, and poor capillary circulation under the nails.
    - **Delayed union** occurs when a fracture does not heal after a reasonable time.
    - **Nonunion** occurs when bone ends look sclerotic and smooth on x-rays.
    - **Malunion** occurs when a fracture unites in an abnormal alignment.
    - **Stiffness** and atrophy of muscles are very common because of immobilization.
    - Early **degenerative joint disease** may result when the fracture line involves a joint surface, and the fracture heals with an incongruous and rough joint surface.

13. **Which fractures are likely to be redisplaced after reduction?**
    - Fracture of both forearm bones
    - Comminuted fractures with third fragment
    - Oblique fractures
    - When swelling decreases and the cast becomes loose

14. **What is the role of the physiatrist in the rehabilitation management of fractures?**
    - The physiatrist should have knowledge of the mechanism of injury, type of fracture, orthopedic treatment received, normal course of healing for that type of fracture, complications, and expected outcomes.
    - Pain management is very important from the patient's point of view. Analgesic administration before physical or occupational therapy is helpful. Narcotics should be discontinued as soon as possible.
    - Good, ongoing, personal communication with the orthopedic surgeon gained by attending orthopedic ward rounds or x-ray conferences is essential. Details of operative findings (e.g., quality of fixation achieved) may be missing in the written operative report. The surgeon also can help in deciding progression through rehabilitation (especially in deciding weight-bearing status).
    - Rehabilitation includes progression through various stages of range of motion (ROM) and strengthening exercises, ambulation training, bracing, home evaluation, adaptive equipment, vocational retraining, and coordination of care.

15. **Which patients require a systematic, holistic approach to fracture rehabilitation?**
    Patients at risk for significant functional impairment or complications:
    - Geriatric patients at risk for falls and with multiple medical problems. Deconditioning secondary to prolonged bed rest or inactivity makes it difficult to achieve independent ambulation and other activities of daily living (ADLs).
    - Multitrauma patients with more than one fracture and/or injury to other systems.
    - Patients with certain fractures (e.g., fractures of the scaphoid) that are notorious for a high incidence of nonunion.
    - Patients with preexisting medical conditions, such as osteoporosis, metastasis, osteogenesis imperfecta, or cardiorespiratory disease.

    Pfeifer M, Sinaki M, Geusens P, et al: Musculoskeletal rehabilitation in osteoporosis: A review. J Bone Miner Res 19:1208–1214, 2004.

16. **Why would you consider a brace in the treatment of a fracture?**
    The brace protects the fracture site, allows ROM exercises and wound dressings, and may facilitate some weight-bearing activities.

KEY POINTS: FRACTURE REHABILITATION

1. Even if a fracture does not require manipulation or operation, rehabilitation is essential for restoration to the premorbid condition.

2. Goals of fracture rehabilitation are to control pain, correct deformity, protect injured tissue, prevent complications, restore ROM, and improve muscle strength.

3. There is no specific timetable for weight-bearing after a fracture. Decisions are based on fracture type, method and quality of fixation, condition of the bone, ability to control weight-bearing, pain, and evidence of bony union.

4. The stages of progression may include complete bed rest, assisted transfer activities, non–weight-bearing ambulation, toe touch, partial weight-bearing, weight-bearing as tolerated, full weight bearing, and, finally, running.

17. **What are some problem fractures in children?**
Supracondylar fracture of the humerus is notorious for complication of Volkmann's ischemic contracture. Dislocation of the head of the radius may be missed initially or recur in cases of Monteggia fracture-dislocation (fracture of the shaft of ulna with dislocation of the head of radius). Metaphyseal and epiphyseal fractures, which involve the growth plate, can lead to premature closure of the epiphysis and a shorter extremity. Osteoporosis from eating disorders and amenorrhea can lead to stress fractures.

18. **How are fractures in children different from those in adults?**
In children, tissues heal well and more rapidly, joints do not get stiff as easily, and the remodeling process commonly corrects deformity. Greenstick fractures, in which the cortex buckles on only one side of the shaft of a long bone, are seen only in children, and epiphyseal injuries may affect growth of a long bone.

19. **What are some common fractures seen in the elderly?**
   - Compression fracture of the spine—due to flexion injury, common in the osteoporotic spine
   - Fracture of the femoral neck
   - Fracture of distal radius—Colles' fracture, often associated with osteoporosis and a fall onto an outstretched arm
   - Fracture of the neck of humerus—may lead to marked limitation of movement in the shoulder joint

20. **How do you manage acute back pain in a patient with osteoporotic vertebral fracture?**
   - Recommend bed rest with gradually increasing activity as tolerated.
   - Relieve pain with analgesics and local heat therapy.
   - Treat constipation, which is common because of use of analgesics and immobility.
   - Avoid kyphotic posture.
   - Provide a brace to support the spine and proper aids (e.g., walker) for ADLs.
   - Enforce ADL training.
   - Avoid resistive/strengthening exercises for 2 months.

21. **Which activities and exercises may lead to fractures in patients with osteoporosis?**
Activities and exercises that involve forceful flexion and twisting of the spine that place high compression loads on the vertebral bodies may lead to compression fractures of the vertebral bodies and should be avoided. These activities and exercises include:
   - Falls
   - Bending forward for prolonged periods
   - Combined flexion and twisting of the spine as in playing tennis or golf
   - Contact sports

22. **What can a patient with osteoporosis do to avoid developing compression fractures of the spine?**
   - Prevent falls.
   - Flex hips and knees to bend down to lift objects.
   - Maintain proper posture and alignment when standing, sitting, or walking.
   - Keep heavy objects close to chest when lifting them or use a safe method of transportation (like tram or train).
   - Extension exercises for the spine and progressive resistive exercises.

23. **Can "hip protectors" prevent hip fractures in vulnerable, elderly patients?**
Hip protectors reduce the impact on bones in the hip region during a fall. Usefulness of hip protectors in preventing hip fractures was studied in 1801 in the frail, elderly population, with mean age of 82 years, by randomly assigning them to a control group and/or to a hip protector group. The authors (Kannus et al) found hip protectors to be useful in preventing hip fractures, whereas others have expressed some doubts. It is different for the susceptible elderly living at home. The rate of compliance for use of hip protectors is low, and their value in reducing costs of medical care is doubtful.

Kannus P, Parkkari J, Niemi S, et al: Prevention of hip fracture in elderly people with use of a hip protector. N Engl J Med 343:1506–1513, 2000.

van Schoor NM, de Bruyne MC, van der Roer N, et al: Cost-effectiveness of hip protectors in frail institutionalized elderly. Osteoporosis Int 15:964–969, 2004.

24. **What is the role of a physiatrist in the management of a pathologic fracture?**
A physiatrist can help manage severe pain and reduce the risk of pathologic fracture during rehabilitation. Concentrate on transfers, ambulation, and other functional activities so the patient can be discharged to her own home or assisted living facility rather than a nursing home.

25. **Where do stress fractures commonly occur?**
Stress fractures are caused by small, repeated stresses. A stress fracture of the 2nd, 3rd, or 4th metatarsal is called a march fracture because it was described in poorly conditioned soldiers after long marches. Soft shoe inserts and well-fitting boots may prevent march fractures in soldiers. Long-distance running and ballet dancing also may lead to march fractures. Other frequent sites for stress fractures include proximal tibia, fibula, neck of femur, and pubic ramus.

26. **Which fractures are missed more often than others on initial evaluation?**
Hairline fractures of the scaphoid may not show on initial x-rays. A history of a fall on an outstretched hand, with pain and tenderness over the anatomic snuff box (radial side of wrist), should be treated as a scaphoid fracture (splinting or casting for 10–15 days) with a repeat x-ray. If fracture is still suspected but not evident, a bone scan or magnetic resonance imaging is warranted. A fracture of the neck of the femur may be difficult to visualize on initial x-rays. Management is similar to suspected fracture of the scaphoid.

27. **What is the common site for fractures in ankylosing spondylitis?**
Osteopenia occurs in ankylosing spondylitis because of immobility and/or local release of cytokines. The most common site for spinal fracture in patients with ankylosing spondylitis is through the intervertebral disc space at levels C5–C6 or C6–C7. It may damage the spinal cord. A minor injury may result in fracture of the spine. Incidence of neurologic deficit is high and may manifest after a delay of 2–30 days. Fracture of the spine with neurologic deficit has a high mortality rate. The spine may fracture at multiple sites.

28. **Does the type of rehabilitation facility influence the patient outcome?**
A skilled nursing facility provides nursing care and some physical and occupational therapy. An inpatient rehabilitation facility is required to provide 3 hours of physical and occupational therapy in one day. These facilities also have nurses and physicians who are familiar with multidisciplinary treatment approaches (Table 49-1).

TABLE 49-1. COMPARISON OF SKILLED NURSING FACILITY AND INPATIENT REHABILITATION FACILITY

	Skilled Nursing Facility	Inpatient Rehabilitation Facility
Average length of stay	36.2 days	12.8 days
Prefracture functional independence measure (FIM) motor score	85.2	85
FIM motor score 2 weeks after fracture	47	70
FIM motor score 12 weeks after fracture	67	80
Percentage of patients discharged home	45.5%	80.1%
Percentage of patients discharged to a nursing home	36.4%	8.1%

Data from Munin MC, Seligman K, Dew A, et al: Effect of rehabilitation site on functional recovery after hip fracture. Arch Phys Med Rehabil 86:367–372, 2005.

WEBSITES

1. American Academy of Family Physicians
   www.aafp.org/afp

2. American Journal of Sports Medicine
   www.sagepub.com

3. Annals of the Rheumatic Diseases
   www. ard.bmjjournals.com/

4. Archives of Physical Medicine and Rehabilitation
   www.archives-pmr.org

5. British Medical Journal
   www.bmj.com/

6. International Journal of Sports Medicine
   www.thieme.de/sportsmed

7. Journal of Bone and Joint Surgery (American)
   www.jbjs.org/

8. Journal of Bone and Joint Surgery (British)
   www.jbjs.org.uk/

9. Journal of Bone and Mineral Research
   www.jbmronline.org/

10. Journal of Orthopedic and Sports Physical Therapy
    www.jospt.org/

11. Journal of Rheumatology
    www.jrheum.com

BIBLIOGRAPHY

1. McFarland EG, Young MA: Biomechanical principles in rehabilitation of fractures. Phys Med Rehabil State Art Rev 9:269–283, 1995.
2. Mehta AJ (ed): Common Musculoskeletal Problems. Philadelphia, Hanley & Belfus, 1996.
3. Mehta AJ (ed): Rehabilitation of Fractures. Physical Medicine and Rehabilitation: State of the Art Reviews, Vol. 9, no. 1. Philadelphia, Hanley & Belfus, 1995.
4. Mehta AJ, Nastasi AE: Rehabilitation of fractures in the elderly. Geriatr Clin North Am 9:717–730, 1993.
5. Young MA, O'Young BJ, McFarland EG: Rehabilitation of the trauma patient: General principles. Phys Med Rehabil State Art Rev 9:185–201, 1995.

CHAPTER 50

REHABILITATION OF SOFT TISSUE AND MUSCULOSKELETAL INJURY

Howard J. Hoffberg, MD, MS, Joanne Borg-Stein, MD, William F. Micheo-Marti MD, Gerold Stucki, MD, MS, and Christoph Gutenbrunner, MD, PhD

1. **What are the soft tissues involved in musculoskeletal (MS) injuries?**
   The soft tissues most commonly involved in MS injuries are muscles, tendons, ligaments, and fascia. Other soft tissues involved can include bursae, tendon and ligament insertions (enthesis), periarticular tissues (e.g., fat), and synovium. Structures that can also be damaged in traumatic and overuse injuries include supporting vascular and lymphatic tissues, as well as visceral organs.

   > Biundo JJ Jr, Mipro RC Jr, Fahey P: Sports-related and other soft-tissue injuries, tendonitis, bursitis, and occupation-related syndromes. Curr Opin Rheumatol 9(2):133–134, 1997.
   > Frontera WR: Epidemiology of sports injuries: Implications for rehabilitation. In Frontera WR (ed): Rehabilitation of Sports Injuries: Scientific Basis. Massachusetts, Blackwell, 2003, pp 3–9.
   > Verdon ME: Overuse syndromes of the hand and wrist: Primary care. Clin Office Pract 23(2):305–319, 1996.

2. **What is the difference between a sprain and strain?**
   A **sprain** is an injury to ligaments. It is usually associated with acute trauma but can also be the result of repeated tensile loads. A **strain** is an injury to the muscle-tendon unit. It may be associated with acute overload or repeated submaximal activity. Acute injuries can be classified from first to third degree, based on severity:
   - **First degree:** Microscopic injury to ligaments or muscle-tendons
   - **Second degree:** Macroscopic injury with fiber continuity (partial tear)
   - **Third degree:** Severe injury with fiber discontinuity (full tear)

   Injury and recovery from soft tissue lesions can be correlated with the inflammatory, fibroblastic, and maturation phases of tissue injury and repair. The injured tissue initially suffers inflammation with localized swelling and erythema, followed by repair in which fibroblasts are present and the tensile load of tissues is reduced for 3–21 days. Finally, the maturation phase occurs, in which collagen fibers are aligned and strength is regained. Repeated stress to the tendons is associated in many instances with degenerative intratendinous changes and not with an inflammatory response. This condition should be described as **tendinopathy**.

   > Frontera WR: Exercise and musculoskeletal rehabilitation: Restoring optimal form and function. Phys Sports Med 31(12):39–45, 2003.
   > Hill C, Riaz M, Mozzam A, et al: A regional audit of hand and wrist injuries. A study of 4873 injuries. J Hand Surg 23(2):196–200, 1998.
   > Maffulli N, Wong J, Almekinders LC: Types and epidemiology of tendinopathy. Clin Sports Med 22:675–692, 2003.

3. **What are the most common causes of MS injury?**
   The epidemiology of MS injury can be affected by several factors, including the causative activity, the patient population, and the age as well as sex of the individuals affected. In our society, trauma is a major cause of morbidity and mortality, with motor vehicle accidents being an important cause of injury with an observed increase in rear-end collisions.

   Work-related activities such as computer use and repeated bending and lifting can be associated with muscle, tendon, and nerve overload. Sports activities are an important cause of knee, back, foot and ankle, and shoulder injury. Military training is also an activity associated with significant MS morbidities.

Balcom TA, Moore JL: Epidemiology of musculoskeletal and soft tissue injuries aboard a U.S. Navy ship. Mil Med 165(12):921–924, 2000.

English CJ, Maclaren WM, Court-Brown C, et al: Relations between upper limb soft tissue disorders and repetitive movements at work. Am J Ind Med 27(1):75–90, 1995.

Versteegen GJ, Kingma J, Meijler WJ, et al: Neck sprain after motor vehicle accidents in drivers and passengers. Eur Spine J 9(6):547–552, 2000.

4. **What variables affect prognosis following an injury?**
    The prognosis for recovery from a soft tissue injury is affected by several factors, including the severity of the injury, appropriate diagnosis and treatment, and compliance with a complete rehabilitation program. Extrinsic factors that may affect prognosis include repeated exposure to sports or work activity, intensity of tasks, and difficulty of sports or work routines. Intrinsic factors that may affect recovery from injury include age and sex of the individual, ligamentous hyperlaxity, lack of flexibility, muscle weakness and imbalance, and anatomic malalignment.

    Frontera WR: Epidemiology of sports injuries: Implications for rehabilitation. In Frontera WR (ed): Rehabilitation of Sports Injuries: Scientific Basis. Massachusetts, Blackwell, 2003, pp 3–9.

    Kibler WB: Rehabilitation of rotator cuff tendinopathy. Clin Sports Med 22:837–847, 2003.

    McGill S. Low Back Disorder: Evidence-Based Prevention and Rehabilitation. Champaign, IL, Human Kinetics, 2002.

5. **What history should be taken in MS trauma?**
    A complete history of MS injury should identify:
    - Clinical symptoms
    - Site of anatomic injury
    - Biomechanical and functional deficits of the individual.

    Clinical symptoms of trauma include pain or sensory deficits, deformity, weakness, or swelling. The site of anatomic injury should include the primary site of tissue damage and associated kinetic chain overloaded structures. Finally, complaints of loss of function as well as change in activity patterns, such as reduced recreational sports participation or modifications in work activity, should be documented.

    Forman TA, Korman SK, Rose NE: A clinical approach to diagnosing wrist pain. Am Fam Phys 72(9):1753–1758, 2005.

    Frontera WR, Micheo WF, Amy E, et al: Patterns of injuries evaluated in an interdisciplinary clinic. PR Health Sci J 3:165–170, 1994.

    Kibler WB: A framework for sports medicine. Phys Med Rehabil Clin North Am 5:1–8, 1994.

6. **What evaluations should be undertaken following MS trauma?**
    The physical examination should identify areas of localized inflammation and tenderness, loss of joint motion, muscle weakness, and imbalance, as well as neurologic and proprioceptive deficits. In addition, diagnostic studies should be ordered to confirm the suspected clinical diagnostic impressions. Diagnostic studies commonly used in the diagnosis and management of soft tissue trauma include x-rays to document associated fractures as well as soft tissue calcifications and swelling; musculoskeletal ultrasound to evaluate soft tissues such as bursae, tendons, ligaments, and nerves; magnetic resonance imaging to evaluate periarticular soft tissues and to assess the extent of soft tissue damage; and electrodiagnostic studies to establish diagnosis and prognosis if a nerve injury is suspected.

    Blankenbaker DG, De Smet AA: MR imaging of muscle injuries. Appl Radiol 33(4):14–26, 2004.

    France JC, Bono CM, Vaccaro AR: Initial radiographic evaluation of the spine after trauma: When, what, where, and how to imagine the acutely traumatized spine. J Orthop Trauma 19(9):640–649, 2005.

    Hodge JC: Imaging of the wrist and hand. GenMed 1(1), 1999: www.medscape.com/viewarticle/408495

7. **What is whiplash?**

Whiplash was first described by Crowe in 1928 as an acceleration-deceleration mechanism of energy transfer from the relatively immobilized torso to the head. Whiplash can occur at an impact speed of 4–5 mph and affects the trapezius, levator scapulae, paraspinal (longus colli), scalene, and sternocleidomastoid muscles. It can commonly affect the zygapophyseal (facet) joints. Facet dysfunction has a prevalence of 30–60% in chronic spinal conditions, with the cervical region having the most frequent symptoms. Severe whiplash to the neck can also include injury to the discs, ligaments, cervical muscles (including tears), vertebral fractures, as well as neurologic sequelae to the sympathetic trunk (vertebral fractures), brachial plexus, cervical roots, and the spinal cord. Whiplash-associated disorders (WAD) can be considered a syndrome of symptoms and signs that may include fatigue, dizziness, paresthesias, spinal pain, nausea, visual symptoms, and jaw pain and must be treated as a biopsychosocial disease (Table 50-1). These symptoms may become persistent in up to 70% of patients, particularly those with headaches and paresthesias.

Allen ME, Weir-Jones I, Motiuk DR, et al: Acceleration perturbations of daily living: A comparison to "whiplash." Spine 19:1285–1290, 1994.

Borenstein D, Weisel S, Boden S: Low Back and Neck Pain: Comprehensive Diagnosis and Management. Philadelphia, W.B. Saunders, 2004.

Ferrari R, Russell A, Carroll L, Cassidy J: A re-examination of the whiplash associated disorders (WAD) as a systemic illness. Ann Rheum Dis 64(9):1337–1342, 2005.

Gunzburg R, Szpalski M: Whiplash injuries. Philadelphia, Lippincott-Raven, 1997.

Kasch H, Bach FW, Stengaard-Pedersen K, Jensen TS: Development in pain and neurologic complaints after whiplash: A 1-year prospective study. Neurology 60(5):743–749, 2003.

Manchikanti L, Boswell MV, Sing V, et al: Prevalence of facet joint pain in chronic spinal pain of cervical, thoracic, and lumbar regions. BMC Musculoskel Disord 5:15, 2004.

TABLE 50-1. SYMPTOMS OF WHIPLASH*

- Neck pain and/or stiffness (60–95%)

- Injuries to the muscles and ligaments (myofascial injuries)

- Head and facial pain with fatigue, irritability, blurry vision, dizziness, tinnitus, and nausea (may be related to a concussion or referral from the neck structures) (60–70%)

- Difficulty swallowing and chewing and hoarseness (may indicate injury to the esophagus and larynx or referral from facial and neck muscles)

- Abnormal sensations (numbness or paresthesias)

- Shoulder and other extremity pain

- Back pain

*May occur either immediately after the injury or several days later.

---

8. **What is the classification of WAD?**

In 1995, the Quebec Task Force Classifications for the Severity of Cervical Sprains formulated the following system:

- **Grade 0:** No neck pain complaints, no physical signs
- **Grade 1:** Neck pain complaints, stiffness or tenderness only, no physical signs
- **Grade 2:** Neck complaints, musculoskeletal signs (decreased range of motion [ROM] and tenderness)
- **Grade 3:** Neck complaints, neurologic signs (weakness, sensory and reflex change)
- **Grade 4:** Neck complaints with fracture and/or dislocation

Other symptoms for grades 1–4 include hearing, visual, and cognitive changes; dysphagia; headache; and temporomandibular joint dysfunction.

Spitzer WO, Skovron ML, Salmi LR, et al: Scientific monograph of the Quebec Task Force on Whiplash-Associated Disorders: Redefining "whiplash" and its management. Spine 20:1S–73S, 1995.

9. **What are the most common diagnostic imaging findings following a cervical trauma?**
The lateral view of cervical spine x-rays often shows a flattening or reduction of the cervical lordosis, which *may* indicate a paraspinal spasm (a protective mechanism to restrict cervical spine motion). The C1–C2 (open mouth or Waters view) x-ray to image the odontoid process is used for acute trauma. Lateral flexion/extension x-ray views identify spinal instability, and oblique x-ray views are used to evaluate the neural foramina, particularly if radiculopathy is suspected. In patients with normal x-rays and neurologic examination, cervical magnetic resonance imaging scans are usually not required. The clinician must be careful in correlating any minor (or pre-existing) abnormalities by diagnostic testing with the patient's presentation.

Borenstein D, Weisel S, Boden S: Low Back and Neck Pain: Comprehensive Diagnosis and Management. Philadelphia, W.B. Saunders, 2004.
Gunzburg R, Szpalski M: Whiplash Injuries. Philadelphia, Lippincott-Raven, 1997.

KEY POINTS: SOFT TISSUE REHABILITATION

1. Tendon, ligaments, and fascia are commonly involved structures in soft tissue injury.

2. Common causes of soft tissue trauma include motor vehicle accidents, work-related activities, and sports participation.

3. Patient complaints associated with soft tissue injury include swelling, pain, stiffness, and loss of function.

4. Pertinent findings in the physician examination are loss of motion and flexibility, muscle imbalance, weakness, and sensory loss, as well as proprioceptive deficits.

5. Treatment goals should be holistic, incorporating pain management with functional outcomes and prevention of complications.

10. **What types of soft tissue problems may result from injuries to the torso?**
Shoulder injuries may affect the rotator cuff, pectoralis, biceps, deltoid, latissimus dorsi, levator scapulae, rhomboid, trapezius, and tricep muscles, as well as the seven joints of the shoulder. Thoracic and rib cage sprains may affect the paraspinal, shoulder girdle, serratus, intercostals, trapezius, and levator scapulae muscles. Involvement of the upper ribs, scalene, and pectoralis muscles may cause a functional thoracic outlet syndrome. Lumbar sprains may affect the quadratus and paraspinal muscles. Pelvic-girdle dysfunction may affect the quadratus lumborum, glutei, piriformis, and iliopsoas, with involvement of the sacroiliac and pubic symphysis joints. This may result in functional leg length discrepancy and scoliosis. Piriformis and gluteal involvement may mimic sciatic-type pain.

Travell J, Simons D: Myofascial Pain and Dysfunction: The Trigger Point Manual, Vol. 2. Baltimore, Williams & Wilkins, 1992.

11. **What is the relationship between myofascial pain and somatic joint dysfunction?**

    The relationship between myofascial pain and somatic joint dysfunction can be characterized by the mnemonic **TART:**

    - **T** = **T**enderness
    - **A** = **A**symmetries of related musculoskeletal structures
    - **R** = **R**estriction of motion
    - **T** = **T**exture abnormalities (in soft tissues)

    Also referred to as somatic dysfunction, myofascial unit and joint dysfunction are caused by an imbalance or overload in the joint-ligament-tendon-muscle-fascia complex, resulting in pain generators from sensitized, small myelinated and free nerve endings or alteration of the large myelinated spindle and Golgi tendon organ afferents (joint proprioception). Somatic dysfunction may affect flexibility, posture, and recruitment and tonus, coordination, and balance of muscles. Both somatic dysfunction (especially the facet joints) and myofascial pain can result in characteristic referral patterns (which may include pain and/or sensory disturbances), autonomic dysfunction (histamine release with vasodilatation), and adrenergic activity (resulting in vasoconstriction, hydrosis and piloerection). Somatic dysfunctions are usually secondary to other pathologies or injuries and should be treated.

    Ferguson LW, Gerwin R: Clinical Mastery in the Treatment of Myofascial Pain. Philadelphia, Lippincott Williams & Wilkins. 2005.

    Greenman P: Principles of manual, 2nd ed. Baltimore, Williams & Wilkins,1996.

    Travell J, Simons D: Myofascial Pain and Dysfunction: The Trigger Point Manual, Vol. 2. Baltimore, Williams & Wilkins, 1992.

12. **Is there a "post-traumatic fibromyalgia"?**

    Post-traumatic fibromyalgia is a controversial subject. Its clinical presentation may represent a chronic multifocal myofascial pain or "widespread pain" syndrome from a traumatic injury. Some patients, including females, patients with genetic predisposition, and patients suffering from chronic sleep deprivation, may also have a predisposition for fibromyalgia. Symptoms become amplified as a result of a lowered pain threshold, alpha-delta sleep disturbances, or psychosocial factors associated with chronic pain and dysfunction.

    It has been postulated that once the peripheral sensitization of the myofascial unit occurs following trauma, irreversible neurotransmitter plasticity in the dorsal spinal cord through alterations of the glutamine-dependent *N*-methyl-aspartate (NMDA) receptors results in central sensitization. Subsequently, the neurotransmitters of the limbic system of the brain are affected. Additional subclinical "trauma" (due to overload of body regions that were not directly involved in the initial trauma or from emotional stress) may activate certain regions of the brain where the aberrant modulation of the pain signals has occurred, resulting in antidromic activation from the brain through the spinal cord to the peripheral nociceptors of the affected tissues. This results in a positive feedback loop perpetuating the soft tissue pain and dysfunction.

    Recently published studies have demonstrated improvement in pain and function if the patient is treated appropriately with selective frequency microamp (subthreshold) current, along with supplements, exercise, and education.

    McMakin C, Gregory W, Phillips T: Cytokine changes with microcurrent treatment of fibromyalgia associated with cervical trauma. J Bodywork Move Ther 9:169–176, 2005.

13. **What is complex regional pain syndrome (CRPS)?**

    Formerly known as reflex sympathetic dystrophy (RSD), CRPS type 1 usually presents in acute extremity injuries (crush or sprain) or may occur with central nervous system (CNS) lesions (i.e., shoulder-hand syndrome following stroke or myocardial infarction) in the *absence* of peripheral nerve injuries. It usually presents in the acute phase with hot, swollen, discolored, sweating limbs, sensitivity to light touch, intolerance of weight-bearing motion, and perceived pain disproportionate to objective findings. Formerly known as causalgia, CRPS type 2 has an associated peripheral nerve injury. The pathophysiology of this disease remains unclear, although disturbances of the sympathetic nervous system and sensory and motor CNS hyperexcitability have been shown (see also Chapter 75).

14. **What are the methods of CRPS treatment?**

The key goals of CRPS treatments include the reduction of pain and lymphedema and the recovery of impaired body functions. Pain management may combine analgesics, short courses of corticosteroids or nonsteroidal anti-inflammatory drugs (NSAIDs), and opioids. Pain and lymphedema may respond to limited courses of oral corticosteroids. Lymphatic massage with compression garments and carbon dioxide baths contribute to pain relief and edema reduction. Blockades of the autonomic nervous system (e.g., the stellate ganglion) can be both diagnostic and therapeutic. Continuous brachial plexus analgesia for 10–14 days, consisting of morphine, clonidine, and bupivacaine, is highly effective for pain relief and chemical sympatholysis in many patients. This must be facilitated with intensive and simultaneous physiotherapy, including ROM and weight-bearing activities, to restore impaired body functions. Physiotherapy may include mirror visual feedback; visual input from a moving, unaffected limb re-establishes the pain-free relationship between sensory feedback and motor execution.

Gradl G, Beyer A, Azad S, Schurmann M: Evaluation of sympathicolysis after continuous brachial plexus analgesia using laser Doppler flowmetry in patients suffering from CRPS I. Anasthesiol Intensivmed Notfallmed Schmerzther 40(6):345–349, 2005 [in German].

McCabe CS, Haigh RC, Ring EF, et al: A controlled pilot study of the utility of mirror visual feedback in the treatment of complex regional pain syndrome (type 1). Rheumatology (Oxford) 42(1):97–101, 2003.

15. **What rehabilitation techniques can be used in musculoskeletal soft tissue trauma?**

In acute injuries, use the **PRICE** (**p**rotection, **r**elative **r**est, **i**ce, **c**ompression, and **e**levation) method. This can be supplemented by analgesics or NSAIDs, splints or supports, soft tissue injections, and manual medicine techniques, such as joint mobilization, manipulation, muscle energy, and strain-counterstrain. Conservative treatments are performed in conjunction with an active exercise program, initially consisting of active ROM and gentle stretching. Once the acute phase has passed, exercise is progressed to strengthening, dynamic stabilization, movement re-education, and improvement of muscular endurance. In resistant or chronic cases, one should consider psychosocial aspects, particularly if the condition affects functional status (activities of daily living, mobility, work, recreational and sexual activities, and sleep).

Lively MW: Sports medicine approach to low back pain. South Med J 95(6):642–646, 2002.

Nyland J, Nolan MF: Therapeutic modality: rehabilitation of the injured athlete. Clin Sports Med 23(2): 299–313, vii, 2004.

Rosen NB, Hoffberg HJ: Conservative management of low back pain. Phys Med Rehabil Clin North Am 9:435–472, 1998.

16. **What other treatments can be used for soft tissue injuries? Are they effective?**

Trigger point injections and dry needling may be utilized to decrease pain and spasm and facilitate rehabilitation. They should *not* be used in isolation, but rather in conjunction with a program stressing muscle flexibility, strengthening, and functional restoration. Proper follow-up after injections to assess the patient's treatment response and ability to progress in the rehabilitation program is essential. There is little evidence to support any beneficial effect of adding corticosteroids to the injection. Lidocaine has been shown to decrease the patient's post-injection soreness. Other physical treatments may include acupuncture, chemodenervation with botulinum toxin, and prolotherapy. Prolotherapy (injections of pro-inflammatory agents to stimulate collagen synthesis) may be particularly helpful in chronic insertional tendinopathy, enthesopathy, or ligamentous sprain. It is always important to address any underlying disc, joint, or nerve root pathology that may be triggering overlying soft tissue and muscle pain in the corresponding myotome.

Cummings TM, White AR: Needling therapies in the management of myofascial trigger point pain: a systematic review. Arch Phys Med Rehabil 82(7):986–992, 2001.

Kamanli A, Kaya A, Ardicoglu O, et al: Comparison of lidocaine injection, botulinum toxin injection, and dry needling to trigger points in myofascial pain syndrome. Rheumatol Int 25(8):604–611, 2005.

Rabago D, Best TM, Beamsley M, Patterson J: A systematic review of prolotherapy for chronic musculoskeletal pain. Clin J Sports Med 15(5):E376, 2005.

17. **What types of treatment can be utilized to prevent recurrence of MS injury and pain?**
Predisposing factors that may result in recurrence include inadequate rehabilitation, muscle imbalance, poor posture or ergonomic habits, as well as "pain memory" or altered neuroanatomic pathways in the CNS as a result of peripheral trauma. Patients should be told that symptoms may recur, and they should be given guidelines indicating when formal treatment is needed (e.g., when symptoms affect function). A daily exercise program, including stretching and postural exercises with adequate reconditioning, supplemented by medication and adaptive equipment, may be necessary. In addition, comprehensive rehabilitation should address, identify, and treat sleep disorders (sleep hygiene) and involve appropriate mental health evaluation, treatment, and pain management skills.

Borg-Stein J, Simons D: Myofascial pain: A focused review. Arch Phys Med Rehabil 83(3 Suppl 1): S40–S49, 2002.

Gerwin RD. A review of myofascial pain and fibromyalgia—factors that promote their persistence. Acupunct Med 23(3):121–134, 2005.

Young MA, O'Young BO, McFarland EG: Rehabilitation of the orthopedic trauma patient: general principles. Phys Med Rehabil State Art Rev 8(1):185–201, 1995.

18. **What are the goals of treatment?**
The main goal of treatment is functional restoration. This includes pain control followed by recovery of ROM, both of individual joints as well as the entire kinetic chain. Muscle strength, endurance, power, and neuromuscular coordination must be normalized. This all facilitates a return to normal functional activities of daily living, occupation, and athletic participation. Importantly, a major goal of treatment is to prevent complications such as residual pain, weakness, atrophy, and a chronic pain disorder.

Borg-Stein J, Simons D: Myofascial pain: A focused review. Arch Phys Med Rehabil 83(3 Suppl 1): S40–S49, 2002.

WEBSITES

1. www.biomedcentral.com

2. www.bottomlinesecrets.com

3. www.mdconsult.com

4. www.medscape.com

5. www.spineuniverse.com

CHAPTER 51

MYOPATHIES: DIAGNOSIS AND REHABILITATION

Nancy E. Strauss, MD, Michelle Stern, MD, and Stanley J. Myers, MD

Please listen to the patient, he's trying to tell you what disease he has.
    —Michael H. Brookes, *A Clinician's Guide to Neuromuscular Disorders, 2nd ed.*

1. **Describe a myopathy and a dystrophy.**
   - A **myopathy** is a muscle disorder that can be attributed to pathologic, biochemical, or electrical changes in muscle fibers or in the interstitial tissue of voluntary muscles. A myopathy can be nonprogressive, slowly progressive, or rapidly progressive. Myopathies can be acquired or inherited.
   - A **dystrophy** is a myopathy that is congenital or inherited and is characterized by progressive degeneration of skeletal muscle fibers. The rate of degeneration outpaces regeneration, and there is connective tissue replacement of muscle fibers. Dystrophies often have a worse prognosis but can be slowly progressive.
   The common feature in all muscle diseases is muscular weakness.

   Gardner-Medwin D: Progressive muscular dystrophy and myotonic disorders. In Walton J (ed): Disorders of Voluntary Muscle, 3rd ed. London, Churchill-Livingstone, 1974, pp 561–613.
   Harper CM: Congenital myopathies and muscular dystrophies. In Brown WF, Bolton CF, Aminoff MJ (eds): Neuromuscular Function and Disease: Basic, Clinical, and Electrodiagnostic Aspects, Vol. 2. New York, W.B. Saunders, 2002, pp 1355–1374.

2. **Describe physical exam findings that may be seen in patients with muscle disease.**
   Usually there is proximal muscle weakness, normal sensation, hyporeflexia, and hypotonia. Muscle imbalance can lead to joint and bony alignment abnormalities. Contractures are usually more common in the lower extremities and progress more rapidly when a wheelchair is used. Inspection of the spine may reveal scoliosis. Impaired strength of trunk and muscles of respiration may be evident when a patient is asked to give a strong cough. Nasal flaring and low-volume nasal voice may result from weakness of respiratory muscles. Myopathic muscle may be atrophic or pseudohypertrophic.

3. **What is pseudohypertrophy?**
   Muscles appear larger due to replacement by fibrous tissue. It commonly occurs in the calves (as well as the thighs and deltoids) in boys with Duchenne's muscular dystrophy (DMD).

4. **How can you test for subtle muscle weakness?**
   Because a significant loss of muscle strength (50%) must be present in order to detect a reduction of absolute strength with manual muscle testing, other assessments must be made to detect weakness. Assessment may include having a patient repeat an activity to demonstrate a decrease in endurance. Observing a patient performing functional activities, such as heel walking, toe walking, hopping, jumping, and stair climbing, aids the examiner in identifying areas of muscle weakness.

5. **What is the Gower's maneuver?**
The patient arises from the floor using the hands placed on the lower extremities to aid in obtaining the upright position. This is due to insufficient proximal lower extremity and trunk strength, especially in the hip and trunk extensors.

6. **Describe the different gait patterns that can occur in myopathy.**
A Trendelenburg, or waddling, gait is a compensation for gluteus medius weakness. A hyperlordotic posture helps to place the center of gravity more posteriorly, thereby compensating for weak hip extensors. Toe-walking increases the extensor moment at the knee, thus compensating for weakness of the quadriceps muscle.

7. **When a muscle disease is suspected, what tests can aid in the diagnosis?**
   - **Creatinine phosphokinase (CPK),** normally found in high concentrations in healthy muscles, may spill into the blood and be elevated in destructive muscle diseases. It is usually highest in DMD/Becker's muscular dystrophy (BMD), and in patients with polymyositis.
   - **Electrodiagnostic testing** shows relatively normal nerve conduction studies with abnormal needle electromyography. Short-duration, low-amplitude complex units with a full recruitment pattern are characteristic. Myotonia is seen in the myotonic disorders.
   - **Muscle biopsy** with biochemical analysis of muscle tissue uses both quantitative and qualitative protein analysis. The muscle chosen should be one that is weak but still functional, and it should not be a muscle that recently was used for needle electromyography, because this may cause erroneous findings of inflammation and fibrosis on pathology.
   - **Genetic/chromosomal analysis** can identify many of the genes responsible for muscle diseases and determine their location and the defect of the particular genes.

8. **What are the major categories of myopathies?**
See Table 51-1.

TABLE 51-1.   MAJOR CATEGORIES OF MYOPATHIES

Classification	Examples
Muscular dystrophy	Becker, Duchenne, myotonic
Congenital	Central core, centronuclear
Metabolic	Myophosphate deficiency, phosphofructokinase deficiency
Mitochondrial	Kearns-Sayre syndrome
Toxic myopathy	Alcohol, statins, steroids
Endocrine	Hypothyroidism, hyperthyroidism
Infectious	AIDS, trichinosis
Inflammatory	Polymyositis, dermatomyositis

9. **List three important factors to consider in categorizing muscle diseases.**
   - Acquired or hereditary?
   - Rapid or slow onset?
   - Course slowly progressive, nonprogressive, or rapidly progressive?

10. **Give an example of an impairment, disability, and handicap as these terms apply to patients with myopathic weakness.**
   - **Impairment:** Abnormal physical exam findings (e.g., hip girdle weakness)

- **Disability:** What the patient cannot do (e.g., inability to negotiate stairs)
- **Handicap:** Social disadvantage that results from the disability (e.g., inability to work secondary to inability to negotiate stairs to enter an office building)

11. **What is the difference between DMD and BMD?**
    Both DMD and BMD are caused by a defect in dystrophin and have the same gene abnormality. Dystrophin is absent in DMD and has an abnormal molecular weight or reduced amount in BMD. BMD has a later onset and a slower rate of progression. Impairment can range from mild to very severe. Death in both DMD and BMD is usually a result of respiratory and cardiac complications.

12. **What is dystrophin?**
    It is a large cytoskeletal protein in the subsarcollemmal lattice that stabilizes the plasma membrane during muscle contractions. Loss of dystrophin leads to an unstable cell membrane and causes the muscle fibers to degenerate and, ultimately, be replaced by fat and connective tissue.

13. **Describe DMD.**
    DMD is usually identified by age 3–4 with gross motor abnormalities manifested by difficulty in running, arising from the floor, stair climbing, and jumping. Lumbar hyperlordosis, genu recurvatum, toe-walking, and pseudohypertrophy of calf muscles, quadriceps, and deltoids are characteristic. Eventually, proximal muscle weakness is accompanied by weakness of nearly all skeletal muscles, sparing extraocular muscles. Other associated features include average intelligence quotient score below normal population, cardiac abnormalities, scoliosis, restrictive pulmonary disease, and orthopedic deformities. Cardiomyopathy is associated with fibrosis and may lead to output failure, pulmonary congestion, and cardiac arrhythmias. DMD can result in death, usually secondary to respiratory complications, between age 20 and 25, but with improved medical management, life expectancy can be longer.

    Brooke MH: A Clinician's View of Neuromuscular Diseases, 2nd ed. Baltimore, Williams & Wilkins, 1986.

14. **When does a patient with DMD typically use a wheelchair?**
    Wheelchair ambulation is usually chosen for safety and energy conservation at approximately age 12. When seated mobility becomes the primary mode of ambulation, contractures will progress. Contractures include equinovarus deformity, knee flexion, hip flexion, elbow flexion, and kyphoscoliosis.

15. **When do patients with DMD usually develop scoliosis?**
    Between the ages of 13 and 15. Scoliosis is rarely a problem until patients require the use of a wheelchair for ambulation. Spinal bracing has not been shown to be effective in preventing scoliosis; however, a well-fitted wheelchair seating support system is important for patient positioning, comfort, and functioning. Spinal surgery should usually be performed before the primary curve becomes greater than 25 degrees and before the vital capacity has been reduced to 50% of predicted.

16. **Describe the pulmonary dysfunction in DMD.**
    Restrictive pulmonary disease is due to weakness of the diaphragm, chest walls, and abdominal muscles. This causes hypoventilation with elevation of CO_2 levels, which can result in morning headache or daytime somnolence. Noninvasive respiratory assistive devices are the preferred form of pulmonary management when possible. Vital capacity consistently drops, and there is CO_2 retention.

17. **What is limb girdle muscular dystrophy (LGMD)/limb girdle syndrome?**

   LGMD includes a group of muscular dystrophies with relatively similar presentation. There is characteristic weakness of hip and shoulder girdle muscles. Onset is usually in the second or third decade, but severity and inheritance mode are variable. There is a clinical heterogeneity of the features. There are many different types of LGMD, most of which can be categorized by their gene abnormality or end product defect.

18. **What are some features of Emery-Dreifuss muscular dystrophy?**

   It is an X-linked relatively slowly progressive myopathy. Contractures may develop before weakness, especially of the elbows, Achilles tendons, and spine. Cardiac conduction defects are common, and pacemaker insertion is often done early, even with evidence of only first-degree heart block, in order to prevent sudden death.

19. **What are the features of facioscapulohumeral muscular dystrophy?**

   At onset, there is usually weakness of the facial (orbicularis oculi and orbicularis oris) or shoulder girdle muscles in the scapular and humeral distributions. There may be prominent winging of the scapula, weakness of the biceps and triceps, but relative sparing of the deltoid (often affecting the right side first). It can later include the anterior tibial and pelvic girdle muscles. Facioscapulohumeral muscular dystrophy is also associated with retinal vascular disease and sensory hearing loss. It is inherited as an autosomal dominant trait on chromosome 4. The age of onset is variable, but it usually presents in the teens.

20. **What is myotonia?**

   A phenomenon associated with a delay of muscle relaxation after contraction. It can be elicited by voluntary muscle contraction, percussion of the muscle, or EMG needle insertion.

21. **Describe the features of type 1 myotonic dystrophy (DM1).**

   DM1 is an autosomal dominant disorder located on chromosome 19. It is caused by the triplet repeat mutation (CTG). DM1 presents primarily with weakness in a distal distribution (hands and feet) but progresses to involve all muscle groups. Associated characteristics include sternocleidomastoid muscle wasting (swan neck appearance), atrophy of temporalis and masseter muscles, elongated facies, ptosis, frontal balding, facial weakness, mental retardation, cataracts, endocrine abnormalities, testicular atrophy, female reproductive abnormalities, smooth muscle abnormalities (with swallowing and pharyngeal musculature weakness), cardiac abnormalities (including arrhythmias), and respiratory abnormalities. A less common form, DM2, has been described.

KEY POINTS: MYOPATHIES

1. Myopathic patients usually have proximal muscle weakness, hypotonia, hyporeflexia, and normal sensation.

2. Respiratory compromise is a serious consequence in certain myopathies.

3. An exercise program for the myopathic patient should be submaximal in intensity, avoid overfatigue, and be carefully supervised.

4. Myotonic dystrophy causes weakness in distal muscles.

5. Key tests in evaluating a patient with a myopathy include serum CPK levels, electromyography, and muscle biopsy.

6. Rehabilitation interventions play a key role in improving quality of life for patients with myopathies.

22. **In which other diseases can myotonia be present?**
    - **Myotonia congenita** (Thomsen's disease) is manifested by muscle stiffness, especially after resting, which loosens up with exercise.
    - **Paramyotonia congenita** commonly involves muscles of the face or hands and is worsened by cold exposure and exercise.

    Myotonia is also seen in Schwartz-Jampel syndrome, acid maltase deficiency, and hyperkalemic periodic paralysis.

23. **Describe features of inflammatory myopathies.**
    Inflammation of muscle may be secondary to an autoimmune dysfunction, infection, or other cause of inflammatory reaction. Dermatomyositis and polymyositis are acquired conditions with significant proximal muscle weakness, commonly including neck flexors. Muscle tenderness and swelling may occur, and weakness spreads. Cardiac and respiratory involvement may occur. These disorders may be associated with collagen vascular disease and malignancy. In dermatomyositis, a skin rash is characteristic, as well as other marked skin changes.

24. **What are the features of inclusion body myositis?**
    Most often occurring in men older than 50 years, inclusion body myositis presents with weakness of the forearm muscles, particularly the finger flexors and wrist flexors. A clue to diagnosis is greater weakness of the finger and wrist flexors than of the wrist extensor. It is a slowly progressive disease and can also involve weakness of the quadricep muscles, ankle dorsiflexors, and dysphagia.

25. **What is McArdle's disease?**
    Caused by phosphorylase deficiency, McArdle's disease usually develops in adolescence and is characterized by cramps after exercise, myoglobinuria, and sometimes muscle weakening. Symptoms disappear after a brief rest and do not recur with continued exercise. This is otherwise called the second-wind phenomenon. Examination can show a muscle contraction that is silent on needle EMG exam.

26. **Describe the features of congenital myopathies.**
    This group of relatively nonprogressive muscle conditions is diagnosed by muscle biopsy. At birth, a hypotonic (floppy) infant will show a delay in motor milestones. Presentation is variable. Examples of congenital myopathies include congenital fiber-type disproportion, central core myopathy, nemaline myopathy, and myotubular myopathy. These conditions are named secondary to histologic findings on muscle biopsy.

27. **What are the goals of a rehabilitation program for the patient with muscle disease?**
    - Prevent and minimize joint contractures.
    - Minimize deleterious effects of immobility and deconditioning.
    - Maintain or improve strength and endurance.
    - Maximize functional mobility.
    - Maximize independence for activities of daily living.

28. **Describe the role of exercise for a patient with muscle disease.**
    Exercise for strengthening must be submaximal, and overfatigue must be avoided. A supervised, submaximal, resistive exercise program in selected patients may result in increased muscle strength without causing overwork weakness. Strength gains may occur in muscles that are not severely dystrophic. Moderate-intensity aerobic exercises may improve cardiovascular performance. High-intensity eccentric muscle contracting may cause increased CPK and muscle soreness. Slowly progressive or nonprogressive diseases have a better chance of a positive

response to high-resistive weight training. Range of motion exercises may slow down progression of contractures. Balance exercises are useful; however, most patients use biomechanical compensatory techniques to stay upright. Energy conservation techniques are vital. Warning signs of overwork weakness include feeling weaker 30 minutes after exercise, excessive muscle soreness 24–48 hours after exercise, severe muscle cramping, and prolonged shortness of breath.

de Lateur BJ, Giaconi RM: Effects on maximal strength of submaximal exercise in Duchenne's muscular dystrophy. Am J Phys Med 58(1):26–36, 1979.

Kilmer DD, Aitkens SG, Wright NC, McCrory MA: Response to high-intensity eccentric muscle contractions in persons with myopathic disease. Muscle Nerve 24:118–187, 2001.

Milner-Brown HS, Miller RG: Muscle strengthening through high-resistance weight training in patients with neuromuscular disorders. Arch Phys Med Rehabil 69:14–19, 1988.

Wagner MB, Katirji B: Rehabilitation management and care of patients with neuromuscular diseases. In Katirji B, Kaminski HJ, Preston DC, et al (eds): Neuromuscular Disorders in Clinical Practice. Boston, Butterworth-Heinemann, 2002, pp 344–363.

29. **Which myopathies are associated with swallowing difficulties?**
Myotonic dystrophy, polymyositis, dermatomyositis, inclusion body myositis, mitochondrial myopathy, oculopharyngeal dystrophy, and DMD.

30. **Describe the benefits of orthoses for patients with muscle disease.**
Orthoses can provide useful external support to help in substituting for weak muscles. They can also improve bony alignment and provide joint stability. Caution must be taken in ordering lower extremity orthoses in patients with disease because (1) the weight of the brace may be too heavy to be carried by the weak muscles, and (2) changing joint alignment and biomechanics may rob the patient of compensatory gait mechanisms and actually arrest ambulation. Lower extremity night splints are often used to provide passive stretch in the lower extremities.

31. **Describe the role of orthopedic surgery for contractures.**
Elective surgery to release contractures must consider benefit versus risk. Surgery may be successful in improving joint alignment and range of motion. However, risks include anesthesia complications (including ventilator dependence) and deconditioning postoperatively, and the need to learn new compensations for biomechanical abnormalities must be considered. If a lower extremity contracture release procedure is performed in a patient with DMD, proper therapy with lower extremity bracing must be initiated quickly to prevent further disuse atrophy and contractures of already weakened muscle.

32. **Describe the role of gait aids and standers for the myopathic patient.**
Gait aids provide upper extremity support and may assist balance but require sufficient upper extremity strength for use. Bilateral canes are helpful in stabilizing the Trendelenburg gait. As the patient weakens further, advancement to bilateral forearm crutches or a platform walker may be required. Standers (such as parapodiums) allow patients with severe lower extremity weakness to be upright, providing support to bilateral lower extremities and trunk. Gait aids provide upper extremity support and may assist balance but require sufficient upper extremity strength for use.

33. **Describe the role of wheelchairs for the myopathic patient.**
When walking becomes unsafe or requires too much energy consumption, a wheelchair or scooter is a liberating device. In wheelchairs, it is an essential principle that the height of the seat be adjusted to permit both arm and leg propulsion. Advantages of a manual chair include lower cost, lighter weight, and ease in folding, transport, and maintenance.

However, if upper extremity strength is not sufficient for propulsion, then a power wheelchair is the preferred option, provided that visual/perceptual safety awareness is sufficient.

Bakker JP, De Groot IJ, Beelen A, Lankhorst GJ: Predictive factors of cessation of ambulation in patients with Duchenne muscular dystrophy. Am J Phys Med Rehabil 81:906–912, 2002.

Brooke MH: A Clinician's View of Neuromuscular Diseases, 2nd ed. Baltimore, Williams & Wilkins, 1986.

WEBSITES

1. Fascioscapulohumeral Muscular Dystrophy Society
   www.fshsociety.org

2. Malignant Hyperthermia Association of the United States
   www.mhaus.org

3. Muscular Dystrophy Association
   www.mdausa.org

4. Myositis Association
   www.myositis.org

5. National Organization of Rare Diseases
   www.rarediseases.org

FRONTIERS AND FUNDAMENTALS IN NEUROREHABILITATION: METHODS TO ENHANCE FUNCTIONAL RECOVERY

Charles E. Levy, MD, and Haim Ring, MD, MSc PM&R

CHAPTER 52

The human brain is a most unusual instrument of elegant and as yet unknown capacity.
—Stuart Seaton

1. **What is "targeted muscle reinnervation"? How does it improve control of a myoelectric prosthesis for a person with a shoulder disarticulation?**
   Typical shoulder disarticulation prostheses are designed to fit very tightly against the rib cage. The prosthesis is driven with separate trunk and scapular motions translated through cables to flex the elbow and open the terminal device. Electric motor-driven prostheses can be controlled with mechanical switches or myoelectrically. Targeted muscle reinnervation includes surgical denervation and the selective reinnervation of a muscle or muscle segment with another nerve to produce a proportionately contracted myoelectric island. For a shoulder disarticulation prosthesis myoelectric control, three islands can be produced by segmentation and reinnervation of the pectoralis with the musculocutaneous, radical, and median nerves. Transcutaneous pickup of the myoelectric signals from the islands detects variable contraction as a way of controlling the prosthesis.

2. **What is constraint-induced movement therapy (CIMT)?**
   CIMT is a physiotherapeutic technique to restore hand function to those with upper limb hemiparesis. Sometimes referred to as **forced use,** it includes time-intensive exercise of the paretic upper limb, usually with restraint of the able upper limb in a mitt or sling.

3. **What is the minimum amount of motion a person must be able to generate in the paretic limb before being enrolled into a CIMT protocol?**
   A minimum motor criterion (MMC) has been set at 20 degrees of voluntary extension of the wrist, 10 degrees abduction at the thumb, and 10 degrees of extension of two fingers in the affected hand repeated three times in 1 minute. This criterion has been established because people with less motion generally respond less robustly. However, in a study of the effects of botulinum toxin for patients with spasticity who could not meet the minimum motor criterion, Levy et al. found that the ability to extend three fingers against gravity predicted positive (though not robust) response. Fritz et al. found that the ability to actively release from a mass flexion grasp predicted success in CIMT in those unable to meet the MMC. Whatever the exact lowest threshold, it appears that having a greater initial movement initially predicts greater response to CIMT.

   Fritz SL, Light KE: Active finger extension predicts outcomes after constraint-induced movement therapy for individuals with hemiparesis after stroke. Stroke 36:1172–1177, 2005.

   Levy CE, Giufridda C, et al: Botulinum toxin A, evidence-based exercise therapy, and constraint-induced movement therapy for upper limb hemiparesis due to stroke: A preliminary study. Am J Phys Med Rehabil [in press].

4. **Describe a typical CIMT regimen.**

Although many variations exist, a generic program would include:

- A restrictive mitt worn over the able hand during 90% of waking hours, preventing its use, and thus encouraging use of the paretic hand.
- Task practice 6 hours/day, 5 days/week, for 2 weeks with the paretic hand. Typical tasks include tossing a bean bag at a target, reaching and grasping objects, stacking blocks, moving blocks from one container to another, turning pages of a magazine, flipping playing cards, writing on and erasing a chalkboard, and feeding.
- The patient is encouraged and expected to use the paretic hand as much as possible throughout the day whether or not he or she is in therapy.

5. **What evidence supports the efficacy of CIMT?**

Numerous small studies have demonstrated the benefit of CIMT for those with upper-limb hemiparesis due to stroke. Most subjects have been enrolled 6 months to 1 year post-stroke, in a period when conventional physiotherapy has failed to achieve further functional improvement. Subjects have benefited in these trials for as many as 18 years after stroke. Significant improvements in strength, active range of motion (AROM), and functional use have been demonstrated. These benefits generally persist long after treatment.

6. **What are the three major theoretical explanations given for the positive effects of CIMT?**

- **Learned nonuse:** The patient experiences failure every time he or she attempts to use the paretic limb: Coffee spills when the individual attempts to drink, the toothbrush is fumbled, and dressing is unsuccessful. Conversely, when the person employs the able hand, tasks are accomplished. In a relatively short time, the patient stops trying to use the plegic hand and learns to rely exclusively on the "intact" one. In time, the necessary precursors for some amount of functional recovery take place, but because the individual no longer tries to use the plegic hand, the individual realizes no gain.
- **Missed practice:** If one wants to acquire a new skill, one must practice, practice, and practice. Performing artists understand that seamless performance demands multiple repetitions of the act. It is sensible that this also applies for the recovery of function following stroke.
- **Latent pathways and branching:** Typical functional use of a limb only requires a subset of corticospinal pathway activation. Approximately 90% of the corticospinal tracts cross over in the medulla, but about 10% do not and are spared in a unilateral cortical stroke or Brown Sequard-type hemisection of the spinal cord. With sufficient facilitation, these **latent pathways** can be activated and functionally utilized; with subsequent activation, **branching** is induced, enhancing the effect.

7. **What is "modified CIMT"?**

A number of trials have reported functional improvement using the principles of CIMT, but with variations in the formula. More than one trial has identified its variation as "modified CIMT," although the protocols of these trials differ. The variances generally involve lesser doses of task practice (as little as an hour per day 5 days per week, or an hour and a half 3 days per week) spread out over longer periods of time (i.e., 10 weeks). Other variations include training individuals in small groups and decreasing the time the mitt or splint is worn in the able hand.

8. **Does CIMT induce neuroplasticity?**

Both functional magnetic resonance imaging and transcortical magnetic stimulation studies in humans have documented changes in cortical activation that correspond with improved motor abilities in upper-limb paresis due to stroke following CIMT.

Levy CE, Nichols DS, Schmalbrock PM, et al: Functional MRI evidence of cortical reorganization in upper-limb hemiparesis treated with constraint-induced movement therapy. Am J Phys Med Rehabil 80:4–12, 2001.

Liepert J, Bauder H, Miltner WHR, et al: Treatment-induced cortical reorganization after stroke in humans. Stroke 31:1210–1216, 2000.

9. **How soon after a stroke can a CIMT therapy be employed?**
   In the postacute phase (approximately 3 months after stroke), CIMT can be helpful to selected patients. However, how close to the time of the stroke a CIMT program can be implemented is yet unknown. Dromerick et al. randomized 20 subjects to receive either a modified course of CIMT or a "traditional" treatment within 14 days of experiencing a stroke. Those who underwent the experimental treatment had better outcomes at 2 weeks; however, no long-term follow-up was performed.

   Dromerick A, Edwards DA, Hahn M: Does application of constraint-induced movement therapy during acute rehabilitation reduce hemiparesis after ischemic stroke? Stroke 31:2984–2988, 2000.

10. **How does electrical stimulation contribute to neuroplasticity in upper limb motor recovery after brain lesions?**
    Even though **cyclic neuromuscular electrical stimulation** (NMES) of the muscle at a set duty cycle while the patient remains largely passive may contribute to voluntary motor recovery, it is probably the least sophisticated application of electrical stimulation. Randomized trials in stroke suggest that this treatment results in greater upper-limb movement but not necessarily improved function. Limitations of cyclic NMES include the fact that a therapist must be present during training, and training typically does not include functional activities in the home environment.

    The NESS H200 (Bioness, Inc., Santa Clara, CA) is a wrist orthosis equipped with five surface electrodes to stimulate the extensor digitorum, extensor pollicis brevis, flexor digitorum superficialis, flexor policus longus, and thenar muscle groups. The orthosis is designed to be easily and independently donned and doffed by hemiplegic individuals and features preset programs to stimulate hand opening and closure. Once programmed, the H200 can be used independently, allowing practice in the natural functional context of home for hours per day. Users are encouraged to practice functional tasks, such as lifting cups to the mouth, with the help of the orthosis. It can also be used with a therapist, in either a preset or externally triggered mode, to engage in functional task practice. In the most extensive test of the H200, 77 individuals with chronic hemiparesis due to stroke exercised two to three times per day with the H200 for a total daily duration of nearly 3 hours for 5 weeks. Significant improvements were seen on the Jebsen-Taylor, Box and Blocks, and 9 Hole Peg tests.

    The NeuroMove NM900 (Zynex Medical, Littleton, CO) is a device that uses electromyography-triggered NMES. The activity of the extensor communis digitorum and carpi ulnaris are monitored, and when a signal at a certain threshold is obtained, electrical impulse is delivered to accomplish finger extension. As the patient improves, the threshold for external assistance is set at a higher level. Small studies have shown improvement in hand function using the NeuroMove in stroke patients.

    Intramuscular systems offer the potential advantages of less pain and improved muscle selectivity and sensitivity. A multicenter trial of an intramuscular system showed improvement in shoulder pain for stroke survivors with shoulder subluxation.

    Alon G, Ring H: Gait and hand function enhancement following training with a multisegmental hybrid-orthosis stimulation system in stroke patients. J Stroke Cerebrovasc Dis 12(5):209–216, 2003.

    Alon G, Sunnerhagen KS, Geurts ACH, Ohry A: A home-based, self-administered stimulation program to improve selected hand functions of chronic stroke. Neuro Rehabil 18:215–225, 2003.

    Ring H, Rozenthul N: Controlled study of neuroprosthetic functional electrical stimulation in sub-acute post stroke rehabilitation. J Rehab Medicine 37:32–36, 2005.

Ring H, Weingarden H: Neuromodulation by functional electrical stimulation (FES) of limb paralysis after stroke. Acta Neurochirurgica 97(Suppl):375–380, 2007.

Yu DT, Chae J, Walker ME, et al: Intramuscular neuromuscular electrical stimulation for poststroke shoulder pain: a multicenter randomized clinical trial. Arch Phys Med Rehabil 85:695–704, 2004.

11. **What other approaches have shown success in restoring function of the upper limb in stroke hemiparesis?**

A number of additional therapies are emerging to encourage upper-limb recovery following stroke.

Robotic devices (i.e., InMotion2, manufactured by Interactive Motion Technologies, Cambridge, MA, a commercial version of the MIT-Manus robot) are appealing because they may offer:

- Precise and reproducible exercise and task practice, free of the variation, boredom, and fatigue involved with human trainers.
- A combination of force, visual, and audio feedback.
- Accurate and reliable performance records.

At this point, robotic therapy has targeted the proximal portions of the upper limb. Although positive effects on strength and motion have been documented, improvement in function has yet to be clearly and consistently demonstrated.

Bilateral arm training with rhythmic auditory cues (BATRAC) is based on the concept that bilateral movement permits interhemispheric facilitation for recovery of limb function. It involves use of a device consisting of T-bar handles mounted in a nearly frictionless track, which allows the patient to either push and pull with both upper limbs in unison or in an alternating fashion, using a metronomic auditory cue. This approach has shown promise in small studies.

Luft AR, McCombe-Walker S, Whitall J, et al: Repetitive bilateral arm training and motor cortex activation in chronic stroke: a randomized controlled trial. JAMA 292:1853–1861, 2004.

12. **Do neurons in the mature central nervous system (CNS) ever regrow?**

Although neurogenesis in the mature CNS is rare, it occurs in at least two regions:

- New neurons for the olfactory bulb are generated in the subventricular zone in the wall of the lateral ventricle and then migrate rostrally to their destinations, where they assume the role of interneurons.
- The subgranular zone of the dentate gyrus gives rise to neocortical granule cells. There is even evidence that damage to granule cells can trigger increased proliferation and recruitment of new granule cells from resident progenitors.

There is, as of yet, no evidence that these processes play a significant role in functional recovery from brain injury. However, their discovery raises the enticing possibility that the brain has latent capabilities for self-repair. There is evidence that neurogenesis may be enhanced by gene therapy or by the application of growth factors.

Abrahams JM, Gokhan S, Flamm ES, Mehler MF: De novo neurogenesis and acute stroke. Are exogenous stem cells really necessary? Neurosurgery 54:150–156, 2004.

13. **Why is it that injured neurons so rarely regenerate in the CNS?**

CNS neurons are capable of extending their axons and branching, although CNS myelin inhibits axonal growth.

14. **What strategies are being employed to overcome barriers to regeneration?**

Regeneration is a multistep process:

1. Injured neurons must survive or be replaced.
2. The damaged or replacement axons must extend their processes to the original targets.
3. The remyelination of the damaged axons must occur.
4. Functional synapses must form.

Stem cells and **fetal tissue** are possible sources for cellular replacement for the damaged CNS. Stem cells are (1) multipotent, (2) can be propagated in vitro, (3) can be genetically tagged with markers or therapeutic genes, and (4) can be directly grafted into the mature CNS. The new cells will have to be able to thrive in the altered environment of the injured CNS and be capable of functional integration into the remaining CNS circuitry.

Neurotrophic factor delivery. Neurotrophins, such as brain-derived neurotrophic factor (BDNF), aid in cell survival and promote axon growth. They are usually combined with growth-promoting cells or matrices to provide the needed permissive substrate. Schwann cells engineered to express BDNF facilitated the regrowth of supraspinal axons across a transected spinal cord. However, axons have difficulty leaving the permissive substrate to reach their targets in the injured CNS. There is some evidence that this may be overcome with induction of neurotrophins in the injured tissue.

Axon guidance and **removal of growth inhibition.** Several growth-promoting molecules have a role in axon guidance, synapse formation and regeneration, and activity-dependent plasticity. After CNS injury, a **gliotic scar** may form. The scar can present both a physical and molecular barrier to regrowth. Growth inhibitory molecules, which are present in the normal CNS, may be re-expressed in the scar. These may include semaphorin III/collapsin I, proteoglycan NG2, chondroitin sulfate, and keratin.

Bridging is a strategy to be applied when a portion of the CNS is lost, a cyst has developed, or extensive scarring exists. A bridge is used to guide axons across these barriers and reintroduce axons into intact parenchyma. Artificial substrates that can act as a scaffold for axon growth are being developed.

15. **If central regeneration is so limited, how does recovery happen?**
Although regeneration to the original target by the original axon is rare, other modes of neuronal rearrangement are more common:
- **Pruning (actually branching):** An uninjured axon grows a new branch to reinnervate the abandoned target. Animal data suggest that when this process occurs, it takes months to reach completion.
- **Collateral sprouting:** A neighboring axon branches to assume the territory of the injured axon. This process can aid in recovery if the contributing neuron is similar to the lost neuron, but this may also lead to dysfunction if the new sprout transmits signals of significant variance to the original. In experimental animals, collateral sprouting is evident within 8 hours of injury and is usually complete within 1 month.
- **Ingrowth:** Takes months to complete. The contributing axon is remote to the injured axon. Because of the distance traversed, the contributing neuron innervates a foreign target, usually with a maladaptive result, and takes months to complete.

16. **Explain "unmasking" as it relates to recovery of function after brain injury.**
Unmasking involves activation of previously "silent" synapses that only begin to express function after injury to primary functional synapses. Bach-y-Rita gives the analogy that if telephone lines direct from New York to San Francisco were irredeemably destroyed, less direct routes from New York to Washington to Denver to San Francisco might be employed. With time and increased demand, the more convoluted route might gain efficiency that rivaled the original. In this way, multisynaptic neural routes might be unmasked and compensate for damaged direct pathways.

Bach-y-Rita P: Central nervous system lesions: Sprouting and unmasking in rehabilitation. Arch Phys Med Rehabil 62:413–417, 1981.

17. **What are the major stimulants used in neurorehabilitation?**
Dextroamphetamine (Dexedrine, GlaxoSmithKline, Research Triangle Park, NC) and methylphenidate (Ritalin, Novartis, East Hanover, NJ) are the major stimulants used in rehabilitation. Modafinil (Mylan Laboratories, Canonsburg, PA) is a recent addition to the category. Cocaine, nicotine, and caffeine are also stimulants used.

18. **What are the histories of amphetamine and methylphenidate?**
    - **Amphetamine** was first synthesized in 1887, and used to treat a wide variety of illnesses, including narcolepsy and depression in the 1930s. In 1936, benzedrine was available over the counter. German Panzer troops used "huge amounts of methamphetamine" during the invasions of Poland, Belgium, and France. American, British, and Japanese forces also used these substances. After World War II, medical interest waned as the abuse potential became better understood. The use of amphetamines declined further with the development of tricyclic antidepressants, starting with imipramine in 1957 and amitriptyline in 1961. Currently, dextroamphetamine is a highly restricted drug, for which the only Food and Drug Administration (FDA)-approved indications are the treatment of narcolepsy and attention deficit hyperactivity disorder. The drug has a half-life of 7–10 hours and reaches peak effect in 2–4 hours.
    - **Methylphenidate** was marketed in 1954 as a mood elevator with less euphoria, addiction, and "rebound letdown" than amphetamines. However, by 1960, cases of abuse and addiction were noted, and by 1962, cases of methylphenidate psychosis were reported. This drug has a half-life of 2–4 hours and reaches peak effect in 1–2 hours.

KEY POINTS: IMPROVED RECOVERY METHODS FOR CENTRAL NERVOUS SYSTEM INJURY

1. Constraint-induced movement therapy, robotic therapy, neuromuscular electrical stimulation, and body weight-suspended treadmill training are improving upper and lower limb recovery.

2. Endogenous and exogenous cellular strategies hold promise to improve recovery from CNS injury.

3. Exercise and physical activity have positive effects on brain neuromodulation and plasticity.

4. Methylphenidate appears to improve speed of processing in individuals with traumatic brain injury.

19. **How do amphetamines and methylphenidate differ?**
    Both drugs increase the availability of dopamine (DA) and norepinephrine (NE). Dextroamphetamine causes direct release of DA and NE, as well as the blockade of catecholamine uptake. However, with dextroamphetamine, the release of dopamine is from a newly synthesized pool that is not calcium dependent, whereas the dopamine released by methylphenidate is probably from a calcium-dependent storage pool. Both drugs affect serotonin in distinct manners.

20. **What other mechanisms might account for the behavioral improvement associated with amphetamine?**
    Evidence suggests that amphetamine coupled with appropriate behavioral therapy initially increases neurite growth, which is then followed by increased synaptogenesis. Animals treated with amphetamine and behavioral therapy showed significant increases in **GAP-43,** an indicator of neuronal sprouting, followed by increases in **synaptophysin** (a presynaptic vesicle protein that can be used to quantify the number of terminals during neuroanatomic remodeling).

21. **Is dextroamphetamine actually helpful for humans with strokes?**
There is not a large body of literature to answer this question. The studies that are available suffer from various drug and behavioral therapy regimens and generally small numbers of subjects. A Cochrane review found that language and motor function may respond to dextroamphetamine but not activities of daily living, depression, or neurologic function. Overall, they conclude that further trials are needed.

    Martinsson L, Wahlgren NG, Hardemark HG: Amphetamines for improving recovery after stroke. The Cochrane Database of Systematic Reviews 4, 2005.

22. **How has methylphenidate been used in rehabilitation?**
In a double-blind, placebo-controlled trial, in acute stroke, methylphenidate was associated with lower scores on depression scales and higher scores on scales of motor recovery. Methylphenidate also appears safe and effective for poststroke depression. In the rehabilitation of patients with acute traumatic brain injury, a single dose of methylphenidate improved working memory, visuospatial attention, and reaction time in a double-blind placebo-controlled trial. Speed of processing and caregiver ratings of attention improved in a 6-week, double-blind, placebo-controlled crossover study in postacute traumatic brain injury (TBI).

    Whyte J, Hart T, Vaccaro M, et al: Effects of methylphenidate on attention deficits in traumatic brain injury: A multidimensional randomized controlled trial. Am J Phys Med Rehabil 83:401–420, 2004.

23. **What is modafinil? How has it been used in rehabilitation?**
Modafinil (Provigil®) is a new member of the stimulant class whose primary application is for sleep disorders. Its mechanism of action has yet to be fully elucidated, but it appears that modafinil is a direct alpha-1 agonist, promotes the release of dopamine in the nucleus accumbens, and inhibits γ-aminobutyric acid (GABA) release in the basal ganglia. It has been used to improve self-esteem in individuals with spinal cord acid injury (SCI), to reduce fatigue in multiple sclerosis, and to elevate mood and decrease sleepiness in myotonic dystrophy.

24. **Are there any human data to support the contention that benzodiazepines inhibit recovery following stroke?**
Goldstein et al. prospectively studied the motor recovery of patients assigned to the control group of a larger study on the effects of GM1 ganglioside on stroke. The control group (which did not receive GM1 ganglioside) was then divided into those who were treated with any "detrimental" drugs (benzodiazepines, dopamine receptor antagonists, α_1-adrenergic receptor antagonists, α_2-adrenergic receptor agonists, phenytoin, and phenobarbital) during their hospital course ($n = 37$) versus those who were not ($n = 57$, the "neutral" group). Of the 37 subjects in the detrimental group, 27 were treated with a benzodiazepine and 8 received dopamine receptor blockers (there also was some overlap). Members of the detrimental drug group displayed significantly greater upper-limb motor impairment and lesser recovery in activities of daily living.

    Limits of this study include: (1) no randomization, (2) those in the "detrimental group" may have had more significant medical or behavioral problems that warranted treatment with the "detrimental" drugs, and (3) the design did not allow determination of the degree to which the individual medications were harmful or whether negative effects were dose related.

    Despite these limitations, use of benzodiazepines and the other "detrimental" drugs should be avoided.

    Goldstein LB: Sygen in acute stroke study investigators: Common drugs may influence motor recovery after stroke. Neurology 45:865–871, 1995.

25. **What is virtual reality?**
Virtual reality (VR) uses advanced technologies, including computers and various multimedia peripherals, to produce environmental experiences that simulate actual environments.

Users are typically provided with visual and audio feedback. In some instances, haptic and olfactory feedback is provided. Advantages of VR include the following:

- Safety
- Repetition
- Augmented feedback
- Precise control of the stimulus
- Precise measurement of the user's response
- Ability to precisely tailor the experience to address the certain goals
- Reproducibility
- Motivation

Realms of application in rehabilitation include upper and lower limb function, wheelchair mobility, balance, activities of daily living, spatial and perceptual deficits, and in a variety of musculoskeletal and neurologic conditions, including stroke, traumatic brain injury, and Parkinson's disease. Models of treatment include training the individual in a video game–type format and teaching by example.

Holden MK: Virtual reality in motor rehabilitation: Review. Cyberpsychol Behav 8:187–211, 2005.

Katz N, Ring H, Naveh Y, et al: Interactive virtual environment training for safe street crossing on right hemisphere stroke patients with unilateral spatial neglect. J Disabil Rehabil 27(20):1235–1243, 2005.

26. What is the relationship between physical activity and exercise, brain-derived neurotrophic factor (BDNF), and neuroplasticity?

Regular exercise is associated with the upregulation of a number of genes that promote plasticity, including BDNF, synaptotagmin 5, and neuronal activity-regulated pentraxin, all which positively impact neuroplasticity. Animal studies suggest that BDNF is a key mediator in synaptic efficacy, neuronal connectivity, and use-dependent plasticity.

BDNF is neurotropic and neuroprotective:

- It promotes the differentiation, neurite expansion, and survival in hippocampal, cortical, striatal, septal, and cerebellar neurons.
- Intraventricular infusion of BDNF protects the hippocampus and cortex from ischemic damage and the septal cholinergic neurons from axotomy-induced loss.

BDNF can enhance neuroplasticity:

- It enhances synaptic transmission and long-term potentiation.
- It stimulates synaptophysin and synaptobrevin synthesis.

Cotman CW, Berchtold NC: Exercise: A behavioral intervention to enhance brain health and plasticity. Trends Neurosci 6:295–301, 2002.

27. What is locomotor training?

Locomotor training, using a body weight support system on a treadmill with manual assistance from trainers, is an experimental intervention to facilitate the recovery of walking in humans after CNS injury. This training has been described by various names, including body weight–assisted training and body weight–supported treadmill training. Using the term *locomotor training* emphasizes the intent of the training over the devices to implement it. The treadmill provides an external rhythmical drive and means to adjust the training speed for stepping. A body weight support system consists of a harness, worn by the patient about his or her pelvis and trunk, which is attached to a system able to precisely adjust the amount of body weight being supported by the system (or conversely, the amount of body weight the limbs must support). The trainers facilitate overall trunk and limb kinematics, timing, and limb loading, which are consistent with the pattern of normal walking.

28. What is central pattern generation?

Central pattern generation refers to the rhythmical right and left, oscillating activity of segmental neural circuitry in the spinal cord. This repetitive, alternating activation of flexors and extensors can occur independently of supraspinal control, producing a gait-like pattern of facilitation and inhibition.

29. **How does locomotor training differ from current practice for the rehabilitation of walking after SCI?**
Conventional gait training following SCI often relies on teaching compensatory strategies, including the use of assistive devices such as canes and walkers. These methods rely on the acquisition of different limb and trunk kinematics, timing, and load-bearing as compared to a typical walking pattern. Locomotor training with body-weight suspension permits gait training in patients with very minimal strength. This treatment allows adjustment of weight support through the limbs, full range of reciprocal motion through the gait cycle, and active movement.

30. **What effect does body weight–supported treadmill training (BWSTT) have on muscle for patients with SCI?**
BWSTT induces an increase in muscle fiber size and brings about increases in muscle oxidative capacity as well as improving lipid profile.

Stewart BG: Treadmill training-induced adaptations in muscle phenotype in persons with incomplete spinal cord injury. Muscle Nerve 30:61–68, 2004.

31. **Is the Lokomat a place to clean laundry?**
Despite the sound of its name, the Lokomat has nothing to do with laundry. In fact, the Lokomat is a driven gait orthosis, consisting of a computer-controlled, motorized treadmill; a weight-suspending harness; and an exoskeletal apparatus that is placed on the patient's legs. Conventional BWSTT is very labor intensive. Up to three therapists are often necessary to facilitate upright posture and normal walking patterns. The Lokomat is automated so that there is no need for human assistance to maintain upright posture and to provide proper stepping. Initial small trials have supported the efficacy of the Lokomat for incomplete spinal cord injury.

Wirz M, Zemon DH, Rupp R, et al: Effectiveness of automated locomotor training in patients with chronic incomplete spinal cord injury: a multicenter trial. Arch Phys Med Rehabil 86:672–680, 2005.

CHAPTER 53

TRAUMATIC BRAIN INJURY: PATHOPHYSIOLOGY, ASSESSMENT, AND MANAGEMENT

Ofer Keren, MD, Robert L. Harmon, MD, MS, and Lawrence J. Horn, MD

The finest piece of mechanism in all the universe is the brain of man.

—Alfred A. Montapert

1. **What is traumatic brain injury (TBI)? How is it differentiated from stroke?**
   TBI is a type of acquired brain injury. Like stroke, TBI may involve brain lesions due to ischemia or hemorrhage. Unlike stroke patients, those with TBI might also sustain direct and indirect forces, producing diffuse brain function impairments. TBI patients tend to have more cognitive, personality, and behavioral impairments than stroke patients.

EPIDEMIOLOGY

2. **What are the incidence and prevalence of TBI? What are two of the most common causes?**
   The estimated incidence rate of mild TBI is 134 per 100,000 persons; of moderate TBI, 15 per 100,000 persons; and of severe TBI, 14 per 100,000 persons. The prevalence is estimated to be between 2.5 million and 6.5 million individuals. The highest incidence occurs among persons 15–24 years of age and 75 years and older. Motor vehicle, bicycle, and pedestrian vehicular accidents account for over half of the TBIs in the United States. Falls are the next most common cause, most often occurring in those under 15 and over 70 years of age.

   Dawudo ST: Traumatic brain injury: Definition, epidemiology, pathophysiology. Available at www.emedicine.com/pmr/topic212.htm

3. **How do drug and alcohol use, use of helmets while riding motorcycles, and use of seat belts impact TBI incidence?**
   Alcohol use associated with motor vehicle accidents may contribute to intracranial hemorrhage following head trauma. Drug use, in general, can impair cognition and reaction time, increasing risk of a motor vehicle accident. Seat belts, motorcycle helmets, and air bags have been shown to significantly decrease head injury risk.

4. **How often is TBI associated with spinal cord injury? With extremity fractures?**
   TBI and spinal cord injury occur together in 25–50% of cases due to traffic accidents. Approximately 10–11% of patients admitted to rehabilitation following TBI have previously unrecognized skeletal trauma, including spine injury. Postinjury spine, pelvis, and extremity x-rays should be obtained. A whole-body bone scan should be considered for skeletally immature patients.

   Young MA, O'Young BJ, McFarland EG: Rehabilitation of the orthopedic trauma patient: General principles. Phys Med Rehabil State Art Rev 9(1), 1995 (entire issue).

PATHOPHYSIOLOGY

5. **What are the principal types of primary injuries resulting from TBI?**
   Primary injuries to the brain occur as a direct result of the forces involved in the traumatic event upon the brain and are not preventable except by preventing the traumatic event itself. These primary injuries include:
   - Contusions and lacerations of the brain surface (typically occurring on the frontal and temporal lobes inferiorly where the brain contacts the base of the skull)
   - Diffuse/regional axonal injury (related to shearing injury disrupting nerve axons in the brain white matter)
   - Diffuse vascular injury resulting in multiple petechial hemorrhages within the brain
   - Contusion or shearing of the cranial nerves (most commonly the olfactory nerve)
   - Tearing of the pituitary stalk (might imply endocrinal impairments).

6. **What are secondary types of injury arising from brain trauma?**
   Secondary damage to the brain results from processes produced by the injuring event but tend to be somewhat delayed in their presentation, suggesting that it may be preventable (at least in theory). The principal types of secondary injuries include:
   - Intracranial hemorrhage (which may be extradural, subdural, subarachnoid, or intracerebral)
   - Brain swelling related to increased cerebral blood volume and/or cerebral edema
   - Increased intracranial pressure
   - Brain damage associated with hypoxia
   - Intracranial infection (particularly with penetrating injuries)
   - Hydrocephalus
   - Neurochemical sequelae leading to neuronal death.

7. **What is diffuse axonal injury (DAI)?**
   DAI is one of the most common and important pathologic features of TBI. The susceptibility of axons to mechanical injury appears to be due to their viscoelasticity and their high organization in white matter tracts. Axons become brittle when exposed to rapid deformations associated with brain trauma. The more appropriate name is *regional axonal injury,* since there are specific areas of the brain that are more prone to damage according to skull anatomy and the trauma mechanism.

8. **What are the different theories that relate to recovery of brain function following brain injury?**
   There are multiple theories regarding recovery of brain function; four of the more common ones are **diaschisis, vicariation, redundancy,** and **behavioral substitution** (Table 53-1). Initially, functional recovery depends on the reversal of ischemia and edema in regions surrounding the areas of neuronal loss. Because areas involved by diaschisis are still intact, there have been attempts to modulate the rate of recovery from this process experimentally and in the clinical setting.

   Albensi BC, Janigro D: Traumatic brain injury and its effects on synaptic plasticity. Brain Inj 17:653–663, 2003.
   Hurley S, Noë A: Neural plasticity and consciousness. Biol Philosophy 18:131–168, 2003.

9. **Describe the neurochemical changes following brain injury.**
   Research suggests that cells die through the processes of necrosis (a rapid and disorganized loss of cellular homeostasis and viability) and apoptosis (a more prolonged and orderly process of cellular breakdown that is genetically regulated). In **necrosis,** acutely after brain injury, large amounts of neurotransmitters are released, particularly excitatory neurotransmitters such as glutamate. Neurotransmitters bind to receptors in neuronal cell membranes, activating postsynaptic ion channels. Excess amounts of ionized calcium enter

TABLE 53-1.	THEORIES REGARDING RECOVERY OF BRAIN FUNCTION
Theory	**Description**
Diaschisis	Following brain injury, there is functional depression in intact areas of the brain at a distance from, but anatomically linked to, the damaged area. The resolution of behavioral deficits would be expected to occur in conjunction with a return of activity in these functionally depressed areas.
Vicariation	Functions are taken over by parts of the brain not originally handling that function.
Redundancy	Recovery of function is based on the activity of uninjured brain regions that normally would contribute to that function.
Behavioral substitution	New strategies are learned to compensate for the behavioral deficit.

the cell this way, as well as through voltage-activated channels, activating phospholipases within the cell. This results in increased arachidonic acid metabolism and the production of free radicals that may damage or destroy the neuronal membrane. The release of intracellular contents may trigger inflammation, leading to damage of neighboring cells. These processes may occur minutes or hours following brain injury.

Cellular degradation through **apoptosis** usually does not lead to the damage of neighboring cells. Necrosis generally occurs in the center of an ischemic area, whereas apoptosis tends to be found in the penumbra. However, there is overlap of these processes in areas of ischemic injury. The release of toxic chemicals from neurons undergoing necrosis may result in apoptosis of other cells. Postacute neurochemical changes relate to alterations in the level and turnover of various neurotransmitters and their receptors. These postacute changes may cause diaschisis-like effects, which were described previously.

10. **What can be used to intervene in this neurochemical process to minimize the adverse effects?**
Drugs can be used to minimize injury in association with acute TBI. Drugs include those that may offer neuroprotection (preventing cellular injury before it occurs) and "rescue" of damaged cells (reversing cellular damage before cell death occurs). Various neurotrophic factors assist in neuronal repair and survival under experimental conditions. Drugs have been produced that block the N-methyl-D-aspartate (NMDA) glutamate receptor in order to minimize glutamate-mediated calcium influx into neurons. Other drugs can minimize inflammation associated with cellular necrosis, including **antioxidants** and **free radical scavengers.**

ASSESSMENT, DIAGNOSIS, AND PROGNOSIS

11. **What are some common evaluation tools used in TBI?**
   - **Acute phase: Glasgow coma scale** (GCS) is scored between 3 and 15, 3 being the worst, 15 the best. It is composed of three parameters: best eye response, best verbal response, and best motor response, as detailed in Table 53-2. A score of 13 or higher correlates with a mild brain injury, a score of 9–12 indicates moderate injury, and a score of 8 or less reflects a severe brain injury. The phrase "GCS of 11" is essentially meaningless; it is important to break the figure down into its components, such as E3V3M5 = GCS 11.
   - **Subacute phase: Disability rating scale** (DRS). One advantage of the DRS is its ability to track an individual from coma to community. Measurement across a wide span of recovery is possible because items in this scale address all three World Health Organization

TABLE 53-2. PARAMETERS OF THE GLASGOW COMA SCALE

Best Eye Response	Best Verbal Response	Best Motor Response
1. No eye opening	1. No verbal response	1. No motor response
2. Eye opening to pain	2. Incomprehensible sounds	2. Extension to pain
3. Eye opening to verbal command	3. Inappropriate words	3. Flexion to pain
4. Eyes open spontaneously	4. Confused	4. Withdrawal from pain
	5. Oriented	5. Localizing pain
		6. Obeys commands

disablement domains. The maximum score is 29 (extreme vegetative state). A person without disability would score zero.
- **Chronic phase:** The **community integration questionnaire** (CIQ) was developed to provide a measure of community integration after TBI. The CIQ consists of 15 items relevant to home integration (H), social integration (S), and productive activities (P). It is scored to provide subtotals for each of these, as well as for overall community integration.
- **Assessments of structure/function:** Assessments of brain structure include studies such as computed tomography/magnetic resonance imaging (CT/MRI), functional MRI/single photon emission computed tomography/positron emission tomography (FMRI/SPECT/PET), electroencephalography (EEG), and evoked potentials, as well as clinical tools such as neuropsychologic evaluations and functional assessments. The **Glasgow outcome scale** is divided into five categories: dead, persistent vegetative state, severe disability, moderate disability, and good outcome. It has been criticized as being relatively insensitive, particularly given the span of the "severe disability" category.

Center for Outcome Measurements in Brain Injury (COMBI): www.tbims.org/combi/list.html

12. **What are the best prognostic indicators for patients following TBI?**
Prognostic indicators related to the injury itself include duration of coma (the shorter the better; >4 weeks is extremely poor), duration of post-traumatic amnesia (the shorter the better; >11 weeks is inconsistent with independent living), and motor response on the GCS (with active posturing, decorticate/decerebrate, or worse representing a fairly clear prognostic demarcation from higher levels of motor function). Other clinical findings, including evidence for brain stem involvement such as dysconjugate gaze or altered pupillary responses, can add power to prognostic indication. The most useful information is often the actual early recovery course a patient demonstrates.

People under 20 years of age generally fare much better than those over 60 with the same kind of injury. Children < 2 years of age are the exception. Between the third and sixth decades, there is not much variability in terms of outcome. Another variable unrelated to the injury itself is the patient's premorbid psychosocial status. An individual with considerable psychological impairment or social disruption can be anticipated to have a relatively poorer outcome from a brain injury than someone without these problems. This is particularly true in the case of significant substance abuse.

Indicators can be divided into three general stages:
- The **first stage** includes indicators useful in the acute care setting. These are most effective in prognosticating life versus death.
- The **second stage** is after the acute phase has passed and the patient has begun involvement in active rehabilitation.
- **Long-term outcome** is best reserved until several months to a year has passed following the injury.

ASSOCIATED INJURIES/COMPLICATIONS/MANAGEMENT

13. **What nerve injuries are commonly associated with TBI?**
    Upper extremity plexopathies may occur as a result of trauma-induced traction, compression, or laceration injuries. Radiculopathies, nerve root avulsions, and nerve root compression are seen. Focal neuropathies associated with heterotopic ossification (e.g., ulnar nerve at the elbow) can occur. TBI-associated spasticity may cause contractures, which also secondarily affect peripheral nerves (e.g., median and ulnar nerve). Multiple trauma may cause fractures and soft tissue injury, resulting in peroneal, median, and ulnar nerve compromise.

    Groswasser Z, Cohen M, Blankstein E: Polytrauma associated with traumatic brain injury: Incidence, nature and impact on rehabilitation outcome. Brain Inj 4:161–166, 1990.

14. **How does the occurrence and management of heterotopic ossification in TBI compare to that in spinal cord injury?**
    Admittedly, as in spinal cord injury, the exact etiology of heterotopic ossification is unknown. One main difference with TBI, however, is in the joint sites involved. Heterotopic ossification involves the upper and lower extremities equally following TBI, whereas the hip and knee are primarily affected following spinal cord injury. The incidence of heterotopic ossification following TBI ranges from 11% to 76%. It most commonly involves the shoulder, elbow, and hip, infrequently occurring at the thigh and knee. Patients at highest risk are those in coma >2 weeks, with spasticity, and with long bone fractures.

    While passive range of motion is advocated (as in spinal cord injury) to decrease the risk of heterotopic ossification, controversy exists as to whether these exercises may actually contribute to ectopic bone formation. One small study of patients with TBI suggested that etidronate disodium may significantly decrease the risk of heterotopic ossification if given early after injury at a dose of 20 mg/kg for 3 months, followed by 10 mg/kg for an additional 3 months. Nonsteroidal anti-inflammatory drugs also have been used, although studies supporting their efficacy in this patient population are lacking.

    Melamed E, Robinson D, Halperin N, et al: Brain injury–related heterotopic bone formation-treatment strategies and results. Am J Phys Med Rehabil 81:670–674, 2002.

15. **How does the management of spasticity associated with TBI differ from that in spinal cord injury?**
    Historically, there has not been much difference. The use of physical agents, splinting, neurolytic and motor point blocks, botulinum toxin injections, and surgical intervention usually follows the same line of decision making regarding management in both patient populations. **Dantrolene sodium** has been considered the oral agent of choice in managing spasticity associated with various forms of brain injury; baclofen and diazepam tend not to be advocated as much because they have side effects that may include sedation and impairment of cognitive function. **Alpha-2 adrenergic agonists**, such as clonidine and tizanidine, have been found to be effective in managing spasticity following various forms of brain injury. **Intrathecal baclofen** therapy is now being used in the management of severe spasticity following brain injuries; while tending to have its main effects on the lower limbs, improved upper limb function with reduction in hypertonicity may also be noted.

16. **What is the most common cause of bladder dysfunction experienced by patients with TBI?**
    Following TBI, the most common cause of bladder dysfunction is uninhibited bladder. The common problem is urinary incontinence or (less frequently) retention. Following TBI, urinary incontinence commonly occurs secondary to impaired cognitive or behavioral functioning with or without overt imaging findings of brain damage. Dyscontrol is common during the acute phase. However, most patients regain control. Urinary incontinence is common after acute TBI

and is associated with poorer functional outcome. Continence problems following severe TBI may be attributable to either organic or psychological factors.

17. **From what kind of insomnia might TBI patients suffer?**
Sleep disturbances after TBI occur in 30–70% of patients. TBI patients most commonly have difficulty falling asleep and maintaining sleep. Sleep disturbances can exacerbate other symptoms such as pain, cognitive deficits, fatigue, or irritability. Potential etiologic factors are lesions of the nervous system as well as general precipitating factors, such as anxiety. Treatment includes psychological intervention and pharmacologic medication such as nonbenzodiazepine hypnotics (e.g., trazodone, zolpidem) or benzodiazepine anxiolytics. The benzodiazepine anxiolytics should be used sparingly, as they can impair cognition. Normal sleep-wake cycles should be established as early as possible to enhance optimal alertness during daylight hours to maximize the patient's participation in rehabilitation and to facilitate the patient's ability to return to work.

Ouellet MC: Insomnia following traumatic brain injury: A review. Neurorehabil Neural Repair 18(4):187–198, 2004.

18. **What cognitive and behavioral changes are commonly seen following TBI?**
Virtually any change in intellectual function or behavior can be observed following brain injury. The most common **cognitive** problems are deficits in attention (inability to concentrate, increased distractibility, or even perseveration) and memory. As with stroke, specific cognitive disorders may emerge that include (but are not limited to) aphasias, agnosias, apraxias, temporal sequencing problems, visual-perceptual and spatial dysfunctions, prosodic deficits, and, with frontal lesions, disorders of judgment, planning, and other metacognitive skills.

The most common **behavioral** problems include impulse control or disinhibition of the dampening system for emotional response to a stimulus (e.g., pseudobulbar affect). The disinhibition may present as anger and violent behavior or as emotional lability. Another problem may be "agitation," which in the early stages of recovery is often related to confusion and post-traumatic amnesia; it is not necessarily related to long-term behavioral changes. More chronic problems include social impropriety, loss of pragmatic skills, low frustration tolerance, and, less commonly, actual violence and aggression.

19. **How might attention abilities be influenced by TBI?**
Disturbances in arousal and attention are most common post-TBI. However, the consensus regarding appropriate evaluation and treatment of attention deficits is limited. Attention is sometimes addressed by the use of dual task paradigms. It has been shown that TBI patients have impaired divided attention when concurrently performing two tasks requiring working memory. Visual attention has many aspects, which may involve different brain locations. Another important aspect of attention, which has received little or no study in TBI populations, is the allocation of attention in space. Although there is no reason to suspect that TBI damage is asymmetrical, there may be an asymmetrical effect on attention, because the attention mechanism itself may be asymmetrical. Some TBI patients benefit from methylphenidate (Ritalin, Novartis, East Hanover, NJ).

20. **Describe appropriate pharmacologic interventions and some behaviorally and environmentally based strategies for patients with disruptive or aggressive behavior.**
Post-traumatic agitation may be present for up to 3 weeks. A survey of brain injury practitioners recommended the following medications: carbamazepine, tricyclic antidepressants, trazodone, amantadine, and beta blockers. **Beta blockers** may be useful in managing post-traumatic agitation, such as in association with central dysautonomia. **Amantadine** and **methylphenidate** may be used when agitated behavior is felt to be related to attention deficits. Amantadine is a dopaminergic agent and NMDA antagonist used to stimulate "initiation" in chronic TBI. It improves and increases activity in the prefrontal cortex, which may benefit the executive

function. There is a significant positive correlation between executive domain scores and left pre-frontal glucose metabolism. **Neuroleptics** and **benzodiazepines** are less commonly used because of concerns related to cognitive impairment and potential slowing of behavioral recovery; these medications tend to be reserved for acute situations in which the patient endangers himself/herself or others.

In some situations, it is tempting to consider sedation rather than treating the patient's "agitated" behavior. Define the undesired behavior in a way upon which all observers can agree. The behavior should be observed in regard to its frequency and associated environmental factors serving as its "triggers." The environment should be modified to remove triggers, if at all possible, and the behavior monitored to see if its occurrence diminishes. Principles of operant conditioning may also be utilized to help extinguish the undesired behavior.

Fugate L, Spacek L, Kresty L, et al: Measurement and treatment of agitation following traumatic brain injury. II: A survey of the Brain Injury Special Interest Group of the American Academy of Physical Medicine and Rehabilitation. Arch Phys Med Rehabil 78:924–928, 1997.

21. **Which anticonvulsant medications are most appropriate for this patient population?**
    Although some TBI patients require anticonvulsants, the current consensus is that anticonvulsant prophylaxis has been overused. Of all hospitalized TBI patients, 5–7% develop seizures. This number may approach 35–50% for more critical patients with penetrating injuries. Evidence supports the use of anticonvulsant prophylaxis and treatment of early seizures occurring within the first week after brain injury. Anticonvulsants are not recommended after 1 week following nonpenetrating TBI in the patient with no history of seizures. Some recommend treating prophylactically in the case of missile or open injuries, which have an association with seizures of approximately 40%. Some have recommended using carbamazepine **or** valproate; these medications may be better tolerated in the brain-injured population. See Chapter 24, Medications: Tools for Wellness and Enablement in Rehabilitation, for further details.

22. **What intracranial complications commonly arise relatively late after TBI?**
    A reduction in the functional recovery rate or a loss of gains may be a subtle but serious sign of a reversible complication. **Post-traumatic hydrocephalus** should be differentiated from **hydrocephalus ex vacuo,** which is the expected ventricular dilatation due to encephalomalacia or loss of brain tissue associated with the brain trauma itself. Shunting of the post-traumatic hydrocephalus can reduce intracranial pressure, which can lead to improved function. **Cerebrospinal fluid fistulas** may occur as a consequence of head trauma, reaching an incidence of 5–11% in patients with basilar skull fractures. **Post-traumatic movement disorders,** such as tremor and Parkinsonism, may be sequelae of injury. Post-traumatic epilepsy may occur relatively late (even years) following injury.

KEY POINTS: FACTORS THAT MEDIATE TBI RECOVERY

1. Resolution of the edema

2. Return of full blood perfusion

3. Resolution of neural suppression by diaschisis

4. Activation of latent pathways

5. Vicariation

6. Redundancy

7. Behavioral substitution

COMA, VEGETATIVE, AND MINIMALLY CONSCIOUS STATES

23. **What is minimally conscious state (MCS)? How does it differ from coma and vegetative state (VS)?**

MCS is a condition of severely altered consciousness in which the person demonstrates minimal but definite behavioral evidence of self/environmental awareness, as opposed to the unresponsive behavior of VS. To diagnose MCS, at least one of the following criteria should be present and occur on a reproducible or sustained basis:

- Follows simple commands
- Gestural or verbal "yes/no" responses (regardless of accuracy)
- Intelligible verbalization
- Movements or affective behaviors that occur in consequent relation to relevant environmental stimulus and are not attributable to reflexive activity

The **vegetative state** is a clinical condition of complete unawareness of the self and the environment accompanied by sleep-wake cycles with either complete or partial preservation of hypothalamic and brain stem autonomic functions (Table 53-3). The diagnosis is based on eye, verbal, and motor responses.

Giacino JT: Disorders of consciousness: Differential diagnosis and neuropathologic features. Semin Neurol 17:105–111, 1997.

TABLE 53-3.   COMPARISON OF CLINICAL FEATURES OF COMA, VEGETATIVE STATE (VS), AND MINIMALLY CONSCIOUS STATE (MCS)

Mental State	Coma	VS	MCS
Eye response	Eyes do not open spontaneously or in response to stimulation	Eyes open spontaneously; sleep-wake cycle resumes; arousal often sluggish, poorly sustained but may be normal	Eyes open spontaneously; sleep-wake cycles*; arousal level ranges from obtunded to normal
Motor response	No evidence of perception, communication ability, or purposeful motor activity (e.g., command following)	No evidence of perception, communication ability, or purposeful motor activity	Reproducible but inconsistent evidence of perception, communication ability, or purposeful motor activity; visual tracking often intact
Verbal response	No evidence of yes/no responses, verbalization, or gesture	No evidence of yes/no responses, verbalization, or gesture	Ranges from none to unreliable and inconsistent yes/no responses, verbalization, and gesture

*Circadian rhythms are important in determining the sleeping and feeding patterns of human beings. There are clear patterns of brain wave activity, hormone production, cell regeneration, and other biological activities linked to this daily cycle.

24. **What are the clinical criteria for emergence from MCS?**

The Aspen Consensus Group on Brain Injury proposed the following clinical criteria for emergence from MCS. One or both should be present:

- Functional interactive communication (ability to answer basic yes/no questions regarding personal/environmental orientation)
- Functional use of objects (demonstrating the ability to appropriately use or discriminate among objects)

Giacino JT, Ashwal S, Childs N, et al: The minimally conscious state: Definitions and diagnostic criteria. Neurology 58:349–353, 2002.

25. **How are a "coma management" program and pharmacotherapy used in managing patients in low-functioning states following TBI?**

There is no clear evidence that any kind of therapy-based program will help end a coma, minimally responsive state, or vegetative state. However, an organized approach to a low-functioning patient permits quantitative assessment of responses to stimuli and early recognition of changes in response to intervention or through spontaneous recovery.

There is a clear indication for preventive therapeutic interventions to maintain the body "in readiness" for the hoped-for neurologic improvement, particularly early on. These measures include basic rehabilitation strategies to manage bowel and bladder function, maintain appropriate nutrition, maintain skin integrity, control spasticity, and prevent contracture formation. If the patient comes out of coma or minimally responsive state, this intervention could permit more rapid participation in an active rehabilitation program and a shorter program length of stay. There is some limited evidence that for individuals who are "destined" to come out of a transient vegetative state or coma, this recovery process may be hastened through the use of pharmacotherapy, particularly dopamine agonists (such as combined levodopa/carbidopa or bromocriptine), amantadine, or tricyclic antidepressants.

Training of the family members/caregivers of a coma patient in an inpatient rehabilitation setting is often justified in order to discharge the patient to a home, which allows a less restrictive and less costly setting.

26. **What is the prognosis for patients in a vegetative state following TBI? What are some of the predictors for the final outcome of severe TBI after prolonged unawareness?**

There is no way to accurately predict the amount of functional recovery expected for a TBI patient in a minimally responsive state, although older age tends to be associated with a poorer outcome. Although some amount of recovery occurs in up to 50% of patients in a vegetative state for about 1 month, the odds of functionally significant recovery decline with the amount of time in a vegetative state. For patients in VS 2–4 weeks after injury, 8–18% remained in this state at 1 year. Data suggest a mortality rate of 15–24% for minimally responsive patients between 1 month and 1 year.

In a recent study, a statistically significant correlation was found with both the Glasgow Outcome Scale and the Barthel Index for the time interval from brain injury to recovery of the following clinical variables: optical fixation, ability to obey commands, spontaneous motor activity, and first safe oral feeding.

Formisano R, Voogt RD, Buzzi MG, et al: Time interval of oral feeding recovery as a prognostic factor in severe traumatic brain injury. Brain Inj 18:103–109, 2004.

KEY POINTS: FOCUSES OF TBI REHABILITATION

1. Assessment of baseline

2. Behavioral management

3. Detailed promotion of neuroplastic recovery

4. Reestablishment of maximal independence

5. Detailed promotion of neuroplastic recovery

6. Return to societal roles

27. **What is the prognosis for a patient who has been in a vegetative state for a year or longer?**
In the mid-1990s, a group of medical societies, including the American Academy of Neurology (AAN), published guidelines defining a vegetative state as "persistent" after a month. The AAN considers those who have been in this condition for a year or longer to have "almost no probability of recovery."

MILD TBI

28. **List the common symptoms experienced by patients with mild TBI (MTBI).**
The symptoms largely parallel those of patients in the more severe portion of the spectrum of traumatic brain injury:
- Headache (the most common complaint; one fairly unique to the more mildly injured patient)
- Vestibular or disequilibrium complaints
- Fatigue, weakness, numbness, and "tingling"
- Sensory deficits relating to hearing, blurred or "changed" vision, smell, and taste dysfunction
- Attention and memory problems
- Irritability and sleep disturbances
- Aggression behavior and other personality changes

29. **What management strategies are available to help patients following MTBI?**
Management of patients with MTBI requires a coordinated team approach. The first management issue pertains to identification and verification of the origin of the presenting signs and symptoms. Although MRI and other imaging studies should be undertaken, much of this documentation occurs through a neuropsychologic assessment. It is important to distinguish individuals who have true organic changes from those with emotional or psychiatric problems or a combination of both. Some physical and secondarily cognitive complaints may be related to injuries of the cranial nerves and craniocervical neurovascular systems. Many complaints can be attributed to musculoskeletal injury of the head and neck. This is particularly true of post-traumatic headache, which nearly always has a musculoskeletal component. Although it is possible, the incidence of overt malingering is not a serious concern.

After a clear idea of a patient's cognitive, emotional, and intellectual state has been established, along with some clarification as to site of origin, evaluation and intervention should target those deficits that are brain-injury related. This may include the use of cognitive compensatory strategies and pharmacotherapy. Education and counseling have a strong role with a psychologist, social worker, or vocational counselor as case managers.

RETURN TO WORK RATE

30. **What percentage of patients with TBI subsequently return to work?**
Reports vary widely, ranging from 12–100%. It would be safe to say that the majority of patients who are able to return to work, about 80%, had mild TBI. For people who have sustained moderate to severe brain injuries, the incidence of returning to work is considerably less. For severe injuries, this has been estimated to be fewer than 20%, perhaps even closer to 10%. The return to work rate for the TBI patient will depend on disablement, prior occupational work requirements, and motivation to return to work.

Franulic A, Carbonel CG, Pinto P, Sepulveda I: Psychosocial adjustment and employment outcome 2, 5 and 10 years after TBI. Brain Inj 18:119–129, 2004.

FUTURE MANAGEMENT

31. **What are the effects of potential biologic supplements on neuroplasticity after TBI?**

    New therapeutic biologic elements in TBI include neurotrophins, growth factors, and cell and tissue neurotransplantation. The goal of these therapies is to reduce the neurologic deficits associated with the trauma as well as to enhance the neuroplasticity processes. These therapies might affect the brain at molecular and cellular levels. The consequences of axonal damage following TBI might, in terms of subsequent deafferentation, potentially induce retrograde cell death and atrophy. The patterns of recovery, involving unconsciousness, post-traumatic confusion/amnesia, and postconfusional restoration, typically occur across the full spectrum of diffuse injury. The patient's long-term recovery may involve more idiosyncratic combinations of dysfunction. The relationship of focal lesions to localizing syndromes may be embedded in the evolving natural history of diffuse pathology. It is noted that injuries with primarily focal pathology do not necessarily follow a comparable pattern of recovery with distinct phases.

WEBSITES

1. www.cdc.gov/ncipc/tbi

2. www.cdc.gov/node.do/id/0900f3ec8000dbdc

3. www.tbindc.org

BIBLIOGRAPHY

1. Boyeson MG, Harmon RL: Acute and postacute drug-induced effects on rate of behavioral recovery after brain injury. J Head Trauma Rehabil 9:78–90, 1994.

2. Cooper PR: Head Injury, 3rd ed. Baltimore, Williams & Wilkins, 1993.

3. Dolce G, Sazbon L (eds): The Post-Traumatic Vegetative State. Stuttgart, Thieme Medical Publishers, 2002.

4. Giacino J, Whyte J: The vegetative and minimally conscious states: current knowledge and remaining questions. J Head Trauma Rehabil 20:30–50, 2005.

5. Horn LJ (ed): Pharmacology and brain rehabilitation. Phys Med Rehabil Clin N Am 8:605–857, 1997.

6. Horn LJ, Zasler ND (eds): Medical Rehabilitation of Traumatic Brain Injury. Philadelphia, Hanley & Belfus, 1996.

7. Kushawha VP, Garland DG: Extremity fractures in the patient with a traumatic brain injury. J Am Acad Orthop Surg 6:298–307, 1998.

8. Rosenthal M, Griffith ER, Bond MR, Miller JD: Rehabilitation of the Adult and Child with Traumatic Brain Injury, 2nd ed. Philadelphia, F.A. Davis, 1990.

9. Zasler ND, Katz DI, Zafonte RD: Brain Injury Medicine: Principles and Practice. New York, Demos, 2007.

CHAPTER 54

STROKE: DIAGNOSIS AND REHABILITATION

Richard L. Harvey, MD, and Elliot J. Roth, MD

Our greatest glory is not in never falling, but in rising every time we fall.
—Confucius (551–479 BC)

1. **What is a stroke?**
   A stroke is an acute neurologic dysfunction of vascular origin, with a relatively rapid onset, causing focal or sometimes global signs of disturbed cerebral function lasting for >24 hours.

2. **What are the causes of stroke?**
   The causes of stroke can be categorized into two major types, hemorrhagic and ischemic. Each type can be further divided into subtypes (Fig. 54-1).

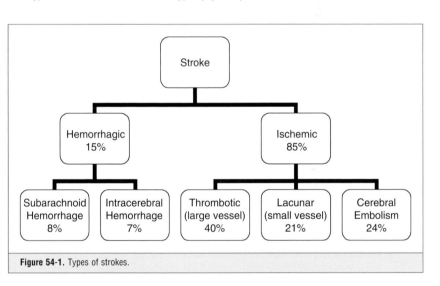

Figure 54-1. Types of strokes.

3. **How many people suffer a stroke annually? What is the prevalence?**
   Approximately 700,000 new strokes occur each year in the United States, with 500,000 being first stroke and 200,000 recurrent stroke. Over 160,000 die each year within 1 month after the stroke, making stroke the third leading cause of death in the United States. Approximately 5.4 million people are alive today who have survived a stroke. Stroke is the second most frequent cause of disability (arthritis is first), the leading cause of severe disability, and the most common diagnosis among patients on most rehabilitation units. Men have a higher incidence of stroke than do women up until age 80, when the incidence reverses. Because stroke deaths are more common at older ages and because women live longer than men, stroke deaths are

more common in women. Blacks have nearly twice the risk of first stroke than whites. The annual cost for stroke care in the United States is over $56 billion.

American Heart Association: Heart Disease and Stroke Statistics—2005 Update. Dallas, American Heart Association, 2005, pp 19–22.

4. **List the modifiable risk factors for stroke.**
   Medical conditions
   - Hypertension
   - Hypercholesterolemia
   - Diabetes mellitus
   - Heart disease and atrial fibrillation
   - Carotid artery disease
   - Previous stroke

   Lifestyle
   - Obesity
   - Smoking
   - Excessive alcohol use (>2 drinks per day)
   - Drug use (cocaine and intravenous drugs)

   The combination of certain metabolic and physiologic risk factors, known as the *metabolic syndrome X*, have also been linked to cardiovascular and stroke risk. These factors include elevated triglycerides, low HDL cholesterol, abdominal obesity, elevated blood pressure, and insulin resistance. Exercise programs that target weight loss may have positive effects on reducing the development of chronic hypertension, hypercholesterolemia, diabetes, and stroke.

   Ninomiya JK, Gilbert L, Criqui MH, et al: Association of metabolic syndrome with history of myocardial infarction and stroke in the Third National Health and Nutrition Examination Survey. Circulation 109:42–46,2004.

5. **What pharmacologic treatments can prevent a stroke in people who have suffered a previous stroke?**
   - **Antiplatelet agents:** The use of aspirin or the combined use of aspirin and dipyridamole can reduce risk of recurrent ischemic stroke by 21–35%. Clopidogrel is an equivalently effective antiplatelet agent for patients who cannot tolerate aspirin.
   - **Anticoagulants:** Warfarin is more effective than antiplatelet therapy for the prevention of secondary stroke in selected cardiac conditions, such as atrial fibrillation and following mechanical valve replacement. Although warfarin is effective at preventing ischemic stroke in other conditions, antiplatelet agents are generally preferred in the prevention of thrombotic and lacunar strokes.
   - **Hydroxymethylglutaryl-CoA (HMG-CoA) reductase inhibitors or statins:** These agents are well tolerated and effectively reduce total and LDL cholesterol. They have also been shown to reduce recurrent ischemic stroke risk in patients with normal cholesterol.
   - **Antihypertensive medications:** Lowering blood pressure even in patients with normal to borderline pressures has a significant effect in reducing recurrent stroke. Angiotensin converting enzyme (ACE) inhibitors or ACE combined with a diuretic have been particularly well tolerated and effective for secondary stroke prevention.

   PROGRESS Collaborative Group. Randomized trial of perindopril-based blood pressure-lowering regimen among 6105 individuals with previous stroke or transient ischemic attack. Lancet 358:1033–1042, 2001.

6. **When is carotid endarterectomy recommended?**
   Patients with between 70% and 99% stenosis of the internal carotid artery benefit from surgical excision of the atherosclerotic plaque (carotid endarterectomy) in centers that have low mortality and morbidity (>3%) associated with this surgical procedure.

7. **List the common neurologic impairments that follow stroke and their frequencies.**
See Table 54-1.

TABLE 54-1. COMMON NEUROLOGIC IMPAIRMENTS FOLLOWING STROKE AND THEIR FREQUENCIES

Impairment	Acute (%)	Chronic (%)
Any motor weakness	90	50
Right hemiplegia	45	20
Left hemiplegia	35	25
Bilateral hemiplegia	10	5
Ataxia	20	10
Hemianopsia	25	10
Visual perceptual deficits	30	30
Aphasia	35	20
Dysarthria	50	20
Sensory deficits	50	25
Cognitive deficits	35	30
Depression	30	30
Bladder incontinence	30	10
Dysphagia	30	10

8. **Describe the symptoms of a complete middle cerebral artery (MCA) stroke.**
The main stem of the middle cerebral artery is derived from the internal carotid artery and supplies the internal capsule, basal ganglia, and the entire lateral convexity of the frontal, parietal, and temporal lobes. Occlusion of the MCA results in symptoms contralateral to the lesion, including complete hemiplegia, hemisensory loss, and homonymous hemianopsia. Strokes in the language dominant (usually left) hemisphere cause aphasia and apraxia (see further discussion). Non-dominant strokes cause hemineglect and visual perceptual deficits.

9. **Describe the symptoms of an upper division MCA stroke.**
The main stem (M1) segment of the MCA supplies the subcortical tissue via the lenticulostriate arteries. Following this, the MCA divides into upper and lower divisions within the insular cortex. The upper division MCA supplies the lateral convexity of the frontal and parietal lobes. Occlusion of the upper division MCA causes contralateral hemiplegia, affecting face and arm more than leg, and modest sensory loss. Strokes in the language-dominant hemisphere cause non-fluent aphasia with good comprehension and apraxia. Nondominant hemisphere strokes cause hemineglect and visual perceptual deficits.

10. **Describe the symptoms of a lower division MCA stroke.**
Hemiplegia is usually absent in lower division MCA strokes, but contralateral homonymous hemianopsia is common. Strokes in the dominant hemisphere cause a fluent aphasia with poor comprehension. Nondominant lower division strokes may cause hemineglect.

11. **Describe the symptoms of an anterior cerebral artery (ACA) stroke.**
The ACA is derived from the internal carotid artery and supplies the medial portion of the frontal and parietal lobes along the interhemispheric cortical surface. Occlusion of the first segment of the ACA between the internal carotid and the anterior communicating artery (the A1 segment) may not cause ischemia because of collateral flow from the contralateral ACA through the anterior communicating artery (ACoA). Occlusion beyond the ACoA (the A2 segment) results in contralateral weakness in the shoulder and leg more than hand and face. Sensory loss follows a similar distribution. Injury to frontal lobe tissue also results in head and eye deviation toward the lesion (away from the hemiplegic limbs), grasp reflex, increased tone called paratonia or gegenhalten (German for "against stop"). Gegenhalten is characterized by a force-dependent increase in resistance to passive range of motion of a limb. Patients with ACA stroke may also have akinetic mutism with reduced initiation of activity, especially on command. When this is severe, the patient may not interact at all with the examiner (abulia), which may sometimes be confused with a global aphasia, although language is intact. Severe gegenhalten and akinetic mutism are more likely to occur with bilateral frontal lobe injury, which can occur when an ACA stroke happens in someone with multi-infarct dementia. Aphasia can be a symptom of a *dominant* hemisphere ACA stroke when the thrombus occludes the recurrent artery of Heubner, a branch off the ACA near the ACoA.

12. **List the common lacunar stroke syndromes.**
Small, deep subcortical strokes ranging from 0.2 to 15 mm^3 in diameter are called lacunes because they have the appearance of "little lakes" on pathologic examination. They are associated with single deep branch arteriolar occlusions, which can occur in the presence of acute or chronic hypertension. The arterioles include the lenticulostriate from the ACA and MCA to internal capsule and basal ganglia, the thalamoperforant from the posterior cerebral artery to the thalamus and midbrain, and the paramedian branches of the basilar artery to pons. The following are the more common lacunar syndromes:
- **Pure motor stroke:** associated with infarcts of the corona radiata, internal capsule, pons, and medullary pyramid.
- **Pure sensory stroke:** associated with thalamic infarcts and infarcts of the thalamocortical projections.
- **Sensorimotor stroke:** probably from thalamic strokes with adjacent internal capsule swelling.
- **Hemichorea-hemiballism:** associated with infarcts in the subthalamic nucleus, striatum, and thalamus.
- **Dysarthria clumsy hand syndrome:** associated with pontine infarcts or the anterior limb of the internal capsule.
- **Hemiataxia:** associated with dorsal pontine infarcts.

Mohr JP: Lacunes. Stroke 13:3–11, 1982.

13. **List brain stem stroke syndromes, their symptoms, and location of lesion.**
See Table 54-2.

14. **Discuss locked-in syndrome.**
Bilateral lesions to the base of the pons stemming from occlusion of the basilar artery can result in complete paralysis of the body, face, and occulomotor nuclei, sparing upgaze. These patients are fully alert but unable to communicate except by eye movements. Rehabilitation goals include maximizing preserved or recovered motor control, establishing a means of communication, reducing need for nursing care, and providing adaptive equipment, including customized wheelchairs. Prognosis for recovery depends on the severity of injury to the brain stem. Long-term stroke survivors with locked-in syndrome living at home report that, for the most part, their quality of life is good.

TABLE 54-2.   BRAIN STEM STROKE SYNDROMES, SYMPTOMS, AND LOCATION OF LESION

Syndrome	Symptoms	Location of Lesion
Weber	Ipsilateral 3rd nerve palsy Contralateral hemiplegia	Base of midbrain

Benedikt	Ipsilateral 3rd nerve palsy
	Contralateral loss of joint position and pain/
	  temperature sensation on face and body
	Contralateral ataxia and choreic movements
		Midbrain
		  tegmentum
		  (between base and
		  4th ventricle)

Millard-Gubler	Ipsilateral 6th and 7th nerve palsy Contralateral hemiplegia	Base of Pons
Medial medullary	Ipsilateral 12th nerve palsy Contralateral hemiplegia	Medial medulla

Wallenberg	Ipsilateral ataxia
	Ipsilateral loss of pain/temperature sensation
	  on face
	Contralateral loss of pain/temperature
	  sensation on body
	Dysphagia
	Dysphonia
	Loss of balance
	Vertigo
	Ipsilateral Horner's syndrome
		Lateral medulla

Adapted from Gilman S, Winans Newman S: Lesions of the brain stem. In Gilman S, Winans Newman S (eds): Manter and Gatz's Essentials of Neuroanatomy and Neurophysiology, 9th ed. Philadelphia, F.A. Davis, 2002, pp 111–118.

KEY POINTS: MOST COMMON CAUSES OF DEATH DURING THE FIRST MONTH AFTER STROKE

1. Stroke itself (progressive cerebral edema, herniation)

2. Aspiration pneumonia

3. Cardiac events (myocardial infarction, sudden death arrhythmia, heart failure)

4. Pulmonary embolism (often occurring 2–4 weeks after stroke)

15. **What is the pattern of typical motor recovery with stroke-related hemiplegia?**
    Patients with acute stroke and severe hemiplegia often initially have limb flaccidity, which is defined as less than normal tone. Later, increased tone or hypertonia appears, which is first noticeable in the lower limb, then subsequently in the upper limb. In some cases, this stage is followed by the development of spasticity, which is a velocity-dependent resistance in stretch of the muscles and is also noticed first in the lower limb and later in the upper limb. Spasticity is seen first in distal muscles crossing the wrist, fingers, and ankle and later is seen in proximal

muscles such as the shoulder, elbow, and hip. Patients who have voluntary movement of the limbs appearing early after stroke are less likely to have severe and disabling spasticity. Voluntary movements usually appear first in proximal muscles, such as those crossing the hip and shoulder, and later in the distal muscles of the hand and foot. The first voluntary movements are also seen in the hip, such as hip extension and adduction. As voluntary movements gain strength, they are often first associated with *synergy* patterns, which are voluntary contractions of a group of limb muscles producing a stereotypical pattern of limb movement. Flexor synergy is usually seen in the upper extremities, and extensor synergy is seen in the lower extremities (Table 54-3). As recovery continues, movements outside of these synergy patterns are possible. Later, isolated joint movements are possible.

TABLE 54-3. LIMB SYNERGY PATTERNS	
Flexor Synergy Pattern (Arm)	**Extensor Synergy Pattern (Leg)**
Shoulder abduction	Hip extension
Shoulder external rotation	Hip adduction
Scapular retraction	Knee extension
Elbow flexion	Ankle plantar flexion
Forearm supination	Ankle inversion
Wrist and finger flexion	

16. **What are the barriers to motor recovery?**
    - Prolonged flaccidity
    - Lack of voluntary movement within 2 weeks
    - Severe spasticity
    - Lack of movement out of synergy patterns
    - Sensory deficits

17. **Compare normal gait to typical hemiplegic gait.**
    - **Time and distance characteristics:** Hemiplegic gait is slower than normal adult gait, and the percent time of the gait cycle spent in stance is *longer* for both the hemiplegic and unaffected sides. Double support time is also longer when compared to normal adult gait. When compared to a normal adult walking at the *same* slower speed as a hemiplegic patient, the percent of gait cycle in stance is the same on the unaffected side but *shorter* on the affected side. Because total stance time on the hemiplegic leg is shorter than normal at equivalent speeds, double support time is also shorter. This stance and double support time reduce weight bearing on the more unstable hemiplegic limb and are compensated by a longer swing time than on the unaffected side.
    - **Kinematics (joint trajectories):** Compared to normal adult gait, hemiplegic patients show less hip flexion at initial contact, less hip extension at toe-off, and more hip flexion at midstance on the affected side. Knee flexion is reduced at toe-off in the hemiplegic limb and through mid-swing. There is excessive ankle plantar flexion at initial contact and mid-swing and reduced plantar flexion at toe-off.
    - **Muscle activity:** There are three different classes of muscle activity during gait cycle in stroke as defined by Knutsson and Richards in 1979:
        - **Type 1:** Excessive activity of calf muscles from early to midstance phase, resulting in excessive plantar flexion, forcing the knee into excessive extension at midstance.

□ **Type 2:** Low levels of muscle activity throughout the stance phase with reduced power at toe-off.

□ **Type 3:** Coactivation of several muscle groups, both plantar flexors and extensors, throughout stance phase and often swing phase as well.

Knutsson E, Richards C: Different types of disturbed motor control in gait of hemiparetic patients. Brain 102:405–430, 1979.

Olney SJ, Richards C: Hemiparetic gait following stroke. Part 1: characteristics. Gait Posture 4:136–148, 1996.

18. **What actions should be taken to prevent medical complications after stroke?**
Because patients with acute stroke can suffer morbidity and mortality from recurrent stroke, aspiration pneumonia, and venous thromboembolism, actions should be taken to prevent these complications.

Prevention of recurrent stroke starts first with risk factor management and modification. Patients who smoke or drink alcohol excessively should be given medical and social support to quit these habits. Hypertension, diabetes, and hypercholesterolemia can be managed with pharmacology, weight control, and exercise. People with stroke need to learn the importance and the role of antiplatelet agents or anticoagulants for the prevention of recurrent stroke.

Aspiration pneumonia will occur in one-third of patients with acute stroke but can be prevented if steps are taken to identify and treat dysphagia. Patients with acute stroke should not be fed orally until a bedside swallow evaluation or screening has been completed. The primary cause of dysphagia in patients with stroke is a delayed swallow trigger and difficulty with oral management of food. Modifying food consistency by thickening liquids or chopping up solids can reduce the risk for aspiration. Patients with severe dysphagia or who have trouble orally ingesting adequate calories are usually better served by providing enteral nutrition through a gastric tube. Fortunately, 80% of patients with dysphagia will improve during recovery and tolerate an oral diet.

Venous thromboembolism will occur in 50% of patients with acute stroke if preventive measures are not applied. Although the risk of pulmonary embolism (PE) is only 1–2%, the risk of death with PE is 50%. By far, the use of subcutaneous heparin (unfractionated– or low–molecular weight) provides the most effective prophylaxis against venous thrombosis, reducing risk to less than 5%. Patients with recent bleeding or bleeding disorders are more safely managed with pneumatic compression devices applied to the lower limbs during bedrest. Knee-high or thigh-high elastic stockings provide a clinically significant risk reduction for venous thrombosis but should not be used in exclusion of heparin or pneumatic compression.

19. **Explain the motor facilitation approaches frequently used in physical rehabilitation with stroke patients.**
Following the World Wars in the United States, many veterans returned home with brain injuries. Early application of physical rehabilitation involved simple strengthening exercises and training in compensatory functional skills. Neurofacilitory therapy developed with a greater understanding of the characteristics of motor impairments after brain injury. The goal of these novel therapeutic approaches was to relearn normal motor control beginning with basic functional movements.

■ **Proprioceptive neuromuscular facilitation (PNF):** Kabat, Voss, and Knott noted in the 1940s and 1950s that functional movements were not performed for the most part with isolated muscle contractions but involved coordinated activity in multiple muscle groups. PNF therapy involves complex trunk and limb movements in spirals and diagonals, such as those used to throw a ball. Mastering such movements can facilitate the performance of functional activities such as walking and feeding.

- **Brunnstrom technique:** Developed by Signe Brunnstrom in the 1950s and 1960s, this is the only neurofacilitory therapy designed specifically for patients with stroke. Brunnstrom noted that the first voluntary movements after stroke are usually those in synergy. She advocated facilitating the strength and control of synergy patterns with the goal of improving functional use of these movements. Because the Brunnstrom techniques work to enhance abnormal synergy patterns, this therapy approach has fallen out of favor.
- **Neurodevelopmental technique (NDT) or Bobath approach:** NDT was originally designed by Berta and Karl Bobath to facilitate motor development in children with cerebral palsy, but it was later applied to patients with stroke and brain injury. This therapy works with patients using developmental patterns of movement (rolling, sitting, crawling, and stepping) to normalize muscle tone, with the goal to enhance normal functional patterns of limb and trunk movement.

Bobath B: Adult Hemiplegia: Evaluation and Treatment, 3rd ed. Oxford, Heinemann, 1990.

Kabt H, Knott M: Proprioceptive facilitation techniques for treatment of paralysis, Phys Ther Rev 33:53–64, 1953.

Lehmkuhl LD, Smith LU, Brunnstrom S: Brunnstrom's Clinical Kinesiology, 4th ed. Philadelphia, F.A. Davis, 1983.

20. **What are the more recently developed approaches to motor relearning in stroke-related hemiplegia?**
    During the 1980s and 1990s, novel therapy approaches began to focus less on neurofacilitory techniques and more on achieving specific functional goals through "task-oriented" motor relearning, a term coined by Sheppard and Carr. These therapies provide direct training in functional tasks using the affected trunk and limbs in order to relearn skilled movements. Two examples include:

- **Constraint-induced movement therapy (CIMT):** First developed and studied by Taub and Wolf in the 1990s, this therapy works to overcome learned non-use of the affected upper limb in chronic stroke survivors who have some residual movement. By *forced use* of the affected arm and hand, patients are able to regain skilled functional movements. CIMT involves restraining the *unaffected* upper limb with a mitt so that the patient is forced to use the *affected* arm and hand for all skilled activities. Combining the use of a restraint with a 2-week course of intensive practice (massed practice of 6 hours a day) and shaping techniques, where functional tasks are broken down into simple components and then combined into more complex activities as the patient gains skill, constitutes CIMT.
- **Body weight–supported treadmill training (BWSTT):** For decades, laboratory cats given experimental complete spinal cord injury demonstrate the ability to perform treadmill walking with their hind limbs when provided with trunk support. This is likely because of intrinsic spinal cord circuitry that signals locomotor patterned movement called the central pattern generator. Using this concept, patients with acute and chronic stroke can benefit from locomotor retraining on a treadmill when provided with partial body weight unloading using an overhead harness system. Because of hemiplegia, patients often need pelvic stabilization and assistance with advancement of the affected leg during training. One limitation of this method is that therapists often fatigue while providing treatment.

Carr JH, Shepherd RB: Neurological Rehabilitation. Optimizing Motor Performance. Oxford, Butterworth Heinemann, 1998.

Taub E, Uswatte G, Pidikiti RD: Constraint-induced movement therapy: A new family of techniques with broad application to physical rehabilitation—a clinical review. J Rehabil Res Dev 36:237–425, 1999.

Visintin M, Barbeau H, Korner-Bitensky N, Mayo NE: A new approach to retrain gait in stroke patients through body weight support and treadmill stimulation. Stroke 29:1122–1128, 1998.

Wolf SL, Winstein CJ, Miller JP, et al: Effect of constraint-induced movement therapy on upper extremity function 3 to 9 months after stroke: The EXCITE randomized clinical trial. JAMA 296:2095–2104, 2006.

21. **What is the role of neuromuscular electrical stimulation (NMES) in stroke rehabilitation?**

    NMES involves applying an electrical current via skin surface electrodes to muscle at levels that cause muscle contraction. Traditionally, this has been provided to trapezius and supraspinatus muscles to reduce the shoulder subluxation often seen after stroke in the affected arm. Correcting shoulder subluxation allows a therapist to provide treatment to an affected arm with the shoulder properly positioned, preventing inadvertent injury. More recently, NMES has been applied to wrist and finger extensors to enhance voluntary hand opening. Modern devices employ electromyographic (EMG) feedback to trigger NMES current. Thus, the patient initiates wrist and finger extension, and if the resultant EMG activity reaches a certain threshold, the NMES current triggers and completes the movement. This is another example of a therapy providing forced use, such that the patient must initiate movement to complete the task. Preliminary studies indicate that EMG-triggered NMES can enhance motor relearning. Pain with electrical stimulation limits the use of this therapy, but this problem may be solved in the future with the use of intramuscular implanted electrodes.

22. **What are the common treatment approaches for spasticity after stroke?**

    Spasticity is a consequence of upper motor neuron injury and is defined as a velocity-dependent increase in resistance of muscle to stretch. Spasticity often complicates stroke recovery by interfering with functional mobility. Pain with movement and painful spasms are complications of spasticity. There are many ways to manage post-stroke spasticity, such as proper positioning, regular muscle stretching, and treating nociceptive stimuli such as a urinary tract infection or stool impaction. Other methods include inhibitory serial casting, oral antispasticity medications, neuromuscular blocks (e.g., phenol or botulinum toxin injections), or implantation of an intrathecal baclofen pump. In some cases, surgical release of a tendon is beneficial, especially when severe spasticity results in soft-tissue and muscle contracture. Selection of a particular intervention is dependent on the patient's clinical presentation, and many can be used in combination. Oral antispasticity agents such as baclofen, tizanidine, dantrolene, and clonazepam are especially useful for painful muscle spasms, but their use for spasticity is limited by sedative effects. Intrathecal baclofen provides excellent spasticity reduction with low doses and causes very little sedation, but it requires the surgical implantation of a pump. Focal spasticity in the upper or lower limb is best managed with chemoneurolysis using intramuscular botulinum toxin or phenol.

    Brashear A, Gordon MF, Elovic E, et al: Intramuscular injection of botulinum toxin for the treatment of wrist and finger spasticity after stroke. N Engl J Med 347:395–400, 2002.

    Meythaler JM, Guin-Renfroe S, Brunner RC, Hadley MN: Intrathecal baclofen for spastic hypertonia from stroke. Stroke 32:2099–2109, 2001.

23. **What are the management strategies for hemiplegic shoulder pain?**

    Approximately 70–80% of patients with stroke and hemiplegia have shoulder pain, contracture, and mechanical dysfunction, making it one of the most common complications of stroke. Causes of hemiplegic shoulder dysfunction are many and can include glenohumeral subluxation, adhesive capsulitis (frozen shoulder), impingement syndromes, rotator cuff tears, brachial plexus traction neuropathies, complex regional pain syndrome ("shoulder hand syndrome," present in up to 25% of patients), bursitis and tendinitis, and central post-stroke pain. Often, there is either a history or radiographic evidence of a preexisting or long-standing shoulder problem, and it is likely that the abnormal mechanical forces resulting from the stroke either exacerbate or manifest the chronic problem. In some patients, pain and loss of range of motion (ROM) are associated with improper positioning or handling, weakness of the shoulder girdle muscles, or spasticity. Shoulder dysfunction has been found to be present more frequently in patients with spastic upper limbs than in those with flaccid upper limbs. Pain and glenohumeral subluxation may occur together or independently, and the extent to which there is a causal relationship between pain and subluxation is unclear.

Treatment of shoulder dysfunction is individualized and primarily consists of proper positioning, consistent and regular stretching (including scapular mobilization), spasticity management, and motor relearning. Additional management can include the use of arm supports, shoulder slings, arm troughs, lap boards, medications, physical modalities (such as heat and cold), and joint injections. The use of shoulder slings is controversial, but if subluxation is the main cause of the shoulder dysfunction, then slings may be helpful. Slings that support the shoulder but allow the arm to remain in a functional position during ambulation are preferred.

24. **What is central post-stroke pain syndrome?**

Previously known as thalamic pain or Dejerine-Roussy syndrome, central post-stroke pain syndrome occurs in less than 5% of stroke survivors. It causes severe and disabling pain, which usually is described by patients as diffuse, persistent, and refractory to many treatment attempts. The most common descriptions of the pain are "burning and tingling," although many experience "sharp, shooting, stabbing, gnawing," and more rarely, "dull and achy" pain. The dysesthesias are often associated with allodynia (pain reaction to mild external cutaneous stimulation) and hyperpathia (exaggerated pain reaction to nociceptive stimulation). Only about 50% of the patients have thalamic strokes; the remainder have cerebrovascular lesions in a variety of locations. A key characteristic is that all patients have lesions involving sensory pathways in the central nervous system, and all have abnormal sensory testing on examination. Clinical management begins with supportive counseling and patient education. Tricyclic antidepressants and anticonvulsant medications (e.g., gabapentin or lamotrigine) have demonstrated efficacy in central pain management.

25. **What are aphasia and apraxia?**

Aphasia is an impairment of language affecting not only spoken language but reading and writing as well. Lesions in the dominant (usually left) hemisphere cause aphasia. The diagnosis of aphasia is dependent on clinical presentation of the language disorder. The clinical examination includes a test of fluency, repetition, naming, comprehension, reading, and writing.

- **Broca aphasia:** Nonfluent with impaired repetition and naming. Comprehension is impaired for complex commands.
- **Wernicke aphasia:** Fluent with multiple errors in word selection, impaired repetition, and naming. Comprehension is severely impaired.
- **Transcortical motor aphasia:** Nonfluent but repeats well. Comprehension is mostly intact.
- **Transcortical sensory aphasia:** Fluent with occasional word selection errors but repeats well. Comprehension is moderately impaired.
- **Conduction aphasia:** Fluent with rare word selection errors but unable to repeat. Comprehension is mostly intact.

Reading and writing are often as impaired as auditory comprehension and oral expression with aphasia. The exception is when patients also have apraxia. Apraxia is a disorder of "praxis" or performance of action. Lesions in the dominant (usually left) hemisphere cause apraxic errors in performance of skilled tasks. Put simply, the stroke causes a neural disconnection between the comprehension of a command and the center that codes for skilled motor output. Thus, when a patient with motor apraxia is asked to perform a certain task (e.g., "brush your teeth"), it can be performed in a clumsy manner or an improper sequence, or it is performed incorrectly altogether. Oral apraxia is common in Broca aphasics and contributes to the lack of fluency. Thus, beyond their language impairment, patients struggle with the oral motor task of producing words. When oral apraxia is more severe than limb apraxia, a patient may write better than he or she speaks. The term *apraxia* is also used in patients with nondominant hemisphere stroke, but here the performance errors are due to visual-perceptual deficits interfering with completion of a motor task rather than a problem of motor control deficits.

26. **What is neglect syndrome?**

Neglect is a disorder of attention. The dominant hemisphere is strongly oriented toward the opposite (usually right) hemispace, whereas the nondominant hemisphere is equally oriented toward both left and right hemispace. Thus, lesions to the left hemisphere do not affect spatial attention, and lesions to the right hemisphere impair attention to the left hemispace. Neglect of the left hemispace includes all sensory modalities, including vision, hearing, and tactile sensation as well as motor orientation to the left side. Different right brain lesions result in different characteristics of neglect:

- **Parietal lobe lesions:** Cause inattention to incoming visual, auditory, and somatosensory information from the left hemispace.
- **Frontal lobe lesions:** Cause impaired exploratory orientation of the left hemispace manifest as right head turning and eye deviation.
- **Cingulate gyrus lesions:** Cause a decreased drive or desire to attend to the left hemispace, regardless of the importance of doing so.

Treatment methods emphasize retraining, substitution of intact abilities, and compensatory techniques. Specific treatment strategies include providing visuospatial cues, fostering awareness of deficits, using computer-assisted training, visual scanning skill training, caloric stimulation, Fresnel prism glasses, eye patching, dynamic stimulation, and optokinetic stimulation.

27. **Describe the frequency and treatment approach for post-stroke depression.**

The incidence of depression after stroke ranges between 10% and 70%, with the best estimates at around 30%. Major depression is present in about one-third of all of those with depression. Post-stroke depression may result from a biologic effect of the brain injury itself, a reaction to the losses caused by the stroke, effects of certain medications, manifestations of certain medical conditions, or a combination of these factors. Participation and functional outcome in rehabilitation are adversely affected by depression.

The choice of treatment depends on the cause and severity of the symptoms. Review of active medications and treating medical illnesses are important first steps. A rehabilitation program that includes therapy for physical and cognitive disabilities, interaction with others, and attention and encouragement from family and staff is often extremely helpful. Many patients respond favorably to more intensive psychotherapy or to the use of antidepressant medications. Although large clinical trials testing the efficacy of antidepressants in the treatment of post-stroke depression are lacking, several small trials have shown that antidepressants may be an important adjunct to the management of depressed mood in stroke survivors.

Hackett ML, Anderson CS, House AO: Management of depression after stroke: a systematic review of pharmacological therapies. Stroke 36:1098–1103, 2005.

28. **Why and how does hydrocephalus occur after stroke?**

Following subarachnoid hemorrhage, blood products that remain in the subarachnoid space may block reabsorption of cerebral spinal fluid (CSF) into the venous sinuses by occluding the arachnoid granulations. These granulations are "one-way valves" that allow passage of CSF into the venous system. If the arachnoid granulations are occluded, CSF will accumulate, resulting in hydrocephalus. This kind of *normal pressure hydrocephalus* can present late in the patient's course (during rehabilitation) and usually requires placement of a ventriculoperitoneal shunt (VPS). Patients with a history of hydrocephalus and VPS can also develop recurrent hydrocephalus if the shunt fails. Patients who decline in function during rehabilitation or fail to reach expected goals should be evaluated by cranial computed tomography (CT) to assess evidence of hydrocephalus. The CT diagnosis of hydrocephalus is supported when ventricles are enlarged and sulci are constricted. Fluid density signal (low signal) in the periventricular brain parenchyma is also suggestive of hydrocephalus.

29. **What are the management strategies for bowel and bladder dysfunction in stroke?**

The incidence of urinary incontinence is 50–70% during the first month after stroke and about 15% after 6 months, a figure comparable to that in the general population. Incontinence may be caused by the brain damage itself (resulting in an uninhibited spastic neurogenic bladder with a synergic sphincter), urinary tract infection, impaired ability to transfer to the toilet or remove clothing, aphasia, or cognitive-perceptual deficits that result in lack of awareness of bladder fullness. Bowel impaction and some medications may exert an adverse effect. Urinary incontinence can cause skin breakdown, social embarrassment, and depression, and it increases the risk of institutionalization and unfavorable rehabilitation outcomes.

The most important therapeutic approach to the stroke-induced neurogenic bladder is the implementation of a timed bladder-emptying schedule. Other important management strategies include treatment of urinary tract infection, regulation of fluid intake, transfer and dressing skill training, patient and family education, and occasionally medications.

Urinary retention is less common but can occur in the presence of diabetic autonomic neuropathy or prostatic hypertrophy. Urinary retention may cause urinary tract infections requiring treatment with catheterization, medication (such as the alpha-adrenergic antagonist tamsulosin), and attention to other primary genitourinary causes.

30. **What signs and symptoms predict a poor functional outcome?**

See Box 54-1.

BOX 54-1. SIGNS AND SYMPTOMS THAT PREDICT POOR FUNCTIONAL OUTCOME

Prior stroke	Unemployed
Urinary incontinence	Cardiac disease
Bowel incontinence	Coma at onset
Depression	Inability to perform activities of daily living
Visuospatial and perceptual deficits	Poor sitting balance
Cognitive deficits	Large cerebral lesions
Delayed acute medical care	Dense hemiplegia
Delayed rehabilitation care	Visual field deficits
Low functional score on admission to rehabilitation	Aphasia
	Increased age
Poor social supports	Other medical comorbidities
Unmarried	

---

31. **How frequently do people with stroke return to work? What factors influence vocational recovery?**

Rates of return to work vary between different studies because of differences in the definition of vocation, differences in age of study participants and length of follow-up, differences in the availability of rehabilitation services, cultural differences in work expectation, and the availability of disability income. In the United States, rates of return to work vary from 11% to 49% within the first year following stroke. Likelihood of return to work is better with white collar, managerial, and professional positions versus blue collar and farming jobs. Younger age, less severe neurologic impairment, absence of aphasia, apraxia, agnosia, or other cognitive and communicative deficits, and better ability to ambulate and perform activities of daily living (ADLs) are positive predictors of return to work.

Saiki S: Disability management after stroke: its medical aspects for workplace accommodation. Disabil Rehabil 22:578–582, 2000.

32. **What are appropriate recommendations for long-term health and fitness after stroke?**
As already described, modifications in diet and appropriate use of medications are critical for prevention of recurrent stroke. Combining these actions with regular exercise can result in better physical strength and aerobic capacity, which can further reduce risk for stroke and cardiovascular disease, and, potentially, improve function.

Studies reveal that progressive resistance strength training is typically well tolerated by stroke survivors and results in increased strength in affected and unaffected muscles. There is also no evidence that strength training worsens spasticity or results in loss of functional ROM in affected limbs. Data suggest that lower limb strength training can improve gait function and potentially improve functional ability and community participation after stroke.

Patients with stroke demonstrate reduced aerobic capacity when compared to age-matched adults. The lower level of cardiovascular fitness found in stroke survivors can limit independence and endurance for regular ADLs. Reasons for reduced aerobic capacity after stroke include reduced physical activity, reduced neural drive in motor systems, and poor motor efficiency. In addition, certain non-neurologic causes may contribute to poor aerobic fitness. These include gross muscle atrophy, change in muscle tissue composition, and increased insulin resistance. Tissue analysis of paretic muscles reveals a relative reduction in the percentage of slow twitch type I muscle fibers that have high oxidative capacity, resistance to fatigue, and sensitivity to insulin-mediated glucose uptake. Consequently, there is an increased relative percentage of fast twitch type II muscle fibers that are used in powerful movement, fatigue quickly, and are less sensitive to the action of insulin. This insulin resistance can contribute to metabolic syndrome or worsen diabetes.

Aerobic training following stroke can be incorporated into a regular exercise routine using a walking program or treadmill training. People with stroke benefit from aerobic training by increasing peak oxygen consumption, lowering oxygen demand at submaximal exercise levels, and increasing peak ambulatory workload capacity. In addition, improved cardiovascular health can further reduce cardiac and stroke risk factors such as hypertension, elevated cholesterol, obesity, and insulin resistance. Patients may also benefit from improved functional performance.

Because stroke survivors are often sedentary prior to stroke, education in the benefits of long-term health and physical fitness is a critical part of comprehensive rehabilitation.

Ivey FM, Macko RF, Ryan AS, Hafer-Macko CE: Cardiovascular health and fitness after stroke. Top Stroke Rehabil 12:1–16, 2005.

WEBSITES

1. National Institute of Neurological Disorders and Stroke: Stroke Information Page
www.ninds.nih.gov/disorders/stroke/stroke.htm

2. National Stroke Association: For Medical Professionals
www.stroke.org/site/PageServer?pagename=MEDPRO

SPINAL CORD INJURY MEDICINE: ACUTE TREATMENT, REHABILITATION, AND PREVENTIVE CARE

Steven A. Stiens, MD, MS, Barry Goldstein, MD, PhD, Margaret Hammond, MD, and James Little, MD, PhD

The truth is that our finest moments are most likely to occur when we are feeling uncomfortable, unhappy or unfulfilled; for it is only in such moments propelled by our discomfort that we are likely to step out of our ruts and start searching for different ways or truer answers.

—M. Scott Peck (1936–2005)

1. **What are some of the important treatments to provide after acute traumatic spinal cord injury (SCI)?**
   - Stabilize the spine in a neutral position, and take plane radiographs of entire spine.
   - Control neurogenic shock with high-flow isotonic IV fluids, with the goal of maintaining systolic blood pressure (SBP) 95–100 with a heart rate of 60–100 bpm.
   - Place Foley catheter and maintain a urine output of 30 mL/hr or more.
   - Start IV methylprednisolone within 8 hours of injury.
   - Provide sequential pneumatic compression to lower extremities.
   - Administer low molecular weight heparin to prevent deep vein thrombosis (DVT) when surgery is complete.

   www.emedicine.com/EMERG/topic553.htm
   Kirshblum SC, Groah SL, McKinley WO, et al: Spinal cord injury medicine 1. Etiology, classification, and acute medical management. Arch Phys Med Rehab 83:S50–S57, 2002.
   Kwon BK, Tetzlaff W, Grauer JN, et al: Pathophysiology and pharmacologic treatment of acute spinal cord injury. Spine J 4(4):451–64, 2004.

2. **What is SCIWORA?**
   Spinal **c**ord **i**njury **w**ithout **r**adiologic **a**bnormality. This condition is commonly seen in young children and older adults. Mechanisms of injury in children include traction in breech delivery, violent hyperextension, or flexion. Predisposing factors in children include large head-to-neck size ratio, elasticity of the fibrocartilaginous spine, and the horizontal orientation of the planes of the cervical facet joints.

   The typical presentation of SCIWORA in the elderly is an acute central cord syndrome after a fall forward and a blow on the head. The ligamentum flavum may bulge forward into the central canal and compromise the sagittal diameter by as much as 50%.

   Essential history in a person with head trauma or neck pain includes identifying any paresthesias or other neurologic symptoms. Flexion and extension films should be done cautiously, only after static neck films have been cleared by a radiologist and only if no neurologic symptoms or severe pains are present. Empirical use of a 24-hour cervical collar with repeat films at resolution of cervical spasm is warranted. Rarely, delayed onset of paralysis may occur because of vascular mechanisms or edema accumulation at the injury site.

   Liao CC, Lui TN, Chen LR, et al: Spinal cord injury without radiological abnormality in preschool-aged children: Correlation of magnetic resonance imaging findings with neurological outcomes. J Neurol Surg 103(1 Suppl):17–23, 2005.

3. **What are the key muscles examined to clinically define the SCI motor level?**
The American Spinal Cord Injury Association (ASIA) has developed standards for neurologic classification (revised in 2000, reprinted 2002) that quantify impairment through objective recording of sensory and motor findings. Because of the multiple segmental innervations of muscles, antigravity strength (3/5 or greater) is considered enough to define a motor level if all muscles listed here have normal 5/5 strength. The **motor level** is the caudal key muscle group that is graded 3/5 or greater, with the segments cephalad graded normal (5/5) strength. A patient is classified as **motor incomplete** if there is voluntary anal sphincter contraction *or* he or she has sensory sacral sparing with sparing of motor function more than three levels below the motor level. The index muscles that define each motor level are listed in Box 55–1.

American Spinal Cord Injury Association: International Standards for Neurological Classification of Spinal Cord Injury. Chicago, ASIA, 2002.
www.asia-spinalinjury.org

BOX 55-1. INDEX MUSCLES THAT DEFINE EACH MOTOR LEVEL

C4—diaphragm	T1—abductor digiti minimi
C5—biceps, brachialis	L2—iliopsoas
C6—extensor carpi radialis (longus and brevis)	L3—quadriceps
C7—triceps brachii	L4—tibialis anterior
C8—flexor digitorum profundus to middle finger	L5—extensor hallucis longus
S1—gastrocnemius, soleus	S2—anal sphincter

---

4. **How is sensory level defined and documented with bedside examination of persons with SCI?**
It is most effective to examine areas of decreased or absent sensation and move toward areas of normal sensation. A **pinprick stimulus** (clean, unused safety pin) is presented lightly to the skin starting at S1 (lateral aspect of the fifth toe), then advanced by dermatome until normal perceived sensation is documented. Results are recorded as 0 = absent, 1 = present but abnormal, or 2 = normal perception sensation (as compared with areas above the lesion). The same process is repeated for **light touch** (brush or cotton). The **zone of partial preservation** is the band of bilateral, altered sensation that separates areas without sensation from those with normal sensation. A patient is described as **sensory incomplete** if sensory function is preserved below the neurologic level and extends through S4–S5.

5. **What is the neurologic level of injury?**
The **neurologic level of injury** is the most caudal level at which *both* motor and sensory modalities are intact on both sides of the body. The motor and sensory levels for SCI are the same in <50% of complete injuries. At spinal cord segments where there is no key muscle that has a sensory dermatome intact (high cervical, thoracic, and sacral levels), the sensory level determines the motor and neurologic levels.

Ho CH, Wuermser LA, Priebe MM, et al: Spinal cord injury medicine. 1. Epidemiology and classification. Arch Phys Med Rehab 88(3 Suppl 1):S49–54, 2007.

6. **Why is sensation most likely to be spared in the perianal area?**
Sacral sparing is due to spinal cord somatotopic organization. Sensory and motor fibers are laminated within the tracts of the spinal cord such that fibers that serve caudal regions are located laterally and closer to the surface. Contusions and spinal cord ischemia produce

relatively more damage to centrally located spinal neurons and axons than those peripherally located within the spinal cord.

7. **What are the most important long tracts in the spinal cord?**
See Table 55-1 and Figure 55-1.

TABLE 55-1. LONG TRACTS IN THE SPINAL CORD		
Tract	Location	Function
Gracile	Medial dorsal column	Proprioception from the leg
Cuneate	Lateral dorsal column	Proprioception from the arm
Spinocerebellar	Superficial lateral column	Muscular position and tone
Pyramidal	Deep lateral column	Upper motor neuron
Lateral spinothalamic	Ventrolateral column	Pain and thermal sensation

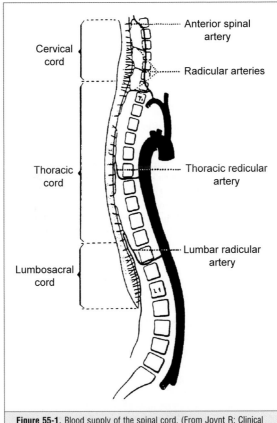

Figure 55-1. Blood supply of the spinal cord. (From Joynt R: Clinical Neurology. Philadelphia, J.B. Lippincott, 1992, with permission.)

8. **Where in the spinal cords are each of the major long tracts located?**
    Figure 55-2 shows the somatotopic organization of the major long tracts of the spinal cord. The dorsal columns have lower-extremity fibers (sacral and lumbar) lying medially, whereas the pyramidal and spinothalamic tracts have lower-extremity fibers lying laterally.

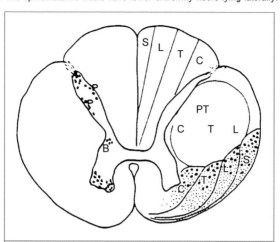

Figure 55-2. Location of major long tracts. Letters represent the lamination of the Funiculus Cuneatus, Funiculus Gracilis, and corticospinal tracts. PT = pyramidal tract, S = sacrum, L = lumbar, T = thoracic, C = cervical. (From Joynt R: Clinical Neurology. Philadelphia, J.B. Lippincott, 1992, with permission.)

9. **What is the artery of Adamkiewicz?**
    The artery of Adamkiewicz, also known as the **lumbar radicular artery,** is a major radicular branch that arises from the aorta and enters the cord between T10 and L3. Although radicular arteries supply each spinal root, typically only this one large artery supplies the low thoracic and lumbar spinal cord via the **anterior spinal artery**. The anterior spinal artery supplies the anterior two-thirds of the spinal cord. It supplies the lumbar and lower thoracic segments, anastomosing with the anterior spinal artery in the lower thoracic region, which is thus the watershed area of the cord. Figure 55-2 shows the blood supply of the spinal cord.

10. **What is the arterial supply of the posterior third of the cord?**
    Paired dorsolateral **posterior spinal arteries** extend the length of the cord and supply the posterior third of the cord through circumflex and penetrating vessels. They arise from the vertebral or posterior inferior cerebellar arteries.

11. **What is the difference between quadriplegia and tetraplegia?**
    It is a matter of medical etymology. *Quadra* is a Latin root meaning four; *tetra* (four) and *plegia* (*plege,* meaning stroke or paralysis) are Greek roots. The compound word *tetraplegia* is more correct because it does not mix Greek and Latin roots.

12. **Name and describe the SCI syndromes. What are their lesions, clinical findings, and common causes?**
    - **Anterior cord syndrome:** The clinical syndrome includes hyporeflexia, atrophy, and variable motor loss, with preservation of position sensation but impaired pinprick (hypalgesia) and temperature sensations. Common causes for these findings are thoracolumbar burst fracture, abdominal aortic aneurysm, and aortic clamping for surgery, which compromise segmental spinal cord circulation.

- **Central cord syndrome:** The clinical constellation includes weakness greater in the arms than legs, lower-extremity hyperreflexia, upper-extremity mixed upper motor neuron and lower motor neuron weakness, and preserved sacral sensation with the potential for preservation of bowel and bladder control. Common causes are spinal stenosis with extension injury, expanding intramedullary hematoma mass, or syrinx.
- **Brown-Séquard syndrome:** This syndrome presents with hemi- or monoplegia or paresis with contralateral pain and temperature sensation deficit. There is a good prognosis for motor recovery progressing from the proximal extensors to distal flexors, although spasticity may compromise total function. Causes include knife wounds to the back and asymmetrically oriented spinal tumors.
- **Posterior cord syndrome:** This uncommon presentation manifests with bilateral deficits in proprioception. The potential causes are vitamin B_{12} deficiency (subacute combined degeneration) and syphilis (tabes dorsalis). B_{12} deficiency can be the cause of late deterioration in gait after SCI.

Petchkrua W, Burns S, Stiens S, et al: Prevalence of vitamin B_{12} deficiency in patients with spinal cord injury or disease. Arch Phys Med Rehabil 84:1675–1679, 2003.

13. **What is the ASIA impairment scale? How are the categories defined?**
The **Frankel classification** was an attempt to separate SCI patients into various functional groups based on sensory and motor sparing. The **ASIA impairment scale,** revised in 2000, is the most contemporary version. It defines distinctions between categories by specifying sensory dermatomes and muscle grades as follows:
- **ASIA A:** Complete (no motor or sensory S4 or S5 function)
- **ASIA B:** Incomplete sensory but no motor function preserved through S4–S5
- **ASIA C:** Motor and sensory function incomplete, with the strength of more than half of the key muscles below the neurologic level having a muscle grade < 3
- **ASIA D:** Motor and sensory function incomplete (motor functional), with at least half of key muscles below the neurologic level having a muscle grade > 3
- **ASIA E:** Normal motor and sensory function

14. **What is the highest complete SCI level that is consistent with independent living without the aid of an attendant?**
C6 complete tetraplegia: An exceptionally motivated individual with C6 tetraplegia demonstrates the capability of and chooses independent living in an accessible environment without the aid of an attendant. A review of outcomes from a subset of people with motor- and sensory-complete C6 SCI revealed that the following percentages of patients were independent for key self-care tasks: feeding 16%, upper body dressing 13%, lower body dressing 3%, grooming 19%, bathing 9%, bowel care 3%, transfers 6%, and wheelchair propulsion 88%. Feeding is accomplished with a universal cuff for utensils. Transfers require stabilization of the elbow extension with forces transmitted from shoulder musculature through the limb as a closed kinetic chain. Bowel care is performed with a suppository insertion wand and Fickle finger for digital stimulation.

Gittler MS, McKinley WO, Stiens SA, et al: Spinal cord injury medicine 3. Rehabilitation outcomes. Arch Phys Med Rehab 83:S65–S71, 2002.

15. **How much motor recovery is expected in a patient with a stable diagnosis of motor and sensory complete traumatic tetraplegia with central spinal cord edema and hematomyelia on MRI?**
Recovery is greatest in muscles supplied within the zone of injury. Less than 30% of SCIs will go from C4 to C5, but >66% of those at C5–C8 gain one root level by 6–12 weeks. The ability to perceive pain from a pin stimulus over the lateral antecubital space (posterior brachial cutaneous nerve) is a good prognostic indicator for eventual recovery of the extensor carpi radialis to 3/5. Eighty-five percent of patients' muscles that demonstrate 1/5 strength initially within the zone of partial motor preservation (myotomes caudal to the neurologic level that remain partially innervated) will achieve >3/5 strength by 1 year. Below the injury zone, only 3%

of patients initially Frankel A (at 72 hours) (same as AIS A) improve to grade D or E on the ASIA impairment scale (AIS). Negative prognostic indicators on MRI include transection, hematomyelia, and edema, but MRI adds little to the clinical exam for prediction of prognosis.

Andreoli C, Colaiacomo MC, Rojas Beccaglia M, et al: MRI in the acute phase of spinal cord traumatic lesions: Relationship between MRI findings and neurological outcome. Radiol Med 110(5–6):636–65, 2005.

Little JW, Ditunno JF, Stiens SA, Harris RM: Incomplete spinal cord injury: Neuronal mechanisms of motor recovery and hyperreflexia. Arch Phys Med Rehabil 80:587–599, 1999.

www.sci-recovery.org

16. **What are the mechanisms of motor recovery after SCI?**
Motor recovery after SCI occurs rapidly during the first and second week, then recovery continues at a slower pace for the first 4 months and slows further thereafter. Initially, recovery could be mediated by central mechanisms (cortical reorganization), such as recruitment of latent pathways (unused until injury). At the injury site, edema and hematomyelia may resolve, reducing secondary injury, neurapraxic block, and demyelination. Within the anterior horn, central synaptogenesis may occur in response to denervation hypersensitivity of the anterior horn cell. Root impingement may resolve with decompression, spinal alignment, and fixation as needed (Fig. 55-3).

Raineteau O, Schwab M: Plasticity of motor systems after incomplete spinal cord injury. Nature Rev 2:263–273, 2001.

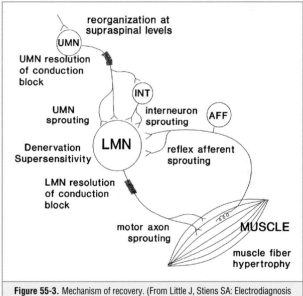

Figure 55-3. Mechanism of recovery. (From Little J, Stiens SA: Electrodiagnosis in spinal cord injury. Phys Med Rehabil Clin North Am 6:263–296, 1995.)

17. **Which are the most common and disabling contractures of the upper extremities after SCI?**
Adduction of shoulder, flexion of elbow, and extension of the metacarpophalangeal (MCP), distal interphalangeal (DIP), and medial interphalangeal (MIP). Helpful contractures are mild flexion of the MCP, proximal interphalangeal (PIP), and DIP. They provide **tenodesis,** which is finger prehension (opposition of the thumb to the index finger), with active wrist extension. Even greater strength can come from a wrist-driven flexor hinge orthosis, which stabilizes the thumb, index, and middle fingers for a tight pincer grasp.

Stiens SA, Kirshblum SC, Groah SL, et al: Spinal cord injury medicine 4. Optimal participation in life after spinal cord injury. Arch Phys Med Rehabil 83:S72–S81, 2002.

18. **A patient with T4 complete paraplegia complains of a pounding headache and was noted to have a blood pressure of 190/100 mmHg, gooseflesh of his trunk and legs, and a paradoxic bradycardia at 50 bpm. What are the diagnosis, pathophysiology, and treatment?**

    Autonomic dysreflexia is an acute hypertensive syndrome, due to a hyperactive reflex sympathetic discharge, often precipitated by viscus distention or noxious stimuli registered below the level of the SCI. The nerve cell bodies for sympathetic outflow are located in the **intermediolateral cell columns,** which run from T1 through L2 bilaterally in the spinal gray matter. Lesions above T6 cut off central modulation of sympathetic discharges. Hypertension, often produced by excessive vasoconstriction, is registered at the carotid baroreceptors, resulting in corrective parasympathetic outflow via the vagus nerve to reduce heart rate and contractility.

    Treatment includes identification and elimination of the cause (commonly urologic obstruction/distention, bowel impaction, skin irritation, ingrown toenail, or intra-abdominal processes). Sit the patient up, and place nitropaste on skin above the SCI level. Should SBP remain elevated greater than 160 mmHg give hydralazine, 10 mg by mouth.

    http://www.aapmr.org/hpl/pracguide/resource.htm#SCI

19. **Why is DVT a pervasive problem after SCI?**

    The primary risks were summarized in 1856 as Virchow's triad:
    - **Venous stasis** (paralysis, spinal shock)
    - **Hypercoagulability** (trauma, tumor as cause for increases in circulating thrombogenic factors)
    - **Vessel injury** (primary trauma or secondary injury due to sensory deficits after SCI).

    The incidence of DVT after SCI ranges from 47–100%, as revealed with various noninvasive surveillance techniques for subclinical disease. The risk is highest during the first 2 weeks to 3 months after SCI, and prevention of clot formation is essential.

    McKinley WO, Gittler MS, Kirshblum SC, et al: Spinal cord injury medicine 2. Medical complications after spinal cord injury: identification and management. Arch Phys Med Rehabil 83: S58–S64, 2002.

20. **What muscle function is typically required to allow community ambulation?**

    At least 3/5 strength in hip flexion bilaterally with at least 3/5 knee extension on one side is required for an effective reciprocal gait pattern to permit community ambulation. Bilateral bracing (ankle-foot orthosis or knee-ankle-foot orthosis) with forearm crutches or a walker maximizes efficiency. The calculation of the sum of bilateral lower-extremity strength measures produces the ASIA lower extremity muscle score (LEMS, normal 50). LEMS correlates with gait velocity, energy expenditure, and peak axial load by arms on crutches. LEMS above 30 is associated with community ambulation.

    Hussey RW, Stauffer ES: Spinal cord injury: Requirements for ambulation. Arch Phys Med Rehabil 54:554–557, 1973.

    Waters RL, Adkins R, Yakura J, Virgil D: Prediction of ambulatory performance based on motor scores derived from standards of the American Spinal Injury Association. Arch Phys Med Rehabil 75:757–760, 1994.

21. **A chronic T2 ASIA B SCI patient mentions that he was unable to tell the difference between a cold and a warm beer by grasping the can with his hand at a recent party. What are your thoughts and actions?**

    This represents a change in temperature perception, which is carried by the superficially located lateral and ventral **spinothalamic tracts**. Afferent fibers enter through the dorsal root and *cross over* to the opposite side of the spinal cord via the anterior commissure, just anterior to the central canal. A differential diagnosis might include progressive post-traumatic syringomyelia (an expanding intramedullary cyst that may originate at the injury site), tethered cord syndrome (progressive spinal cord dysfunction due to stretch or traction of the cord), myelopathy, radiculopathy, plexopathy, or peripheral neuropathy.

The patient should be questioned about shooting pain with sneezing or coughing, Valsalva maneuver, or heavy lifting, which all may increase subarachnoid pressures. The exam should include neck flexion to assess the presence of **Lhermitte's sign** (a sudden electric-like shock extending down the spine with head flexion), pinprick/touch sensation, reflexes, and strength. Further evaluation includes electrodiagnostic testing and MRI.

http://www.mscisdisseminationcenter.org/

22. **What are the treatment and outcome for progressive post-traumatic syringomyelia?**
Conservative measures include avoidance of high-force isometric contractions, Valsalva maneuver, head elevation at night, and maintenance of the neck in a neutral position. Surgical shunting may be associated with shunt obstruction and syrinx reaccumulation.

Sgouros S, Williams B: A critical appraisal of drainage in syringomyelia. J Neurosurg 82:1–10, 1995.

23. **How can an acute abdomen be diagnosed in a person with an SCI?**
Patient history may be as subtle as anorexia, and examination findings may be as nondescript as an elected pulse or BP. Key symptoms, although not always present, include anorexia, nausea, restlessness, changes in spasticity, nonlocalized abdominal pain, and shoulder pain in the person with tetraplegia. Signs may include elevated pulse rate (although bradycardia may exist if autonomic dysreflexia is present), fever, and spasticity. Abdominal tenderness is not common in individuals with a level above T5. Rapid diagnosis with laboratory studies (complete blood count [CBC], amylase) and imaging studies is warranted to improve on the all-too-common delays in diagnosis. A resultant 10–15% mortality rate exists in this population. A person with an injury level above T6 may experience autonomic dysreflexia, vague nonlocalized abdominal discomfort, increased spasticity, and a rigid abdomen. A level between T6 and T10 may allow for localization with abdominal wall inflammation. Levels lower than T12 spare sympathetic splanchnic outflow, and responses are normal.

Charney KJ, Juler GL, Comarr AE: General surgery problems in patients with spinal cord injuries. Arch Surg 110:1083–1088, 1975.

KEY POINTS: SPINAL CORD INJURY MEDICINE

1. Sacral sparing occurs with central lesions of the spinal cord (contusion, ischemia, tumor). Sensory symptoms tend to descend as the lesion expands.

2. Brown-Séquard syndrome presents with unilateral paresis on the side of the spinal cord lesion and contralateral pain and temperature sensation deficit. A common cause is a stab in the back causing a hemisection that interrupts descending motor tracts and ascending spinothalamic tracts that have crossed the spinal cord.

3. The most common tumors of the spinal cord are astrocytomas, ependymomas, and oligodendrogliomas.

4. The most common tumors that metastasize to the spinal cord are breast, lung, gastrointestinal, lymphoma/myeloma, and prostate. They all cause extramedullary compression that can respond to emergent radiation therapy and steroids or surgical decompression.

24. **What is Charcot spine? Why would someone with SCI have it?**
    Jean M. Charcot was a French neurologist who treated many syphilitics. He described osteoarthropathy from trauma in people with **tables dorsalis** (syphilitic posterior column deterioration) who lacked protective sensation.

    Because of their spinal trauma and analgesia below the level of injury, those with SCI are particularly prone to this insensate joint destruction. After spinal fixation, the fusion mass acts as a lever, contributing to hypermobility at the joint caudal to the fusion. The joints themselves can be a pain source that trigger autonomic dysreflexia or a nidus of infection after hematogenous spread.

    Bayley JC, Cochran TP, Sledge CB: The weight-bearing shoulder: The impingement syndrome in paraplegics. J Bone Joint Surg 69A:676–678, 1987.

25. **A 17-year-old, newly SCI-injured, muscular man with C6 incomplete tetraplegic complains of lethargy and abdominal cramping. What could it be?**
    Immobilization hypercalcemia should be considered. Symptoms of hypercalcemia can be remembered with the mnemonic "**stones, bones, and abdominal groans.**" Other symptoms include lethargy, nausea, and anorexia.

    The diagnosis is made with measurement of the total serum calcium adjusted for the total protein. Serum ionized calcium is also elevated and is a more accurate test. The 24-hour calcium excretion normally should be <250 mg. Treatment includes mobilization, rehydration with saline, and treatment with furosemide (which enhances Ca^{2+} secretion in the loop of Henle). Calcitonin can be used in resistant cases.

26. **What are some of the complications patients with SCI develop as they age?**
    The leading cause of rehospitalization is urinary tract infections and other diseases of the urinary system. For patients with SCI levels in the range of C1–C8, respiratory problems and pneumonia are common. Those with paraplegia have a high incidence of pressure ulcers. Weight gain is a problem that is related to inactivity and contributes to metabolic syndrome, including the triad of obesity, glucose intolerance, and lipoprotein abnormalities. Shoulder pain is associated with age, increased weight, and overhead reaching during transfers. Treatment consists of steroid injection if severe and acute. A shoulder protection program that limits overhead reaching, stretches anterior muscles, and strengthens posterior shoulder stabilizers is beneficial.

    Chiodo AE, Scelza WM, Kirshblum SC, et al: Spinal cord injury medicine. 5. Long-term medical issues and health maintenance. Arch Phys Med Rehabil 88(3 Suppl 1):S76–S83, 2007.
    Groah SL, Stiens SA, Gittler MS, et al: Preserving wellness and independence of the aging spinal cord injured: A primary care approach for the rehabilitation medicine specialist. Arch Phys Med Rehabil 83: S82–S89, 2002.

27. **A 64-year-old woman with T2 SCI complains of a gradual reduction in endurance and dizziness and palpitations while pushing her wheelchair up a long hill to her office. What are your thoughts?**
    Evaluation should include blood pressure, objective upper-extremity strength assessment with myometry, electrocardiogram (ECG), and laboratory studies, including CBC and electrolytes. A drop in blood pressure with exercise suggests coronary ischemia. Silent cardiac ischemia is common after SCI because of blocks in cardiac pain perception with lesions above T5. Coronary narrowing can be detected by doing Persantine thallium testing of dynamic cardiac perfusion. Patients with SCI are at high risk for coronary artery disease due to inactivity, lower high-density lipoproteins (HDL), tendency toward hyperglycemia, and the risk for obesity.

    Sipski ML, Richards JS: Spinal cord injury rehabilitation: State of the science. Am J Phys Med Rehabil 85:310–342, 2006.
    Stiens SA, Johnson MC, Lyman PJ: Cardiac rehabilitation in patients with spinal cord injuries. Phys Med Rehabil Clin North Am 6:263–296, 1995.

WEBSITES

1. www.nim.nih.gov/medlineplus/spinalcordinjuries.html

2. www.ninds.nih.gov/disorders/sci/sci.htm

3. www.spinal-cord.org

4. www.spinalinjury.net

BIBLIOGRAPHY

1. Blackwell T, Krause J, Winkler T, Stiens S: A Desk Reference for Life Care Planning for Persons with Spinal Cord Injury. New York, Demos, 2001.

2. Hammond M (ed): Medical Care of Persons With Spinal Cord Injuries. Department of Veterans Affairs, US Gov Printing #557-463: http://vaww1.va.gov/vhi/docs/SCIfinal.pdf

3. Kirshblum SC, Groah SL, McKinley WO, et al: Spinal cord injury medicine 1: Etiology, classification, and acute medical management. Arch Phys Med Rehabil 83:S50–S57, 2002.

4. Lin V: Spinal Cord Injury Medicine: Principles and Practice. New York, Demos, 2003.

5. McKinley WO, Gittler MS, Kirshblum SC, et al: Spinal cord injury medicine 2. Medical complications after spinal cord injury: Identification and management. Arch Phys Med Rehabil 83:S58–S64, 2002.

6. Priebe MM, Chiodo AE, Scelza WM, et al: Spinal cord injury medicine. 6. Economic and societal issues in spinal cord injury. Arch Phys Med Rehabil 83(3 Suppl 1):S84–S88, 2007.

7. Scelza WM, Kirshblum SC, Wuermser LA, et al: Spinal cord injury medicine. 4. Community reintegration after spinal cord iniury. Arch Phys Med Rehabil 88(3 Suppl 1):S71–S75, 2007.

CHAPTER 56

MOVEMENT DISORDERS: CLASSIFICATION AND TREATMENT

Kenneth H. Silver, MD, and Paul Fishman, MD, PhD

Never confuse motion with action.

–Benjamin Franklin (1706–1790)

1. **How can we categorize the involuntary movement disorders into general types?**
   Involuntary movement disorders can usually be classified as those characterized by too little movement *(hypokinetic)* or too much movement *(hyperkinetic)* (Box 56-1).

BOX 56-1. CLASSIFICATION OF INVOLUNTARY MOVEMENT DISORDERS

Hypokinetic

Parkinson's disease

Parkinson-like conditions

Progressive supranuclear palsy

Drug-induced multisystem atrophy (includes Shy-Drager syndrome, nigral-striatal degeneration, olivopontine-cerebellar degeneration)

Lewy body disease

Cortical-basal ganglionic degeneration

Hyperkinetic

Tremors

Tics

Tourette's syndrome

Dystonia (generalized and focal)

Dyskinesia

Chorea (including Huntington's disease)

Hemiballismus

Myoclonus

Asterixis

Parkinson's disease (tremor)

KEY POINTS: OTHER CONDITIONS THAT CAN LOOK LIKE PARKINSON'S DISEASE

1. Drug-induced parkinsonism

2. Progressive supranuclear palsy

3. Multisystem atrophy (including Shy-Drager syndrome)

4. Multiple head trauma (parkinsonism pugilistica)

2. **What are the major clinical features of Parkinson's disease (PD)?**
    Parkinsonian patients commonly show a **resting tremor, bradykinesia** (slowness of movement), and a form of increased muscular tone called **rigidity**. Other common features include a reduction in facial movements resulting in **masked facies, stooped posture,** and reduction of the amplitude of movements **(hypometria)**. Also seen are changes in speech to a soft monotone **(hypophonia)** and small, less legible handwriting **(micrographia)**. Walking becomes slower, stride length is reduced, and pivoting is replaced with a series of small steps **(turning "en bloc")**.

KEY POINTS: MAJOR CLINICAL FEATURES OF PARKINSON'S DISEASE

1. Resting tremor

2. Bradykinesia and muscle rigidity

3. Stooped posture and postural instability

4. Abnormal gait (small steps, turning "en bloc," freezing)

5. Hypophonia

3. **Who gets Parkinson's disease?**
    PD is a disease of older people, although it is reported that up to 10% of idiopathic PD begins by age 40. Approximately 1% of those over age 65 have PD, with an incidence of 20 in 100,000 in the general population and a prevalence of 1–1.5 million cases in the United States. The cause of PD is unknown, but people with a history of exposure to pesticides and herbicides (such as farm workers) appear to be at increased risk. Between 5% and 10% of PD cases may have an inherited basis with five identified genes at this time (alpha synuclein, parkin, DJ-1, PINK-1, LRRK-2).

    Dombovy M, Pippin B: Rehabilitation concerns in degenerative movement disorders of the central nervous system. In Braddom RL (ed): Physical Medicine and Rehabilitation, 2nd ed. Philadelphia, W.B. Saunders, 2000, pp 1164–1176.
    Gancher S: Parkinson disease in young adults, 2005, eMedicine website: www.emedicine.com/neuro/topic635.htm

4. **How does Parkinson's disease usually begin?**
    The most common initial symptom is **resting tremor,** which usually goes away when the limb is in motion. The tremor usually begins in the hand, while head tremor (titubation) is unusual. Activities that involve other limbs, such as walking, usually increase the tremor. Patients may feel clumsy or weak, as well as slow and stiff. They will have noticed that certain normal activities such as dressing (particularly buttoning), shaving, cutting food, and writing are more difficult. Family members may misinterpret the patient's appearance and feel that he or she is "depressed" (however, there *is* an increased incidence of depression among patients with PD).

5. **Which drugs are used to treat Parkinson's disease?**
    Anti-Parkinson medications work either by replacing dopamine (levodopa), acting as a postsynaptic (dopamine) agonist, or reestablishing the dopamine/acetylcholine balance in the striatum (anticholinergics) (Box 56-2). A guiding principle is to start L-dopa treatment in patients with symptoms that interfere with the performance of activities of daily living (ADLs) despite other treatment. A resting tremor alone does not *usually* impede function.

BOX 56-2. DRUGS TO TREAT PARKINSON'S DISEASE

Dopaminergic agents
Carbidopa/levodopa (Sinemet)
Dopamine agonists
Apomorphine (Apokyn)
Bromocriptine (Parlodel)
Pergolide (Permax)
Pramipexole (Mirapex)
Ropinirole (Requip)
Rotigotine patch (pending approval as of early 2007)

Catechol-*O*-methyl transferase (COMT) inhibitors
Entacapone (Comtan, Stalevo in combination with carbidopa/levodopa)
Tolcapone (Tasmar)

Monoamine oxidase B (MAO-B) inhibitors
Rasagiline
Selegiline (Eldepryl)

Anticholinergics
Trihexyphenidyl (Artane)
Benztropine
Ethopropazine

Amantadine (Symmetrel)

6. **What are the common side effects of PD medications?**
The most common side effects of L-dopa are **nausea, abdominal cramping,** and **diarrhea**. These side effects are significantly reduced when L-dopa is given in combination with carbidopa. Dopamine agonists, in general, cause nausea more frequently than the L-dopa/carbidopa combinations.
  All anti-Parkinson drugs cause **postural hypotension,** which can reach symptomatic levels. This can be treated with salt supplements and salt-retaining mineralocorticoids (fludrocortisone [Florinef]) or the α-adrenergic agonist, midodrine (ProAmatine).
  Virtually all anti-Parkinson drugs can cause **confusion,** hallucinations, and even psychosis. Cognitively impaired patients and those with psychiatric illness are most at risk.

7. **What are the surgical options for treating or controlling PD?**
Patients with moderate to severe motor symptoms, despite optimal medical management, can benefit from surgery. Three different brain regions that are potential sources of the tremor in Parkinson's disease (thalamus, globus pallidus interna [GPI], and subthalamic nucleus [STN]) can be targets for **stereotactic-guided surgery**. Although the traditional approach was to make a permanent destructive lesion, the majority of patients undergo implantation of a **deep brain stimulator** (DBS). A DBS to the thalamus is very effective for relief of severe tremor, whether caused by PD or essential tremor. These adjustable and programmable devices interfere with the activity of overactive brain areas in PD. A DBS is most commonly placed in the STN with resultant improvement in severity and duration of L-dopa off time. DBS has an additional effect of reduction of dyskinesia and is approved for refractory dystonia as well.

Several types of experimental surgical therapies for PD are in clinical trials, including gene therapy and implantation of stem cells. Complications of surgery include brain hemorrhage and infection as well as device failure. Experimental surgical treatments may have unexpected problems such as the dyskinesias seen in fetal transplantation patients, even off L-dopa.

Tagliati M: Surgical treatment for Parkinson disease, 2004, eMedicine website: www.emedicine.com/neuro/topic573.htm

8. **Describe some of the symptoms seen in advanced PD.**
    More advanced patients can also have loss of action of L-dopa at times not simply related to end-of-dose **(on-off syndrome),** which can be very abrupt (freezing). Attempts to improve symptoms by increasing medications seem to overshoot, resulting in the induction of involuntary jerking and twisting movements **(dyskinesias).** Advanced patients move frequently from periods of relative immobility ("off" or akinesia) to normal mobility ("on") to abnormal movements that interfere with voluntary movements ("on" with dyskinesias). **Postural changes** such as stooping with the development of permanent kyphosis can occur after years of Parkinson's disease. Loss of postural stability is common in advanced PD, even in the L-dopa "on" state. Dementia and depression are common with advanced disease, as is dysphagia with increased aspiration risk.

9. **What are the causes of disability in Parkinson's disease?**
    Social isolation, often caused by changes in physical appearance, is common in Parkinson's patients. Even in mildly affected patients, many physical activities require additional effort to perform. This leads to declining efficiency at work and, in many cases, abandonment of many forms of leisure activities. **Manual dexterity** is invariably impaired as Parkinson's worsens, affecting many ADLs such as dressing, cutting food, writing, and handling small objects (e.g., coins).

    Walking becomes impaired as the disease progresses. Postural alterations include increased neck, trunk, and hip flexion, which, coupled with a decrease in righting oneself and equilibrium reactions, lead to balance deficits and an increased risk of falling. Slowing of gait is typically seen, with difficulty turning and a tendency toward short, shuffling steps. Tripping may occur on irregular surfaces. The patient tends to stagger backward **(retropulsion)** when pushed from the front and forward **(propulsion)** when pushed from behind. Patients have a gait similar to very elderly persons: Attempts to increase speed result in more rapid stepping but not in increased stride length. Worsening proximal muscle rigidity significantly reduces trunk rotation and arm swing.

    Speech impairment in Parkinson's patients results in soft, monotonic, virtually mumbled speech. Advanced patients will have **dysphagia** as well and are at risk of silent aspiration. **Drooling** is more a result of decreased frequency of spontaneous swallowing rather than an increase in saliva production.

10. **What is the rationale for rehabilitation in PD?**
    Rehabilitation for PD should be functionally based, identifying and prioritizing problem areas, such as degree of rigidity and bradykinesia or postural control, and how these symptoms interfere with ADLs. This can be done objectively using established scales for Parkinson's disease, such as the Unified Parkinson's Disease Rating Scale (UPDRS). It is important to note not only which tasks can be performed, but also how much time is required to perform them. The general pattern of gait, including walking speed and distance, should be gauged. Forward and backward stepping, as well as the ability to navigate obstacles, needs to be checked. Fine motor tasks such as writing should be periodically assessed. Measurements need to be recorded for restrictions in joint mobility, particularly hips, knees, shoulders, and trunk. Analysis of equilibrium is important and should include tandem walking. Because of the difficulty

Parkinson's patients have in performing complex movements, evaluation should include the ability to perform simultaneous and sequential tasks.

Unified Parkinson's Disease Rating Scale: www.mdvu.org/pdf/updrs.pdf

11. **Which physical therapy (PT) strategies are useful for the Parkinson's patient?**
    In general, patients need to be counseled to maintain a reasonable level of activity at all costs, as physical exertion becomes more difficult with disease progression and the risk of deconditioning increases. More complex disability will often require the attention of the rehabilitation team.

    The typical habitus of the Parkinson's patient is a stooped posture with flexed upper extremities, minimal trunk rotation, and a shuffling gait with a narrow base of support. Exercises focus on proper body alignment (upright posture) and postural reflexes (response to dynamic balance challenges). Although symptoms caused by the disease itself (rigidity, bradykinesia, and tremor) are not generally amenable to specific physiotherapies, the secondary manifestations of loss of extremity and axial range of motion (ROM) and deconditioning, which in turn contribute to deficits in gait, balance, and transfers, are often responsive to PT.

12. **Describe PT strategies to help with postural problems in Parkinson's disease.**
    Hip extensions while standing are important, offsetting the tendency toward forward trunk flexion; performing hip extension while standing is stressed. Pelvic-tilt exercises for the low back and stretching the pectoral and iliopsoas muscles will assist in maintaining normal postural alignment. A variety of stretching exercises for the arm, leg, and trunk, performed either by the therapist or at home, can offset the tendency to lose joint ROM from the rigidity and bradykinesia. These may include passive and active-assisted stretching combined with relaxation techniques and can include shoulder-girdle exercises with a broomstick handle or a pulley to stretch the arms and trunk. Back flexion and extension exercises can be useful in improving balance and posture in sitting and standing. Quadriceps and hip extensor strengthening also can assist the patient in being able to climb stairs or arise from a sitting surface.

13. **Which PT strategies should be considered to help with gait difficulties?**
    Frenkel's exercises for coordination of foot placement are helpful to maintain accurate lower-extremity positioning during the gait cycle. Wobbleboard or balance-feedback trainers can be used to improve body alignment and postural reflexes. The tendency to topple backward can be addressed with heel lifts as well as by assistive mobility devices.

    Stationary bicycles, arm ergometers, and treadmills can help to restore diminished reciprocal limb motions and increase step length. Proper heelstrike should be emphasized, as should adequate arm swing and trunk rotation during ambulation. The tendency to freeze in narrow and complicated spaces can be reduced with visual targets, such as the tip of a walking stick or markers on the floor. Some patients prevent freezing by counting rhythmically as they walk or by humming marching music. When frozen, relaxing back on the heels and lifting the toes, as well as raising the arms from the sides with sudden movements, can help restore locomotion.

    The difficulty in arising from sitting surfaces can be addressed with elevated sitting surfaces (chair, toilet) and strategically placed grab rails/bars (bed, bathtub). Small mats and rugs that can trip the shuffling patient should be removed.

14. **Discuss the use of wheelchairs and walkers for patients with PD.**
    The patient may eventually need a wheelchair. An effort should be made to keep the person with PD ambulatory as long as feasible to minimize the development of contracture, stiffness, and deconditioning that attends further immobilization. Although wheeled walkers are useful in assisting ambulation, particularly by preventing backward instability, patients with significant postural deficits may prefer more stable devices (such as a shopping cart or walking behind a wheelchair). Some wheeled walkers have been designed specifically for Parkinson's patients. They have added weight to lower their center of gravity. Handbrakes are essential in such devices to ensure control, and patients must have the arm/hand dexterity and cognition to use them.

15. **Which occupational therapy strategies can help people with PD?**

Occupational therapy can provide vital input for maintaining the home, vocational, leisure, and transportation capabilities of the patient. **Adaptive equipment** is provided when deficits in upper-extremity control limit efficient and safe function. For instance, plate guards or specialized dishes prevent food from sliding off; plates can be weighted or made more adherent to the table. Cups and utensils can have large handles and also may be weighted to dampen excessive motions caused by tremor. Swivel forks and spoons can help compensate for loss of ROM. Buttons on clothing can be replaced with Velcro or zipper closures.

Other **environmental aids** can help keep the person with Parkinson's disease productive at work. Workplace adaptations to accommodate for Parkinson's-related impairments and disabilities may include equipment to support writing (built-up pens and forearm supports) and typing skills (electronic keyboards and computerized scanning and pointing devices), as well as power mobility devices (scooters or wheelchairs). Many patients can retain driving ability, although the slowing of motor responses as the disease worsens may place these patients at risk when driving. Occupational therapists (or other qualified therapists) can play a critical role in **assessment and retraining of driving skills,** particularly extremity reaction timing and visual field scanning. Families should be counseled to have the patient undergo driver's testing and training earlier, when mobility and ADL performance begin to suffer, rather than later when accidents will more likely occur.

16. **How can the speech therapist intervene in PD?**

The hypokinetic dysarthria seen in patients can be addressed with **diaphragmatic breathing exercises** and improved posture and flexibility, which increase vital capacity. The prevalence and type of swallowing disorder of the Parkinson's patient vary. The patient often has trouble with oral bolus formation, as well as loss of coordination between oral and pharyngeal stages of swallowing. Tongue and mandibular movement and range are commonly limited. After proper **swallowing assessment,** strategies can include using smaller portions taken more frequently, altering food textures and consistencies to maximize safe oropharyngeal function, optimizing head and neck position during swallow, facilitating oral and pharyngeal movement and reflexes, and performing exercises to increase facial and lingual strength and ROM.

HYPERKINETIC MOVEMENT DISORDERS

17. **What is tremor? How can it be classified?**

Tremors, the most common form of involuntary movement disorders, are characterized by rhythmic oscillations of a body part. Tremors can be classified as to the situation in which they are most prominent (i.e., with movement or maintained posture or at rest). Tremors at rest are predominantly PD or Parkinson like (i.e., associated with neuroleptics) (*see* Box 56-3).

Hallett M: Classification and treatment of tremor. JAMA 266:1115–1117, 1991.

18. **Are physiologic tremors worrisome?**

No. They are usually of no clinical significance and often increase or are precipitated by emotional stress, aggravated by fatigue, hypoglycemia, thyrotoxicosis, exercise, alcohol withdrawal, and fever, and can be drug induced (caffeine, theophylline, lithium, amiodarone). They can be treated by educating the patient to avoid precipitating conditions.

19. **How are other tremors treated?**

Essential tremor (ET) is the most common cause of tremor, affecting up to 6% of the population. The most useful medication in treating ET, task-specific tremor, and action tremor is **propranolol** (40–240 mg). Other beta blockers have fewer side effects but are less effective. The anticonvulsant **primidone** is also effective but commonly causes sedation and confusion with initial treatment. Other antitremor drugs with reported efficacy include the benzodiazepine

---

BOX 56-3. CLASSIFICATION OF TREMORS

Postural tremors
Physiologic tremor
Essential (familial, senile) tremor
Tremor with basal ganglial disease
Cerebellar postural tremor
Tremor with peripheral neuropathy
Post-traumatic tremor
Alcoholic tremor

Kinetic tremors
Cerebellar tremor
Rubral tremor

Task-specific tremors
Writing tremor
Vocal tremor
Orthostatic tremor

---

alprazolam and the anticonvulsants gabapentin and topiramate. Some patients may benefit from injections of botulinum neurotoxin into selected muscles.

Measures to reduce or alleviate anxiety are useful, as are strategies to control oscillation excursion with weights or other mechanical compensations. Treatment is usually unsatisfactory for intention tremor, but, again, weighting the limb can be of limited assistance. Severe, disabling tremor can be significantly and, at times, dramatically improved with stereotactic thalamotomy or implantation of a DBS.

20. **What is the physiologic basis for tics?**
    This is largely unknown. Tics are sustained nonrhythmic muscle contractions that are rapid and stereotyped, often occurring in the same extremity or body part during times of stress. Tics have not been known to cause physical impairment but may have obvious social consequences and handicaps.

    Tics can be seen as representing a spectrum of disease from **transient** tic disorder (duration < 1 year) to **chronic** tic disorder (duration > 1 year), manifesting as either vocal or motor tics, but not both.

21. **What is the most socially disabling aspect of Gilles de la Tourette's syndrome?**
    Probably the involuntary use of obscenities **(coprolalia)** as well as obscene gestures **(copropraxia),** although such behavior may be mild and transient and occurs only in a minority of afflicted persons. **Tourette's syndrome** is characterized by motor and vocal tics lasting for more than 1 year. Other features of this hereditary disease include vocal and motor tics, echolalia, loud cries, and yips, with some affected individuals having few symptoms while others can be socially disabled. Emotional and learning problems during childhood are common in those affected.

    Neuroleptics, most commonly pimozide and haloperidol, are most predictably effective, but sedation limits their use. Behavioral manifestations can respond to psychotherapy, and anxiety can be addressed with relaxation exercises and biofeedback.

22. **What common features of dystonias distinguish them from other movement disorders?**

Dystonias are slow, sustained contractions of muscles that frequently cause twisting movements or abnormal postures. The disorder resembles athetosis but shows a more sustained isometric contraction. When rapid movements are involved, they are usually repetitive and continuous. The movements are a result of simultaneous co-contraction of agonists and antagonists and can interfere with speed, smoothness, and accuracy of movements in the affected body part.

Dystonia often increases with emotional or physical stress, anxiety, pain, or fatigue and disappears with sleep. Symptom severity can vary throughout the day. Patients often develop methods to self-inhibit or diminish the dystonic movements by changing posture or touching the affected body part.

Moberg-Wolff EA, Thiyaga-Rajah A, Santiago-Palma J, Banna SA: Dystonias, 2004. On eMedicine website: www.emedicine.com/pmr/topic235.htm

Pentland B: Parkinsonism and dystonia. In Greenwood R, Barnes M, McMillan T, Ward C (eds): Neurological Rehabilitation. London, Churchill Livingstone, 1993, pp 474–485.

23. **How are the dystonias classified?**

See Box 56-4.

BOX 56-4. CLASSIFICATION OF DYSTONIAS

Focal dystonia
Torticollis (neck)
Blepharospasm (periorbital)
Oromandibular (mouth or jaw)
Writer's or occupational cramp (arm or leg)

Segmental dystonia
Cranial
Brachial
Crural

Other dystonias
Generalized dystonia (includes dystonia musculorum deformans)
Multifocal dystonia
Hemidystonia

---

24. **What causes dystonias? How are they treated?**

The most common dystonias are usually idiopathic. Some patients have inherited or metabolic disorders such as **dystonia musculorum deformans, Wilson's disease** (degeneration of liver and basal ganglia), and **lipid storage diseases**. Patients with certain neurodegenerative diseases can exhibit dystonia, such as Parkinson's, Huntington's, and Leigh's diseases. Dystonias can have acquired causes such as perinatal brain injury, carbon monoxide poisoning, or encephalitis. Focal brain disease involving the basal ganglia, such as stroke, tumor, or local trauma, can cause dystonia on the contralateral body side. Spinal cord disorders such as syringomyelia or tumor can cause segmental or focal dystonia.

Detection and correction of an underlying abnormality (drug-induced, structural cause) are the first steps in dystonia treatment. Anticholinergics are the most effective oral agents for both generalized and focal dystonias. Baclofen, carbamazepine, and clonazepam are sometimes helpful. Focal dystonias are now commonly treated with botulinum toxin.

25. What is spasmodic torticollis? How is it treated?

Spasmodic torticollis is the most common type of focal dystonia. It affects most frequently the sternocleidomastoid, trapezius, scalenes, and posterior neck muscles in an asymmetric pattern. Patients are predominantly women in their forties or fifties. The movement can be tonic or intermittent. The head usually rotates to one side or the other but also can assume a predominantly forward **(antecolic)** or backward **(retrocolic)** position. Improvement of symptoms often occurs with the use of certain gestures of the hands to various head or facial sites (e.g., lightly touching the chin with a finger). Symptoms are worsened by prolonged standing or walking or under conditions of stress or fatigue. Associated pain is common and can either be an initial presentation or develop over time. Complete or partial remissions can occur. Social stigmatization is a major concern, as are functional impairments, which can include driving, reading, or activities that involve looking down and using the hands.

Rehabilitation management can include pain control, stretching tight musculature, and trigger point injections. Although some suggest exercises to strengthen contralateral, uninvolved muscles and reciprocally inhibit involved ones, others feel such exercises worsen symptoms. Biofeedback has been used but is not routinely effective. The mainstay of treatment, as with the other focal dystonias, remains pharmacologic intervention, especially intramuscular injection of botulinum toxin.

26. What features are characteristic of writer's cramp?

Writer's, or occupational, cramp involves the dominant hand and wrist and appears during certain activities, such as writing, typing, or playing a musical instrument. The many appellations referring to the precipitating activity include writer's cramp, pianist's hand, telegrapher's cramp, or "chapter-writer's spasm." It presents with onset of a specific activity as an uncontrollably tight grip, accompanied by flexion of the wrist. It may be associated with jerking or sustained movements. Usually, other coordinated movements of that extremity are normal. Often the symptoms present in a certain posture or position—for instance, a patient may be able to write at a blackboard, but not seated at a desk.

Therapy is directed at re-educating muscle movement patterns and maintaining ROM. Enlarging or changing the contour of grasped objects, such as built-up pens, is useful. Relaxation exercises are helpful, as can be splinting, minimizing, or inhibiting dystonic postures. Therapy can also be directed at teaching contralateral hand use.

27. Which movement disorder is associated with chronic neuroleptic therapy?

Tardive dyskinesia (TD) is a condition characterized by involuntary, choreiform movements of the face and tongue associated with chronic neuroleptic medication use. Common movements include chewing, sucking, mouthing, licking, "fly-catching movements," and puckering or smacking (buccal-lingual-masticatory syndrome). Choreiform movements of the trunk and extremities can also occur, along with dystonic movements of the neck and trunk. TD occurs in up to 20% of patients treated chronically with neuroleptics (dopamine antagonists) and probably represents hypersensitivity of dopamine receptors and overactivity of the dopamine system resulting from long-term dopamine-receptor blockade. Duration of treatment, dose, and age are risk factors for its development. Similar movements can also be seen in the elderly without exposure to dopamine-blocking drugs. Resolution of TD after neuroleptic drugs are withdrawn is slow and incomplete, with half of TD patients still symptomatic a year after drug discontinuation.

28. Can TD be treated or prevented?

The incidence of TD has been dropping significantly since the introduction of the so-called atypical neuroleptics, such as clozapine, risperidone, and olanzapine. These drugs, unlike haloperidol, have antipsychotic actions that do not solely depend on dopaminergic pathways. The original atypical antipsychotic, clozapine, remains unsurpassed in its antipsychotic potential and lack of extrapyramidal side effects, but its use is limited by a high incidence of agranulocytosis. Benzodiazepines such as **clonazepam** are the most useful medications for suppression of the movements. The partial dopamine agonist tetrabenazine has been effective in treating TD and may soon be available in the United States on a compassionate-use basis. Because the symptoms are most prominent at rest, activity (including chewing gum) can be of some value to patients. Some have suggested value in oral desensitization when hyperreactivity to sensory stimuli exists. Other rehabilitation strategies have not been proven useful.

29. **What causes ataxia? How can it be treated?**
Along with intention tremor and dysmetria, ataxia is usually associated with cerebellar disease. Common causes include stroke, multiple sclerosis, and acute and chronic toxicity (alcohol most commonly). Slowly progressive ataxia may represent a group of hereditary disorders, some of which are diagnosed with genetic testing. Unexplained ataxia can be an autoimmune manifestation of an otherwise occult malignancy (ovarian, breast, small-cell carcinoma).

Response to drug therapy has been poor, with many agents touted as useful (propranolol, isoniazid, carbamazepine, clonazepam, tryptophan, buspirone, thyroid-stimulating hormone). The mainstay of treatment for ataxia is occupational therapy to help learn compensatory techniques for performing basic self-care and occupational activities, and assessing the benefits of weighted bracelets or similar devices to dampen the oscillations. Gait training and education in the use of assistive devices for walking can prevent falls and enhance mobility in the ataxic individual.

30. **How do athetosis, chorea, and ballismus differ?**
See Table 56-1.

TABLE 56-1. COMPARISON OF ATHETOSIS, CHOREA, AND HEMIALLISMUS	
Disease	**Features**
Athetosis	Slow, writhing, repetitious movements Can lead to bizarre postures Usually affects face and upper extremities Often secondary to other neurologic disorders (e.g., stroke, tumor)
Chorea	Nonstereotyped, unpredictable, jerky movements Usually involves oral structures, can involve any or all body parts Can be associated with any central neurologic disease; most familiar is Huntington's disease
Hemiballismus	Extremely violent flinging of unilateral arm and leg Usually secondary to bleed or infarct in subthalamic nuclei; less often from abscess or tumor

31. **Is Huntington's disease (HD) treatable? Who is at risk?**
Chorea means "to dance," and the gait in these patients takes on an ataxic, dancing appearance. Unfortunately, HD is a terminal disorder involving involuntary, choreiform movements that are abrupt and purposeless. It is associated with a progressive dementia. It is an autosomal, dominant hereditary disorder affecting 4–6 persons in 100,000. It reached the public's attention as afflicting Woody Guthrie, a well-known American folk singer. Diagnosis can be made with

certainty with genetic testing, and genetic counseling of newly diagnosed individuals is essential, particularly for asymptomatic individuals.

Symptom onset can range from childhood to the eighth decade, although most individuals become affected after age 30. The abnormal movements begin in the fingers, toes, and facial regions, often with dysarthria, teeth grinding, and facial grimacing. Along with the choreiform movement, progressive dementia and emotional/behavioral abnormalities are seen. Intellectual impairment and psychosis invariably occur and progress rapidly to become the most disabling features.

The pathology of HD includes degeneration of the basal ganglia, particularly the caudate nucleus. There is no treatment proven to reduce the progression of disease, but experimental therapies to reduce the toxicity of the associated abnormal protein (polyglutamine) are in clinical trial. Symptomatic relief is indicated, especially for the abnormal movements, depression, and psychosis. Rehabilitation techniques that involve improving coactivation and trunk stability, rhythmical stabilization, and traditional relaxation techniques (including biofeedback) have been mentioned as reasonable treatment strategies.

Rosenblatt A, Ranen N, Peyser C: A Physician's Guide to the Management of Huntington's Disease, 2nd ed. New York, Huntington's Disease Society of America, 1999.

32. What causes myoclonus? Is it common?

Myoclonus is one of the most common involuntary movement disorders of central nervous system origin. It is characterized by sudden, jerky, irregular contractions of a muscle or groups of muscles. It can be subdivided into myoclonus that is *stimulus-sensitive* **(reflex myoclonus)** or *non–stimulus-sensitive*, which occurs at rest **(spontaneous myoclonus).**

Etiologically, myoclonus can be **physiologic** (occurring in normal persons while falling asleep or walking or with anxiety, such as sleep jerks and hiccups); **essential** (increasing with activity, sometimes disabling but without neurologic deficit); **epileptic** (associated with generalized seizures, as in juvenile myoclonic epilepsy); or **symptomatic** (part of a more widespread neurologic disorder, such as an encephalopathy or stroke). **Spinal myoclonus** involves a group of muscles innervated by a certain spinal segment (segmental myoclonus) and can be associated with spinal cord disease (i.e., trauma or multiple sclerosis) and tumors.

A number of drugs have been used to treat myoclonus and can be effective in some situations. These include clonazepam and valproate; however, the newer anticonvulsant levetiracetam (Keppra) has also been useful in several forms of myoclonus.

33. What types of movement disorders can be psychogenic?

Psychogenic movement disorders mimic the entire spectrum of organic movement disorders, including tremor, dystonia, myoclonus, and parkinsonism (in decreasing order of frequency). In one series of 842 patients with movement disorders, 28 (3.3%) were diagnosed as having some type of psychogenic movement disorder, most commonly tremor. Psychogenic movement disorders can also occur in conjunction with organic movement disorders. Psychogenic etiologies should be considered when the onset, course, or manifestations are unusual. There is often an association with prior psychiatric disease, particularly depression, and most patients will have other pseudoneurologic symptoms (e.g., weakness or sensory loss). Treatment approaches include psychotherapy, placebo treatment, or behavioral management as used in other types of conversion disorders.

Factor R, Podskalny G, Molho E: Psychogenic movement disorders. Frequency, clinical profile, and characteristics. J Neurol Neurosurg Psychiatr 59:406–412, 1995.

Schrag A, Lang A: Psychogenic movement disorders. Curr Opin Neurol 18:399–404, 2005.

WEBSITES

1. American Parkinson Disease Association
   www.apdaparkinson.org

2. Michael J. Fox Foundation
   www.michaeljfox.org

3. Movement Disorder Society
   www.movementdisorders.org

4. Parkinson's Disease Foundation
   www.pdf.org

5. We Move
   http://wemove.org

CHAPTER 57

MULTIPLE SCLEROSIS: CLINICAL PATTERNS, SYMPTOM MANAGEMENT, AND REHABILITATION

Seema Khurana, DO, Rory J. O'Connor, MD, and Jan Lexell, MD, PhD

The course of life is unpredictable, no one can write his autobiography in advance.
— Abraham J. Heschel (1907–1972)

1. **What are the demographics of multiple sclerosis (MS)?**
   One-quarter to one-half million people in the United States have MS, and approximately 8000 new cases are diagnosed each year. Symptoms typically begin between ages 20 and 50 in 90% of cases; the peak age is 33 years. MS is twice as common in whites and females. Residing in a temperate climate is also an associated factor. The incidence of MS increases at higher latitudes. Identical twin concordance is 30%. The lifetime risk of a female child whose mother has MS is 5% (fifty-fold higher than the general population).

   > http://members.aol.com/MSInfoCen2/geodistr.htm
   > Sadovnick AD, Ebers GC: Epidemiology of multiple sclerosis: A critical overview. Can J Neurol Sci 20:17–29, 1993.

2. **What is the pathophysiology of MS?**
   MS is characterized by plaques of central nervous system (CNS) white matter demyelination with lymphocytic invasion scattered throughout the brain, spinal cord, and optic nerves. New evidence suggests there is also axonal damage and brain atrophy. Many environmental and genetic factors have been implicated in the cause of the disease. There are many other factors suggested to trigger the disease.

   > www.clevelandclinicmeded.com/diseasemanagement/neurology/multsclerosis/multsclerosis.htm#pathophysiology
   > O'Riordan JI, Thompson AJ, Kingsley DP, et al: The prognostic value of brain MRI in clinically isolated syndromes of the CNS. A 10-year follow-up. Brain 121:495–503, 1998.
   > Herndon RM: Medical hypothesis: Why secondary progressive multiple sclerosis is a relentlessly progressive illness. Arch Neurol 59:301–304, 2002.

3. **What patterns of disease are seen in MS?**
   There are typically four patterns of MS:
   - **Relapsing-remitting MS** is the most common, with approximately 85% of people presenting with this pattern. Episodic relapses occur approximately once per year with recovery and a stable phase between relapses. Recovery may be incomplete, and disability accumulates over time. Ten percent of patients have a benign course with no disability or mild disability.
   - Half of patients with relapsing-remitting MS change patterns after 10–20 years to **secondary progressive MS** (a gradual neurologic deterioration without acute relapses).
   - Ten to 15% have **primary progressive MS**. This pattern shows a gradual but continuous neurologic deterioration.
   - **Progressive-relapsing MS** occurs in less than 5% of cases and involves gradual but continuous neurologic deterioration with superimposed relapses. Death may occur in weeks to months.

Lublin FD, Reingold SC: Defining the clinical course on multiple sclerosis: Results of an international survey. Neurology 46:907–911, 1996.
www.med.harvard.edu/publications/On_The_Brain/Volume05/Number4/MSf.html

4. What diagnostic tools are used to diagnose MS?

- Using **standard magnetic resonance imaging (MRI)**, 80–90% of patients diagnosed with MS have evidence of plaques. These hyperintense lesions are most common in periventricular white matter, corpus callosum, brain stem, optic nerves, and spinal cord. Standard MRI alone cannot make the diagnosis of MS.
- **Enhanced fluid-attenuated inversion-recovery (FLAIR) MRI** improves differentiation of plaques from normal structures such as cerebrospinal fluid.
- Nonconventional techniques, such as **magnetic transfer imaging (MTI),** are more sensitive and specific for MS lesions. MTI with gadolinium may detect white matter lesions in those patients who have a negative MRI scan.
- Interocular latency difference on **visual evoked potential testing** is the most sensitive indicator of optic nerve dysfunction. The most common somatosensory evoked potential abnormality with MS is increased interpeak latencies.

Filippi M, Rocca MA, Minicucci L: Magnetic transfer imaging in patients with definite MS and negative conventional MRI. Neurology 52:845–848, 1999.
Trip SA, Miller DH: Imaging in multiple sclerosis. J Neurol Neurosurg Psychiatr 76:11–18, 2005.

5. Does psychological stress play a role in relapses?

There is clear evidence that psychologically stressful life events play a role in relapses. However, it is not clear what type of stressful events are involved. It is likely that connectivity within the neuroendocrine system induces these exacerbations.

Mohr DC, Hart SL, Julian L, et al: Association between stressful life events and exacerbation in multiple sclerosis: A meta-analysis. BMJ 328:731, 2004.

6. What is Lhermitte's sign?

A transient, short-lasting sensation related to neck movement felt in the back of the neck, lower back, or other parts of the body. The sensation is mainly caused by neck flexion and usually induces an electric type of sensation.

Al-Araji AH, Oger J: Reappraisal of Lhermitte's sign in multiple sclerosis. Mult Scler 11(4):398–402, 2005.

7. What are important prognostic signs in MS?

Unfortunately, a poor prognosis is easier to predict than a good prognosis. Signs associated with **poor prognosis** include male gender, initial presentation over age 35, initial motor or cerebellar dysfunction, a rapid progression of disease, and initial symptoms being polysymptomatic. **Better prognostic factors** include female gender, age less than 35, initial sensory signs or optic neuritis, sudden onset with good recovery and long remissions, and complete and rapid remission of initial symptoms.

8. What MRI and evoked potential findings are seen in MS?

With standard MRI, 80–90% of patients diagnosed with MS have evidence of plaques. These hyperintense lesions are most common in periventricular white matter, corpus callosum, brain stem, optic nerves, and spinal cord. Standard MRI alone cannot make the diagnosis of MS. See question 4 for additional tools.

Interocular latency difference on visual evoked potential testing is the most sensitive indicator of optic nerve dysfunction. The most common somatosensory evoked potential abnormality with MS is increased interpeak latencies.

Filippi M, Rocca MA, Minicucci L: Magnetic transfer imaging in patients with definite MS and negative conventional MRI. Neurology 52:845–848, 1999.

9. **What outcome measures are used in MS?**

The most widely used MS outcome measure has been the **expanded disability status scale** (EDSS), which is based on Kurtzke's original disability status scale introduced in 1955. The EDSS is not a unidimensional scale; it mixes pathology, impairments, and activity limitations. In addition, it exhibits poor targeting, low interrater reliability, and low responsiveness.

There is increasing interest in using patient-based outcome measures as clinical measures in MS. Several psychometrically sound measures of functional ability and quality of life have been developed, including the **multiple sclerosis impact scale** (MSIS) and the **Hamburg quality of life questionnaire in multiple sclerosis** (HAQUAMS). Both of these questionnaires can be completed by the patients themselves or by interview. Both have good reliability, construct validity, and responsiveness.

Gold SM, Heesen C, Schulz H, et al: Disease specific quality of life instruments in multiple sclerosis: Validation of the Hamburg Quality of Life Questionnaire in Multiple Sclerosis (HAQUAMS). Mult Scler 7:119–130, 2001.

Hobart J, Freeman J, Thompson A: Kurtzke scales revisited: The application of psychometric methods to clinical intuition. Brain 123:1027–1040, 2000.

Hobart J, Lamping D, Fitzpatrick R, et al: The Multiple Sclerosis Impact Scale (MSIS-29): A new patient-based outcome measure. Brain 124:962–973, 2000.

10. **How do you design a rehabilitation program to maximize beneficial MS outcome with inpatient or outpatient rehabilitation?**

Studies show that **inpatient rehabilitation** has a beneficial effect on activity and participation in both relapsing-remitting and progressive MS. In addition, there are improvements in health-related quality-of-life perception. After discharge, as the neurologic status worsens, the physical and psychological benefits of rehabilitation may last greater than 6 months, but diminish without ongoing therapies.

Outpatient therapies, therefore, play an important role in the management of MS. Patti et al demonstrated that a 6-week program of outpatient rehabilitation improved physical and psychological parameters in patients with primary and secondary progressive MS. For patients with relapsing-remitting MS, intravenous corticosteroids combined with rehabilitation significantly improves outcomes, with an effect lasting at least 3 months.

Freeman JA, Langdon DW, Hobart JC, et al: Inpatient rehabilitation in multiple sclerosis: Do the benefits carry over in the community? Neurology 52:50–56, 1999.

Liu C, Playford ED, Thompson AJ: Does neurorehabilitation have a role in relapsing-remitting multiple sclerosis? J Neurol 250:1214–1218, 2003.

Patti F, Ciancio MR, Cacopardo M, et al: Effects of a short outpatient rehabilitation treatment on disability of multiple sclerosis patients—a randomised controlled trial. J Neurol 250:861–866, 2003.

Craig J, Young CA, Ennis M, et al: A randomised controlled trial comparing rehabilitation against standard therapy in multiple sclerosis patients receiving intravenous steroid treatment. J Neurol Neurosurg Psychiatry 74:1225–1230, 2003.

11. **Can patients with MS benefit from exercise?**

Caution must be taken when prescribing physical activity, because symptoms may temporarily worsen with increased core temperature on exposure to heat or physical exercise. Programs are therefore designed to activate working muscles but avoid overload. Exercise evaluation and prescription must account for fatigue, spasticity, ataxia, and incoordination, as well as neurologic deficits already present in MS. Emphasis should be placed on maintenance of general conditioning. Maximizing passive and active range of motion is critical. Aerobic training improves fitness and quality of life.

The best exercise for the task is often the task itself. Design of an exercise plan for MS patients should focus on centered goals, range limitations, and strength deficits.

Functional levels and key task deficits in interaction with current state-of-the-art adaptive equipment should all be used to devise an individualized program. The program should include prescribed activity throughout the day (lifestyle exercise). Range of motion should be independent whenever possible, and include family or attendant assistance as needed for the unobtainable. Specific tasks (transfers, dressing, driving) should be attempted with assistance. If needed, subcomponents of actions can be broken down for repetitive practice. Backup options should be identified for anticipated variations in functional performance.

Brown TR, Kraft GH: Exercise and rehabilitation for individuals with multiple sclerosis. Phys Med Rehab Clin N Am 16:513–555, 2005.

12. How can fatigue be assessed and treated in MS?

Fatigue is the subjective lack of physical or mental capacity to perform usual activities and is one of the most common complaints made by patients living with MS. Studies have shown that 78–87% of people with MS experience fatigue. The subjective experience of fatigue does not correlate with the objective physical symptoms or neurologic impairments. **MS-related fatigue** has been described as a time-consuming and all-absorbing phenomenon that involves the whole human being. Fatigue in MS may be misunderstood and misinterpreted by both relatives and professional staff. Several different scales, such as the **fatigue severity scale, fatigue descriptive scale,** and **fatigue impact scale,** are used for assessment. In evaluating the patient, ensure sleep hygiene, rule out medical problems such as hypothyroidism or infection, and evaluate ongoing medication that may exacerbate fatigue (e.g., baclofen, carbamazepine). Nonpharmacologic management is generally the most effective treatment. Both physical and occupational therapy will be helpful to train the patient in energy-conservation techniques and work simplification. An evaluation should be made for adaptive equipment needs. Based on evidence from controlled trials, amantadine and modafinil have been shown to be effective in the management of fatigue caused by MS.

Fatigue is worsened by heat, as well as by physical exertion and heavy meals that may increase core temperature. Therapies should be scheduled with this in mind. Patients should be warned about not being able to lift themselves out of a hot bath because of profound muscle weakness.

LaBan MM, Martin T, Pechur J, Sarnacki S: Physical and occupational therapy in the treatment of patients with multiple sclerosis. Phys Med Rehabil Clin N Am 9:603–614, 1998.

Olsson M, Lexell J, Soderberg S: The meaning of fatigue for women with multiple sclerosis. J Adv Nurs 49:7–15, 2005.

Rammohan KW, Rosenberg JH, Lynn DJ, et al: Efficacy and safety of modafinil (Provigil) for the treatment of fatigue in multiple sclerosis: A two centre phase 2 study. J Neurol Neurosurg Psychiatry 72:179–183, 2002.

www.mult-sclerosis.org/fatigue.html

www.nationalmssociety.org/Sourcebook-Fatigue.asp

13. What is Uhthoff's phenomenon?

Uhthoff's phenomenon refers to visual problems that occur in persons with MS that are brought on during periods of increased body temperature. The usual history is of "black spots" appearing in the visual fields of one or both eyes while the person is exercising, in the sauna, taking a hot shower, or experiencing fever. This phenomenon is felt to reflect areas of impaired but still functioning myelin that breaks down in transmitting electrical impulses when the surrounding fluid heats up.

14. How is spasticity managed in MS?

Spasticity is seen in approximately 55% of MS patients. It can cause pain, disrupt sleep, and impair volitional movement and daily activities. Conversely, spasticity may play a role in the ability to transfer, stand, and ambulate. Therefore, the decision to treat spasticity must consider all potential risks and benefits. Causes for an increase in tone must be determined before initiating treatment. The most common causes of increases in spasticity are urinary tract infections, constipation, and pressure sores.

Typical patterns of activity limitation in MS include an inconsistent variety of impairments such as touch, position sense, dexterity, and strength deficits. Movement is dampened by excessive tone, overflow motor activation patterns, and unintentional agonist-antagonist cocontraction. Treatment is functionally focused and applied in the context of lifestyle. The mainstay of stretching is performed in the morning to get started and at night to prevent spasms. Stretching is followed by active range of motion and active-assisted exercise. Oral medications (baclofen, Valium, tizanidine, clonazepam, clonidine) are introduced sparingly, focusing dosing at times of higher tone or functional need. The combination of up to three oral agents and focal injections for peripheral neurolysis, botulinum toxin, and dorsal root rhizotomy may be necessary. Baclofen pump installation achieves improvement in control without mental status compromise.

The first line of treatment involves daily positioning, stretching, and splinting. The next addition is an oral agent. Baclofen is usually used first when oral agents are needed. It is started at 5–10 mg/day, with the dose titrated every 5–7 days. Other oral medications include dantrolene, diazepam, clonidine, clonazepam, tizanidine, gabapentin, and cycloheptadine. Botulinum toxin injections are most effective for focal spasticity. Intrathecal baclofen or phenol are options when other medications are ineffective. These treatments are most effective for lower-extremity spasticity.

Paisley S, Beard S, Hunn A, Wight J: Clinical effectiveness of oral treatments for spasticity in multiple sclerosis: A systematic review. Mult Scler 8:319–329, 2004.

Richardson D: Physical therapy in spasticity. Eur J Neurol 9(Suppl 1):17–22, 2002.

15. **When should you suspect bladder dysfunction? What are the patterns of dysfunction and their treatment?**
Because of the constellation of white matter lesions from MS that can occur throughout the central nervous system (CNS), all patterns and combinations of bladder dysfunction may present, including frontal uninhibited detrusor contraction, upper motor neuron parasympathetic hyperreflexia, and upper motor neuron pelvic floor spasticity. Lower motor neuron patterns, such as atonic bladder and pelvic floor laxity, are less common. Early symptoms of urgency and detrusor spasm can be blunted with oxybutynin or tolterodine in intermittent or sustained release.

Symptomatic bladder dysfunction occurs in most patients with MS. The severity of dysfunction is not related to the age of the patient or duration of disease, but urologic complaints are strongly related to the degree of disability. Bladder hyperreflexia and hyporeflexia may occur. The most common urodynamic lesion found in MS is detrusor hyperreflexia. Unfortunately, symptoms do not differentiate between failure to retain and failure to empty. In addition, bladder dysfunction may change over the course of the disease. Periodic urodynamics should be considered.

First, urinary tract infections should be ruled out and, if needed, treated with appropriate antibiotics. Intermittent catheterization is recommended for patients with failure to empty. Nighttime bladder dysfunction can be treated with low-dose oral antidiuretic hormone (Desmopressin). Detrusor hyperreflexia can be treated with oxybutynin (Ditropan) or tolterodine (Detrol). Botulinum toxin intravesically is a new promising and effective treatment for severe and disabling bladder dysfunction.

Dasgupta R, Fowler CJ: Sexual and urological dysfunction in multiple sclerosis: Better understanding and improved therapies. Curr Opin Neurol 15:271–278, 2002.

Sahai A, Khan M, Fowler CJ, Dasgupta P: Botulinum toxin for the treatment of lower urinary tract symptoms: A review. Neurourol Urodyn 24:2–12, 2005.

KEY POINTS: IMPORTANT FEATURES OF MULTIPLE SCLEROSIS

1. MS is the most common cause of neurologic disability in adults of working age.

2. MS is a relapsing-remitting or progressive cause of motor, sensory, and cognitive impairments.

3. MS is a clinical diagnosis, which is supported by radiologic, laboratory, or nerve conduction studies.

4. Rehabilitation plays an important role in the management of all forms of MS and can prevent further deterioration.

---

16. **How is incoordination treated?**

Incoordination is an umbrella term for motor dysfunction that does not stem from lack of strength. Through history and examination the clinician strives to dissect the following: decreased dexterity from corticospinal changes, sensory proprioceptive deficits, apraxia, and ataxia. Incoordination is a common problem in MS and ranges from mild tremor to severe ataxia. Cerebral outflow tremors are the most common type. Therapy is aimed at compensatory strategies. Weighted cuffs to dampen incoordination may diminish the amplitude of tremor but are not well tolerated. Visualization of the activity with a mirror, establishment of other sensory cues, and proprioceptive neuromuscular facilitation are helpful. **Frankel's exercises**, originally described to treat tabes dorsalis, are used to treat incoordination and ataxia. They require a high degree of concentration and frequent repetition and therefore may not be appropriate for all MS patients. **Carbamazepine** has been reported to reduce the severity of tremors at doses of 400–600 mg/day. Isoniazid, propanolol, primidone, clonazepam, and gabapentin have all been used with varying success. Stereotactic ventrolateral thalamotomy has benefited select patients.

Alusi SH, Aziz TZ, Glickman S, et al: Stereotactic lesional surgery for the treatment of tremor in multiple sclerosis: A prospective case-controlled study. Brain 124:1576–1589, 2001.

17. **How are mobility limitations treated in MS?**

Seventy-five percent of MS patients have varying degrees of mobility limitations. Treatment requires a comprehensive evaluation. Weakness, fatigue, spasticity, and incoordination may all limit mobility and require treatment. Gait evaluation should be made on varying terrains, elevations, and stairs. Evaluation of deficiencies will guide the therapy prescription. The need for orthotics and assistive devices should be considered. Increasing the width of the ambulatory base with a cane or lightweight walker often improves the safety of ambulation. A top cap that decreases friction when the foot drags across the floor can be considered for patients with foot-drop.

Wiles CM, Newcombe RG, Fuller KJ, et al: Controlled randomise crossover trial of the effects of physiotherapy on mobility in chronic multiple sclerosis. J Neurol Neurosurg Psychiatry 70:174–179, 2001.

18. **What affective disorders are seen in MS?**

The prevalence of depression in people with MS is 50%, which is 3–10 times higher than in general medical populations. Subsyndromal depression has a point prevalence of 48% and is a risk factor for major depression. Symptoms of MS may mimic depression (e.g., fatigue, weight loss). However, depression in MS often presents with irritability or undue worry about symptoms. Rating scales to measure depression in MS should reflect this by avoiding an overreliance on somatic symptoms. The Beck Depression Inventory (BDI) is the best outcome measure. A BDI greater than or equal to 10 indicates depression in this population. Any answers indicating suicidal intent should be taken seriously, because suicide is 7 times more likely in people with MS than the age-matched general population. Anxiety is also a common feature in MS. Approximately 15% of patients with MS and depression have a history of alcohol abuse.

Pathologic affect, however, can cause considerable distress. It occurs in nearly 10% of patients with MS and is associated with frontal lobe involvement. Tricyclic antidepressants or selective serotonin reuptake inhibitors (SSRIs) appear to be effective.

Psychotherapy and cognitive behavioral therapy have been shown to be as effective as SSRIs. In bipolar affective disorder, valproic acid may be better than lithium, which has the potential to increase tremor. If sedation is required, clonazepam can be tried. For psychotic symptoms a newer neuroleptic, such as olanzapine, is often useful.

Feinstein A, Feinstein K: Depression associated with multiple sclerosis. Looking beyond diagnosis to symptom expression. J Affect Disord 66:193–198, 2001.

Mohr DC, Boudewyn AC, Goodkin DE, et al: Comparative outcomes for individual cognitive-behavior therapy, supportive-expressive group psychotherapy, and sertraline for the treatment of depression in multiple sclerosis. J Consult Clin Psychol 69:942–949, 2001.

Sadovnick AD, Remick RA, Allen J, et al: Depression and multiple sclerosis. Neurology 46:628–632, 1996.

19. **What cognitive impairments are seen with MS?**
Varying degrees of cognitive impairment are seen in MS, even early in the disease. It appears to be more significant in chronic progressive MS than in relapsing-remitting MS. Approximately half of MS patients are affected, and up to 7% are severely impaired. There is no correlation between disease duration or extent of physical disability and cognitive impairment; however, Bone and colleagues demonstrated a correlation between plaque load and dementia. MRI changes correlate with changes on several psychometric tests.

The most frequent cognitive deficits seen in MS are in short-term memory, abstract reasoning, executive functions, and delayed processing. Frontal lobe dysfunction is commonly seen, including initiation, insight, and planning. Prefrontal disconnection may exhibit itself as inappropriate behavior, excessive talking, and poor judgment.

Neuropsychological assessment should be offered to MS patients with cognitive decline. Subsequent counseling and cognitive rehabilitation are important to reduce the effects of cognitive deficits on activities of daily living (ADLs).

Bone G, Ladurner G, Dinichauser L, et al: Cognitive disturbances and MRI findings in MS. J Neuroimag 3:169–172, 1993.

Feinstein A, Ron M, Thompson AJ: A serial study of psychometrics and MRI changes in multiple sclerosis. Brain 116:569–602, 1993.

Rao SM, Leo GJ, Ellington L, et al: Cognitive dysfunction in multiple sclerosis. II. Impact on employment and social functioning. Neurology 41:692–696, 1991.

20. **What is the effect of MS on patients' ability to perform ADLs?**
As the disease progresses, the ability to perform personal activities of daily living (P-ADLs), such as toileting, dressing, eating, grooming, ambulation, and bathing, as well as instrumental activities of daily living (I-ADLs), such as communication, cooking, housekeeping, shopping, and transportation, is reduced. Limitations in ADL performance in MS have a great impact on personal independence, quality of life, and on social roles and the well-being of patients' families. With a mean disease duration of 15 years, approximately one third of patients remain fully independent in ADLs and approximately 30% require assistance with dressing, bathing, feeding, stair-climbing, driving a car, or using public transportation. MS patients can be independent in P-ADLs but still have limitations in I-ADLs, which is not evident from assessments of P-ADLs alone. Assessments of both P-ADLs and I–ADLs are therefore needed to assist MS patients in their strive to maintain a high level of independence.

Finlayson M, Winkler Impey M, Nicolle C, Edwards J: Self-care, productivity and leisure limitations of people with multiple sclerosis in Manitoba. Can J Occup Ther 65:299–308, 1998.

Mansson E, Lexell J: Performance of activities of daily living in multiple sclerosis. Disabil Rehabil 26:576–585, 2004.

McDonnell GV, Hawkins SA: An assessment of the spectrum of disability and handicap in a population in multiple sclerosis: A population-based study. Mult Scler 7:111–117, 2001.

21. What is the effect of MS on patients' families?

MS can have a significant impact on family finances, particularly if the wage earner in a household becomes unable to work. Not only is there loss of income, but also the costs of medical care can produce a substantial economic burden on families. Quality of life is lower for the spouses of people who have MS of longer duration, greater disease severity, and unstable clinical course.

Children of parents with MS find it particularly difficult to cope with the complexities of the condition. In addition, parents often neglect to explain to their children the etiology of the condition, leaving many worried that it is contagious. Simple educational interventions could contribute to enhancing children's understanding of their parents' condition.

Aronson KJ: Quality of life among persons with multiple sclerosis and their caregivers. Neurology 48:74–80, 1997.

Catanzaro M, Weinert C: Economic status of families living with multiple sclerosis. Int J Rehabil Res 15:209–218, 1992.

Cross T, Rintell D: Children's perceptions of parental multiple sclerosis. Psychol Health Med 4:355–360, 1999

22. What is the impact of MS on employment?

Work is an important part of most MS patients' lives, and preserving their ability to participate in the workplace can promote quality of life, ease financial burden on individuals, and reduce the cost of MS to society. Specific workplace adaptations and vocational rehabilitation programs can facilitate patients to remain in employment, as can more general interventions such as mobility aids, fatigue-management programs, and strategies to compensate for cognitive impairments.

Kraft GH: Rehabilitation still the only way to improve function in multiple sclerosis. Lancet 354:2016–2017, 1999.

O'Connor RJ, Cano SJ, Ramio L, et al: Factors influencing work retention for people with multiple sclerosis: Cross-sectional studies using qualitative and quantitative methods. J Neurol 252:892–896, 2005.

23. What type of pain is seen in MS?

Until recently, MS was considered a painless disease; however, we now know that more than half of all MS patients experience pain, that there are different types of pain, and that all types of pain can be severe. Acute types of pain in MS are trigeminal neuralgia, episodic facial pain, paroxysmal pain in arms and legs, and headache. Two percent of MS patients experience trigeminal neuralgia. It occurs 400 times more often in MS patients than in the general population. Treatment of trigeminal neuralgia and episodic/paroxysmal pain includes carbamazepine, baclofen, phenytoin, gabapentin, or lamotrigine. Chronic pain of neurogenic origin is common in MS patients and is described as burning, tingling, or tickling. Older tricyclic antidepressants, particularly amitriptyline, are effective in many patients, often in combination with transcutaneous electrical nerve stimulation (TENS). Gabapentin up to or above 2400 mg for long-term use, or 3600 mg for short-term use, is usually well tolerated and effective. Spasms and cramps can also be very painful. Treatment is the same as for spasticity.

Ehde DM, Gibbons LE, Chwastiak L, et al: Chronic pain in a large community sample of persons with multiple sclerosis. Mult Scler 9:605–611, 2003.

24. How does MS affect pregnancy and vice versa?

MS does not appear to affect a woman's fertility, risk of spontaneous abortion, or congenital malformations. However, caution should be taken by women considering pregnancy, because many medications taken for MS are or may be teratogenic. The consensus on risk of relapse during pregnancy is that it is not increased and may be decreased in the third trimester. The relapse rates in the 6 months after pregnancy, however, may be two to three times the nonpregnant rate. Pregnancy does not appear to have an adverse effect on long-term outcome and disability.

Damek P, Schuster EA: Pregnancy in multiple sclerosis. Mayo Clin Proc 72:977–989, 1997.

25. What is the relationship between optic neuritis and MS?

The Optic Neuritis Study Group followed more than 400 optic neuritis patients for more than 5 years. Those who were more likely to develop MS were white, female, had a history of vague neurologic symptoms at the time of presentation with the optic neuritis, had a family history of MS, or had a positive MRI finding. Fifty-one percent of those with three or more lesions on MRI at the time of the original presentation developed MS.

Optic Neuritis Study Group: Visual function 5 years after optic neuritis. Arch Ophthalmol 115:1545–1552, 1997.

26. What immunomodulators are licensed for use in treating MS?

Immunomodulation is used in MS to prevent disability caused by disease progression and to reduce the frequency, severity, or duration of relapses. Interferon betas, glatiramer acetate, and mitoxantrone can be prescribed for patients with relapsing-remitting MS, and, in the case of mitoxantrone, secondary progressive and relapsing-progressive MS.

Interferon beta was first approved in 1993, and three formulations are currently available for use. It is postulated that interferons exert their effects by inhibiting leukocyte proliferation, modulating cytokine production, and inhibiting T-cell migration across the blood–brain barrier. Common side effects include flu-like symptoms, injection site reactions, and elevations in liver function tests. Labs should be drawn every 3–6 months.

Glatiramer acetate is an amino acid complex developed to mimic the antigenic portion of myelin. It is postulated to promote anti-inflammatory cytokine production and possibly inhibit antigen presentation. Side effects are generally mild and similar to the interferons. No blood tests are needed for monitoring.

Mitoxantrone is an anthracycline-based chemotherapeutic agent. It inhibits DNA synthesis and repair, thereby reducing the population of immunologically active cells. It has the potential to cause severe side effects, including cardiotoxicity and leukemia.

Martinelli BF, Rovaris M, Capra R, et al: Mitoxantrone for multiple sclerosis. Cochrane Database Syst Rev 4:CD002127, 2005.
Munari L, Lovati R, Boiko A: Therapy with glatiramer acetate for multiple sclerosis. Cochrane Database Syst Rev 1:CD004678, 2004.
Rice GP, Incorvaia B, Munari L, et al: Interferon in relapsing-remitting multiple sclerosis. Cochrane Database Syst Rev 4:CD002002, 2001.
Rizvi SA, Agius MA: Current approved options for treating patients with multiple sclerosis. Neurology 63(Suppl 6):S8–S14, 2004.

27. What new medications are on the horizon?

Natalizumab is a monoclonal antibody currently under investigation for the treatment of exacerbations of MS. It acts against integrins, which are adhesion molecules involved in multiple immune cell interactions. It has a rare side effect of progressive multifocal leukoencephalopathy. Other monoclonal antibodies are presently at a trial stage.

Cyclophosphamide has been demonstrated to reduce contrast-enhancing lesions on MRI and may have a role as a rescue treatment for patients who do not respond to interferons. Similarly, **methotrexate** was shown to decrease number of relapses and reduce overall disability.

A range of other putative inflammatory inhibitors have been tested. These include simvastatin, minocycline, and mycophenolate.

Killestein J, Polman CH: Current trials in multiple sclerosis: Established evidence and future hopes. Curr Opin Neurol 18:253–260, 2005.

28. **Should cannabinoids be used in the management of MS?**
Many patients with MS believe that cannabis ameliorates muscle spasticity; however, this is not borne out by placebo-controlled studies. Cannabinoid receptors are found throughout the CNS, as well as the peripheral immune system, leading to the conclusion that cannabinoid agonists may potentially modulate the neurologic effects of MS or modulate pathologic immune mechanisms.

The largest randomized, controlled trial of cannabinoids in MS enrolled more than 600 patients but found no evidence that cannabinoids reduce muscle spasticity. Patients reported that they felt better while taking the active medication, but because of the side effects, there was a degree of unmasking.

Killestein J, Hoogervorst EL, Reif M, et al: Safety, tolerability, and efficacy of orally administered cannabinoids in MS. Neurol 58:1404–1407, 2002.

Zajicek J, Fox P, Sanders H, et al: Cannabinoids for treatment of spasticity and other symptoms related to multiple sclerosis (CAMS study): Multicentre randomised placebo-controlled trial. Lancet 362:1517–1526, 2003.

WEBSITES

1. MS Association of America
www.msaa.com

2. MS Consortium
mscare.org

3. The MS Foundation
www.msfocus.org

4. www.mult-sclerosis.org

5. National MS Society
www.nationalmssociety.org

CHAPTER 58

MOTOR NEURON DISEASE: CLASSIFICATION, DIAGNOSIS, AND REHABILITATION

Michael Hatzakis, Jr., MD, Gregg D. Meekins, MD, and Arthur A. Rodriquez, MD

> *These are the times when all of us have much to be thankful for and much to be thoughtful about, times when it is particularly good to feel the warm, strong clasp of a friend's hand and so, this Christmas more than ever, we say Merry Christmas.*
>
> —Eleanor and Lou Gehrig

1. **What is a motor neuron disease?**

   Motor neuron disease (MND) results in weakness and muscle wasting. These diseases include those that affect the upper (corticobulbar and corticospinal) motor neurons and/or the lower (bulbar and spinal) motor neurons. MNDs are classified based on the location of the pathophysiologic involvement.

2. **Describe the classification of the motor neuron diseases.**
   - Upper motor neuron disorders
     - Primary lateral sclerosis
     - Familial (hereditary) spastic paraplegia
     - Lathyrism
   - Combined upper and lower motor neuron disorders
     - Sporadic amyotrophic lateral sclerosis (ALS)
     - Familial ALS
     - Familial ALS/MND with frontotemporal dementia
     - Familial ALS/MND, Parkinson's disease, and frontotemporal dementia
     - Western Pacific ALS–parkinsonism-dementia complex
     - Polyglucosan body disease
   - Lower motor neuron disorders
     - Spinal muscular atrophies
     - Benign focal spinal muscular atrophy (Hirayama's disease)
     - X-linked bulbospinal muscular atrophy (Kennedy's disease)
     - Infantile progressive bulbar palsy (Fazio-Londe, Brown–Vialetto–van Laere syndrome)
     - Progressive muscular atrophy
     - Poliomyelitis and post-polio syndrome
     - Monoclonal gammopathy and MND
     - Cancer and MND
     - HIV and MND
     - Radiation lower motor neuron syndrome

3. **What is known about the pathophysiologic causes of MNDs?**

   Pathogenic mechanisms for motor neuron injury include toxic or environmental exposures, infection, inflammation, oxidative stress, excitotoxicity, genetic predisposition, and other unknown factors. **Radiation-induced injury** to motor neurons generally occurs as a late complication between 6 months and 10 years after exposure and with doses exceeding 60 Gy. Pathologic findings include focal necrosis, axon loss, and fibrinoid necrosis of vessel walls.

The exact mechanism for motor neuron injury in sporadic ALS is unclear, but its etiology is likely multifactorial. **Familial ALS** accounts for approximately 5–10% of cases of ALS, mostly with an autosomal-dominant inheritance pattern. ALS in association with Parkinson's disease and frontotemporal dementia is associated with mutations in the microtubule-associated tau protein on chromosome 17, resulting in the formation of insoluble aggregates, which lead to cell injury.

Direct infection and injury to anterior horn cells are seen as a consequence of the polio enterovirus. HIV infection has been associated with ALS, progressive muscular atrophy, and segmental limb atrophy; although the mechanisms of cell injury are unclear.

4. **How is the poliomyelitis virus transmitted?**

   Poliomyelitis is usually contracted orally. Once in the body, the virus replicates in the lymphoid tissues of the pharynx and intestine and then spreads to the regional lymphoid tissues, resulting in a viremia and nonspecific illness. Viremia is the most accepted mechanism for direct nervous system exposure to the virus. The reason for the virus's selective affinity for certain cells, such as the motor neurons, is unknown, but it may relate to specific receptors on their cell membranes. It is possible to get polio more than once because the offending virus has three antigenically distinguishable forms.

5. **Is it true that most people who had polio in the past didn't even know they had the disease?**

   Yes. The poliovirus is an extremely infectious agent, but only a fraction of those infected have any symptoms. The disease progresses to central nervous system (CNS) involvement with paresis or paralysis in only 1–2% of cases. In 4–8% of cases, only a nonspecific illness is noted by the individual, and in the others, the infection is not apparent.

6. **How does weakness occur after polio infection? What are the mechanisms for recovery?**

   In histologic studies of motor neurons of monkeys with acute paralytic poliomyelitis, nearly all (96–97%) of the motor neurons of severely paralyzed limbs were affected by the virus during the acute infection. Approximately half of these motor neurons died during the early convalescent period, and the other half survived. A good correlation was found between the proportion of destroyed motor neurons and the severity of paralysis. With death of the motor neurons, **Wallerian degeneration** occurs, and the muscle fibers associated with those neurons become "orphaned," resulting in motor weakness. Some recover by reinnervation of muscle cells by axonal sprouts from neighboring branches of alpha motor neurons.

7. **Why is it that polio patients often required several years to plateau in their functional recovery?**

   Survivors commonly recovered muscle strength gradually in muscles not completely paralyzed. Some lucky individuals ultimately recovered to a point of minimal or no residual dysfunction. Improvements in function often began in the first weeks but could continue for several years after the acute illness. The mechanisms of recovery include both resolution of dysfunction of partially damaged motor neurons and reinnervation of denervated muscle fibers by surviving motor units, with muscle hypertrophy following reactivation.

8. **Which is the most common presenting form of MND in adults? Who is the iron man who died of it?**

   ALS, or Lou Gehrig's disease, is the most common adult form of MND and was named after the New York Yankees' first baseman, who died from this disorder. Gehrig played first base for the Yankees from 1923 to 1939, batting after Babe Ruth, and had a lifetime batting average of 0.340 and a record 23 grand slams. He was best known as the "iron man" for playing in 2130 consecutive games.

ALS is a disease with progressive injury and death of both pyramidal (upper motor) neurons and bulbar and anterior horn (lower motor) neurons. Approximately 3–10% of individuals with ALS have frontotemporal dementia. Overall, 30–50% of individuals show signs of cognitive impairment, suggesting ALS may have more widespread effects on the CNS. Presenting symptoms with ALS vary, with combinations of upper and lower motor neuron involvement and with diffuse or segmental bulbar and/or limb weakness. Death usually results from complications of the bulbar and/or respiratory involvement.

9. **What are the prevalence and incidence of ALS?**
   The incidence of ALS is approximately 1.6–2.4 cases per 100,000 population, but it may increase with age. For instance, in a study in southwestern Ontario, the incidence increased to 7.4 cases per 100,000 population by the eighth decade, with an average age at diagnosis of 62 years. Half of patients with ALS are between ages 50 and 70. The average survival from time of diagnosis is approximately 2.5 years, with shorter life expectancy with later age of onset. Approximately 10% of patients have a slower disease course with life expectancy greater than 10 years. The male-to-female ratio varies from 1.2:1 to 1.6:1.

10. **Describe the typical clinical features of ALS.**
    The typical complaint is weakness. The most common findings at the time of initial examination include **atrophy, weakness, spasticity** (upper motor neuron), and **fasciculations** (lower motor neuron). Additionally, muscle stretch reflexes can be depressed in regions where there is primarily lower motor neuron involvement or where atrophy is so advanced that upper motor neuron signs cannot be found. Otherwise, it is common to find brisk muscle stretch reflexes in areas of muscle atrophy. On occasion the patient may present with only mild spasticity, suggesting a purely upper motor neuron disorder (e.g., spastic dysarthria or facies, or both, with no detectable lower motor neuron signs). Muscle cramping is also a frequent complaint.
    In general the most striking feature of ALS is the focal, often asymmetrical, onset of **weakness,** which then spreads to adjacent areas of the body. **Spasticity** can be disabling and make ambulation difficult. The **bowel and bladder sphincters** are spared in this disease, except for constipation related to inactivity or poor nutritional intake. Sensation is generally spared, although paresthesias and decreased vibratory sensation can be found in up to 25% of patients.

11. **What are some of the characteristic features that, when present, weigh against the diagnosis of ALS?**
    Signs that, when present, weigh against a diagnosis of ALS include sensory signs and symptoms, voluntary eye movement abnormalities, and bowel and bladder incontinence. Classic ALS includes degeneration and/or complete loss of motor neurons in the brain stem and spinal cord areas corresponding to the muscle atrophy and degeneration of the large pyramidal neurons in the primary motor cortex and the pyramidal tracts, thus leaving intact the ascending sensory tracts. The **nucleus of Onuf** (the nucleus controlling the striated muscles of the pelvic floor and the bowel and bladder sphincters) is preserved, explaining why bowel and bladder functions are also preserved.

12. **What other MNDs besides poliomyelitis are found in children?**
    - **Acute infantile spinal muscular atrophy** (Werdnig-Hoffmann disease) is an autosomal recessive disorder with an estimated incidence of 1 in 15,000 to 1 in 25,000 live births. The disease is apparent at birth in one third of the children and is usually diagnosed by age 3 months. Survival averages 6–9 months from diagnosis and does not exceed 3 years. Severe hypotonia, weakness, and resultant delays in motor milestones dominate the clinical picture. The infants characteristically lie motionless with the lower limbs abducted in the frog-leg position. Fasciculations of the tongue are almost pathognomonic for the disease. Death usually results from respiratory failure.
    - **Chronic infantile spinal muscular atrophy** (chronic infantile Werdnig-Hoffmann disease) is much more slowly progressive than the acute form of the disease. Clinical signs are

usually present by age 3 years, but occasionally appear as early as 3 months. This disease has variable progression, with the average age of death being over 10 years. It also has an autosomal recessive inheritance.

- **Juvenile proximal spinal muscular atrophy** (Kugelberg-Welander disease) is characterized by slowly progressive weakness and atrophy of the proximal limb and girdle musculature. It is usually transmitted as an autosomal recessive disorder (type III proximal hereditary motor neuropathy) but also has an autosomal dominant form (type IV juvenile proximal hereditary motor neuropathy). The clinical onset can occur anytime between childhood and the seventh decade of life (in the adult form, type V proximal hereditary motor neuropathy), but it usually occurs between ages 2 and 17. Both the juvenile and adult forms of this disease begin with symmetrical atrophy and weakness of the pelvic girdle and proximal lower limbs, then progress to involvement of the shoulder girdles and upper arms.

- **Progressive bulbar paralysis of childhood** has two forms, **Fazio-Londe disease** and **Brown–Vialetto–van Laere syndrome**. Both cause a slowly progressive weakness of the muscles of the face, tongue, and pharynx. Fazio-Londe disease, which has been described rarely since 1925, produces bilateral deafness as the first symptom. This occurs between 18 months and 31 years of age (average onset, 12 years). Cranial nerve palsies usually appear approximately 4–5 years later. Survival may exceed two decades. Inheritance is apparently autosomal recessive.

- **Distal spinal muscular atrophy** (spinal form of Charcot-Marie-Tooth disease) has several forms, with different inheritance patterns: (1) **autosomal recessive** juvenile mild (onset, 2–10 years of age) and juvenile severe (onset, 4 months to 20 years), and (2) **autosomal dominant** in the juvenile (onset, 2–20 years) and in the adult (onset, 20–40 years). Life expectancy is normal except in some severe juvenile cases. Clinical features include weakness and atrophy, which usually start distally in the legs.

13. **What is post-polio syndrome?**
Post-polio syndrome is essentially a diagnosis made by exclusion in polio survivors. A good definition of post-polio syndrome has been given by Halstead and Rossi (1987) and is based on five criteria:
1. A confirmed history of paralytic poliomyelitis
2. Partial to fairly complete neurologic and functional recovery
3. A period of neurologic and functional stability of at least 15 years' duration
4. Onset of two or more of the following health problems since achieving a period of stability: unaccustomed fatigue, muscle and/or joint pain, new weakness in muscles previously affected and/or unaffected, functional loss, cold intolerance, new atrophy
5. No other medical diagnosis to explain these health problems

14. **What are the most frequent complaints of patients with post-polio syndrome?**
In general, new musculoskeletal and neuromuscular symptoms. Table 58-1 lists the most frequent new health and ADL problems of post-polio individuals, whether they were seen in a post-polio clinic or responded to a national survey. The most prevalent new health-related complaints were fatigue, muscle or joint pain, and weakness. The most prevalent new ADL complaints were difficulties with walking and stair-climbing.

15. **Why do post-polio individuals lose strength as they age?**
There is no empirical evidence that the loss of strength is directly related to poliomyelitis. All individuals lose motor neurons and strength with age, and those who have a reduced number of motor neurons because of the poliovirus infection are at greater risk of losing strength. Imagine a normal individual with 100 motor neurons and a post-polio survivor with 10 motor neurons for a given muscle group. If one motor neuron is lost per year, it is clear that the post-polio survivor will decline more quickly. Some also suggest that motor neurons damaged by the poliovirus may age prematurely as a result of the increased metabolic demand.

TABLE 58-1. NEW HEALTH AND ADL PROBLEMS IN POST–POLIO PATIENTS

Symptom	Halstead* (*n* = 539)	Halstead[†] (*n* = 132)	Agre[‡] (*n* = 79)
New health problems			
Fatigue	87%	89%	86%
Muscle pain	80	71	86
Joint pain	79	71	77
Weakness			
Previously affected muscles	87	69	80
Previously unaffected muscles	77	50	53
Cold intolerance	—	29	56
Atrophy	—	28	39
New ADL problems			
Walking	85	64	—
Stair-climbing	83	61	67
Dressing	62	17	16

*Halstead LS, Rossi CD: New problems in old polio patients: Results of a survey of 539 polio survivors. Orthopedics 8:845–850, 1985.
[†]Halstead LS, Wiechers DO (eds): Research and Clinical Aspects of the Late Effects of Poliomyelitis. White Plains, NY, March of Dimes Birth Defects Foundation, 1987.
[‡]Agre JC, Rodriguez AA, Sperling KB: Symptoms and clinical impressions of patients seen in a postpolio clinic. Arch Phys Med Rehabil 70:367–370, 1989.

16. **Is it possible for individuals with clinically normal muscles to be affected by the post-polio syndrome?**
Yes, it is possible that an individual who had up to 80% of his or her motor neurons affected by polio in a given muscle to have recovered to full muscle strength and later have this muscle weakened by the post-polio syndrome, because of the abnormal number of motor units. This is because a smaller percentage of anterior horn cells innervate many more muscle fibers.

17. **Outline the evaluation of a patient with a possible MND.**
As with all diseases, the initial assessment to determine the diagnosis includes obtaining a detailed history, performing a good physical examination, and obtaining appropriate laboratory tests.
- History
  - Major complaints of the patient (and/or parents)
  - Pattern of weakness (in general, MNDs produce proximal weakness, whereas neuropathic disorders cause distal weakness, often accompanied by sensory abnormalities)
  - Age of onset and rate of progression
  - Family history
- Physical examination
  - Visual inspection for muscular atrophy, muscular hypertrophy, and fasciculations
  - Sensory examination (sensory loss is very rare in motor neuron diseases but common in neuropathic disorders)
  - Muscle stretch reflexes
  - Manual muscle testing using a grading of 0–5
  - Range-of-motion (ROM) testing to detect contractures

□ Functional assessment
- Laboratory studies
  □ Nerve conduction studies
  □ Electromyography (EMG)
  □ Other evaluations, depending on the clinical presentation of the patient (to look for rare disorders, diabetes mellitus, thyrotoxicosis)
  □ Urinalysis (to check for heavy metal intoxication, such as lead or mercury)
  □ Muscle biopsy

18. **How are electrodiagnostic studies helpful in diagnosing ALS? What are the classic features of ALS on electrodiagnostic testing?**

It is of primary importance in the diagnosis of ALS to ensure that no treatable or nonfatal disorder accounting for the patient's signs and symptoms is overlooked (*see* question 21). Electrodiagnostic studies are used to exclude the presence of an axonal or demyelinating disease, such as chronic inflammatory demyelinating polyneuropathy, or a neuromuscular junction disorder, such as myasthenia gravis. Needle EMG sampling must be performed, especially in the weakest muscles, in at least three levels (cervical, lumbar, and sacral) or two levels and bulbar musculature (most commonly, tongue). Classic features seen on EMG sampling of muscles are the presence of fibrillations, positive sharp waves, and motor unit action potential changes typical of reinnervation, with fasciculations and decreased recruitment.

The **El Escorial criteria** for a definitive diagnosis of ALS specify concomitant clinical evidence of upper motor neuron disease (hyperreflexia, spasticity) and electrodiagnostic evidence of upper and lower motor neuron abnormalities (reduced recruitment, large motor unit action potentials, and fibrillations) in at least three of the four possible levels of the neuraxis (bulbar, cervical, thoracic, lumbosacral) in the absence of electrophysiologic or neuroimaging evidence of another explanation for weakness. No major criteria are without controversy, and the diagnosis of ALS is no exception.

Some electromyographers prefer the **Lambert criteria,** which include fasciculations as a major finding, suggesting lower motor neuron involvement, and specify nerve conduction studies with normal sensory studies and motor conduction not less than 70% below the lower limit of normal in severely affected muscles.

19. **List some disorders that may mimic an MND.**

See Box 58-1.

BOX 58-1. DISORDERS THAT MAY MIMIC MOTOR NEURON DISEASE	
Cervical spondylosis	Myositis
Motor polyradiculopathy	Myopathies
Chronic inflammatory demyelinating polyneuropathy	Myasthenia gravis
	Stroke
Multifocal motor conduction block	Paraneoplastic syndromes
Spinal muscular atrophy syndromes	Mononeuropathies
Focal amyotrophy	Parkinson's disease
Primary lateral sclerosis	Syndrome of benign fasciculations
Multiple sclerosis	

20. **What are the general principles of rehabilitation management of a patient with a motor neuron disorder?**

- **Prospective care:** Preventative and maintenance treatment is provided, as for all patients.

- **Expectant care:** Includes education and decision-making based on the anticipated progress. Patient-centered interdisciplinary rehabilitation is carried out on an ongoing outpatient basis. Plans for certain activities, when patients are still able to carry them out, need to occur early in the rehabilitation course. Mobility aids provided should allow some adaptation as capabilities decline. Plans for or against assistive ventilation need to be made early, as bulbar symptoms and cognitive changes can affect communication.

21. **How should the treatment of a patient with MND be approached?**
The primary goal in treating patients with MNDs is to assist the patient in the maintenance of function, independence, and quality of life for as long as possible. With the knowledge of disease progression, many of the complications of this disease may be prevented with good expectant care. Therapeutic interventions for the treatment of pain, decline of swallowing function, soft-tissue tightness, deformity, scoliosis, weakness, and respiratory dysfunction can minimize complications and maximize the patient's ability to function. Functional training for locomotion, dressing, eating, and other ADLs can prolong the independent or partial independent phase of disease progression. An emphasis should be placed on interdisciplinary care.
Drug therapy for ALS is limited. A recently developed drug such as **riluzole (Rilutek),** an antiglutamate agent, may be effective in slowing the progression of the disease. It has been found to improve survival in patients with **bulbar onset disease,** but the effects generally are small compared with its side effects, which include asthenia, not to mention being costly to administer.

22. **What are a few of the prognostic indictors for patients with ALS?**
Survival is typically 3–5 years from onset of symptoms. Approximately 10–16% live more than 10 years. Poorer prognostic indicators include more severe disease at onset, older age at onset, female sex, and bulbar onset. Electrodiagnostic indicators of poor prognosis include profuse spontaneous fibrillations, sharp waves, and low-amplitude compound muscle action potentials.

23. **Is pain a common problem in patients with MNDs?**
Pain is uncommon in the early presentation of ALS. Pain also is not often a major problem, except in patients with acute poliomyelitis, who may have severe muscle pain.
Control of pain for individuals with ALS can usually be accomplished by both physical and pharmacologic treatments. The heat treatments, along with stretching, are useful in the acute stages to control pain and maintain ROM. Nonsteroidal anti-inflammatory drugs may also be used. Many patients, however, may have mechanical pain related to weakness, contracture, or deformity. Muscle cramps and stiffness related to spasticity may be treated with baclofen, with care taken not to cause fatigue or loss of function.

KEY POINTS: FEATURES OF MOTOR NEURON DISEASES NOT TO BE MISSED

1. Motor neuron diseases do not affect sensation.

2. Classic features that present most commonly in motor neuron disease are atrophy, weakness, spasticity, and fasciculations.

3. Mean survival is generally 5 years.

4. Survival is not necessarily improved with any treatment, but quality of life can be improved.

5. Electrodiagnostic features include denervation, reduced recruitment, large-amplitude motor units, and fasciculations.

24. **What are approaches to treat sialorrhea?**

Individuals with MNDs typically have impaired saliva management. The first priority is to determine if the patient is suffering sialorrhea or thickening of mucus production. Thickening of mucus can be treated by improvement of hydration and with medications. Management of sialorrhea begins with methods to reduce production of saliva. Pharmacologic means include drugs such as glycopyrrolate (Robinul), amitriptyline (Elavil), or benztropine (Cogentin). Individuals with sialorrhea can be given suction machines if saliva production is a problem. For thick mucus production, manually and mechanically assisted techniques can improve mobilization of saliva. One such device is an insufflator-exafflator to extract excess mucus. Individuals with ALS may retain the ability to cough, but it is often ineffective.

25. **How are muscle contractures treated?**

Muscle contracture is a common problem in patients with MNDs. The best treatment is **prevention.** Contractures usually first occur at muscles that span two joints with the joints in the flexed position. Common sites include the shoulder adductors, elbow flexors, forearm pronators, finger adductors, hip flexors or internal rotators, knee flexors, ankle plantar flexors, and foot invertors.

   Physical treatment includes passive, active-assistive, and active ROM, depending on the condition of the patient, usually after the application of superficial heat. Modalities can be used safely, as individuals with motor neuron disease have spared sensation; thus, application of heat and ice can be used as long as the patient can effectively communicate temperatures too high or low. When preventing or correcting shortening of a muscle that spans two joints, it is important to ensure that the muscles are stretched at both joints that they cross. Also, splinting and casting can be used to treat contracture. Surgery is only rarely needed. Appropriate positioning can aid in the prevention of deformity.

26. **How does one treat deformity in patients with motor neuron disorder?**

Malalignment of body segments leads to contracture and deformity; therefore, appropriate **prospective treatment** is needed to prevent or minimize the development of contracture or deformity. Appropriate stretching, bracing, and positioning can help prevent contractures. As truncal and spine-stabilizing muscles become weak, it is vital to assure the individual with an MND has appropriate seating and support. For instance, a child sitting in a large wheelchair with a sling-type seat can result in hip misalignment. Such improper seating will lead to contracture and subsequent scoliotic deformity. The minimal wheelchair prescription should include a firm seat, with adequate lumbar, truncal, and arm support. Also, thoracolumbosacral orthotic devices can help to prevent progressive scoliotic deformity in patients with significant weakness of the trunk.

   Some patients with post-polio syndrome place significant stress on the knee while ambulating. This can cause the development of either genu valgus and/or genu recurvatum deformity, which is usually treated with a knee-ankle-foot orthosis.

27. **How is scoliosis managed?**

Prevention and management of scoliosis comprise one of the major goals in the management of neuromuscular disease. Scoliosis occurs with increasing age and with advancing disability. Usually, the paraspinal muscular weakness is symmetrical, and although the child is ambulatory, the development of scoliosis is uncommon; however, once the child becomes nonambulatory, scoliosis develops rapidly. Most children with MND develop a collapsing, paralytic type of scoliosis.

   The initial approach to managing scoliosis is to order the most appropriate **wheelchair,** which must be measured for each individual. A symmetrical sitting posture with adequate upper- and lower-extremity support must be maintained; the sling seat should be avoided because it permits asymmetrical pelvic rotation. A solid foam-padded seat cushion can be used to level the pelvis during sitting in the early stages. Children tolerate **sitting-support orthoses** until the curve reaches >40 degrees. At that point, a relatively rapid progression continues that generally cannot be managed orthotically, and surgery may be indicated. Current literature supports using a surgical approach before ventilatory capacity (VC) drops below 50% of age-adjusted expected values. This literature suggests greater postsurgical morbidity and mortality once VC drops below 50%.

28. **What is the approach to strengthening and exercise for individuals with MND?**
Strengthening exercises must be prescribed judiciously and followed carefully. It is generally accepted that vigorous, fatiguing, or progressive resistive exercise may cause further weakness and muscle fiber degeneration. Low-intensity, nonfatiguing, and submaximal exercise may be beneficial for maintenance or improvement in muscle strength and cardiorespiratory fitness, as well as positive psychological effects. Weakness is also treated with appropriate orthotic devices for support. Post-polio patients with grade 4 out of 5 muscle strength have improved strength with resistive exercise without apparent harm. Exercise should be prescribed carefully in muscles with less than 3 out of 5 strength.

29. **How does one treat the patient with ventilatory difficulty?**
Early signs and symptoms of carbon dioxide retention hypoxia include difficulty with sleeping, nighttime dyspnea, nightmares, and daytime somnolence. Ventilatory aids (e.g., cuirass or plastic wrap) enhance ventilation in the recumbent position. In the later stages of MND, oral positive-pressure ventilation, pneumobelt, or cuirass ventilators can be used throughout the day, powered by the wheelchair battery. Tracheostomy is rarely needed, and its use is somewhat controversial.

30. **How is dysphagia in MND detected and treated?**
Individuals with MND and dysphagia are at increased risk of suboptimal caloric and fluid intake, worsened muscle atrophy, weakness, and fatigue. Symptoms of dysphagia include jaw weakness, fatigue, drooling, choking on food, and slow eating. Early techniques include modification of food and fluid consistency and coaching and training by a speech therapist guided by barium swallow examination. As dysphagia progresses, gastrostomy or jejunostomy tubes are indicated if conservative management does not maintain a safe level of caloric intake. If dysphagia is developing, placement of a feeding tube should occur before the vital capacity falls to 50% of the age-predicted normative value.

31. **Discuss the approach to end-of-life issues with the individual with MND.**
It is important to establish an open environment of communication with patients with progressive MNDs. It is important that patients and their families understand the progression of the impairments and the potential risks of not treating specific conditions such as dysphagia. It is also vital to discuss plans for end of life, such as hospice care and relief of pain and dyspnea. Provide supportive care for depression and anxiety. It is important to review advance care directives with patients and their families well ahead of significant functional impairment.

BIBLIOGRAPHY

1. Agre JC, Rodriquez AA, Tafel JA: Late effects of polio: Critical review of the literature on neuromuscular function. Arch Phys Med Rehabil 72:923–931, 1991.
2. Agre JC: The role of exercise in the patient with post-polio syndrome. Ann NY Acad Sci 753:321–334, 1995.
3. Agre JC, Mathews DJ: Rehabilitation concepts in motor neuron diseases. In Braddom RL (ed): Physical Medicine and Rehabilitation. Philadelphia, W.B. Saunders, 1996, pp 955–971.
4. Daube JR: Electrodiagnostic studies in amyotrophic lateral sclerosis and other motor neuron disease. Muscle Nerve 23:1488–1502, 2000.
5. Dumitru D: Electrodiagnostic Medicine. Philadelphia, Hanley & Belfus, 1995.

6. Francis K, Bach JR, DeLisa JA: Evaluation and rehabilitation of patients with adult motor neuron disease. Arch Phys Med Rehabil 80:951–963, 1999.

7. Halstead LS, Grimby G (eds): Post-Polio Syndrome. Philadelphia, Hanley & Belfus, 1995.

8. Halstead LS, Rossi CD: Post-Polio Syndrome: Clinical experience with 132 consecutive outpatients. Birth Defects Orig Artic Ser 23(4):13–26, 1987.

9. Halstead LS, Rossi CD: New problems in old polio patients: Results of a survey of 539 polio survivors. Orthopedics 8(7):845–850, 1985.

10. Hudson AJ: The motor neuron diseases and related disorders. In Joynt RJ (ed): Clinical Neurology, Vol 4. Philadelphia, J.B. Lippincott, 1991, pp 1–35.

11. Joerg-Patrick S: Neuromuscular disorders in systemic malignancy and its treatment. Muscle Nerve 18:636–648, 1995.

12. Kottke FJ: Therapeutic exercise to maintain mobility. In Kottke FJ, Lehmann JF (eds): Krusen's Handbook of Physical Medicine and Rehabilitation, 4th ed. Philadelphia, W.B. Saunders, 1990, pp 436–451.

13. Krivickas LS: Amyotrophic lateral sclerosis and other motor neuron diseases. Phys Med Rehabil Clin N Am 14:327–345, 2003.

14. Miller RG, Rosenberg JA, Gelinas DF, et al: Practice parameter: The care of the patient with amyotrophic lateral sclerosis (an evidence-based review): Report of the Quality Standards Subcommittee of the American Academy of Neurology: ALS Practice Parameters Task Force. Neurology 52:1311–1323, 1999.

15. Przedborski S, Mitsumoto H, Rowland LP: Recent advances in amyotrophic lateral sclerosis research. Curr Neurol Neurosci Rep 3:70–77, 2003.

16. Sinaki M: Exercise and rehabilitation measures in amyotrophic lateral sclerosis. In Tsubaki T, Yase Y (eds): Amyotrophic Lateral Sclerosis [Excerpta Medica International Congress series 769]. Amsterdam, Elsevier Science, 1988, pp 343–368.

17. Subcommittee on Motor Neuron Diseases/Amyotrophic Lateral Sclerosis of the World Federation of Neurology Research Group on Neuromuscular Diseases and the El Escorial "Clinical Limits of Amyotrophic Lateral Sclerosis" Workshop Collaborators. El Escorial: World Federation of Neurology criteria for the diagnosis of amyotrophic lateral sclerosis. J Neurol Sci 124(suppl):96–107, 1994.

18. Swash M: An algorithm for ALS diagnosis and management. Neurology 53(suppl 5):S58–S62, 1999.

19. Van Den Berg-Vos RM, Van Den Berg LH, Visser J, et al: The spectrum of lower motor neuron syndromes. J Neurol 250:1279–1292, 2003.

XII. MEDICAL COMPLICATIONS IN REHABILITATION

HAZARDS OF PHYSICAL INACTIVITY

CHAPTER 59

*Eugen M. Halar, MD, Steven A. Stiens, MD, MS, and
Kathleen R. Bell, MD*

Misery acquaints a man with strange bedfellows.

—William Shakespeare (1564–1616), *The Tempest*

1. **Describe the adverse effects of bed rest and physical inactivity on the organs and systems.**
   See Table 59-1.

TABLE 59-1. NEGATIVE EFFECTS OF BED REST, IMMOBILITY, AND MICROGRAVITY ON ORGAN SYSTEMS

Organ System	Negative Effects
Muscles	Disuse atrophy, weakness, muscle stiffness, decline in mobility function
Joints	Contracture, loss of ROM, decline in mobility and ADLs
Bone	Osteoporosis, heterotopic ossification, fractures
Cardiovascular	Decline in VO_{2max}, stroke volume, cardiac reserve; dehydration, resting and postexercise tachycardia; orthostatic intolerance, deconditioning, risk factor for coronary artery disease, thromboembolism
Respiratory	Diminished diaphragmatic and chest movements while supine, change in regional blood perfusion, impaired coughing and secretion clearance, aspiration, atelectasis, pneumonia; pulmonary embolisms
Gastrointestinal	Gastroesophageal reflux, loss of appetite, slowed nutrient absorption, anorexia, malnutrition (hypoproteinemia), constipation
Urinary tract	Incomplete bladder emptying and urinary retention in supine position; incontinence, calculi formation, infections
Skin	Decubitus ulcer, maceration, monilial infection
Neurologic	Peripheral nerve compression, balance impairment
Psychological	Depression, disorientation, anxiety, hallucinations, sleep-wake cycle disruption, decreased pain tolerance, sensory deprivation
Metabolic/ hormonal	Decreased metabolic rate, calcium loss, immobilization hypercalcemia, nitrogen loss, impaired glucose utilization, increased insulin resistance, alteration in androgen and spermatogenesis and electrolyte imbalance

ADL = activities of daily living, ROM = range of motion.
Browse NL: The Physiology and Pathology of Bedrest. Springfield, IL, Charles C. Thomas, 1965.
Deitrick JR, Whedon GD, Shorr E: Effects of immobilization on various metabolic and physiologic functions of normal men. Am J Med 4:3–6, 1948.
Halar EM, Bell KR: Immobility and inactivity. In DeLisa JA, Gans BM, Walsh NE, et al (eds): Physical Medicine and Rehabilitation: Principles and Practice, 4th ed. Philadelphia, Lippincott Williams & Wilkins, 2005, pp 1447–1467.

2. **What is disuse atrophy? What structural and functional changes occur in the muscle?**

Disuse atrophy is the reduction of muscle mass and strength resulting from the lack of muscle use. The main structural changes include a decrease in diameter and size of muscle fibers, reduced compliance to stretch, reduced number of sarcomeres in series and peak tetanic tension, relative increase of connective tissue, weakness, and reduction of endurance and fitness.

Berg HE, Dudley GA, Haggmark T, et al: Effects of lower limb unloading on skeletal muscle mass and function in humans. J Appl Physiol 70:1882–1885, 1991.

3. **How can I prevent and treat muscle atrophy and weakness?**

By providing a combination of progressive resistive exercises for strength and flexibility to antigravity muscles and by functional training in mobility, muscle atrophy can be prevented and treated. The lack of weight-bearing can reduce the soleus muscle weight by 37%, but adding only 1 hour per day of mobility training reduces this decline to 22%. Total loss of muscle weight due to immobility is greater for legs than for arms: 11.9% versus 4%. Exercise promotes specific gene expression and the formation of specific proteins called myogenic regulatory factors (MRFs). One of them, myogenin, prevents atrophy and promotes muscle fiber hypertrophy.

Brown M, Hasser EM: Weight-bearing effects on skeletal muscle during and after simulated bed rest. Arch Phys Med Rehabil 76:541–546, 1995.
LeBlanc A, Rowe R, Evans H, et al: Muscle atrophy during long duration bed rest. Int J Sport Med 18(Suppl):S283–S334, 1997.

4. **What is needed to maintain optimal muscle strength?**

A muscle must regularly exert at least 50% or more of its maximum strength in order to preserve and maintain its normal strength and avoid atrophy. The rate of decline resulting from immobility is approximately 15% off the baseline strength per week.

Fitts RH, McDonald KS, Schluter JM: The determinants of skeletal muscle force and power: Their adaptability with changes in activity pattern. J Biomech 24:111–122, 1991.

5. **What is a joint contracture?**

Joint contracture is a limitation of passive joint range of motion (ROM) resulting from a reduction in muscle fiber length and its compliance to stretch and restrictions caused by structural changes of the connective (collagen) tissue in the muscle, tendons, ligaments, joint elements (capsule), and skin. For example, in the case of knee flexion contracture, hamstring shortening is usually associated with an increase in synovial adhesions and a decrease in synoviocyte proliferation with increased fibroblasts in the posterior capsule of the knee.

Trudel G, Jabi M, Uhthoff HK: Localized and adaptive synoviocyte proliferation: Characteristics in rat knee joint contractures secondary to immobility. Arch Phys Med Rehabil 84:1350–1355, 2003.

6. **What five factors accelerate contracture formation in an immobilized limb?**

The mnemonic **BITES** lists these factors nicely:
- **B** = Bleeding, fibrin deposition, and fibrosis
- **I** = Inactivity, Infection
- **T** = Tissue trauma (acute and chronic) and subsequent fibrosis
- **E** = Edema; slower healing, fibrosis
- **S** = Systemic disease (e.g., diabetes, connective tissue disorders)

7. **How can functional (optimal) length of muscle and collagen fibers be maintained?**

Coiled collagen fibers, if not stretched regularly, become fixed in the shortened position. New cross-links are formed between the fibers, making collagen fibers more packed and stiff, leading to contracture. Lack of stretch decreases and repetitive stretch increases the number of sarcomeres per muscle fiber. In addition, static stretch even of short duration partially prevents atrophy of type 1 muscle fibers in denervated muscles.

Sakakima H, Yoshida Y: Effect of short duration static stretching on the denervated and reinnervated soleus muscle: Morphology in the rat. Arch Phys Med Rehabil 84:1339–1342, 2003.

Karpakka J, Vaananen K, Orava S, Takala TE: The effects of preimmobilization training and immobilization on collagen synthesis in rat skeletal muscle. Int J Sports Med 11:484–488, 1990.

KEY POINTS: SIGNIFICANCE OF STRETCHING AND LOADING

1. During child growth, muscle fibers elongate by adding new sarcomeres to the end of myofibrils.

2. In adults, muscle fiber is also capable of adding or losing sarcomeres in series to regain a new functional length as a response to stretch and loading.

3. Stretching is a powerful stimulus for muscle protein synthesis, production of sarcomeres, and for maintaining the optimal cross-links arrangement and length of collagen fibers.

4. Lack of stretching produces the loss of sarcomeres in series, shortening of muscle, collagen fibers, and resting muscle belly length, leading to stiffness and contracture.

8. **What are methods to prevent or treat contractures?**

- Stretch, stretch, and hold: The longer the better (repetitive or static stretch during ROM and flexibility exercises)
- Control spasticity: Medication, chemodenervation, and neurolysis interventions
- Early mobility: Encouraging functional activities
- Heat for joints and muscles (ultrasound, paraffin, warm hydrotherapy during stretch)
- Dynamic splints (spring-loaded assistance to push in direction of preferred range)
- Serial casting and static splinting
- Surgical tendon release
- Enhancing muscle strength of the opposing muscles (electrical stimulation, strength exercises)

Means KM: Rehabilitation of joint contractures. In Grabois M (ed): Physical Medicine and Rehabilitation: The Complete Approach. Malden, MA, Blackwell Science, 2000, pp 859–870.

9. **What physical factors prevent osteopenia by stimulating osteoblastic activity?**

Muscle pull and weight-bearing are important factors in activating osteoblasts and preventing immobilization osteoporosis. The distribution and density of collagen fibers is affected with stretch and loading, signaling osteoblasts to increase bone production (via piezoelectric effect). This can be very localized. For instance, persons with rotator cuff injury and an immobilized arm demonstrate a localized bone loss that is proportional to degree of impairment.

Bailey DA, McCulloch RG: Bone tissue and physical activity. Can J Sport Sci 15:229–239, 1990.

LeBlank A, Schneider VS, Evans J, et al: Bone mineral loss and recovery after 17 weeks of bed rest. J Bone Miner Res 5:49–57, 1999.

10. **Why do patients often complain of backache after prolonged confinement to bed?**

    Their intervertebral joints are stiffer, their paraspinal muscles are weaker, and their vertebrae are more osteoporotic, all of which dispute the effectiveness of bed rest as a therapy option for low back pain.

    Deyo RA, Diehl AK, Rosenthal M: How many days of bed rest for acute low back pain? N Engl J Med 315:1064–1092, 1986.

    Sinaki M, Wahner HW, Bergstrath EJ, et al: Three year controlled randomized trial of the effect of dose-specific loading and strengthening exercises on bone mineral density of the spine and femur in nonathletic physically active women. Bone 19(3):233–244, 1996.

11. **How does bed rest affect urination and defecation?**

    Difficulty with swallowing in a horizontal position limits fluid intake. In addition, decreased antidiuretic hormone levels result in dehydration. The recumbent position limits positions for successful urination and defecation. All these factors lead to constipation and poor appetite, compounding the problem.

12. **What happens to plasma volumes during bed rest?**

    The initial response to recumbence is mobilization of the blood into the chest and abdomen (central fluid shift) with an increase in venous return, cardiac preload, cardiac output, and myocardial work. During protracted bed rest there is a progressive decline in blood volume because of lowered production of aldosterone and antidiuretic hormones and cardiac output. The decrease in plasma volume is greater than the reduction in red cell mass, resulting in increased viscosity. Increased viscosity and hypovolemia greatly enhance the risk for thromboembolisms.

    Coyle EF, Hemmert MK, Coggan AR: Effects of detraining on cardiovascular responses to exercise: Role of blood volume. J Appl Physiol 60:95–99, 1986.

    Greenleaf JE: Physiological responses to prolonged bed rest and fluid immersion in humans. J Appl Physiol 57:619–633, 1984.

13. **What is the most common cause of sudden, unexpected death in hospitalized patients?**

    Acute pulmonary embolism.

14. **What is the orthostatic reflex? Why is it lost during bed rest?**

    The orthostatic reflex occurs when an initial drop in blood pressure upon assuming an upright position is detected at the carotid baroreceptors, which signal the medullary sympathetic center to trigger vasoconstriction in the muscular layers of the small arterioles. Like all muscles, these muscles become atrophic from disuse when the body remains horizontal or weightless. A combination of this effect and hypovolemia results in orthostatic hypotension, resulting in syncope, falls, and injuries. The NASA space program targets this and other complications of weightlessness for astronauts by including a carefully planned exercise routine. Devices using harnesses can simulate gravity and provide resistance for muscle. The terrestrial health care system for astronauts has not yet been fully adapted for bed-confined patients.

    National Space Biomedical Research, or Human Adaptation and Countermeasures Office of NASA, Johnson Space Center: Research on Space Exercise Programs. University of Washington; Northwest Science & Technology, 2001, pp 6–8.

KEY POINTS: UNDERLYING MECHANISMS OF MUSCLE RESPONSE TO PHYSICAL ACTIVITY

1. Skeletal muscle cells, osteoblasts, fibroblasts, and smooth muscle cells are activated by mechanical stresses.

2. Muscle cells are highly responsive to functional demands; loading produces hypertrophy, disuse produces atrophy.

3. Mechanical tension generates specific gene expression (i.e., myosin isoform for muscle phenotype). Myosin heavy chain gene expression formulates the encoding for adaptation to a given type of physical activity.

4. Stretch is an important factor in production of more actin and myosin and adding new sarcomeres in series.

5. Active muscle produces growth factors (i.e., IGF-1 and FGF) that control tissue repair and remodeling of skeletal and cardiac muscle.

6. Increase in production and consumption of IGF-1 in the muscle upon overloading provides the evidence for a link between mechanical stimulus and activation of gene and growth factors' responses.

15. **How do external pressures experienced during bed rest cause skin break down?**
Capillary filling pressures fall from 35 mmHg at the arterial end to 18 mmHg at the venous portion, or approximately 0.5 psi. To maintain perfusion and avoid collapse of skin capillaries, the external pressure therefore must be kept below 0.5 psi. This means that a 150-lb patient in bed requires a minimum of 300 sq in. of skin area for support. The good news is that this much area is, in fact, available on the dorsum of the trunk and extremities of a recumbent person. The bad news is that persons with impaired bed mobility or hip and knee contractures, placed on prolonged bed rest on typical hospital mattresses, are at a significantly higher risk for developing pressure sores. Cranking up the head of the bed further exacerbates the problem by adding shear stresses to the skin over the sacrum, producing a "preshear" sore condition.

16. **Are any organs and systems helped by bed rest?**
Some diagnoses or injured body parts may benefit from short-term bed rest such as long bone fractures, acute congestive heart failure (since bed rest decreases afterload, increases venous return, and decreases metabolic rate), severe acute myocardial infarctions, sepsis, and acute trauma. Strict immobilization is no longer a requirement for patients with acutely inflamed joints.

17. **Can exercise keep you "young"?**
Regular exercise as a part of an active lifestyle can maintain strength and flexibility, as well as improve balance and basic physical functions. It also reduces falls, glucose intolerance, hypertension, mineral bone loss, depression, and cognitive decline. The cliché, "use it or lose it," applies to all ages.

Bortz WM: Disuse and aging. JAMA 248:1203–1208, 1982.

Clark LP, Dio MD, Barker WH: Taking to bed: Rapid functional decline in an independent mobile older population living in an intermediate-care facility. J Am Geriatr Soc 38:967–972, 1990.

http://nihseniorhealth.gov/exercise/toc.html

Yaffe B, Barnes D, Nevitt M, et al: A prospective study of physical activity and cognitive decline in elderly women. Arch Intern Med 161:1703–1708, 2001.

18. **What can be gained from a regular training and exercise program?**
See Table 59-2.

TABLE 59-2. BENEFITS OF REGULAR TRAINING AND EXERCISE PROGRAM	
System	Benefits
Cardiovascular	Boosts VO_{2max}, functional reserve and stroke volumes, lowers heart rates with prolonged use, and improves cardiovascular fitness
Musculoskeletal	Increases blood supply, number of capillaries, mitochondria, and utilization and availability of oxygen; improves balance, strength, and endurance Delays the onset of anaerobic metabolism
Metabolic and endocrine	Improves glucose utilization; reduces triglycerides, LDL, body weight and associated complications Delays the onset of type 2 diabetes mellitus
Nervous	Reduces depression, delays dementia onset, increases motor units recruitment and firing rate, prevents side effects of inactivity and social isolation
Cancer	Improves life expectancy, reduces fatigue

Blair SN, Kampert JB, Kohl HW Jr., et al: Influence of cardiorespiratory fitness and other precursors on cardiovascular disease and all-cause mortality in men and women. JAMA 276:205–210, 1996.
Rovio S, Kareholt I, Helkala EL, et al: Leisure-time physical activity at midlife and the risk of dementia and Alzheimer's disease. Lancet Neurol 4:705–711, 2005.
American College of Sports Medicine: www.acsm.org

19. **List seven common strategies for minimizing the harmful effects of bed rest and inactivity.**
   - Minimize duration of bed rest.
   - Maximize activity and stimulation.
   - Prescribe exercise in bed (prone propulsions, Therabands and resistive exercises, yoga positions).
   - Encourage early mobilization (sitting and standing at bedside, using the bedside commode, walking to the bathroom) and training program.
   - Prescribe functional progressive mobility training (bed mobility, transfers, ambulation, stair-climbing).
   - Prescribe isotonic, isokinetic strengthening exercises to antigravity muscles.
   - Enhance mental stimulation, artistic interests, and socialization.

20. **Imagine a patient with T3 American Spinal Injury Association (ASIA) paraplegia on bed rest for healing a stage 3 ischial pressure ulcer. List all potential interventions to prevent the complications of immobility.**
   - Position the patient's bed near a window to allow maximal light exposure.
   - Order a prone gurney for "ambulation" and prone arm ergometry.
   - Change position in bed every 2 hours.
   - Use an alternating pressure air mattress "topper" for the bed.
   - Apply emollients to unbroken skin.

- Prescribe Thera-Band resistance strengthening exercises, emphasizing elbow extensors, shoulder depressors, and hand strength.
- Use sequential compression devices and elastic compression stocking for prevention of edema and thromboses.
- Use passive ROM to the lower extremities and ankle splints.
- Utilize side-lying bowel care and intermittent catheterization along with generous fluid intake.
- Promote the use of incentive spirometry every 2 hours and during the "commercial" breaks on television.
- Provide adapted bedside computer access; schedule bedside "parties" with regular visits from friends and relatives.

CHAPTER 60

METABOLIC BONE DISEASE: ASSESSMENT AND MANAGEMENT

Charles E. Levy, MD, Patricia Graham, MD, and Gulseren Akyuz, MD

The tragedy of osteoporosis is that it's largely avoidable.
—Robert P. Heaney, MD, in *Surgeon General's Report on Bone Health: Prevention Is Key*, 2004

1. Which disorders are considered metabolic bone diseases?
The major metabolic bone disease seen by physiatrists is osteoporosis, but this category also includes Paget's disease, osteomalacia, renal osteodystrophy, hyperparathyroidism, osteogenesis imperfecta, and osteopetrosis.

2. What is peak bone mass? When is it achieved?
Peak bone mass (PBM) is the highest level of bone mass achieved as a result of normal growth. It typically occurs between ages 20 and 30 for cortical bone and likely earlier for trabecular bone, with variation at specific skeletal sites. For example, PBM of the femoral neck is achieved in the 17th year, whereas the lumbar vertebrae usually reach their maximum between ages 18 and 24 years. Bone mineral density (BMD) is generally accumulated through adolescence, after which it declines at variable rates depending on anatomic location.

3. What happens to PBM at menopause?
Starting around the fourth or fifth decade of life, bone mass declines at a rate of 0.3–0.5% per year. In the 5–7 years following menopause, bone loss accelerates up to 10 times the initial rate, with vertebral loss most prominent. The cumulative loss of bone mass ranges from 20–30% in men and 40–50% in women.

4. What is the difference between osteoporosis and osteomalacia?
Osteoporosis is a progressive disease of bone, characterized by a reduction in bone mass caused by an imbalance between bone formation and bone resorption. In osteoporosis, normally mineralized bone is present in decreased density. In contrast, the amount of bone tissue in **osteomalacia** is normal (or increased), but there is reduced mineral content to the organic component ratio, leading to "softening" of bone.

The World Health Organization defines osteoporosis relative to an established BMD reference (e.g., female, Caucasian, age 20–29). Osteoporosis is defined in terms of standard deviations from this norm, and reported as a T-score for adults. It may be diagnosed in postmenopausal women and in men ages 50 and older if the T-score of the lumbar spine, total hip, or femoral neck is below the mean by 2.5 standard deviation (SD) or more.
- **Normal:** T-score > 1.0 SD below young adult mean (YAM)
- **Osteopenia:** T-score between 1.0 SD and 2.0 SD below YAM
- **Borderline osteoporosis:** T-score between 2.0 SD and 2.5 SD below YAM
- **Osteoporosis:** T-score ≥ 2.5 SD below YAM
- **Severe osteoporosis:** T-score > 2.5 SD below YAM with fragility fracture

5. Is osteoporosis a significant problem only in women?
No. The lifetime risk of fracture is more than 40% for women > age 50. However, it is estimated that men account for 20% of patients with osteoporosis. Although men have

fractures later in life (after age 80), once diagnosed with osteoporosis, they are 2–5 times more likely to have a second fracture than women, because men have a greater number of comorbidities at that age.

Bone Health and Osteoporosis: A Report of the Surgeon General. Washington, DC, USDHHS, PPHS, Office of the Surgeon General, 2004.

6. **How significant are osteoporotic fractures in people with spinal cord injury (SCI)?**
Up to one third of patients with long-term SCI report fractures. Complication rates are as high as 40%. Internal fixation can be unstable, and delayed fracture healing is often seen.

7. **What are the symptoms of osteoporosis?**
Osteoporosis is largely asymptomatic until the occurrence of a catastrophic event, which will likely be a fracture of a vertebra (50%, usually an anterior compression fracture), hip (25%), or other site (e.g., wrist, tibia, humerus). Fractures of the spine occur most commonly in the low thoracic (T8–T12) or upper lumbar (L1–L2) vertebrae. Each complete compression fracture causes approximately 1 cm loss in height. In severe cases with multiple fractures, height loss may be 10–20 cm. After a first osteoporotic compression fracture, risk increases 2–5 times for a second fracture, usually superior to the first. Fractures of isolated vertebral bodies at T4 or higher are unusual and may suggest malignancy. This accumulation of compression fractures can lead to postural deformities and pain.
- Dorsal kyphosis and exaggerated cervical lordosis ("dowager's hump")
- Chronic thoracic or low back pain, nuchal myalgia
- Abdominal protrusion, gastrointestinal discomfort
- Restricted excursion of the thoracic cage, pulmonary insufficiency and pneumonia

8. **How serious is the problem of hip fracture in osteoporosis?**
In the United States, approximately 17.5% of women will ultimately sustain a hip fracture (compared to 6% of men) and will account for a large percentage of the anticipated $12.2–17.9 billion spent each year in direct medical costs. Most hip fractures in osteoporotic individuals require operative management, with a resulting 2.8–4.0 increase in mortality in the first 3 months after the fracture and a 1-year morbidity rate of 14–36%. Hip protectors (undergarments with extra padding overlying the region of the femoral head) lower the risk of hip fracture with falls.

Office of the Surgeon General: Bone Health and Osteoporosis: A Report of the Surgeon General. Washington, DC, USDHHS, PPHS, Office of the Surgeon General, 2004.

9. **What factors help predict who will sustain a hip fracture?**
- Caucasian postmenopausal women
- Taller, thinner women
- Lower bone density
- Poor self-rated health
- History of hyperthyroidism or maternal hip fracture
- Treatment with anticonvulsants (phenytoin), barbiturates, or long-acting benzodiazepines
- High caffeine intake
- Inactivity (<4 hours on one's feet)
- Inability to rise from a chair without using one's arms
- Resting tachycardia
- Poor depth perception; poor perception of visual contrast

10. **Classify pain mechanisms caused by compression fractures.**
Pain mechanisms in osteoporosis can be classified as mechanical or chemical:
Mechanical causes
- Bone or joint distortion because of direct or indirect structural disruption
- Compression of nerves or soft tissue
- Mechanical stress on weak bone

Chemical causes

- Local endogenous algesic mediators such as histamine, serotonin, quinine, and substance P are released and activated because of vertebral collapse or microfractures.

11. **How is osteoporosis classified?**
    See Table 60-1.

TABLE 60-1. CLASSIFICATION OF OSTEOPOROSIS

Classification	Clinical Course	Remarks
Primary		
Involutional type I (postmenopausal)	Predominantly trabecular bone loss in axial skeleton	Affects women only within menopause, lasting 15–20 yr
Involutional type II (age associated)	Proportional loss of trabecular and cortical bone	Affects men or women over age 65
Idiopathic juvenile	Ages 8–14, self-limited (2–4 yr)	Normal growth; consider secondary forms
Idiopathic young adult	Mild to severe, self-limited (5–10 yr)	
Secondary (type III)	Dependent on underlying cause	Usually reversible to some extent after treatment of the primary disease
Endocrine		
Gastrointestinal		
Bone marrow disorders		
Connective tissue disorders		
Malnutrition		
Female athlete triad		
Lymphoproliferative diseases		
Medications		
Cadmium poisoning		
Others		
Regional		
Complex regional pain syndrome (reflex sympathetic dystrophy)	Three overlapping clinical stages: typical course lasts 6–9 mo, followed by spontaneous or assisted resolution	Radiographic changes may occur in first 3–4 wk, showing patchy demineralization of affected area; triple-phase bone scan shows increased uptake in involved extremity before radiographic changes; brief tapering dose of corticosteroids often warranted
Transient regional osteoporosis	Localized, migratory, predominantly involves hip, usually self-limited (6–9 months)	Rare; diagnosis by clinical suspicion, radiograph, and bone scan; treatment similar to that for complex regional pain syndrome

12. **What is the female athlete triad?**

Female athlete triad is a combination of disordered eating, amenorrhea, and osteoporosis. Inadequate caloric intake during periods of increased training can result in depleted fat stores; associated estrogen depletion can then disrupt menses and predispose the athlete to decreased BMD and fracture. Sports most associated with the triad include figure skating, gymnastics, diving, ballet, and distance running. Up to 62% of female college athletes have disordered eating. The incidence of secondary amenorrhea in the general population is approximately 5%, but that increases to 10–20% in athletes and as high as 50% in elite athletes.

Kaziz K, Iglesias E: The female athlete triad. Adolesc Med 14:87–95, 2003.

13. **How is the female athlete triad diagnosed and treated?**

Early screening of metabolic, psychological, and training risk factors is recommended to prevent osteoporotic fractures. Disrupted menses that return to normal in off-season (i.e., summer break) should be investigated within the first 3 months, before resumption of accelerated training activities, as should weight loss below goal weight and first incidence of stress fracture or overuse injury. The differential diagnosis of amenorrhea includes pregnancy; dysfunction of the hypothalamus, pituitary, ovaries, or uterus; and endocrine malfunction (hypothyroidism, Cushing's syndrome). If bone pain is unrelieved with rest, nonsteroidal anti-inflammatory drugs (NSAIDs), and other conservative measures and radiographs are negative, bone scan or magnetic resonance imaging (MRI) is recommended. Proper shoes may reduce stress to bones and other soft tissues. Education and monitoring by a dietician can help the athlete maintain goal weight in a healthy fashion.

Treatment includes diet modification, hormone monitoring during periods of disrupted menses, proper training regimens, and counseling to correct distorted body image. Hormone-replacement therapy should be considered early to increase BMD in females with amenorrhea, although even with this treatment, irreversible bone loss can occur.

Hobart JA: The female athlete triad. Am Fam Physician 61:3357–3364, 3367, 2000.
Otis CL, Drinkwater B, Johnson M, et al: American College of Sports Medicine Position Stand. Med Sci Sports Exerc 29:i–ix, 1997.

14. **Describe the history and physical examination for osteoporosis.**

Assess risk factors: nutritional insufficiencies, endocrine or gastrointestinal disease, alcoholism, medications known to affect bone (e.g., corticosteroids, certain anticonvulsants, immunosuppressants), and secondary amenorrhea (anorexia and extreme exercise). Look for anorexia, cushingoid appearance, hypogonadism, goiter, inflammatory disease, gynecomastia, and chronic obstructive pulmonary disease (COPD) (barrel chest, distant breath sounds, and wheezes).

15. **What about falls?**

In the **history,** check for:
- The number, frequency, circumstances, and environment of falls
- Fragility fracture history of the patient and family members older than age 50
- Loss of height, posture, balance, weakness
- Sensory deficits
- Status of sensorium
- Medication list (e.g., sedatives)
- Urinary incontinence
- Visual deficits
- Need for ambulatory assistive device
- Home safety profile
- Depression/agitation

In the **physical exam,** check for:
- Cardiac arrhythmias (syncope)
- Weakness

- Proprioception/position sense
- Posture (e.g., forward leaning) contractures
- Gait and balance
- Memory and concentration
- Inflammatory or degenerative disease

16. **What laboratory tests are warranted?**
The medical work-up is aimed at determining the cause and extent of osteoporosis:
   - **Basic serum chemistries** should be done to evaluate possible renal, hepatic, hyperthyroid, and hypercholesterolemia contributions to low BMD. These include renal function panel, total protein (nutritional status), cholesterol panel, hepatic enzymes, and thyroid function panel.
   - **Complete blood count and erythrocyte sedimentation rate** (ESR) are used to rule out inflammatory processes and anemias associated with malignancies.
   - **Serum testosterone** levels (in men) are tested to rule out hypogonadism.
   - **Urinalysis** screens test for proteinuria caused by nephrotic syndrome and low pH as a result of renal tubular acidosis.
   - **Evaluate calcium homeostasis** with measurements of 24-hour urinary levels of calcium and creatinine and serum levels of ionized calcium, phosphorus, intact parathyroid hormone, and vitamin D, 25-hydroxy.
   - **Urine pregnancy test** and **serum female hormone levels** (luteinizing hormone [LH], follicle-stimulating hormone [FSH], estradiol, drawn between days 2 and 4 of regular menstrual cycle onset) and prolactin levels can evaluate amenorrhea, which may be exercise induced.
   - **Serum and urine markers of bone resorption,** such as urine N-telopeptide and serum bone-specific alkaline phosphatase, quantify bone turnover rates and can be used to establish baseline. Repeat markers in 3 months can provide first indication of treatment efficacy (i.e., lowered bone turnover level).

17. **What are codfish vertebrae?**
Codfish vertebrae refer to a radiographic finding caused by expansion of the intervertebral discs into the superior and inferior vertebral end plates, causing an exaggerated bioconcavity. Fuller Albright, a pioneer in metabolic bone disease, noted in 1948 that this bioconcavity resembled the vertebrae of codfish, which are naturally bioconcave.

18. **How is bone mass assessed?**
   - **Dual energy x-ray absorptiometry** (DXA) remains the World Health Organization's (WHO) gold standard for bone mass assessment. BMD > 2.5 SD below the mean correlates with osteoporotic fractures. Lateral radiographs of the thoracic and lumbar spine are recommended with moderate to severe degenerative arthritis of the spine; sclerosis, scoliosis, and calcium spurs can falsely elevate BMD T-scores. Vertebrae with compression fractures must be eliminated when evaluating BMD of L1–L4 vertebrae.
   - **Quantitative computed tomography** (QCT) separately measures cortical and cancellous bone and true BMD. However, radiation exposure is hundreds of times greater than for DXA, and QCT is relatively expensive.
   - **Micro QCT** (3DCT) provides three-dimensional views that give information about bone density, trabecular microfractures, microcallus formations, trabecule count, thickness, and organization shapes.
   - **High-resolution magnetic resonance imaging** (HRMRI) provides three-dimensional views of trabecular bone and information about microarchitectural structure. It determines the bone volume, trabecule count, trabecular space, and thickness.
   - **Fourier transform infrared spectroscopy** (FTIRS) analyzes slim sections (5 μm) of bone tissue. It provides information about bone matrix such as crystallization, collagen structure, heterogeneity, and distribution.

- **Bone biopsy,** usually of the iliac crest, is invasive, and analysis is time consuming, so that it is generally reserved as a research tool. In renal osteodystrophy and osteomalacia, bone biopsy can be important in management.

19. **What are the indications for measurement of bone density?**
According to the International Society of Clinical Densitometry (ISCD), the following are indications for measurement of bone density:
   - Women aged 65 and older
   - Postmenopausal women under age 65 with other risk factors
   - Men aged 70 and older (especially those who have fallen from a standing height)
   - Adults with a disease or condition associated with low bone mass or bone loss
   - Adults taking medications associated with low bone mass or bone loss (e.g., glucocorticoids, phenytoin, cyclosporine)
   - Anyone being considered for pharmacologic therapy for bone loss
   - To monitor treatment effect on osteoporosis
   - Anyone in whom evidence of bone loss would lead to treatment
   - Women discontinuing estrogen therapy

20. **What are the ISCD guidelines for DXA measurement of BMD?**
   - **Spine:** Use posteroanterior L1–L4 views for spine BMD measurement. If only one valuable vertebra remains after excluding other vertebrae, diagnosis should be based on a different valid skeletal site. Anatomically abnormal vertebrae may be excluded from analysis (i.e., compression fracture) if there is more than a 1.0 T-score difference between the vertebra in question and adjacent vertebrae. When vertebrae are excluded, the BMD of the remaining vertebrae is used to derive the T-score. Lateral spine should not be used for diagnosis but may have a role in monitoring.
   - **Hip:** Use femoral neck or total proximal femur T-score, whichever is lowest.
   - **Forearm:** BMD should be measured if hip and/or spine cannot be measured or interpreted, if the patient has hyperparathyroidism, or if the patient is extremely obese (over the weight limit for DXA table, approximately 300 lb).

21. **What are the ISCD guidelines for measurement of BMD in pediatric populations?**
T-scores are not used in people younger than 20 years; Z-scores should be used instead. Z-scores are based on age-matched norms. A Z-score of -2.0 or lower is defined as "below the expected range for age," and a Z-score above -2.0 is "within the expected range for age." Z-scores should be population specific when adequate reference data are available. Spine and total body are the preferred skeletal sites for measurement. Changes may be required with growth of the child. Diagnosis of osteoporosis in children should not be made by Z-score alone. The value of BMD in predicting fractures in children is not clearly determined.

22. **Explain the role of serial BMD measurements.**
Serial BMD testing is used to determine whether treatment should be started in untreated patients or changed in treated patients. Intervals between BMD testing should be individualized. Typically, one year after initiation or change of therapy is appropriate, with longer intervals once therapeutic effect is established.

23. **What new standard for establishing the threshold for osteoporosis screening and treatment is likely to replace the present WHO criteria?**
The WHO criteria are based on DXA T-score only. The **absolute fracture risk,** first elucidated by Kanis et al, will establish screening and treatment thresholds for the individuals at highest risk for fracture compared with the general population. In addition to standard DXA T-score, other factors are taken into account, such as sex, gender, age, history of previous falls and fragility fractures, presence of medications that might impair sensorium or increase

risk of low bone mineral density, low body mass index, and present activity level, among others. This integrated approach assesses for the long-term (10-year) probability of hip fracture and is based on the concept that not all fractures are created equal (i.e., 1 hip fracture = 4 vertebral fractures = 20 other fractures, such as a Colles' fracture at the wrist).

Kanis JA, Black D, Cooper C, et al: A new approach to the development of assessment guidelines for osteoporosis. Osteoporos Int 13:527–536, 2002.

24. Who was Julius Wolff? What is Wolff's law?

Wolff, a professor of surgery at the University of Berlin, published *The Law of Bone Remodeling* in 1892, stating that static stress to a bone—whether it be compression, tension, or shear—would cause bone to remodel along mathematically predictable lines. Wolff collaborated with Professor Culman, a mathematician from Zurich who developed a method of analyzing the structural stresses in various components of bridges, building frames, and cranes. To test Wolff's supposition, Culman assigned his students the task of drawing the stresses on a particular hypothetical crane, which, unbeknownst to the students, was shaped to resemble the human femur. The students' vectors closely resembled the trabeculae of the actual femur, thus confirming what was later called Wolff's law. In essence, this law states that mechanical use (weight-bearing) results in increased cortical bone mass and strength, whereas disuse leads to bone atrophy.

25. How is exercise used as a preventative measure in osteoporosis?

Physical activity may (1) enhance bone strength by optimizing BMD and improving bone quality and (2) reduce the risk of falling. The mechanostat theory provides a basis for the benefits of exercise, noting the relationship between the intensity of bend or strain on bone and the adaptation of bone to that stimulus. In this model, whenever activity falls below a certain threshold, bone resorption exceeds bone formation. In contrast, net gains of bone occur only when the intensity of loading is increased above the physiologic loading zone. This model accounts for the bone loss observed during immobilization and the increased bone mass of elite athletes.

26. What is the relationship between immobilization and osteoporosis?

Following extended immobilization (either external such as for fractures or self-imposed because of pain), evidence of osteopenia can be noted on x-rays within 2–3 months.

27. Describe exercise considerations for osteoporosis.

The National Osteoporosis Foundation Scientific Advisory Board's *Position Paper on Exercise and Osteoporosis* (1991) describes five important principles of therapeutic exercise for osteoporosis:

1. **Principle of specificity:** Activities should stress sites most at risk for fracture, and skeletal protection should be provided for those areas with severe loss of bone mass.
2. **Principle of progression:** A progressive increase in intensity is required for continued improvement.
3. **Principle of reversibility:** The positive effects of an exercise program will be lost if stopped.
4. **Principal of initial values:** Those with an initial low capacity will have the greatest functional improvement.
5. **Principle of diminishing returns:** There is a limit to improvements in function, and as the limit is approached, greater effort is needed for increasingly smaller gains.

Exercise programs in the elderly should improve muscle strength and balance and be safe, frequent, regular, and sustained. A program of walking, sitting, and standing exercises or water aerobics provides a good start. The height of a bicycle seat, saddle style, and handle-bar height and style should be adjusted for an upright spinal alignment. Swimming is unlikely to improve BMD but provides chest expansion, spinal extension, and low-impact cardiopulmonary fitness. A home exercise program should include deep breathing, back-extension exercises, pectoral stretching, and isometric exercises to strengthen the abdomen and avoid kyphosis.

Srivastava M, Deal C: Osteoporosis in elderly: Prevention and treatment. Clin Geriatr Med. 18: 529–555, 2002.

28. **What are the benefits of tai chi?**
Tai chi is associated with a lesser rate of BMD loss in postmenopausal women. Tai chi practitioners report decreased falls and associated injuries.

> Chan K, Qin L, Lau M, et al: A randomized, prospective study of the effects of Tai Chi Chun exercise on bone mineral density in women. Arch Phys Med Rehabil 85:717–722, 2004.
> Wolf SL, Barnhart HX, Kutner NG, et al: Reducing frailty and falls in older persons: An investigation of Tai Chi and computerized balance training. Atlanta FICSIT Group. Frailty and injuries: Cooperative studies of intervention techniques. J Am Geriatr Soc 44:489–497, 1996.

29. **Which back exercises should be avoided?**
Exercises performed with the spine in flexion predispose osteoporotic women to vertebral compression fractures (as do sudden rotational movements such as an overly vigorous golf swing or tennis serve).

30. **Why is bracing used for vertebral compression fractures? What bracing options are available?**
For **acute pain,** the reduction of spinal motion allows paraspinal muscles to cease painful guarding and also provides a physical barrier to reinjury, allowing earlier resumption of activity after injury.

For **chronic back pain,** bracing substitutes for weak muscles, reduces ligamentous strain, and offers some protection against the occurrence of new fracture. Bracing options, from least to most restrictive, include:
1. **Elastic binders,** which act as a reminder to restrict motion and also increase intra-abdominal pressure
2. The heat-moldable plastic **thoracolumbar orthosis** (TLO), shaped to the patient's contours and then applied in an elastic support, fabricated by a physical therapist; this takes only minutes to fabricate and is generally a less expensive option
3. The hyperextension **thoracolumbosacral orthosis** (TLSO), such as the Jewett and CASH (cruciform anterior sternal hyperextension)
4. Custom-molded **plastic body jacket**
Continued use of spinal orthotics is discouraged because of the increased likelihood of weakening and atrophy of trunk muscles and decreased spinal mobility. **Posture-training supports** (small pouches containing weights up to 2 lb suspended by loops from the shoulders), positioned just below the inferior angle of the scapula to counteract the tendency to bend forward, are worn for 1 hour twice a day.

KEY POINTS: OSTEOPOROSIS

1. Osteoporosis is largely a treatable, preventable progressive disease that affects both men and women.

2. Osteoporosis is asymptomatic until a fracture occurs, usually in the spine (50%) or hip (25%). The fracture also may occur elsewhere (e.g., wrist, tibia, femur).

3. Dual energy x-ray absorptiometry (DXA) is the single standard by which to assess bone density and fracture risk. Bone mineral density > 2.5 standard deviations below the mean correlates with osteoporotic fractures.

4. Exercise, gait training, home modifications, and hip protectors reduce the risk of falls and fractures and enhance bone health and quality of life.

31. **What home modifications should be considered?**
- Elimination of throw rugs
- Nonskid tape of different colors on the outer edges of steps

- Improved lighting
- Stair rails
- Elimination of loose cords and clutter
- In the bathroom and shower: Nonskid mats, grab bars, transfer tub benches
- Entry ramps
- Anticipating emergencies: Easy access to emergency phone numbers, a fire exit plan, fire and smoke alarms

Other strategies and devices to reduce vertebral compressive forces include:

- Carrying heavy items at waist height and close to the body (consider backpacks)
- Repositioning desks, files, and telephones closer to spare trunk flexion
- Pacing
- Alternating tasks that demand sitting with those that require standing
- Wheeled carts
- Rotating platforms (e.g., lazy Susans)
- Swiveling, wheeled office chairs with a lumbar support
- Electronic can openers, knives, and mixers
- Lightweight cups and bowls
- Levered door closures
- Long-handled reachers, shoehorns, sock aids, and sponges

32. **What are the goals of pharmacology in osteoporosis?**
    - Slowing or reversal of the underlying disease process
    - Pain control

33. **Discuss the options for pain control for vertebral compression fractures.**
    Back pain resulting from a vertebral compression fracture usually resolves in 4–6 weeks. **Bed rest,** although helpful initially, should be limited. Modalities such as **moist heat** and **massage** may alleviate symptoms.

    Nonsteroidal anti-inflammatory drugs (NSAIDs) and COX-2 **inhibitors** are often helpful but carry risks of peptic ulcers and renal and cardiac disorders. Smaller doses are often appropriate for the elderly. Opioids offer acute pain relief but slow gastrointestinal motility, cause constipation, can impair cognition (fall risk), and create drug dependence.

34. **What cytokines and colony-stimulating factors activate the development of osteoblasts and osteoclasts?**
    Osteoblasts
    - Interleukin-1
    - Tumor necrosis factor
    - Parathyroid hormone
    - 1,25-dihydroxy vitamin D_3
    Osteoclasts
    - Interleukins-1, -3, -6, and -11
    - Granulocyte-macrophage colony-stimulating factor
    - Macrophage colony-stimulating factor
    - Tumor necrosis factor
    - Leukemia-inhibiting factor
    - Stem cell factor

35. **What are bisphosphonates? How do they work?**
    All bisphosphonates (alendronate, risedronate, ibandronate, and pamidronate) are phosphatase-resistant analogs of pyrophosphates, which inhibit bone resorption. The bisphosphonates bind to hydroxyapatite, preventing its dissolution and impairing osteoclast function resulting in a reduction of osteoclast activation. Oral alendronate (Fosamax) and risedronate (Actonel) can be dosed daily or weekly. Both increase BMD and reduce vertebral and nonvertebral fractures

in women with osteoporosis. Ibandronate (Boniva) is approved for oral (daily or once per month) and intervenous dosing (every 3 months). It increases BMD at the hip, but its effect on fracture reduction is unknown. Treatment with bisphosphonates should be supplemented with calcium and vitamin D. Side effects include gastrointestinal problems, abdominal or musculoskeletal pain, nausea, heartburn or irritation of the esophagus, and itching or rash.

36. What role does calcitonin play in the treatment of osteoporosis?

Calcitonin directly inhibits osteoclastic activity, reducing bone resorption so that vertebral bone mass is increased. Calcitonin is unique among osteoporosis therapies in that it provides analgesia for acute and chronic pain of vertebral compression fractures, and decreases vertebral fracture incidence (although it is unclear if there is benefit for the hip). It may be administered subcutaneously, intramuscularly, or nasally. A high incidence of nausea, transient facial flushing, and inflammatory reaction is associated with injected calcitonin, but these drop dramatically with nasal administration. Concurrent adequate intake of vitamin D and calcium is essential.

Silverman S: Calcitonin. Clin Geriatr Med 1:381–394, 2003.

37. What are SERMs?

SERMs are selective estrogen receptor modulators. Raloxifene binds to estrogen receptors, activating certain estrogen pathways while blocking others, thus decreasing bone resorption. Raloxifene may offer extraskeletal benefits to selected patients (e.g., those with elevated lipids or high breast cancer risk); however, its effects on bone are much less robust than the bisphosphonates. Bazedoxifene and lasodoxifene are new-generation SERMs.

38. Are there any treatments based on parathyroid hormone?

Teriparatide (Forteo) is a parathyroid hormone analog that is of benefit when administered parenterally (subcutaneously, daily). It is an anabolic agent that stimulates new bone formation and is currently used to treat patients who are at very high risk for (recurrent) fracture, are intolerant of bisphosphonates, or who have advanced osteoporosis. Its use beyond 2 years is not recommended.

39. What is strontium renelate?

The element strontium was used as therapy for osteoporosis in the 1950s, but it fell out of favor because of concerns about mineralization defects. Recent studies have yielded more promising results. Strontium ranelate (Protelos) stimulates bone production by transforming preosteoblasts to osteoblasts and by increasing the activity of osteoblasts. It decreases bone resorption by reducing the formation and the activity of osteoclasts. It increases BMD at the hip, femoral neck, and lumbar spine, and decreases both vertebral and nonvertebral fractures in postmenopausal women with osteoporosis.

Reginster JY, Seeman E, De Vernejoul MC, et al: Strontium ranelate reduces the risk of nonvertebral fractures in postmenopausal women with osteoporosis: Treatment of Peripheral Osteoporosis (TROPOS) Study. J Clin Endocrinol Metab 90:2816–2822, 2005.

40. How are estrogens and interleukin-6 connected in the pathophysiology of postmenopausal osteoporosis? How does this apply to hypogonadal men?

Estrogens inhibit the genetic transcription of interleukin-6. Therefore, loss of estrogens leads to greater amounts of interleukin-6, leading to increased numbers of osteoclasts. Ultimately, the homeostasis of bone formation and resorption are disrupted, favoring bone loss. **Androgens** exert a similar influence on interleukin-6 as estrogens.

41. What are the effects of hypogonadism and testosterone for men?

Late-onset hypogonadism is a risk factor for spinal osteoporosis. Men with idiopathic hypogonadism have BMDs more than two standard deviations below the mean. Although it is evident that severe male hypogonadism can cause osteoporosis, the effect of moderate decreases in testosterone levels in aging men on rates of bone loss is uncertain. **Testosterone** replacement improves BMD in men with established testosterone deficiencies and in men without known testosterone deficiency but established vertebral fractures or who are receiving corticosteroids. Studies of testosterone replacement in older men with low bioavailable testosterone levels have demonstrated maintenance of femoral neck BMD and improvement of spinal BMD in men with total testosterone levels below 200 ng/dL. However, testosterone increases prostate size and may even promote the development of occult prostate cancer. Thus, testosterone is not approved solely for treatment of osteoporosis.

Kenny AM, Prestwood KM: Osteoporosis. Pathogenesis, diagnosis, and treatment in older adults. Rheum Dis Clin North Am 26:569–591, 2000.

42. **How much calcium should be consumed daily by different age groups?**
See Table 60-2.

TABLE 60-2. OPTIMAL CALCIUM REQUIREMENTS RECOMMENDED BY THE NATIONAL INSTITUTES OF HEALTH CONSENSUS PANEL	
Age Group	Optimal Daily Intake (mg)*
Birth–6 mos	400
6 mos–1 yr	600
1–5 yrs	800
6–10 yrs	800–1200
11–24 yrs	1200–1500
Men: 25–65 yrs	1000
Women: 25–50 yrs	1000
Postmenopausal women on estrogens: 50–65 yrs	1000
Postmenopausal women not on estrogens: 50–65 yrs	1500
Men and women > 65 yrs	1500
Pregnant and nursing women	1200–1500

Matkovic V (ed): Osteoporosis. Physical Medicine and Rehabilitation Clinics of North America, Vol. 6, no. 2. Philadelphia, W.B. Saunders, 1995.
*The actual diet should be tailored to individual preferences. For example, 1 oz of Swiss cheese = 1 cup of milk = 1 cup of yogurt = 1 oz of calcium-enriched orange juice = approx. 300 mg of calcium.

WEBSITES

1. National Institutes of Health
health.nih.gov/result.asp/488

2. Medline Plus: Osteoporosis
www.nlm.nih.gov/medlineplus/osteoporosis.html

PRESSURE ULCERS: ASSESSMENT AND TREATMENT

CHAPTER 61

Michael M. Priebe, MD, and Richard Salcido, MD

Persons who rest on their laurels get pressure ulcers.
—Theodore Cole, MD, Professor Emeritus, University of Michigan

1. **An axiom in the prevention and treatment of pressure ulcers is "where there is no pressure, there is no pressure ulcer." Why does pressure cause ulceration?**
   The reason is tissue ischemia. When tissues are compressed between a bony prominence and an external surface, capillaries are compressed and blood flow is obstructed. This leads to ischemia, reperfusion injury, infarction, and, ultimately, tissue necrosis.

2. **How much pressure is too much?**
   In his classic 1961 study of the etiology of pressure ulcers, Kosiak found a clear relationship between pressure and time in producing tissue injury in the muscle tissues of dogs. Sustained low pressure for up to 4 hours did not cause tissue injury, but high pressure for only 2 hours produced moderate injury. He also found that alternating pressure resulted in less tissue injury than the equivalent amount of constant pressure. How much pressure is too much? We don't really know. *In general, the more pressure applied, the shorter the duration needed to produce tissue injury.* Therefore, rather than relying on absolute pressure measurements, we focus on pressure management and perform pressure relief frequently.

   Kosiak M: Etiology of decubitus ulcers. Arch Phys Med Rehabil 42:19–29, 1961.

3. **Which tissues are most sensitive to pressure?**
   Tissues vary in their sensitivity to pressure. Muscle is the most sensitive, whereas skin is most resistant to pressure-induced ischemia. Therefore, pressure-induced ulcers typically involve the deep tissue first. Superficially, the affected area appears as an area of induration, erythema, and warmth, but with intact skin. Within a few days to a week, even with complete pressure relief, the wound may open and reveal a deep crater.

   Daniel RK, Priest DL, Wheatley DC: Etiologic factors in pressure sores: An experimental model. Arch Phys Med Rehabil 62(10):492–498, 1981.
   Salcido R, Donofrio JC, Fisher SB, et al: Evaluation of ibuprofen for pressure ulcer prevention: Application of a rat pressure ulcer model. Adv Wound Care 8(4):30–32, 34, 38–40, 1995.

4. **If muscle is the most sensitive tissue to pressure, why do surgeons use muscle flaps (myocutaneous flaps) to close large pressure ulcers?**
   Myocutaneous flap procedures are based on the basic surgical principle of eliminating dead space. Myocutaneous flaps do not provide a "cushion" but rather provide well-vascularized tissue to fill the dead space left after resection of a pressure ulcer. Another benefit of a myocutaneous flap is that the surgeon is often able to move the suture line—a very vulnerable region caused by the formation of scar tissue—away from the site of maximum pressure.

5. **How do shear and friction contribute to pressure ulcer formation?**
   Shear and friction theoretically cause superficial tissue ischemia by kinking capillaries in the dermis that are oriented perpendicularly to the surface of the skin. This is worsened by the

presence of pressure. This combination often results in a superficial pressure ulcer. The presence of significant shear forces reduces by half the amount of pressure needed to disrupt blood flow in the dermis.

Dinsdale SN: Decubitus ulcers: Role of pressure and friction in causation. Arch Phys Med Rehabil 55:147–154, 1974.

6. **What are the major objectives of pressure management to prevent pressure ulcers?**
   - Use pressure-reducing support surfaces in bed and chair to protect soft tissues.
   - Provide even distribution of pressure across the entire weight-bearing surface.
   - Increase the weight-bearing surface by utilizing body surfaces that can tolerate more pressure for weight distribution (e.g., the posterior thigh during sitting).
   - Minimize shear forces through good positioning in chair or bed. Specifically, avoid the following postures: a "slouched" posture with posterior pelvic tilt while sitting in the wheelchair, or sitting in bed with the head of the bed at a 30- to 45-degree angle.
   - Perform frequent pressure relief.

7. **What are six important elements of assessing a pressure ulcer?**
   1. Anatomic location
   2. Stage
   3. Size (length, width, depth, wound area)
   4. Tissue quality (wound bed, necrosis, undermining, sinus tracts)
   5. Exudate (volume, quality, odor)
   6. Wound margins/surrounding tissue (induration, erythema, cellulitis)

   Consortium for Spinal Cord Medicine Clinical Practice Guidelines: Pressure ulcer prevention and treatment following spinal cord injury: A clinical practice guideline for health-care professionals. J Spinal Cord 24 Med (Suppl 1):S40–S101, 2001.

8. **At what anatomic sites are pressure ulcers most likely to develop?**
   Pressure ulcers develop most commonly over areas of bony prominence. The most common sites include the sacrum, coccyx, ischia, trochanter, heel, and malleoli. The locations on the list may change order, depending on the patient population (e.g., spinal cord injury [SCI] or geriatric) and the time after injury (e.g., acute SCI or chronic SCI).

9. **What is the difference between a sacral ulcer and a coccygeal ulcer?**
   Sacral ulcers are located over the sacral prominence and are caused by lying supine in bed. Coccygeal ulcers are located over the coccyx and are caused by poor posture in which there are shearing forces and pressure over the coccyx. This commonly occurs while sitting in bed semireclined or sitting in a wheelchair with a slouched posture. These ulcers can coalesce into a single ulcer, but attempts should be made to differentiate them because the etiologies and, therefore, the treatments are different.

10. **What does a pressure ulcer location tell us?**
    The location tells us what caused the pressure ulcer and allows for focused interventions for treatment and prevention. Location is often predictable and depends on the individual's activity level. Persons who spend much or all of the day lying in bed most often develop pressure ulcers over the sacrum, trochanters, and heels. Persons who are sitting develop pressure ulcers over the ischia, coccyx, and trochanters.

11. **How does sitting exert pressure on the trochanters?**
    The trochanters bear weight during sitting, and the weight borne is particularly increased in the presence of pelvic obliquity. These trochanteric ulcers tend to develop posterior to the greater trochanter rather than directly lateral to it (which is seen in side-lying ulcers). Use of a

wheelchair with a sling seat that is overstretched may also contribute to trochanteric pressure ulcers.

12. **How are pressure ulcers staged?**
    Figure 61-1 summarizes the four stages of pressure ulcers, as defined by the National Pressure Ulcer Advisory Panel.

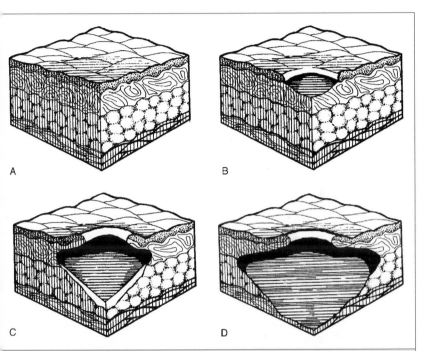

Figure 61-1. The four stages of pressure ulcers. *A,* Stage I: Nonblanchable erythema of intact skin, the heralding lesion of skin ulceration. Erythema does not last for more than 30 minutes. *B,* Stage II: Partial-thickness skin loss involving the epidermis and/or dermis. The ulcer is superficial and presents clinically as an abrasion, blister, or shallow crater. *C,* Stage III: Full-thickness skin loss involving damage or necrosis of subcutaneous tissue that may extend down to, but not through, underlying fascia. The ulcer presents clinically as a deep crater with or without undermining of adjacent tissue. *D,* Stage IV: Full-thickness skin loss with extensive destruction, tissue necrosis, or damage to muscle, bone, or supporting structures (e.g., tendon or joint capsule) (Figures courtesy of Michael M. Priebe, MD; National Pressure Ulcer Advisory Panel: Pressure ulcers prevalence, cost and risk assessment: Consensus development conference statement. Decubitus 2:24–28, 1989.)

13. **What is the best treatment for a pressure ulcer?**
    Every patient is different and every wound is unique. There are, however, four basic principles to guide treatment. You can treat any pressure ulcer using these principles.
    - **Prevention is paramount.** Careful attention to risk factors allows early detection of persons at risk for developing a pressure ulcer. Preventive efforts are ongoing and must continue once a wound is healed.
    - **Correct the underlying systemic and systematic factors that initially led to the development of the ulcer.** Biologic, psychosocial, and environmental problems must be

addressed to maximize healing. These problems may include poor nutritional status, anemia, osteomyelitis, poor vascular supply to the wound region, poor posture, inappropriate equipment, anxiety, and depression. A complete evaluation is necessary to determine which of these are most critical to address initially.

- **Wounds must be adequately débrided before healing can occur.** Wounds with necrotic debris in the wound bed do not heal properly. It is necessary to remove the dead tissue as the first step in pressure ulcer care. Chronic, nonhealing pressure ulcers may also benefit from débridement to stimulate the acute wound–healing cascade.
- **Maintain a moist wound environment.** A moist environment provides the optimal conditions for cell migration and mitosis. A dry wound impedes the healing process. Many products are available to assist in maintaining a moist wound environment.

Priebe MM, Martin M, Wuermser LA, et al: The medical management of pressure ulcers. In Lin VW (ed): Spinal Cord Medicine: Principles and Practice. New York, Demos, 2003, pp 567–590.

14. **What is the difference between an eschar and a scab?**
    - An **eschar** is the tough, leathery matter covering a wound. It is necrotic skin and subcutaneous tissue and is not a beneficial natural dressing. Eschars should be removed. An eschar harbors bacteria and prevents the formation of granulation tissue and epithelialization of the wound. An eschar also prevents adequate wound staging.
    - A **scab** is dried serum that covers a superficial wound. Conventional wisdom indicates that a scab may be the body's way of laying down a natural dressing or a matrix for healing and usually maintaining a clean and moist environment for a superficial wound bed. If there is cellulitis, or if it is unclear whether the dry matter is a scab or an eschar, remove it.

15. **What is the fastest way to débride a necrotic pressure ulcer?**
    The fastest, and often the most effective, way is surgical, or "sharp," débridement. Small wounds may be débrided at the bedside, but extensive wounds should be débrided in the operating room, especially if hemostasis will be difficult to maintain, or anesthesia is needed. Débridement is often necessary early in the management of stages III and IV pressure ulcers and is mandatory in the face of advancing cellulitis or sepsis.

    Ayello EA, Cuddigan JE: Debridement: Controlling the necrotic/cellular burden. Adv Skin Wound Care 17(2):66–75; quiz, 76–78, 2004.

16. **What is meant by autolytic débridement?**
    Autolytic débridement is utilizing the body's own enzymes to degrade dead tissue. This is accomplished by placing an occlusive dressing over the wound and allowing the wound fluid to collect under the dressing. The wound fluid, which is full of enzymes, helps to soften the eschar and begins the separation of healthy from nonviable tissue, making sharp débridement easier. Be very careful, though, because if the wound is infected, an abscess can be created by covering the wound with an occlusive dressing.

17. **True or false: You can put anything on a pressure ulcer except the patient, and it will heal.**
    True and false. The human body is amazing in its ability to heal itself, often in the face of continued injury or insult. However, many agents used historically in wound care actually delay healing. Povidone-iodine, hydrogen peroxide, acetic acid, and sodium hypochlorite, commonly used to cleanse wounds, are cytotoxic to human fibroblasts and delay wound healing. The cellular toxicity of these agents may exceed their antibacterial potency.

18. **How often should a "wet-to-dry" dressing be changed?**
    It is important to determine why the dressing is being used. If the wound requires débridement, "wet-to-dry" dressings are appropriate and should be removed when dry, usually twice or three times a day depending on the environment. The dressing material should be removed dry

(not moistened before removal) and any attached matter pulled out of the wound to clean it. These dressings nonselectively débride wounds, meaning that healthy tissue may also be damaged as you remove necrotic tissue.

19. **Under what conditions is the application of "wet-to-moist" dressing most appropriate?**
If the wound is clean and the goal is to maintain a moist wound environment, wet-to-moist dressings are appropriate. These should be changed before they dry out—usually at a minimum of three or four times a day. Remember, wet-to-dry dressings should only be used for débridement and discontinued or changed to wet-to-moist once the wound bed is clean.

20. **What is the difference between wet-to-moist dressings and the various forms of new fangled wound dressings?**
The real difference is ease of care. Because wet-to-moist dressings need to be changed every 6–8 hours, nursing care costs and burden of care can escalate rapidly. Newer dressings, although generally more expensive, can often be changed once a day or less. This decrease in the number of applications offsets the increased cost of the dressing. Regardless of the dressing chosen, the same principles apply—correct the underlying factors, adequately débride the wound, and provide a moist wound environment for healing.

21. **How does one select among the many different types of dressings?**
Although there are hundreds of different dressings on the market, the use of one dressing from each of the following four major classes of dressings can allow one to effectively manage just about any pressure ulcer.
   - Transparent membranes are best for superficial, minimally draining wounds.
   - Hydrocolloids are good for superficial wounds with minimal to moderate drainage.
   - Foam dressings are appropriate for superficial, heavily draining wounds.
   - Alginate products can be used in either superficial or deep wounds with moderate to heavy drainage.
     However, don't forget about saline and gauze. Wet-to-moist dressings have been used for years to heal pressure ulcers.

22. **Provide a simplified algorithm for treatment of pressure ulcers.**
See Figure 61-2.

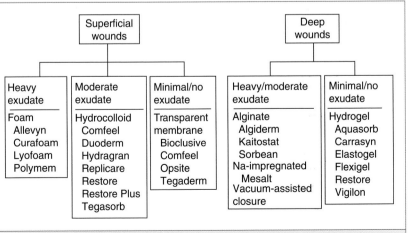

Figure 61-2. Simplified algorithm for the treatment of pressure ulcers. (Courtesy of Michael M. Priebe, MD.)

23. **What does one do if the wound isn't healing after a couple of weeks?**
If a wound shows no signs of healing, it is likely that there are underlying factors that have not been completely addressed. Go back and carefully evaluate each of the factors related to the wound for that patient. Usually, the problem is not that one has chosen the wrong dressing, but that one has failed to identify and correct an underlying factor such as malnutrition, osteomyelitis, or inadequate blood supply.

Cuddigan J, Frantz RA: Pressure ulcer research: Pressure ulcer treatment. A monograph from the National Pressure Ulcer Advisory Panel. Adv Wound Care 11:294–300, 1998.

KEY POINTS: PRINCIPLES OF PRESSURE ULCER CARE

1. Prevention is paramount in management and should be addressed continually.

2. Correct the *underlying* medical, biologic, environmental, and psychological factors that initially led to the development of the ulcer and prevented it from healing.

3. Wounds must be adequately débrided before healing can occur.

4. Maintain a moist wound environment to maximize wound healing.

24. **Why is the patient's serum albumin sometimes low in the presence of proper nutritional support?**
The most common reason is inadequate protein intake. However, there may be other reasons. Serum albumin is an acute phase reactant, which decreases during times of acute illness. Albumin may also be lost through a highly exudative wound. The serum prealbumin, which indicates whether there is adequate protein intake, can differentiate between excess protein loss (normal prealbumin) and inadequate protein intake (low prealbumin). Its half-life is much shorter than albumin and, therefore, represents a more up-to-the-minute evaluation of nutritional intake.

24. **How much protein is needed to heal a pressure ulcer?**
Recommendations for protein requirements for persons with pressure sores range from 1.5–2.0 grams of protein/kilogram of ideal body weight/day. The key is to substitute protein calories for carbohydrate and fat calories, not just add them. Obesity can become a significant problem for patients with decreased activity and increased caloric intake during the prolonged healing time.

Thompson C, Fuhrman MP: Nutrients and wound healing: Still searching for the magic bullet. Nutr Clin Pract 20(3):331–347, 2005.

25. **How is osteomyelitis underlying a pressure ulcer diagnosed?**
The gold standard for diagnosis of osteomyelitis is pathologic findings in a bone biopsy. Plain radiographs can be helpful, but changes on x-ray develop late in the course of osteomyelitis. Bone scans are rarely useful because of the high false-positive rate in the presence of a pressure ulcer. Magnetic resonance imaging has been shown to be sensitive and specific for osteomyelitis underlying a pressure ulcer. However, only the bone biopsy can also give culture information to guide antibiotic selection.

Darouiche RO, Landon GC, Klima M, et al: Osteomyelitis associated with pressure sores. Arch Intern Med 154:753–758, 1994.

WEBSITES

National Pressure Ulcer Advisory Panel
www.npuap.org/about.htm

CHAPTER 62

NEUROGENIC BLADDER: PATHOPHYSIOLOGY, DIAGNOSIS, AND REHABILITATION

Inder Perkash, MD, MS

The length of a film should be directly related to the endurance of the human bladder.
—Alfred Hitchcock (1899–1980)

1. **How is neurogenic bladder defined?**
   A bladder is considered neurogenic if there are impairments in function that result from abnormalities in the peripheral or central nervous system (CNS). Voluntary control problems include sensory problems, inability to perceive bladder fullness, inability to voluntarily initiate micturition, and incontinence. The result is urinary retention and/or incontinence. Neurologic disorders can affect the brain, brain stem, spinal cord, or peripheral nerves to cause these problems.

2. **What are the neural pathways linking the bladder to the CNS?**
   The organizational center for micturition in the brain is localized in the **pontine-mesencephalic reticular formation.** Lesions above this level (suprapontine) are usually associated with **detrusor hyperreflexia,** whereas intrapontine supraconal lesions are always associated with **detrusor–sphincter dyssynergia.** The micturition center in the spinal cord is localized primarily in the intermediolateral region of **spinal cord segments S2–S4,** with S3 being the most important nerve root for bladder innervation.
   The human bladder is supplied by both the parasympathetic (motor and sensory) and the sympathetic nervous systems. The **pelvic parasympathetic nerves** (S2–S4) innervate the detrusor muscle and carry both motor and sensory fibers. Preganglionic parasympathetics extend from the spinal cord to the synapse with postganglionic fibers in the bladder wall. Preganglionic fibers originate in the spinal cord, and postganglionic fibers originate in the bladder wall and innervate the bladder through short loops. The urethra traverses the pelvic floor, which includes the periurethral and external and urethral sphincters innervated by the **pudendal nerves** (S1–S4). The innervation of most of the striated muscles of the pelvic floor, including those of the periurethral and anal sphincter, is through the pudendal nerve arising from S1–S4.

3. **Describe the physiology of micturition.**
   The first sensation of filling occurs at approximately 100 mL and a feeling of fullness is perceived at 300 mL. This feeling of fullness is registered at the frontal parietal cortex. The filling bladder can be ignored and micturition inhibited, or it can be resolved with a voluntary void. The bladder is very compliant and may accommodate high urine volumes of more than 500 mL, because of the passive viscoelastic properties and beta-adrenergic sympathetic stimulation. Therefore, both inhibition and initiation are under voluntary control of the cerebral cortex, and continence is achieved. However, during sudden vigorous activities such as jumping, coughing, or dancing, continence is maintained reflexively via the conus with the **holding reflex.**

4. **How does a spinal cord injury (SCI) tip the balance?**

   The pelvic floor becomes spastic, making the holding reflex hyperactive. Complete spinal cord injury above the conus prevents sensations and voluntary bladder control. As the bladder fills and pressures rise, sudden reflex detrusor contractions attempt to force urine out. Reflex contractions of the pelvic floor (external urethral sphincter) prevent the void, resulting in urine retention or intermittent leakage when the sphincter relaxes (detrusor–sphincter dyssynergia).

5. **What is the role of sympathetic innervation of the bladder and bladder neck?**

   Motor and sensory sympathetic nerves originate in the **intermediolateral cell columns** of spinal cord segments T11–L2 and promote urine storage and continence. These nerves traverse the paravertebral ganglia to the hypogastric plexus to the bladder wall, bladder neck, and posterior urethra.

   The bladder wall (fundus or body) primarily exhibits **beta-adrenergic receptors** and responds to norepinephrine by relaxing. There is also an abundance of beta-adrenergic receptors at the bladder base, which includes the upper trigone and vesicoureteral junction. This helps bladder storage by relaxing the detrusor muscle.

   The bladder neck (vesicoureteral junction) is predominantly supplied with **alpha-adrenergic fibers.** There is a high density of alpha-adrenergic receptors along the bladder neck, particularly in males. This helps to prevent retrograde ejaculation and also helps close the bladder neck during bladder filling. Because alpha-adrenergic activity leads to closure of the bladder neck, alpha-adrenergic blockers (alpha-adrenergic antagonists) usually are used to improve voiding by relaxing the bladder neck.

6. **What basic bedside neurourologic assessments provide initial clinical data for urologic management?**

   The **history** should elicit specific impairments in bladder sensation, storage, and voiding. The **general neurologic examination** should localize the primary neural lesion. **Rectal examination** is used to evaluate sphincter tone and voluntary strength, bulbocavernous reflex, and the prostate gland for benign or malignant enlargement. In women, **vaginal examination** may reveal cystocele, rectocele, uterine support, and the course of the urethra. Toe plantar flexors (S2) and hip external rotator (S1) strength provide information about the integrity of sacral spinal cord segments that also supply the external urethral sphincter (S2).

   An **abdominal examination** is important to feel for a distended bladder, as well as palpation before and after attempted voiding. In patients with SCI, attempted voiding can be promoted by **suprapubic tapping** over the bladder, **Valsalva maneuver,** and **Credé** (suprapubic pressure). However, objective evaluation of micturition problems can be accomplished only by urodynamic testing.

   Postvoid residual (PVR) measurements are made by allowing the patient's bladder to fill naturally to capacity and then having the patient attempt to void voluntarily in a natural position (standing or sitting). Measurement of the voided volume is compared with the residual volume obtained by catheterization or ultrasound. A PVR > 100 mL or more than about 20% of the total voided urine is considered abnormal.

7. **How is a routine urodynamic evaluation done?**

   The term **video urodynamics** refers to the simultaneous pressure flow studies with fluoroscopic visualization of the lower urinary tract. Similar studies can also be done using transrectal ultrasonography to simultaneously visualize the lower urinary tract.

   Cystometry (CMG) is the recording of intravesical pressures during bladder filling. It requires introduction of a catheter through the urethra and slow filling of 20–50 mL/min of water at body temperature. During bladder filling, intravesical pressure usually does not rise above 20 cm H_2O before bladder contraction. Compliance decreases and pressure increases at smaller volumes in patients with an overactive bladder. Detrusor–sphincter dyssynergia and repeated urinary tract infections (UTIs) can lead to bladder wall stiffness caused by detrusor hypertrophy or fibrosis, which reduces compliance and may contribute to reduced bladder capacity. PVR can increase because of outflow obstruction.

8. **What is detrusor compliance?**
Compliance is defined as the increase in bladder pressure per unit of volume introduced and is calculated by the change in volume divided by the change in pressure (Δ V/Δ P). The detrusor wall is composed of roughly equal amounts of muscle and collagen. When the collagen is more abundant, the elasticity decreases, the detrusor becomes stiffer, and the pressure rises faster during filling. Hypertrophic, spastic (neurogenic) detrusor muscle can lead to compliance as well.

   Wyndaele JJ, Madersbacher H, Kovincha A: Conservative treatment of the neuropathic bladder in spinal cord injured patients. Spinal Cord 39:294–300, 2001.

9. **What is detrusor–sphincter dyssynergia?**
The normal process of voiding includes a balanced synergy of simultaneous bladder wall contraction and sphincter relaxation. Detrusor–sphincter dyssynergia is a pathologic hyperactive holding reflex characterized by the presence of involuntary pelvic floor urinary sphincter contraction and increased electromyographic (EMG) activity during detrusor (bladder wall) contraction. This is observed in patients with spinal cord lesions below the pons and is absent in those with intracranial lesions. In patients with partial neurologic lesions, it is sometimes difficult to differentiate involuntary sphincteric activity such as dyssynergia from voluntary contractions to inhibit micturition. A careful evaluation is therefore required to diagnose detrusor–sphincter dyssynergia in a patient with a normal neurologic examination.

10. **How are the bulbocavernous reflex and sacral evoked potential tested? Why?**
The bulbocavernous reflex is a polysynaptic (S2–S4), crossed sacral withdrawal reflex and a nociceptive reflex of very constant latency. Clinically, it can be tested by squeezing the glans or clitoris and feeling the contraction of the anal sphincter muscle. This reflex is present in all normal persons and in SCI patients with lesions above the conus. The bulbocavernous reflex can also be recorded objectively by stimulating the dorsal nerve of the penis and picking up the EMG response (50–200 μV) in the anal sphincter muscle or from the perineal striated muscle.
   The **sacral-evoked response** can be obtained either by stimulating the dorsal nerve of the penis with a ring electrode or by placing a stimulating needle on the left or right side of the bulbocavernosus muscle in the perineum to define a unilateral lesion. The **first latency** (about 12 m/sec) can be recorded over T4–L1 on the back, which represents the sensory peripheral conduction time. The **central conduction time** can be recorded at the scalp, which is usually 50 msec. Patients with previously diagnosed neurologic disease and those with subtle abnormalities on neurologic screening are candidates for this type of evaluation. Sacral-evoked potential testing and somatosensory-evoked potential testing should not be used as screening tests but rather as objective measurements of the location, presence, and nature of afferent penile sensory dysfunction. The findings of such testing can aid in anatomic localization of the lesion as peripheral, sacral, or suprasacral.

11. **Which type of neurourologic dysfunction is typically found in patients with upper motor neuron lesions?**
The pattern of vesicourethral dysfunction depends on the site of the spinal lesion and any preexisting or associated disease, such as diabetes mellitus, radiculopathy, and ethanol abuse, which can reduce detrusor contraction. Prostate enlargement and urethral stricture can cause obstruction. Initially after an acute spinal injury, there is widespread autonomic paralysis **(spinal shock phase),** which often recovers by 3–6 weeks but can take longer. The reappearance of reflexes below the level of injury heralds the end of the spinal shock. The bladder can easily become overdistended due to preventing the return of reflex detrusor contraction. Later, the

appearance of detrusor–sphincter dyssynergia leads to intermittent voiding (squirting of urine alternating with retention of urine). Bladder emptying can then be accomplished with intermittent catheterization. Baseline urodynamic testing is usually performed 6–8 weeks after acute injury, when the changes in function associated with recovery and reflex return have been stabilized.

Intermittent catheterization can be started as early as 7–15 days after injury. Fluid intake may need to be restricted to <1500 mL/day. The bladder is drained with a straight catheter (Foley size 14 or 16) every 4 hours with a target bladder volume of no more than 500 mL. After the establishment of bladder reflex, the patient is evaluated objectively with urodynamic monitoring of intravesical voiding pressures (leak pressure). A **cystometrogram (CMG)** may need to be repeated to evaluate the effect of anticholinergics on voiding pressures. Persistently high voiding pressures (>40–50 cm H_2O) with sustained rise during CMG may necessitate a further increase in the dosage of anticholinergics.

To start, patients are given oxybutynin (Ditropan), 2.5–5 mg two or three times per day, to lower intravesical pressure to <40–50 cm H_2O. Patients who do not tolerate regular oxybutynin, particularly because of dryness of the mouth, can be given either longer-acting oxybutynin or tolterodine. There is some evidence that tolterodine may have less effect on muscarinic receptors in the salivary glands. This helps to achieve continence between catheterizations; therefore, patients do not have to wear external drainage and leg bags.

Wyndaele JJ, Madersbacher H, Kovincha A: Conservative treatment of the neuropathic bladder in spinal cord injured patients. Spinal Cord 39:294–300, 2001.

12. **What is the best way to provide bladder drainage in patients with acute spinal cord injury?**
During the first 7–14 days, an indwelling catheter should be left in the bladder for drainage to prevent inadvertent overdistention. A small catheter (F14 or F16) is recommended, which prevents urethral irritation and allows periurethral secretions to drain easily around it. Most patients who have severe injuries require an indwelling catheter to monitor fluid intake and output because they are on intravenous fluids.

Silver JR, Doggart JR, Burr RG: The *reduced* urinary output after spinal cord injury: A review. Paraplegia 33:721–725, 1995.

Van Kerrebroeck PE, Amarenco G, Thuroff JW, et al: Dose-ranging study of tolterodine in patients with detrusor hyperreflexia. Neurourol Urodyn 17:499–512, 1998.

13. **Which method provides optimal long-term drainage of the neurogenic bladder?**
Patients who have a reflex bladder, particularly tetraplegics, cannot catheterize themselves but can wear an external drainage condom. These patients should be considered for surgical reduction of outflow obstruction. Transurethral sphincterotomy (TURS), or stenting of the urethral sphincter, reduces outflow resistance to enable voiding at low pressure. This also helps to reduce the autonomic dysreflexia triggered by detrusor–sphincter dyssynergia.

A patient with a small retractile penis with reflex bladder may be considered for a penile implant to allow a better water seal of the condom catheter. Other patients who cannot self-catheterize and have a small retractile penis may need an indwelling catheter or suprapubic cystostomy.

In female patients who cannot self-catheterize and are incontinent, vesical or supravesical diversion, such as a suprapubic cystostomy or bowel pouch, may be considered. Continent reservoirs that can be catheterized through sites on the abdomen are also available. Currently, such patients are also considered for dorsal root (rhizotomy) and sacral motor root electrical stimulation to permit functional electric stimulation for voiding.

Perkash I: Long-term urologic management of the patient with spinal cord injury. Urol Clin North Am 20:423–434, 1993.

Perkash I: Contact laser sphincterotomy: Further experience and longer follow-up. Spinal Cord 34:227–233, 1996.

KEY POINTS: NEUROGENIC BLADDER

1. The term *neurogenic bladder* refers to organ level dysfunction (impairment) that results from central or peripheral nervous system damage.

2. The pelvic parasympathetic nerve (S2–S4) innervates the detrusor muscle (bladder wall) with motor and sensory fibers. S3 is usually the major nerve.

3. The somatic mixed pudendal nerve (S2–S4) includes motor and sensory fibers and innervates the pelvic floor, which includes the external anal sphincter. S2 is the key nerve.

4. Detrusor–sphincter dyssynergia is the simultaneous contraction of the detrusor (bladder wall) and external anal sphincter (pelvic floor), which generates excessive bladder pressures (>50 cm H_2O).

5. Detrusor–sphincter dyssynergia occurs with lesions of the spinal cord above the conus. Persistent high-pressure voiding (with pressures beyond 50 cm H_2O) is associated with hydronephrosis and deterioration of renal function over the years.

6. Supraconal bladder dysfunction is associated with bilateral paralysis of toe movement, hyperreflexic phasic stretch reflexes of the gastrocsoleus muscles (SI), and positive bulbocavernosus and anocutaneous reflexes.

14. **Describe the usual protocol for urologic follow-up of patients with spinal cord injury.**

    Patients with SCI are monitored with annual ultrasounds of the kidneys, ureters, and bladder to detect renal parenchymal loss, hydronephrosis, and stones. The annual risk for bladder stones is 4% with indwelling catheters. Blood urea nitrogen (BUN) and serum creatinine (Cr) levels are compared with previous years. Levels of serum creatinine, which is a muscle metabolite, may be normally as low as 0.5 mg/dL in some tetraplegics who lack muscle mass. **Radionuclide renal perfusion imaging** is used to evaluate glomerular filtration and renal plasma flow. This is done if needed to further quantify renal function.

    If hydronephrosis of the kidneys or ureters is noted or deterioration of the renal function is found, a full work-up, including **CT scanning with dye or intravenous urogram** and **voiding cystourethrogram** may be needed. **Cystoscopic examination** is also done to evaluate outflow obstruction and/or to rule out other bladder problems such as tumors. A cystoscopic examination with visualization and biopsy to detect bladder cancer is recommended for patients who have been heavy smokers or who have used chronic indwelling catheters for years.

    Ord J, Lunn D, Reynard J: Bladder management and risk of bladder stone formation in spinal cord injured patients. J Urol 170(5):1734–1737, 2003.

    Yang CC, Clowers DE: Screening cystoscopy in chronically catheterized spinal cord injury patients. Spinal Cord 37(3):204–207, 1999.

15. **What bladder problems are seen in patients with brain injury?**

    Following head injury or other intracranial lesions, the bladder is hyperreflexic, but there is no dyssynergia. Initially, there may be retention of urine, and patients can be managed with an indwelling catheter followed by intermittent catheterization every 4–6 hours. Some patients may have an enlarged prostate, which may require treatment later. Involuntary leakage of urine can be controlled with a small dosage of oxybutynin or tolterodine. Inadequate voiding caused by internal sphincter resistance can be improved with the use of alpha blockers such as **terazosin,** an alpha-receptor antagonist, starting with a dose of 1 mg at night and titrating up to an effective dose (1–5 mg twice daily). Effectiveness of this therapy on voiding needs to be assessed with postvoid residual measurements, with gradually increasing the dose as needed over several days. All autonomic drugs are gastrointestinal irritants and therefore should be given with meals. Initially, patients may not tolerate the prolonged postural hypotension, so they are given a low dose until they get used to the drug.

In patients with intracranial lesions such as parkinsonism, the bladder also is hyperreflexic. The use of drugs (anticholinergics) to manage tremors may lead to retention of urine. In all such patients with detrusor hyperreflexia, a transurethral resection of the prostate can sometimes result in permanent incontinence. There is also some evidence that oxybutynin is more lipid-soluble and thus may have higher concentration in the brain. This might influence reversible short-term memory problems.

Perkash I: Intermittent catheterization failure and an approach to bladder rehabilitation in spinal cord injury patients. Arch Phys Med Rehabil 59:9–17, 1978.

Perkash I: Long-term urologic management of the patient with spinal cord injury. Urol Clin North Am 20:423–434, 1993.

Sugiyama T, Park YC, Jurita T: Oxybutynin disrupts learning and memory in the rat passive avoidance response. Urol Res 27:393–395, 1999.

16. **What are the common urinary tract complications of neurogenic bladder? How can they be prevented?**
   - The earliest changes in the bladder are noticed as **trabeculations** seen inside an irregular, thickened bladder wall and even small diverticuli, seen on voiding cystographic studies.
   - **Vesicoureteral reflux** has been recorded in 10–30% of poorly managed patients. The presence of reflux is a serious complication because it leads to pyelonephritis and renal stone disease.
   - **Severe bladder outflow obstruction** can result in bilateral hydronephrosis and hydroureters and even an overdistended areflexic bladder.
   - Repeated **bladder infections** can lead to bladder wall changes and marked reduction in the compliance of the bladder.

   All of these bladder wall changes can be prevented to some extent by adequately draining the bladder at a pressure below 40 cm H_2O, either by intermittent catheterization along with the use of anticholinergic drugs or by timely surgical relief of the outflow obstruction.

   Perkash I: Controlling UTIs in patients with spinal cord injuries: Maintaining low intravesical voiding pressures is crucial. J Crit Illness 11(Suppl):41–48, 1996.

17. **How common are UTIs in patients with SCI?**
   UTIs and their sequelae are the most frequent medical complications experienced by patients with spinal cord injury. In persons who have long-term indwelling catheters or suprapubic catheters, the presence of bacteriuria is almost universal. The incidence of bacteriuria is reduced significantly in patients who can perform intermittent self-catheterization. Repeated UTIs have been associated with bladder biolayer (similar to biofilm on ureteral catheters) on the bladder wall.

   Reid G, Kang YS, Lacerte M, et al: Bacterial biofilm formation on the bladder epithelium of spinal cord injured patients. II: Toxic outcome on cell viability. Paraplegia 31:494–499, 1993.

18. **What constitutes a significant UTI in a patient with SCI?**
   A significant UTI is one accompanied by a 1.5°F rise in body temperature with positive urine microbial culture and a large number of pus cells. Ordinary spun urine showing >5–10 pus cells/high-power microscopic field is considered to indicate tissue infection. If this is observed in patients on intermittent catheterization, it may require treatment. In the absence of fever, an asymptomatic infection may not be treated in patients with indwelling or suprapubic catheters. The urine culture can be obtained by introducing a new clean catheter to avoid cultures from the old biofilm.

   Cardenas DD, Hooton TM: Urinary tract infection in persons with spinal cord injury. Arch Phys Med Rehabil 76:272–280, 1995.

19. What preventive measures can be taken to reduce the risk of UTIs?

Patients wearing external condom drainage with voiding pressures <50 cm H_2O, particularly following TURS, are relatively safe from UTIs, but they need to clean the external drainage bag and tubing with 6% bleach. A daily thorough washing will clean the appliances. Personal hygiene with showering and adequate cleaning of the perineum and a daily cleaning of the cushion cover may reduce pelvic floor colonization and subsequent anterior urethral heavy colonization and contamination.

20. List the drugs used in the management of bladder problems and their desired effects.

Options for pharmacologic manipulation of bladder function are outlined in Table 62-1. Tolterodine and oxybutynin as anticholinergics are available to manage detrusor hyperreflexia. Most of the autonomic drugs that change arteriolar tone also seem to have effect on the bladder neck (e.g., alpha agonists constrict the bladder neck and alpha blockers relax the bladder neck).

In the human bladder (detrusor muscle) there are muscarinic receptors (M2 and M3). M3 receptors, compared with M2, are small in number but are mainly responsible for bladder contraction. Antimuscarinic drugs (oxybutynin, tolterodine, darifenacin, solifenacin, and trospium chloride) are the five major drugs currently available to manage detrusor hyperreflexia and to help reduce bladder voiding pressures. Comparative clinical studies have shown that

TABLE 62-1. PHARMACOLOGIC MANIPULATION OF BLADDER FUNCTION		
Desired Functional Change	**Drug**	**Mode of Action**
Improve bladder emptying Facilitate bladder contraction (muscarinic action)	Bethanechol (clinically used)	Limited indications. It should not be used with outlet obstruction or in suspected coronary disease. It can be used in selected patients along with alpha-sympathetic blockers and in patients with atonic or hypotonic bladder.
Decrease outlet resistance	Prazosin, terazosin, doxazosin (clinically used) Phenoxybenzamine (mutagenic in laboratory animals) Tamsulosin (newer selective blocker)	Alpha-adrenoceptor blockers improve voiding by opening bladder neck.

Continued

TABLE 62-1. PHARMACOLOGIC MANIPULATION OF BLADDER FUNCTION—CONT'D

Desired Functional Change	Drug	Mode of Action
Reduce bladder contraction Increase outlet resistance	Atropine, propantheline, oxybutynin, tolterodine, trospium, chloride, darifenacin, solifenacin, phenylephrine, ephedrine	Anticholinergic action (antimuscarinic action) Sympathetic agonist response, alpha-adrenergic receptors
Improve bladder storage and increase outlet resistance	Tricyclic antidepressants	Central and peripheral anticholinergic effects and enhancement of alpha-adrenergic effect on bladder base and proximal urethra.

oxybutynin and solifenacin may be marginally more effective than tolterodine, although the latter seems to be better tolerated. Dry mouth and constipation are still major problems for patient compliance with all of them because of widespread existence of M3 receptors, particularly in the salivary glands.

Schwantes U, Topfmeier P: Importance of pharmacological and physicochemical properties for tolerance of antimuscarinic drugs in the treatment of detrusor instability and detrusor hyperreflexia—chances for improvement of therapy. Int J Clin Pharmacol Ther 37:209–218, 1999.

BIBLIOGRAPHY

1. Gray GJ, Yang C: Surgical procedures of the bladder after spinal cord injury. Phys Med Rehabil Clin North Am 11:57–72, 2000.
2. Perkash I: Urologic diagnostic testing. In Lennard TA (ed): Pain Procedures in Clinical Practice, 2nd ed. Philadelphia, Hanley & Belfus, 2000, pp 66–74.
3. Rutkowski SB, Middleton JW, Truman G, et al: The influence of bladder management on fertility in spinal cord injured males. Paraplegia 33:263–266, 1995.
4. Stohrer M, Goepel M, Kondo A, et al: Standardization of terminology in neurogenic lower urinary tract dysfunction, with suggestions for diagnostic procedures. Neurourol Urodyn 18:139–158, 1999.
5. Yang CC, Cardenas DD: Bladder management in women with neurologic disabilities. Phys Med Rehabil Clin North Am 12(1):91–110, 2001.

CHAPTER 63

NEUROGENIC BOWEL DYSFUNCTION: EVALUATION AND ADAPTIVE MANAGEMENT

Steven A. Stiens, MD, MS, Lance L. Goetz, MD, and Jonathan Strayer, MD

This is a fundamental principle of medicine, that whenever the stool is withheld or is extruded with difficulty, grave illnesses result.

—Maimonides (1135–1204)

1. **How are the large intestine and pelvic floor innervated?**

   Colonic peristalsis is orchestrated by a series of nerve cells that link the brain to the colonic mucosa (Fig. 63-1). The **vagus** (vagabond) nerve wanders from the brain stem and innervates the gut all the way to the splenic flexure of the colon. The **nervi erigentes** (inferior splanchnic nerve) carries pelvic parasympathetic fibers from the S2–S4 conal spinal cord levels to the descending colon and rectum. The descending colon receives sympathetic innervation from the **hypogastric nerve** (L1–L3). The enteric nervous system includes unmyelinated fibers from postganglionic parasympathetic ganglia and interneurons that coordinate peristalsis. **Auerbach's (intramuscular, or myenteric) plexus** is located between the circular and longitudinal muscle layers, and **Meissner's (submucosal, or under the mucosa) plexus** relays

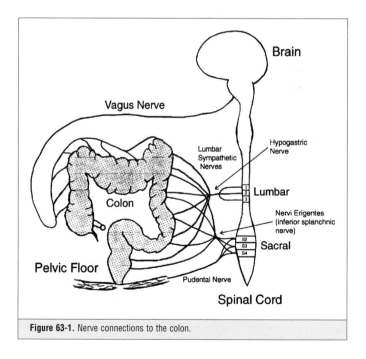

Figure 63-1. Nerve connections to the colon.

sensory and local motor responses. The external anal sphincter is supplied by the somatic **pudendal nerve** (S2–S4), which innervates the pelvic floor.

Stiens SA, Fajardo NR, Korsten MA: The gastrointestinal system after spinal cord injury. In Lin V (ed): Spinal Cord Injury Medicine: Principles and Practice. New York, Demos, 2003, pp 321–349.

2. **What is the "law of the intestine"?**
   In 1899, two English physiologists, W.M. Bayliss and E.H. Starling, reported that whenever the intestinal wall is stretched or dilated, the nerves in the myenteric plexus cause the muscles above the dilation to constrict and the muscles below the dilation to relax, propelling the contents toward the anus.

   http://med.plig.org/2/8.html

3. **What is the normal physiologic sequence of steps that lead to defecation?**
   Reflex activity
   1. **Giant migratory contractions** start at the cecum and advance stool through the colon to the rectum.
   2. Stool distends the rectum as the internal sphincter relaxes **(rectal inhibitory or sampling reflex),** which triggers a conscious "urge."
   3. Contraction of the external anal sphincter and puborectalis muscle retains stool **(holding reflex).**
   Voluntary activity
   1. Relaxation of the external anal sphincter and puborectalis releases stool.
   2. Contraction of the levator ani, external abdominals, and diaphragm, combined with glottic closure, elevates intra-abdominal pressure and propels stool out.

4. **What nervous system lesions produce the various patterns of neurogenic bowel dysfunction?**
   Neurogenic bowel is a term that relates colon dysfunction (constipation, incontinence, and discoordination of defecation) to lack of nervous control.
   - The **upper motor neuron (UMN) bowel** results from a spinal cord lesion above the conus medullaris and typically manifests as fecal distention of the colon, overactive segmental peristalsis, hypoactive propulsive peristalsis, and a hyperactive holding reflex with spastic external anal sphincter constriction that requires mechanical or chemical stimulus to trigger reflex defecation.
   - The **lower motor neuron (LMN) bowel** results from a lesion that affects the parasympathetic and somatic pudendal cell bodies on axons at the conus, cauda equina, or inferior splanchnic nerve and the pudendal nerve. LMN bowel findings include low descending colonic wall tone and a flaccid pelvic floor and anal sphincter. No spinal cord–mediated reflex peristalsis occurs. Slow stool propulsion is coordinated by the myenteric plexus alone, and incontinence is common with movement. The denervated colon produces a drier, rounder (scybalous) stool because the prolonged transit time results in increased absorption of moisture from the stool.

   Stiens SA, Biener-Bergman S, Goetz LL: Neurogenic bowel dysfunction after spinal cord injury: Clinical evaluation and rehabilitation management. Arch Phys Med Rehabil 78:S86–S102, 1997.

5. **What is the internal anal sphincter? How does it fit into the anal sphincter mechanism?**
   The internal anal sphincter is the thick layer of colonic smooth muscle that surrounds the anal canal at the distal rectum. It is the major contributor to the resting pressure of the closed anal canal. Closure is maintained by tonic excitatory sympathetic (L1, L2) discharges. Anal dilatation by stool **(rectoanal inhibitory reflex)** or digital stimulation inhibits internal sphincter tone. Those experienced in bowel care are frequently able to palpate an increase in internal sphincter tone after defecation, which is a clinical sign that defecation is over and bowel care

should be completed. The **anal sphincter mechanism** includes the internal anal sphincter, external anal sphincter, and the puborectalis muscle that wraps around the distal rectum to kink it forward toward the pubis to maintain continence.

6. **What is the difference between a bowel program and bowel care?**
   Although the terms are frequently interchanged, the most correct usage is as follows:
   - A **bowel program** is the individualized comprehensive management plan for prevention of the problems that come with neurogenic bowel dysfunction. A bowel program has a variety of components, which include diet, fluid intake, physical activity, medications, and consistent scheduled bowel care.
   - **Bowel care** is the individualized procedure for initiating and completing a bowel movement. It is the process for assisted defecation. Bowel care may include any or all of the following steps: preparation, positioning, checking for stool, inserting rectal stimulant medications, digital rectal stimulation, manual evacuation, recognizing completion, and clean-up.

   Stiens SA, Biener-Bergman S, Goetz LL: Neurogenic bowel dysfunction after spinal cord injury: Clinical evaluation and rehabilitation management. Arch Phys Med Rehabil 78:S86–S102, 1997.

7. **How is digital stimulation done?**
   Digital rectal stimulation is a technique for inducing reflex peristaltic waves of the colon to evacuate stool. The procedure is performed by gently introducing the entire gloved and lubricated finger into the rectum. Moving the finger in a circular pattern opens the external anal sphincter by providing a stretch stimulus that reduces spastic tone and outflow resistance. Rotation of the gloved finger in a firm circular manner produces stimulation, maintaining contact with the rectal mucosa, and dilates the proximal rectum. It is important to continually maintain contact with the mucosa. Rotation is continued until the bowel wall relaxes, flatus passes, stool comes down, or the internal sphincter constricts. This maneuver activates peristalsis locally (coordinated by the myenteric plexus) and stimulates conal-mediated reflex peristalsis. Ideally, digital stimulation should require no more than 1 minute to generate peristalsis, but the procedure can be repeated every few minutes as needed to aid in stool evacuation.

8. **Describe the bowel care used to facilitate reflex defecation for a person with a UMN bowel.**
   Persons with UMN injuries need a scheduled trigger of defecation every 1–3 days because they are unable to feel the stool in the rectum or to voluntarily initiate defecation. A person with spinal cord injury (SCI) must regularly trigger bowel movements in order to predictably eliminate stool and avoid colonic overdistention. The defecation reflex is stimulated digitally with a finger (or assistive device) inserted in the rectum (digital stimulation) and/or with appropriate stimulant medication.

   The initial stimulant medication trigger is typically a suppository, enema, or mini-enema, which is placed against the mucosa in the upper rectum and produces a mucosal contact stimulus that initiates conus-mediated reflex peristalsis. The stimulant medication is placed against the mucosa in the upper rectum. After the active ingredients dissolve and disperse, stool flow begins and is augmented as necessary with digital stimulations. These stimulations are repeated every 5–10 minutes if no stool passes. End of bowel care is signaled by cessation of gas and stool flow, palpable internal sphincter closure, or the absence of stool from the last two digital stimulations. Patients frequently "sense" the end of defecation. This sensation signaling the end of bowel care is possibly mediated by visceral afferents or partial sacral sparing of anal afferents.

9. **What events and intervals mark the progress of the bowel care?**
   See Figure 63-2.

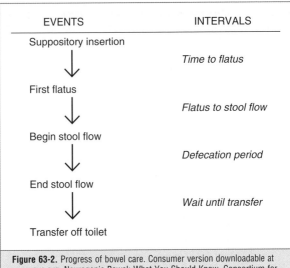

Figure 63-2. Progress of bowel care. Consumer version downloadable at www.pva.org. Neurogenic Bowel: What You Should Know, Consortium for Spinal Cord Medicine, 1999.

10. What is the gastrocolic response?

Feeding induces increased propulsive colonic motility mediated by cholinergic motor neurons. Some have referred to this increase in gut motility as the **gastrocolic reflex,** but the mechanism may not be exclusively neural and has yet to be conclusively defined. Proposals include central vagal mediation, intrinsic colon pathways, and humoral mediation via cholecystokinin or gastrin. This increase in peristalsis is facilitated by a fatty or proteinaceous meal and blunted by atropine. Some investigators have reported that the gastrocolic response is less robust yet still present after SCI.

Sun EA, Snape WJ, Cohen S, et al: The role of opiate receptors and cholinergic neurons in the gastrocolic response. Gastroenterology 82:689–693, 1982.

11. Describe the techniques to produce defecation and maintain continence in persons with LMN bowel dysfunction.

Persons with LMN injuries often have more difficulty with their bowel care because of low anal sphincter tone and the absence of spinal reflex peristalsis. The rectum must be cleared of stool frequently, usually one or more times per day, to prevent leakage of stool that cannot be retained by the patulous external sphincter. Rectal stimulant medications are not generally recommended for patients with LMN bowel, because the absence of a spinal cord–mediated reflex peristalsis limits their effectiveness. Some patients wear tight underwear or bicycle pants to support the pelvic floor and help retain stool.

The LMN bowel care procedure usually consists of removing stool with the finger **(manual evacuation)** and using digital stimulation to increase peristalsis. Continence is improved by modulation of stool consistency with a high-fiber diet. Plant fibers such as psyllium hydromucilloid "regularize" stool by absorbing and retaining excess water in order to prevent dry, hard stool.

12. What if the bowel care routine becomes excessively long, dependent, or complicated by autonomic dysreflexia or intractable bleeding hemorrhoids?

Some persons with long histories of SCI may have limited ability to independently manage their own bowel care, develop difficulty in maintaining continence, or evolve excessively long ineffective bowel routines with insufficient results. A **colostomy** offers independent bowel management, less incontinence, and reduced bowel care time, with an improvement in quality of life. A colostomy is generally an elective procedure and is usually reversible, although people with SCI who elect colostomy seldom have it reversed. Colostomies are often considered if severe bilateral grade 3 pressure ulcers are present.

Living With a Colostomy website: www.ostomy.fsnet.co.uk

13. **How can complications related to the neurogenic bowel be prevented?**
Complications include hemorrhoids, impaction, colonic diverticuli, rectal prolapse, perirectal abscess, megacolon, and colon cancer. Current prevention strategies include a high-fiber diet to maintain a soft stool. Supporting the pelvic floor with a gel or air cushion to distribute pressure over the entire perineal surface prevents the enlargement of hemorrhoids and maintains closure of the anal sphincter.

Following a regular schedule of bowel care sessions is important, even if stool elimination does not occur each time. Missed bowel care can contribute to excessive stool buildup, which makes the stool drier and more difficult to eliminate. Retained stool can overstretch the colon wall, reducing the effectiveness of peristalsis and resulting in longer bowel programs with poor results. Hemorrhoids can be prevented through frequent digital stimulations (to minimize the time necessary for the bowel program) and by avoiding constipation.

Gore RM, Mintzer RA, Calenoff L: Gastrointestinal complications of spinal cord injury. Spine 6:536–544, 1981.

14. **What laxative preparations should be avoided as chronic medication? Which are preferred?**
   - Chronic use of stimulant laxatives that are **anthraquinone derivatives,** such as senna, aloe, and cascara preparations, should be avoided because they may cause neuropathic damage to the myenteric plexus. Pigments from these laxatives also can stain the colonic mucosa (melanosis coli).
   - **Stool softeners or osmotic agents,** such as docusate sodium, sorbitol, milk of magnesia, polyethylene glycol (PEG), and mineral oil, are preferred.
   - **Daily fiber supplements** that contain cellulose, polysaccharide, or psyllium can improve stool consistency if adequate fluid intake is maintained.
   - **Chronic suppository use** is not known to cause colonic complications. Attempts to wean from bisacodyl suppositories to glycerine or to rely solely on reflex emptying from digital stimulation can be made over time.

Muller-Lisser SA, Kamm MA, Scarpignato C, Wald A: Myths and misconceptions about chronic constipation. Am J Gastroenterol 100:232–242, 2005.
Ramkumar D, Rao SSC: Efficacy and safety of traditional medical therapies for chronic constipation: Systematic review. Am J Gastroenterol 100:936–971, 2005.

15. **What medications are used to augment the bowel program?**
Oral agents
   - Fiber supplements such as psyllium hydromucilloid and calcium polycarbophil maintain stool moisture and bulk.
   - Docusate sodium is a surface-acting emulsifying agent that lubricates and maintains stool moisture.
   - Oral prokinetic agents such as metoclopramide and cisapride have been used to assist with acute hypomotility syndromes. However, serious cardiac arrhythmias with cisapride caused its withdrawal from the market. Oral or IV erythromycin has been shown to be a useful prokinetic agent for temporary use among critically ill patients.
Suppositories to trigger defecation
   - Glycerin—mild stimulus, lubricating

- Bisacodyl (phenolphthalein derivative)—a polyphenolic molecule that produces colonic mass action on contact and provides a stronger chemical stimulus; bisacodyl may be compounded with a vegetable oil or with a potentially faster-acting polyethylene base
- CO_2-generating suppositories—produce reflex defecation in response to colon dilatation; not uniformly reliable in persons with SCI

Enemas to trigger defecation

- **Enemeez** mini-enemas are rapid acting. They contain docusate sodium, polyethylene glycol, and glycerin (with or without benzocaine), which can reduce the incidence of autonomic dysreflexia by locally anesthetizing the rectal wall.
- Bisacodyl enemas with a water base are available as well.
- Large-volume enemas (i.e., 300 mL in volume), such as glycerine and mineral oil combination, saline, or soap suds, vary in use at different facilities and are poorly studied. These should be reserved for patients who are refractory to other medications.

Berne JD, Norwood SH, McAuley CE, et al: Erythromycin reduces delayed gastric emptying in critically ill trauma patients: A randomized, controlled trial. J Trauma 53(3):422–425, 2002.

House JG, Stiens SA: Pharmacologically initiated defecation for persons with spinal cord injury: Effectiveness of three agents. Arch Phys Med Rehabil 78:1062–1065, 1997.

16. **How can diarrhea in patients with neurogenic bowel be managed?**
Diarrhea can be related to gastrointestinal infection, food intolerance, or use of antibiotics (most common treatment for a urinary tract infection). Treatment in these patients is similar to that for patients without a neurogenic bowel and includes antidiarrheal agents, laboratory evaluation for infectious causes (including *Clostridium difficile,* when indicated), and discontinuation of offending agents. Commonly, diarrhea alternating with constipation is related to partial bowel obstruction with flow of diarrhea around an impaction. A rectal exam is essential in evaluating these patients and may relieve the obstruction. Higher impactions are revealed by stool-filled loops of bowel on plain radiographs and require complete evacuation of the bowel, usually with oral magnesium citrate preparations.

KEY POINTS: NEUROGENIC BOWEL DYSFUNCTION

1. Discover patient's past bowel habits.
2. Use examination to define pattern of defecation dysfunction.
3. Design a bowel program that can overcome impairments, build on past successes, and maximize life participation.
4. Specify frequency and methodology for bowel care.
5. Review patient outcome data.

17. **What is a continent appendicocecostomy stoma? What good is it for bowel care?**
The Malone, or antegrade continence enema (ACE), procedure surgically produces a catheterizable stoma that enters the cecum for self-administration of antegrade enemas to initiate bowel care. Through an 8-cm incision in the right lower quadrant, the appendix is localized and brought to the surface of the abdomen to form a stoma by amputating the tip to expose the lumen. The appendix is sewn into place and the stoma can be covered with a bandage. Bowel care is performed by catheterizing the cecum through the appendix, then

infusing 100–400 mL of saline to trigger defecation. Bowel care is completed in the classic manner of repeated digital rectal stimulation in order to promote peristalsis and liberate stool and enema liquid. The Malone procedure has been successful on many patients with spina bifida and a few with SCI.

Yang CC, Stiens SA: Antegrade continence enema for the treatment of neurogenic constipation and fecal incontinence after spinal cord injury. Arch Phys Med Rehabil 81:683–685, 2000.

18. **What is the importance of serotonin in gut function? What is tegaserod?**
It is now known that nearly all of the serotonin in the body resides in the gut, and serotonergic activity stimulates gut motility. Serotonin agonists such as tegaserod (Zelnorm) had been FDA approved only for short-term use and have been used for short-term treatment of irritable bowel syndrome and chronic constipation. Although they do not improve sensation of the need for defecation, serotonin agonists have generated interest for use in persons with SCI. The FDA has determined that tegaserod marketing should be discontinued due to increased risk for stroke, unstable angina, and myocardial infarction for those who use the drug. Patients who have been successfully treated with tegaserod have the option to continue the medication after documented education about the risks. Side effects, including dizziness, headache, and diarrhea, are common. Of course, it does nothing to improve sensation of the need for defecation, which is lacking in persons with SCI.

Layer P, Keller J, Mueller-Lissner S, et al: Tegaserod: Long-term treatment for irritable bowel syndrome patients with constipation in primary care. Digestion 71(4):238–244, 2005; Epub, July 12, 2005.
Read NW, Gwee KA: The importance of 5-hydroxytryptamine receptors in the gut. Pharmacol Ther 62(1–2):159–173, 1994.
www.fda.gov/cder/drug/infopage/zelnorm/zelnorm_QA_2007.htm

19. **What is the pulsed irrigation evacuation (PIE)?**
This relatively new device is used for bowel evacuation in persons who have difficulty using more conservative measures. PIE has been used in hospital settings and by persons at home. The system delivers warm water in a palatial fashion to act like a "superenema." Some SCI centers have used PIE in bowel preparation for procedures or for persons with chronic severe obstipation. Long-term efficacy data are unavailable.

Accidents Stink!: Bowel Care 202 (a 50-minute comedy film demonstrating bowel care). www.conceptsinconfidence.com, 1-800-822-4050.
www.piemed.com

20. **What is the point of all this effort?**
Social continence! Education of clinicians, patients, and caregivers is essential. We all must be "brethren in the bowel." To more fully participate in public life, persons with SCI need to develop mastery over their bowels. After all, accidents stink!

WEBSITES

1. www.bowelcontrol.org.uk

2. Neurogenic Bowel Management in Adults with Spinal Cord Injury
www.guideline.gov/summary/summary.aspx?ss=15&doc_id=850&nbr=394

BIBLIOGRAPHY

1. King R, Biddle A, Braunschweig C, et al: Clinical practice guidelines: Neurogenic bowel management in adults with spinal cord injury: Guideline group, consortium for spinal cord medicine. Washington, DC, Paralyzed Veterans of America, 1998.

2. Lisenmeyer TA, Stone JM, Stiens SA: Neurologic bladder and bowel management. In DeLisa JA (ed): Rehabilitation Medicine: Principles and Practice, 3rd ed. Philadelphia, J.B. Lippincott, 2005, pp 1619–1644.

3. Stiens SA, Braunschweig C, Cowel JF, et al: Clinical practice consumer guideline: Neurogenic bowel: What you should know—a guide for people with spinal cord injury: Consortium for spinal cord medicine. Washington, DC, Paralyzed Veterans of America, 1999.

4. Stiens SA, King J: Neurogenic bowel management. In Braddom R (ed): Physical Medicine and Rehabilitation, 3rd ed. Philadelphia, W.B. Saunders, 2007, pp 637–649.

5. Stiens SA, Pidde T, Veland B, David M: Accidents Stink: Bowel Care 202 [video]. PVA Education and Training Foundation, 2002. http://conceptsinconfidence.com/, 2002, [1-800-424-8200].

CHAPTER 64

COMMUNICATION AND SWALLOWING IMPAIRMENTS: ASSESSMENT AND REHABILITATION

Donna C. Tippett, MPH, MA, CCC-SLP, Kenneth H. Silver, MD, and Jeffrey B. Palmer, MD

Think like a wise man, but communicate in the language of the people.
—William Butler Yeats (1865–1939)

1. **Explain how speech and language are different.**
   - The term ***speech*** refers to motor acts that result in the production of sounds through the coordination of muscles involved in respiration, phonation, resonance, and articulation.
   - The term ***language*** refers to the symbolic organization of sounds into meaningful and purposeful words and sentences to represent thought.

2. **Who should be referred for a speech-language pathology evaluation?**
   Anyone with a suspected communication or swallowing impairment should be referred for a speech-language pathology evaluation. The effects of communication and swallowing problems can be minimized, and sometimes eliminated, with proper evaluation and treatment. If there is a question regarding the appropriateness of a referral, speech-language pathologists can perform a screening before giving a lengthy assessment. It is appropriate to obtain a speech-language pathology consultation within 24–48 hours after an individual is admitted to the hospital for an acute event, especially if dysphagia is suspected. Indications of dysphagia include drooling, "squirreling" of food in the mouth, gurgly voice after swallowing, and coughing after swallowing. Orders for speech-language pathology consultations are increasingly part of the admitting orders and are included on stroke pathways.

3. **Discuss some of the causes of communication disorders and dysphagia.**
   The etiologies of these disorders may be **developmental** (e.g., language delay secondary to mental retardation, dysarthria secondary to cerebral palsy) or **acquired** (e.g., aphasia following left hemisphere stroke, cognitive/communicative impairment following traumatic brain injury, dysarthria associated with multiple sclerosis, alaryngeal speech following laryngectomy, dysphagia secondary to brain stem stroke).

4. **What influences prognosis and candidacy for speech-language intervention?**
   It is difficult to make a definitive statement regarding candidacy for speech-language treatment given the diversity of patient populations and disorders seen by speech-language pathologists. However, it is usually true that treatment should be deferred for patients who are obtunded, sedated, or very ill (*see* Table 64-1).

5. **How are aphasias classified?**
   There is no universally accepted nomenclature, and several schemes use different names for the same combination of symptoms (e.g., Wernicke's aphasia = receptive aphasia = syntactic aphasia). The advantages and disadvantages of aphasia classification continue to be debated in the literature, although one clear benefit is efficient communication among clinicians. The syndrome classification system, associated with the **Boston school of aphasia**, relies on an

TABLE 64-1. PROGNOSTIC FACTORS FOR SPEECH-LANGUAGE INTERVENTION

Variable	Prognostic Value
Age at onset of disorder	The older the patient, the poorer the prognosis
General health	The healthier the patient, the better the prognosis
Motivation and cooperation	High degrees of motivation and cooperation are favorable prognostic signs
Environmental factors	Family support can facilitate carryover of treatment objectives
Etiology	Progressive diseases are associated with poorer outcomes, but treatment may still be indicated to facilitate communication and swallowing via compensatory strategies
Initial speech-language pathology evaluation	Responsiveness to diagnostic treatment is a favorable outcome variable

examination of fluency, comprehension, repetition, and word finding to make the diagnosis (Fig. 64-1). As more is learned about brain structure and function, new types of aphasias are being identified. One recently recognized type is subcortical aphasia. This type of aphasia is associated with injuries to areas of the brain previously not identified with language and language processing (e.g., internal capsule, putamen, thalamus).

KEY POINTS: COMMON TYPES OF APHASIAS

1. **Fluent** or **Wernicke's aphasia:** Difficulty comprehending spoken or written language; speaking with words that are frequently unnecessary, misspoken, or even made up (neologisms)

2. **Nonfluent** or **Broca's aphasia:** Difficulty expressing oneself, either orally or in writing, often with slow, labored, telegraphic output

3. **Global aphasia:** Profound loss of ability to comprehend or express language

4. **Conduction aphasia:** Poor repetition relative to impairments in comprehension and expression

5. **Anomic aphasia:** Difficulty with word retrieval or word finding in oral and written expression; speech output characterized by vague circumlocutions; comprehension is well preserved

6. **Transcortical aphasia:** Repetition is preserved; comprehension and expression are impaired to varying degrees, depending on the location and extent of brain damage (transcortical motor, transcortical sensory aphasia, transcortical mixed)

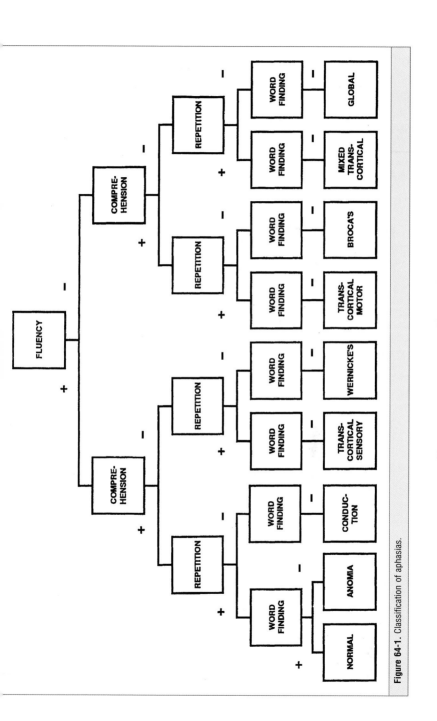

Figure 64-1. Classification of aphasias.

6. **How can the clinician distinguish fluent versus nonfluent aphasia?**
   Aphasias are often difficult to classify in practice. It is most important for a physician to recognize that a language problem is present and to initiate a referral to speech-language pathology. Fluent aphasias localize to the temporal area of the brain and may not be associated with a hemiparesis, making some people think that the individual is psychotic. However, these patients often have a hemianopsia or other subtle neurologic deficit. Nonfluent aphasias are associated with more anterior lesions, are near the motor strip, and are usually associated with a right hemiparesis, so the diagnosis of a left hemisphere lesion (e.g., cerebrovascular accident, tumor, abscess) is readily apparent.

7. **Explain the common terminology associated with aphasia.**
   See Table 64-2.

TABLE 64-2. COMMON TERMS ASSOCIATED WITH APHASIA		
Term	**Definition**	**Example**
Neologism	Substitutions of entirely invented words for correct ones	"Poofle" for "doctor"
Semantic paraphasia	Word substitutions belonging to the same semantic class	"Chair" for "table"
Phonemic paraphasia	Substitutions of one sound for another	"Fable" for "table"
Telegraphic speech	Speech output includes substantive words (e.g., nouns, verbs) and omits grammatical modifiers	"Girl eat cake"
Agrammatism	Sparse, hesitant groping speech limited to the most essential content words	
Echolalia	Meaningless repetition of other's utterances	
Palilalia	Pathologic repetition of syllables or sounds; associated with degenerative brain diseases	

8. **Describe the typical communication deficits seen in patients with right cerebral hemisphere damage.**
   These patients demonstrate relatively **intact language** but **impaired communication abilities**. Key features are insensitivity to context (i.e., missing nuances and subtleties), difficulty organizing information in a meaningful way (e.g., answering questions with tangential, unnecessary information), difficulty "reading" facial expressions and gestures, inability to understand figurative language, lack of affect, caustic sense of humor, impulsivity, left neglect, denial of deficits, better performance on structured than on open-ended tasks, and writing errors (e.g., omission/preservation of strokes, letters, or words; perseveration of strokes, letters, and words; failure to dot i's and cross t's; extra capitalization).

9. **Describe the typical communication deficits seen in patients with traumatic brain injury.**
Cognitive/communication problems that result from traumatic brain injury vary widely. The degree of deficit depends on multiple factors, including the location and severity of brain injury, as well as an individual's personality, and preinjury abilities. Cognitive/communication impairments include problems attending and concentrating, learning and remembering new information, organizing thoughts, making appropriate decisions, and interpreting figurative expressions. Insight regarding deficits is often diminished, necessitating the need for supervision to ensure safety. Social communication skills may be compromised, such as, turn taking and topic maintenance during conversation. Language deficits may be present, such as difficulty in finding the words to convey meaning.

10. **Should individuals with dementia be referred for a speech-language pathology evaluation and treatment?**
Both direct and indirect interventions can be beneficial to individuals with dementia. Direct interventions are those in which the speech-language pathologist intervenes with patients individually or in groups. Examples include repeated exposure to previously known information, facilitated recall, learning-by-doing systems, and multisensory stimulation. Indirect intervention includes caregiver training in communication strategies to optimize communication (e.g., simplified syntax, slower rate of speech, yes/no questioning), modification of the physical environmental modification (e.g., minimize distractions, increase lighting), and development of routines (e.g., seating assignments in the dining room). If there is the additional presentation of swallowing problems, the speech-language pathologist can ensure safe swallowing through compensatory strategies and/or diet alteration. The goal of intervention is to create strategies to preserve communication and cognitive functioning, as well as quality of life for as long as possible.

Hopper T: Indirect intervention to facilitate communication in Alzheimer's disease. Semin Speech Lang 22(4):305–315, 2001.
Tomoeda CK: Comprehensive assessment for dementia: A necessity for differential diagnosis and management. Semin Speech Lang 22(4):275–289, 2001.

11. **Define apraxia of speech.**
Apraxia is a disorder of the execution of learned movement that cannot be explained by weakness, incoordination, sensory loss, or lack of attention to commands. Apraxias include those of **construction, dressing, gait,** and **speech. Apraxia of speech** is characterized by highly variable and unpredictable substitutions of sounds, often unrelated to intended sounds, blockages and repetitions similar to stuttering, and slow, effortful output secondary to reduced capacity to program the positioning of speech muscles and the sequencing of muscle movements for the volitional production of sounds. There is no significant weakness, slowness, or incoordination of speech muscles in reflexive or automatic acts.

12. **What is agnosia?**
Agnosia is a disorder of recognition that may occur in any of the major sense modalities despite adequate perception in these modalities (e.g., audition, vision, tactile sensation). An auditory agnosia is an inability to match an environmental noise with its sound source. For example, a patient may not be able to recognize a watch from its ticking but can identify a watch placed in his hand. A visual agnosia is an inability to identify an object on visual confrontation. For example, a patient may not be able to identify his wife when shown a picture but can describe her appearance (e.g., blonde hair, blue eyes).

13. **How are the dysarthrias classified?**
Dysarthria is a **speech impairment,** not a language impairment like aphasia. Individuals with dysarthria are often difficult to understand and may have "slurred speech." They do not

have problems with listening, reading, writing, or spoken language (e.g., vocabulary, grammar). As with the aphasias, the dysarthrias can be classified in a variety of ways—age at onset, etiology, cranial nerve involvement, and speech component involvement. A well-known classification system is the Mayo Clinic approach, which reflects neuroanatomic and neurophysiologic bases for dysarthrias. Six types of dysarthrias are described based on perceptual features:

- Flaccid (in bulbar palsy)
- Spastic (in pseudobulbar palsy)
- Ataxic (in cerebellar disorders)
- Hypokinetic (in parkinsonism)
- Hyperkinetic (in dystonia and chorea)
- Mixed (in disorders of multiple motor systems, such as multiple sclerosis)

14. **How is speech production assessed?**
    Speech production is assessed by three major approaches. First, speech production can be assessed by examining nonspeech and speech aspects of each component of oral motor function in a systematic fashion (Table 64-3). The functional component approach includes the respiratory mechanism, larynx, velum/pharynx, tongue, lips, face, teeth, and jaw. Next, speech production can also be assessed by using commercially available tests. Finally, speech intelligibility is rated at single-word and connected-speech levels. Physicians can assess speech production briefly by asking patients to repeat words and phrases, rapidly produce words such as "Topeka" or "buttercup" to test speech diadochokinesis, and by rating the intelligibility of conversational speech.

    Netsell R, Daniel B: Dysarthria in adults: Physiologic approach to rehabilitation. Arch Phys Med Rehabil 60:502–508, 1979.

TABLE 64-3. NONSPEECH AND SPEECH TESTS OF ORAL MOTOR FUNCTION

Components	Nonspeech Tasks	Speech Tasks
Respiratory mechanism	Breathing rate at rest	Maximum sustained phonation
Larynx	Elevation with swallow	Ability to change pitch
Velum/pharynx	Velar position at rest	Maintenance of oral/nasal contrasts
Tongue	Lingual range of movement	Lingual articulation
Lips, face, and teeth	Facial symmetry	Labial articulation
Jaw	Mandibular strength against resistance	Mandibular assist for articulation

15. **How can individuals who have undergone laryngectomy speak?**
    Alaryngeal speech can be produced by the following means:
    - **Esophageal speech:** Air is trapped in the mouth or pharynx, propelled into the esophagus, and then released. Air flows through the upper esophageal sphincter, resulting in a belchlike sound.
    - **Artificial larynx:** There are two types of artificial larynges: an external type that is placed against the neck and an intraoral type. Both types are battery powered and produce a mechanical sound.

- **Tracheoesophageal puncture (TEP):** A small puncture is surgically created through the common wall between the trachea and the esophagus. A small, one-way shunt valve is inserted into this puncture. To speak, the individual inhales air through the tracheostoma and into the lungs and then covers the stoma with a finger. Air from the lungs is directed from the trachea, through the shunt valve, and into the esophagus. The esophagus vibrates, creating a sound source for speech.

With all of these methods, sound is shaped into words by the tongue, teeth, lips, and jaw.

16. **What are some communication alternatives to natural speech?**
    Alternatives can be divided into oral and nonoral options. A familiar oral option is the use of an electrolarynx by a laryngectomee. Electrolarynges are also useful short-term communication options for individuals who have tracheostomy tubes with inflated cuffs. Nonoral options include handwriting, gesture, and augmentative communication systems, which range from simple alphabet and picture boards to sophisticated computer systems. Amer-Ind is a gestural communication system based on American Indian hand signals that can be used with stroke patients. Augmentative communication systems can facilitate communication between caregivers, family members, and intubated or tracheostomized patients in intensive care settings.

17. **How can individuals with tracheostomy and ventilator dependency communicate orally?**
    Unidirectional speaking valves can restore oral communication for individuals with tracheostomy. A unidirectional speaking valve allows inhalation to occur at the level of the tracheostomy and exhalation through the larynx, mouth, and nose. Valve candidates must have generally intact laryngeal structure and function (e.g., valves cannot be used with individuals who have had a laryngectomy). The cuff of the tracheostomy tube must be deflated when a valve is used. Some valves are designed to be used in-line with ventilator circuitry. Recent studies have shown that ventilator-dependent individuals can achieve excellent oral communication via cuff deflation alone.

    Hoit JD, Banzett RB, Lohmeier HL, et al: Clinical ventilator adjustments that improve speech. Chest 124(4):1512–1521, 2003.
    Prigent H, Samuel C, Louis B, et al: Comparative effects of two ventilatory modes on speech in tracheostomized patients with neuromuscular disease. Am J Respir Crit Care Med 167(2):114–119, 2003.
    Suiter DM, McCullough GH, Powell PW: Effects of cuff deflation and one-way tracheostomy speaking valve placement on swallow physiology. Dysphagia 18(4):284–292, 2003.
    Tippett DC (ed): Tracheostomy and Ventilator Dependency: Management of Breathing, Speaking and Swallowing. New York, Thieme, 2000.

18. **Describe the stages of swallowing.**
    It is customary to divide the process of swallowing into three or four stages; however, these divisions are arbitrary.
    - The **oral preparatory stage** includes placement of food in the mouth and creation of a cohesive "bolus." This stage is not always considered separately and may be included in the oral stage of swallow.
    - The **oral stage** includes propulsion of the bolus into the pharynx by the tongue.
    - The **pharyngeal stage** includes initiation of the swallow response, velopharyngeal apposition, elevation and anterior movement of the larynx, epiglottic tilt, closure of the larynx, pharyngeal constriction, and opening of the cricopharyngeus.
    - In the **esophageal stage,** boluses are moved through the esophagus into the stomach by peristalsis.

    Logemann JA: Evaluation and Treatment of Swallowing Disorders. Austin, TX, PRO-ED, 1998.

19. **Does the presence of a gag reflex indicate that swallowing function is preserved?**

    There is a widespread misconception that the presence or absence of the gag reflex can predict swallowing function. The gag reflex is commonly tested as an indicator of swallowing function, and individuals without gag reflexes are often referred for swallowing evaluations. However, the gag reflex is a protective reflex to keep foreign material from entering the foodway and airway.

    It is **not** related to swallowing function. The gag reflex can be absent in individuals who swallow normally, and intact in individuals with dysphagia. Presence or absence of the gag reflex is difficult to assess because the response can be diminished with repeated attempts at elicitation.

    Davies AE, Kidd D, Stone SP, MacMahon J: Pharyngeal sensation and gag reflex in healthy subjects. Lancet 345(8948):487–488, 1995.

    Leder SB: Videofluoroscopic evaluation of aspiration with visual examination of the gag reflex and velar movement. Dysphagia 12(1):21–23, 1997.

20. **Define the terms *laryngeal penetration, aspiration,* and *silent aspiration*.**

    - **Laryngeal penetration** is the entrance of food, liquid, and/or secretions in the airway to the level of the true vocal folds.
    - **Aspiration** is the passage of food, liquid, and/or secretions in the airway through the level of the true vocal folds.
    - The term **silent** refers to the absence of any outward sign of difficulty (e.g., choking, coughing, throat clearing, watery eyes).

    Rosenbek JC, Robbins JA, Roecker EB, et al: A penetration-aspiration scale. Dysphagia 11(2):93–98, 1996.

21. **How useful is the bedside swallowing study?**

    The bedside swallowing study provides useful information about speech/oral motor status, oral stage of swallow, level of alertness, appropriate position for feeding, and ability to self-feed. Information from the bedside examination is used to determine if and how an instrumental examination should be conducted. There are limitations, however, particularly regarding pharyngeal events. Experienced dysphagia clinicians have been shown to miss aspiration 40% of the time at the bedside in individuals who were subsequently shown to aspirate on videofluoroscopy. This is because aspiration can be "silent," that is, without any outward indication such as coughing or throat clearing. Numerous studies have been conducted to identify clinical correlates of aspiration that improve our ability to predict the occurrence of this phenomenon. However, the bedside evaluation is not adequate for determining the physiologic basis for dysphagia and is usually not adequate for planning treatment. Instrumental evaluation is required for these purposes.

    Daniels SK, Ballo LA, Mahoney MC, Foundas AL: Clinical predictors of dysphagia and aspiration risk: Outcome measures in acute stroke patients. Arch Phys Med Rehabil 81(8):1030–1033, 2000.

    Logemann JA, Lazarus C, Jenkins P: The relationship between clinical judgment and radiographic assessment of aspiration. Presented at the American Speech-Language-Hearing Association Annual Meeting, Toronto, November, 1982.

    Rosenbek JC, McCullough GH, Wertz RT: Is the information about a test important? Applying the methods of evidence-based medicine to the clinical examination of swallowing. J Commun Disord 37(5):437–450, 2004.

    Tohara H, Saitoh E, Mays KA, et al: Three tests for predicting aspiration without videofluorography. Dysphagia 18(2):126–134, 2003.

22. **What is the videofluoroscopic swallowing study?**

    A **videofluoroscopic swallowing study** (VFSS) is a radiographic evaluation conducted by a speech-language pathologist and physician (radiologist or physiatrist) (Table 64-4). Patients are given liquid and solid foods impregnated with barium. Various maneuvers may be tried to facilitate safe, effective swallowing. Logemann (1998) developed the "modified barium swallow study" in which specific food types and amounts are used. The VFSS should go beyond identifying the presence or absence of aspiration. Impairments of each stage of swallow and the mechanism of laryngeal penetration/aspiration must be described. From this information, recommendations for intervention are based. The esophagus should be imaged whenever feasible, unless the risk of aspiration is too great or the patient cannot be positioned to examine the esophagus.

Logemann JA: Evaluation and Treatment of Swallowing Disorders. Austin, TX, PRO-ED, 1998.

TABLE 64-4.   COMPONENTS OF THE VIDEOFLUOROSCOPIC SWALLOWING STUDY

Study Quality	Results	Recommendations
Unacceptable	Pass versus fail No aspiration versus aspiration	
Adequate	Safe with purees; aspirates thin liquids	Recommend thickening liquids
Optimal	Premature loss of liquid boluses over the base of tongue; incomplete epiglottic tilt; silent laryngeal penetration and aspiration of liquids; diminished pharyngeal constriction; retention of puree boluses and subsequent overflow aspiration; improved airway protection using neck flexion when drinking liquids and using effortful swallow with purees	Recommend the compensations of neck flexion and effortful swallow; recommend swallowing rehabilitation to increase pharyngeal constriction

KEY POINTS: INDICATIONS FOR A VIDEOFLUOROSCOPIC SWALLOWING STUDY

1. When a swallow impairment is suspected, or if an individual is at high risk for dysphagia

2. When the clinical examination is insufficient to answer relevant questions

3. When nutritional and respiratory issues are of concern

4. When medical diagnosis is not established

5. When the direction for swallowing rehabilitation needs to be established

23. How do we identify and treat esophageal phase swallowing disorders?
Esophageal dysphagia may result from neuromuscular disorders, motility abnormalities, and intrinsic or extrinsic obstructive lesions. Webs, rings, or strictures of the esophagus can obstruct the lumen and might require dilatation. Esophageal motor disorders include conditions of either hyperactivity (e.g., esophageal spasm) or hypoactivity (e.g., weakness). Either of these can lead to ineffective peristalsis with retention of material in the esophagus after swallowing, and subsequent regurgitation back into the pharynx and aspiration. Methods to

assess esophageal dysfunction include barium-contrast esophagography with or without video recording, endoscopy, manometry, and scintigraphy.

24. **What is the fiberoptic endoscopic evaluation of swallowing?**
    A **fiberoptic endoscopic evaluation of swallowing** (FEES) involves passing an endoscope transnasally into the hypopharynx so that the foodway and airway can be observed before and after, but not during, the moment of swallowing. The image is blocked or "whited out" at the moment of swallow by the pharynx closing around the endoscopic tube. Solids and liquids are dyed green to improve visualization. FEES was first described by Langmore et al. (1988) and can be performed at the bedside by a speech-language pathologist. A modification of the FEES is the FEESST, which includes laryngopharyngeal sensory testing.

    Aviv JE: Sensory discrimination in the larynx and hypopharynx. Otolaryngol Head Neck Surg 116(3): 331–334, 1997.

    Langmore SE, Schatz K, Olsen N: Fiberoptic endoscopic examination of swallowing safety: A new procedure. Dysphagia 2(4):216–219, 1988.

25. **How much aspiration is too much?**
    The relationship between dysphagia, aspiration, and aspiration pneumonia is complex. Dysphagia and aspiration are necessary, but not sufficient, conditions for the development of aspiration pneumonia. Important risk factors are dependency for oral feeding, dependency for oral care, number of decayed teeth, tube feeding, more than one medical diagnosis, number of medications, and smoking. Aspiration of refluxed gastric contents is particularly injurious to the lung, as pH $\leq$ 2.4 destroys lung tissue.

    Langmore SE, Terpenning MS, Schork A, et al: Predictors of aspiration pneumonia: How important is dysphagia? Dysphagia 13(2):69–81, 1998.

    Yoneyama T, Yoshida M, Ohrui T: Oral care reduces pneumonia in older patients in nursing homes. J Am Geriatr Soc 50(3):430–433, 2002.

26. **What are some common compensations and exercises for dysphagia?**
    Recommendations for swallowing compensations and exercises are made by speech-language pathologists based on the results of bedside and instrumental swallowing evaluations (Table 64-5).

27. **Does electrical stimulation improve swallowing function?**
    Electrical stimulation to improve swallowing has received a great deal of attention in the clinical and research realms of dysphagia treatment. Freed et al. (2001) described the use of synchronized electrical stimulation of the thyrohyoid musculature through surface electrodes placed on the neck to treat dysphagia resulting from reduced laryngeal elevation. There are several concerns regarding the internal and external validity of this study. Burnett et al. (2003) used intramuscular stimulation of the mylohyoid, thyrohyoid, or geniohyoid muscles to study 15 healthy male volunteers and concluded that paired stimulation of these muscles should be evaluated in detail during swallowing as a possible means of augmenting laryngeal elevation and improving airway protection in patients with dysphagia. At this time, electrical stimulation remains controversial. Clinicians should defer use of this technique until there is additional sound research to support it.

    Burnett TA, Mann EA, Cornell SA, Ludlow CL: Laryngeal elevation achieved by neuromuscular stimulation at rest. J Appl Physiol 94(1):128–134, 2003.

    Coyle JL: Critical appraisal of a treatment publication: Electrical stimulation for the treatment of dysphagia. Perspect Swallowing Disord 11:12–15, 2002.

    Freed ML, Freed L, Chatburn RL, Christian M: Electrical stimulation for swallowing disorders caused by stroke. Respir Care 46(5):466–474, 2001.

    Humbert IA, Poletto CJ, Saxon KG, et al: The effect of surface electrical stimulation on thyolaryngeal movement in normal individuals at rest and during swallowing. J Appl Physiol 101(6):1657–1663, 2006.

    Ludlow CL, Humbert I, Saxon K, et al: Effects of electrical stimulation both at rest and during swallowing in chronic pharyngeal dysphagia. Dysphagia 22(1):1–10, 2007.

TABLE 64–5. SWALLOWING COMPENSATIONS AND EXERCISES

Swallowing Compensations	Purposes
Neck flexion	Prevent premature spillage over base of tongue; increase airway protection by widening the vallecula and putting the epiglottis in a more overhanging position
Head/neck rotation	Decrease retention of boluses by turning head/neck to the weaker side, closing off that side, and directing boluses to the stronger side
Mendelsohn maneuver	Sustain laryngeal elevation during swallow to increase airway protection
Supraglottic swallow	Adduct vocal folds to achieve improved airway protection
Masako maneuver	Protrude tongue through central incisors to increase pharyngeal constriction
Swallowing Exercises	**Purposes**
Shaker exercises	Head-raising exercises to augment opening of the cricopharyngeus
Lingual range of movement and strength against resistance exercises	Improve oral manipulation and control of boluses
Yawning exercises	Increase movement of the back wall of the throat
Falsetto exercises	Increase laryngeal elevation
Thermal/tactile stimulation	Improve initiation and timing of swallow response

WEBSITES

1. American Speech-Language-Hearing Association
   www.asha.org

2. Brain Injury Association of America
   www.biausa.org

3. Dysphagia Research Society
   www.dysphagiaresearch.org

4. National Aphasia Association
   www.aphasia.org

5. National Center for Neurogenic Communication Disorders
   http://cnet.shs.arizona.edu

6. National Institute of Neurological Disorders and Stroke (NINDS)
   www.ninds.nih.gov

CARDIAC REHABILITATION: RISK FACTOR REDUCTION, EXERCISE RESUMPTION, AND LIFESTYLE MODIFICATION

Yehoshua A. Lehman, MD, Steven A. Stiens, MD, MS, Gabi Zeilig, MD, and Ira G. Rashbaum, MD

CHAPTER 65

To resist the frigidity of old age one must combine the body, the mind and the heart—and to keep them in parallel vigor one must exercise, study and love.

–Karl von Bonstetten (1745–1832)

1. Who can benefit from cardiac rehabilitation (CR)?

Patients who have physiologic, functional, and psychosocial deficits related to impairments of the cardiovascular system can benefit from CR. This includes patients with the following diagnoses or cardiovascular conditions: ischemic heart disease, recent myocardial infarction, post–coronary artery bypass graft (CABG) surgery, postpercutaneous transluminal coronary angioplasty (PTCA), post–coronary artery stent, post–cardiac transplant, post–heart valve replacement, post–heart valve repair, stable angina, and congestive heart failure.

Bartels MN, Whiteson JH, Alba AS, Kim H: Cardiopulmonary rehabilitation and cancer rehabilitation. I. Cardiac rehabilitation review. Arch Phys Med Rehabil 87(3 Suppl 1):S46–S56, 2006.

2. What are the overall goals of the CR process?

- To reduce myocardial ischemia and the risk of infarction or sudden death
- To maximize cardiovascular capacity and fitness
- To maximize exercise tolerance and activities of daily living (ADL) performance
- To establish a patient-controlled and safe aerobic exercise program
- To provide guidelines for safe activities and work
- To control risk factors for coronary artery disease (CAD)
- To help patients cope with perceived stressors
- To utilize energy conservation and work simplification
- To improve quality of life

Agency for Health Care Policy and Research: Cardiac Rehabilitation Guidelines Panel: Cardiac Rehabilitation. Clinic Practice Guidelines no. 17. Rockville, MD, AHCPR, 1995, AHCPR publication no. 96-0672.

3. Describe the phases of the CR process.

The CR intervention sequence integrates into the classic medical continuum of care and management of any illness: prevention, acute care (medical/surgical), and rehabilitation. The typical patient referred for CR has sustained a myocardial infarction and/or undergone CABG. CR has, therefore, typically been divided into three sequential phases that bring the patient out of acute care:

- **Phase I:** Inpatient phase from hospital admission to hospital discharge (**phase IA:** medical/surgical/cardiac unit; **phase IB:** inpatient rehabilitation unit)
- **Phase II:** Outpatient training phase includes aerobic conditioning, reacquisition of full activity, risk factor management, and lifestyle changes

- **Phase III:** Maintenance phase, with patient-monitored continuation of the aerobic exercise program, risk-reduction strategies, and activity/work modifications

These phases represent a timeline for the process of intervention. It is important to recognize that many interventions continue through the phases on an ongoing basis and that the application of CR interventions should be tailored to the needs of each individual.

Halar EM (ed): Cardiac rehabilitation. Phys Med Rehabil Clin North Am 6(1), 1995 (entire issue).

4. **What are possible contraindications for entry into inpatient or outpatient exercise programs?**
   According to the American College of Sports Medicine, they are:
   - Unstable angina
   - Resting systolic blood pressure (BP) $\geq$ 200 mmHg
   - Resting diastolic BP $\geq$ 100 mmHg
   - Orthostatic BP drop or drop during exercise training of > 20 mmHg
   - Moderate to severe aortic stenosis
   - Acute systemic illness or fever
   - Uncontrolled atrial or ventricular dysrhythmias
   - Uncontrolled sinus tachycardia (120 bpm)
   - Uncontrolled congestive heart failure
   - Third-degree atrioventricular (AV) block
   - Active pericarditis or myocarditis
   - Recent embolism
   - Thrombophlebitis
   - Resting ST displacement (>3 mm)
   - Uncontrolled diabetes
   - Neurologic and orthopedic problems that prohibit exercise

5. **What are the foci of intervention during phase I, the inpatient phase of CR?**
   - Early ambulation and ADL training under supervision
   - Alleviation of anxiety and depression
   - Reassurance to reestablish patient's control of self
   - Patient education regarding rationale for treatment and exercises
   - Medical evaluation of cardiac injury, electrocardiogram (ECG) and enzyme changes, imaging
   - Development of a team knowledge base of the patient's previous activities and work and life roles, as well as current personal goals that he or she wants to achieve during CR
   - Establish modifiable risk factor reduction strategies
   - Assessment of cardiovascular function and impairments
   - Establish level of the risk for development of complications; risk stratification
   - Prescription and education with guidelines for activity and work after discharge

6. **Describe the relationship between heart rate, stroke volume, cardiac output, aerobic capacity, and the anginal threshold.**
   - The **maximum heart rate** (HR) is defined as the maximum HR obtained on an exercise stress test. It decreases with age and can be estimated for the normal population by subtracting the patient's age in years from 220.
   - **Stroke volume** (SV) is the amount of blood ejected with each ventricular contraction and increases with exercise to become maximum at 50% over the basal HR (resting HR).
   - **Cardiac output** (CO) equals HR × SV and relates directly to the total body oxygen consumption ($\dot{V}O_2$) because all O_2 consumed is delivered to the body tissues via the blood.
   - **Maximum aerobic capacity** ($\dot{V}O_{2max}$) is the greatest rate ($\dot{V}O_2$ mL/kg body mass/min) of O_2 consumption a person is capable of metabolizing, and it relates directly to maximum work output in watts. One way to understand and calculate $\dot{V}O_{2max}$ is to use the formula SV × HR × (arterial−venous O_2 difference), which integrates the delivery and extraction of O_2. Thus an

increase in CO, the product of SV × HR, and/or increase in arteriovenous O_2 difference increases the $\dot{V}O_{2max}$. The $\dot{V}O_{2max}$ decreases with age, inactivity, and after a myocardial infarction.

- The **anginal threshold** is defined as the CO at which myocardial O_2 demand exceeds O_2 delivered. An ischemic myocardium is not capable of maintaining the same cardiac workload, which results in a fall in CO, $\dot{V}O_{2max}$, and/or BP.

Franklin B: American College of Sports Medicine: Guidelines for Exercise Testing and Prescription, 6th ed. Indianapolis, ACSM, 2000.

7. **What are the risk factors for atherosclerotic coronary artery disease?**
The significant **risk factors** for developing CAD are age, male sex, elevated total cholesterol, elevated low-density lipoprotein (LDL) cholesterol, low level of high-density lipoprotein (HDL) cholesterol, elevated systolic or diastolic BP, diabetes, obesity, sedentary lifestyle, cigarette smoking, stress, family history of premature coronary disease, and ECG evidence of left ventricular hypertrophy.

From the risk factors reported in the Framingham study of 1984, one can define the **modifiable risk factors** as hypertension, cigarette smoking, hypercholesterolemia, inactivity, low HDL cholesterol (<35 mg/dL), obesity, hypertriglyceridemia, diabetes mellitus, and stress.

There is strong evidence that risk factor modification can cause regression of the atherosclerotic process. For example, a prospective study of patients randomized to a control group and monotherapy with simvastatin, lovastatin, colestipol, or niacin for cholesterol control demonstrated coronary atheroma regression, lower rates of CABG, and reduced mortality rates. Meta-analysis studies of randomized control trials of CR programs consisting of exercise training and risk factor management have demonstrated a 10% reduction in the 3-year mortality rate.

KEY POINTS: CARDIAC REHABILITATION

1. The maximum heart rate (HR) is defined as the maximum HR obtained on an exercise stress test, and can be estimated subtracting the patient's age in years from 220.

2. Stroke volume (SV) is the amount of blood ejected with each ventricular contraction and increases with exercise to become maximum at 50% over the basal HR (resting HR).

3. Cardiac output (CO) equals HR × SV and relates directly to the total body oxygen consumption ($\dot{V}O_2$), because all O_2 consumed is delivered to the body tissues via the blood.

4. Maximum aerobic capacity ($\dot{V}O_2$) is the greatest rate ($\dot{V}O_2$ mL/kg body mass/min) of O_2 consumption a person is capable of metabolizing, and it relates directly to maximum work output in watts.

8. **What are the major goals of phase II, the outpatient phase of CR?**
Besides continuing the goals of phase I CR, the major goals of phase II are as follows:
- To achieve cardiovascular conditioning and fitness via an aerobic exercise training program
- To achieve control of modifiable risk factors using psychosocial and pharmacologic interventions and lifestyle changes
- To achieve an early return to work

During phase II of the CR program, the patient will be educated to self-monitor for the appropriate level of exercise, work, or activities via HR monitoring and/or rating of perceived exertion and receive psychosocial support to reduce anxiety and depression. The CR phase II should result in improvements in $\dot{V}O_{2max}$, lowering of HR for a given exercise or workload, and reduced systolic BP and have beneficial peripheral effects on improvement of O_2 extraction/

utilization by skeletal muscle. It will also result in reduction of anxiety and depression and improved coping mechanisms.

Lakkat T, Venalainen J, Rauramma R, et al: Relation of leisure-time, physical activity, and cardiorespiratory fitness to the risk of acute myocardial infarction in men. N Engl J Med 330:1549–1554, 1994.

9. List the five major parts of a CR exercise prescription.

- **Modality:** The American College of Sports Medicine recommends that the exercise modality be "any activity that uses large muscle groups, that can be maintained for a prolonged period, and is rhythmic and aerobic in nature."
- **Intensity:** Either prescribed by target HR, rating of perceived exertion, or metabolic equivalents. It is usually 60–70% of $\dot{V}O_2$ for healthy patients.
- **Duration:** Depends on the mode and intensity of exercise. Usually it is 20–45 minutes initially and later may increase to 60-minute sessions.
- **Frequency:** While in the hospital daily and at least three times weekly while in the aerobic training and maintenance phases, usually skipping a day between intensive sessions.
- **Rate of progression:** Depends on the patient's individual tolerance, progress, endurance, needs, and goals.

10. What is the purpose of a warm-up period?

The warm-up period, usually lasting 5–10 minutes, increases the intensity of exercise gradually from rest to the desired intensity level and also stretches the major muscles that will be used. This warm-up decreases the risk of cardiovascular problems (i.e., delay in onset of angina) and prevents sprain or strain injuries. Some patients, such as those with cardiac transplants and congestive heart failure, need longer periods of warm-up before proceeding to the more intensive aerobic exercises.

11. What is the purpose of a cool-down period?

It allows gradual reduction of cardiac work and redistribution of blood from muscles and extremities to internal organs. A gradual reduction of exercise intensity with continued body movements maintains venous return; prevents pooling of blood in the lower limbs, postexercise hypotension, and end-organ insufficiencies; and promotes continuous dissipation of heat.

12. What are the major interventions of phase III, the maintenance phase of CR?

Phase III has the same goals as phase II (the training phase), except that the program is monitored by the patient and/or family. The program continues outside the CR center, in a community-based setting or wherever the patient feels comfortable. The members of the CR team (i.e., physician, therapist, nutritionist, psychologist, social worker) may be available to assist and advise the patient as needed. The patient continues the level of exercise program achieved and self-monitors his or her own exercises and activities in order to avoid overexertion. Periodic evaluations should be done to monitor the patient's progress and tolerance and maintenance of previously achieved goals. Before beginning or changing the exercise program, the patient should check with his or her doctor.

Ornish D, Brown S, Scherwitz L, et al: Can lifestyle changes reverse coronary heart disease? The Lifestyle Heart Trial. Lancet 336:129–133, 1990.

13. Which changes in lifestyle for CAD are beneficial?

Aggressive lifestyle changes in respect to control of hypertension and smoking, dieting with <10% of total calories from fat, combined with 3 hours of aerobic exercise per week as well as stress management have been demonstrated to produce clinically significant regression in coronary atherosclerosis, as documented by coronary arteriography. In the Lifestyle Heart Trial Study, patients on the American Heart Association–recommended diet of <30% fat showed progression of their coronary atherosclerosis on repeat catheterization. Such studies suggest that conventional recommendations for patients with CAD are not sufficient to abate or reverse the disease process.

A CR dietary program should provide the metabolites needed for muscle adaptation with exercise, reduce risk factors associated with lipids and body fat content, and establish a body habitus that minimizes cardiac work, thus maximizing functional independence. In an attempt to approach this dietary ideal, the amount as well as the content of the diet needs to be calculated. The incidence of myocardial infarction in depressed patients is significantly greater, and depression after myocardial infarction increases morbidity and mortality; thus, pharmacologic and psychological intervention are both important components of CR. Adequate social support enhances recovery of patients and is a buffer against stresses.

14. **What factors cause reduced cardiovascular capacity after spinal cord injury (SCI)?**
Reduced exercise capacity in SCI patients is multifactorial. These factors include impaired autonomic nervous system control of the cardiovascular system; altered hormonal effects on the cardiovascular system; loss of the muscle pump causing decreased venous return, muscle weakness, and/or atrophy; altered respiratory system; small size of cardiac chambers; greater use of type II over type I muscle fibers; and sedentary lifestyle.

15. **What modes of aerobic exercise training can be used in SCI patients?**
Wheelchair propulsion, arm ergometry, wheelchair cycling using an arm crank, functional electrical stimulation (FES), and hybrid exercise (arm ergometry combined with lower-extremity FES).

16. **Should patients with congestive heart failure be excluded from CR?**
No. Stabilized and compensated patients with congestive heart failure are capable of achieving an increase in functional capacity up to 20%. Slow progression in the intensity and duration of each exercise session, applied for at least 3 months and thereafter continued with a maintenance program, has demonstrated a significant improvement in functional capacity in these patients.

17. **What about cardiac transplant?**
Because of denervation of the heart, the HR increases only in response to changes in circulating catecholamines. Intervention in transplant recipients includes a longer warm-up, slowly progressive endurance exercise at 50–60% of maximum HR, followed by longer cool-down periods. Cardiac transplant patients are characteristically very deconditioned and need conditioning and CR programs.

18. **What about other patients under rehabilitative care who may have risk factors for coronary disease and cardiac complications?**
The list of patients is enormous and includes geriatric patients, those with stroke, those with a previous history of cardiac abnormalities, etc. These patients should be rehabilitated within the guidelines of cardiac precautions.

Pang MYC, Eng JJ, Dawson AS: Relationship between ambulatory capacity and cardiorespiratory fitness in chronic stroke. Influence of stroke—specific impairments. Chest 127:495–501, 2005.

19. **What are the recommendations for a general exercise program for stroke survivors?**
- **Aerobic exercise:** Large-muscle activities such as walking, treadmill, stationary cycle, combined arm–leg ergometry, arm ergometry, seated stepper. *Intensity:* 40–70% heart rate reserve; 40–70% peak oxygen uptake; 50–80% maximal heart rate; 11–14 (6–20 scale) rating of perceived exertion (RPE). *Duration:* 20–60 min/session (or multiple sessions). *Frequency:* 3–7 days/week.
- **Strength:** Circuit training, weight machines, free weights, isometric exercise. *Intensity:* 1–3 sets of 10–15 repetitions of 8–10 exercises involving the major muscle groups. *Frequency:* 2–3 days/week.

- **Flexibility:** Stretching. *Intensity:* 2–3 days/week (before or after aerobic or strength training). *Duration:* Hold each stretch for 10–30 seconds.
- **Neuromuscular:** Coordination and balance activities. *Duration:* 2–3 days/week (consider performing on same day as strength activities).

  Gordon NF, Gulanick M, Costa F, et al: Physical activity and exercise recommendations for stroke survivors. Stroke 35:1230–1240, 2004.

20. **What is the gold standard for evaluating cardiorespiratory fitness?**
    Measurement of maximal oxygen consumption ($\dot{V}O_{2max}$) during the maximal exercise test.

    Skerker R: Review and update. The aerobic exercise prescription. Crit Rev Phys Med Rehabil 2:257–271, 1991.

21. **What are the most suitable modalities for assessment of the cardiorespiratory fitness of individuals with chronic stroke and residual disabilities?**
    - The cycle ergometry provides a better estimation of $\dot{V}O_{2max}$ than the 6 minute walk test (MWT), since the 6 MWT is also influenced by other factors such as balance, strength, and spasticity problems found in chronic stroke patients.
    - The treadmill with harness support could be a valid alternative.

    Pang MYC, Eng JJ, Dawson AS: Relationship between ambulatory capacity and cardiorespiratory fitness in chronic stroke. Influence of stroke-specific impairments. Chest 127:495–501, 2005.

WEBSITES

American Heart Association

1. www.americanheart.org/presenter.jhtml?identifier=1200000

2. www.nlm.nih.gov/medlineplus/tutorials/cardiacrehabilitation/htm/index.htm

BIBLIOGRAPHY

1. Agency for Health Care Policy and Research: Cardiac Rehabilitation Guidelines Panel: Cardiac Rehabilitation. Clinic Practice Guidelines no. 17. Rockville, MD, AHCPR, 1995, AHCPR publication no. 96-0672.
2. Franklin B: American College of Sports Medicine: Guidelines for Exercise Testing and Prescription, 6th ed. Indianapolis, ACSM, 2000.
3. Gordon NF, Gulnick M, Costa F, et al: Physical activity and exercise recommendations for stroke survivors. Stroke 35:1230–1240, 2004.
4. Halar EM (ed): Cardiac rehabilitation. Phys Med Rehabil Clin North Am 6(1): 1995, (entire issue).
5. Hansen D, Dendale P, Berger J, Meeusen R: Rehabilitation in cardiac patients: What do we know about training modalities? Sports Med 235(12):1063–1084, 2005.
6. Lakkat T, Venalainen J, Rauramma R, et al: Relation of leisure-time, physical activity, and cardiorespiratory fitness to the risk of acute myocardial infarction in men. N Engl J Med 330:1549–1554, 1994.
7. Ornish D, Brown S, Scherwitz L, et al: Can lifestyle changes reverse coronary heart disease? The Lifestyle Heart Trial. Lancet 336:129–133, 1990.
8. Pang MY, Eng JJ, Dawson AS, et al: Relationship between ambulatory capacity and cardiorespiratory fitness in chronic stroke. Influence of stroke-specific impairments. Chest 127:495–501, 2005.
9. Pashkow F, Dafoe W (eds): Clinical Cardiac Rehabilitation: A Cardiologists Guide, 2nd ed. Baltimore, Williams & Wilkins, 1999.
10. Skerker R: Review and update. The aerobic exercise prescription. Crit Rev Phys Med Rehabil 2:257–271, 1991.
11. Zwisler AD, Schou L, Soja AM , et al, for the DANREHAB group: A randomized clinical trial of hospital-based, comprehensive cardiac rehabilitation versus usual care for patients with congestive heart failure, ischemic heart disease, or high risk of ischemic heart disease (the DANREHAB trial)—design, intervention, and population. Am Heart J 150(5):899.e7–899.e16, 2005.

CHAPTER 66

PULMONARY REHABILITATION: IMPROVING DYSPNEA, ENDURANCE, AND WELL-BEING

John R. Bach, MD, and Heakyung Kim, MD

Keep your fears to yourself, but share your inspiration with others.
—Robert Louis Stevenson (1850–1894)

People who want to make a living from the treatment of nervous patients must clearly be able to do something to help them.
—Sigmund Freud, MD (1856–1939)

1. **List the two basic categories of respiratory diseases.**
   - Intrinsic versus mechanical
   - Obstructive versus restrictive

   Intrinsic or obstructive disease results in **oxygenation impairment,** and patients are normally eucapnic or hypocapnic, despite hypoxia. Patients with mechanical dysfunction of respiratory muscles, lungs, or chest wall have **ventilatory impairment** causing retention of CO_2, which causes hypoxia secondarily.

   Bach JR: Management of Patients with Neuromuscular Disease. Philadelphia, Hanley & Belfus, 2004.

VENTILATORY IMPAIRMENT (CO_2 RETENTION)

2. **List the diseases causing ventilatory impairment that are amenable to respiratory rehabilitation.**
   Ventilatory impairment can result from any neuromuscular or skeletal disorder that causes respiratory muscle dysfunction without oxygenation impairment from lung intrinsic disease. Patients with diagnoses listed in Box 66-1 are often candidates for physical medicine alternatives to endotracheal intubation or ventilatory support and airway secretion management via indwelling airway tubes.

3. **What do patients with primarily ventilatory impairment need in order to benefit from noninvasive respiratory interventions?**
   Patients who can benefit most from physical medicine and general rehabilitation interventions must have the following:
   - Ability to be able to cooperate and learn
   - Preservation of adequate bulbar-innervated muscle function to use equipment and techniques that can optimize general physical functioning, including the various inspiratory and expiratory muscle aids and oximetry feedback that can optimize pulmonary function.

   In general, only patients with advanced, averbal bulbar amyotrophic lateral sclerosis and spinal muscular atrophy type 1, without adequate parental involvement, can require tracheostomy to prolong survival.

> **BOX 66-1. CONDITIONS CAUSING VENTILATORY IMPAIRMENT AMENABLE TO PHYSICAL MEDICINE INTERVENTION**
>
> - Myopathies
> - Muscular dystrophies
> - Dystrophinopathies (Duchenne and Becker dystrophies)
> - Other muscular dystrophies (limb-girdle, Emery-Dreifuss, facioscapulohumeral, congenital, childhood autosomal recessive, and myotonic dystrophy)
> - Sleep-disordered breathing (including obesity hypoventilation)
> - Non–Duchenne myopathies (congenital and metabolic myopathies, polymyositis, myasthenia gravis)
> - Neurologic disorders
> - Spinal muscular atrophies
> - Motor neuron diseases
> - Kyphoscoliosis
> - Poliomyelitis
> - Chronic obstructive pulmonary disease
> - Traumatic tetraplegia and other myelopathies
> - Neuropathies (phrenic neuropathies, Guillain-Barré syndrome)
> - Multiple sclerosis

4. **State the seven most common errors in evaluating and managing patients with ventilatory impairment.**
   1. Misinterpretation of symptoms that are caused by hypercapnia and inspiratory muscle weakness
   2. Failure to do spirometry with the patient supine and to monitor maximum insufflation capacity
   3. Use of arterial blood gas analyses instead of oximetry and noninvasive CO_2 monitoring
   4. Administration of oxygen, periodic intermittent positive-pressure breathing (IPPB), continuous positive airway pressure (CPAP), or inadequate bilevel positive airway pressure (BiPAP) when noninvasive respiratory muscle aids are indicated
   5. Use of methylxanthines and any other respiratory medications on an ongoing basis without evidence of bronchospasm
   6. Failure to prevent acute respiratory failure and hospitalization
   7. Resort to tracheostomy when peak cough expiratory flows exceed 3 L/sec

5. **Name the clinical parameters critical for monitoring patients with neuromuscular disease.**
   - Vital capacity (VC) and maximum insufflation capacity (MIC) via spirometry
   - Peak cough flows (PCF), unassisted and assisted
   - Oxyhemoglobin saturation (SpO_2) via oximetry
   - End-tidal carbon dioxide ($EtCO_2$) via capnography

6. **What is the maximum insufflation capacity?**
   The MIC is the maximum volume of air that a patient can hold with a closed glottis. It correlates with bulbar-innervated muscle function and pulmonary compliance. It can be provided by the "air stacking" (holding with a closed glottis) of consecutively delivered volumes of air from a volume ventilator or manual resuscitator or by glossopharyngeal breathing (GPB).

7. **What are respiratory muscle aids?**
   The respiratory muscles can be aided by applying manual or mechanical forces to the body or intermittent pressure changes to the airway. The devices that act on the body include the

negative-pressure body ventilators (NPBVs), which create atmospheric pressure changes around the thorax and abdomen; body ventilators and forced exsufflation devices, which apply force directly to the body to mechanically displace respiratory muscles; and devices that apply intermittent pressure changes directly to the airway.

Bach JR: Update and perspectives on noninvasive respiratory muscle aids. Part 1: The inspiratory muscle aids. Chest 105:1230–1240, 1994.

Bach JR: Update and perspectives on noninvasive respiratory muscle aids. Part 2: The expiratory muscle aids. Chest 105:1538–1544, 1994.

8. **What are the ideal inspiratory muscle aids for long-term daytime use?**
    Mouthpiece intermittent positive pressure ventilation (IPPV) and the intermittent abdominal-pressure ventilator (IAPV) are both very effective for daytime use. For **mouthpiece IPPV,** a mouthpiece is mounted near the mouth, adjacent to the sip-and-puff, tongue, or chin controls for a motorized wheelchair, where the patient can easily grab it approximately 2–10 times a minute as needed for full ventilatory support.

    The **IAPV** intermittently inflates an air sac contained in a corset or belt worn beneath the patient's outer clothing. Inflation by a positive-pressure ventilator moves the diaphragm upward, causing a forced exsufflation. During deflation, the abdominal contents and diaphragm fall to the resting position, and inspiration occurs passively. Because it depends on gravity, a trunk angle of at least 30 degrees from horizontal is necessary for the IAPV to be effective. The IAPV augments tidal volumes by 250–1200 mL. Patients with < 1 hr of ventilator-free breathing ability often prefer to use the IAPV when sitting rather than use noninvasive methods of IPPV.

Bach JR, Alba AS, Saporito LR: Intermittent positive pressure ventilation via the mouth as an alternative to tracheostomy for 257 ventilator users. Chest 103:174–182, 1993.

Bach JR, Baird JS, Plosky D, et al: Spinal muscular atrophy type I: Management and outcomes. Pediatr Pulmonol 34:16–22, 2002.

9. **What are the ideal inspiratory muscle aids for nocturnal use?**
    - **Nasal IPPV delivered via CPAP masks (nasal interfaces)** has become the most popular method of noninvasive nocturnal ventilatory support. At least three or four different nasal interfaces should be tried by each patient to determine which ones are preferred. Many patients use different styles on alternate nights to vary skin contact pressure.
    - **Mouthpiece IPPV with Lipseal retention** (Respironics International, Murrysville, PA) is a more effective but generally less preferred method of nocturnal ventilatory support. With the Lipseal mouthpiece, IPPV can be delivered during sleep with less insufflation leakage, and with little risk of the mouthpiece falling out of the mouth. However, speaking clearly is difficult.

Bach JR: A comparison of long-term ventilatory support alternatives from the perspective of the patient and care giver. Chest 104:1702–1706, 1993.

10. **How can airway secretions be best eliminated in this population?**
    At least 3 L/sec of expiratory flow is necessary to bring airway secretions out of the airway and into the mouth. However, whether using a ventilator or not, patients with primarily ventilatory impairment are often unable to generate adequate peak cough flows without assistance. With the use of an insufflation to >1.5 L and with a properly timed abdominal thrust, PCF can usually be increased to 3–7 L/sec. When scoliosis, abdominal distention, trauma, moderate bulbar muscle dysfunction, or obesity interfere with manually assisted coughing, a mechanical insufflator-exsufflator can be used to provide more than 4 L/sec of peak expiratory flow with cough.

Gomez-Merino E, Bach JR: Duchenne muscular dystrophy: Prolongation of life by noninvasive respiratory muscle aids. Am J Phys Med Rehabil 81:411–415, 2002.

11. **What is a mechanical insufflator-exsufflator?**

A mechanical insufflator-exsufflator (e.g., CoughAssist mechanical in-exsufflation, or MI-E, "Cough Machine," Cofflator [J.H. Emerson, Cambridge, MA]) is a device that clears bronchopulmonary secretions by applying positive pressure to the airway, and then rapidly shifting to negative pressure. The rapid shift produces a high expiratory flow, simulating a cough with PCFs of greater than 4 L/sec. These pressures are delivered via mask, endotracheal tube, or tracheostomy tube to be effective. Full lung expansion and complete emptying are required in 4–8 seconds. This usually necessitates machine pressures of approximately 40 to –40 cm H_2O. A concomitant abdominal thrust is applied during the exsufflation with negative pressure phase.

12. **When do you use a mechanical insufflator-exsufflator?**

Patients with neuromuscular disorders, high spinal cord injury, traumatic brain injury, or cerebral palsy, who have less than 5 L/sec PCF of manually assisted or unassisted cough flows or severe fatigue, can benefit from its use. Relative contraindications are bullous emphysema, pneumothorax, pneumomediastinum, recent barotrauma, impaired consciousness, or inability to communicate.

13. **Describe the symptoms and signs of hypoventilation (hypercapnia).**

Fatigue, shortness of breath, morning or continuous headaches, sleep awakenings with shortness of breath, poor concentration, frequent nightmares, and symptoms and signs of heart failure, such as lower limb swelling, irritability, anxiety, decreased libido, frequent arousal from sleep to urinate, impaired intellectual function, depression, excessive weight loss, muscle aches, and memory impairment.

14. **Which factors decrease blood oxyhemoglobin saturation (SaO_2)?**

- Hypoventilation causing hypercapnia
- Airway obstruction (usually mucus)
- Intrinsic lung disease (such as atelectasis or pneumonia)

Under normal conditions, hemoglobin in red blood cells rapidly binds oxygen and fully saturates. Alveolar impairments that prevent full exposure of the blood to freshly inhaled air prevent full saturation. Oximeters that measure pulse and blood SpO_2 are increasingly inexpensive, and oximetry should be considered a **fourth vital sign**. If airway mucus encumberment (especially to the extent that causes oxyhemoglobin desaturation) is not cleared and SpO_2 is not returned to normal ($>94\%$) in a timely manner, pneumonia develops.

15. **Discuss the use of oximetry in initiating noninvasive IPPV.**

Introduction to, and use of, mouthpiece or nasal IPPV (noninvasive ventilatory assistance or support) can be facilitated by oximetry feedback. An SpO_2 alarm may be set at 94%. CO_2 will normalize, and the patient sees that by taking deeper breaths, the SpO_2 will exceed 94% within seconds. The patient is instructed to maintain the SpO_2 >94% all day and can achieve this by increasing unassisted breathing rate and volumes and supplementing this by mouthpiece or nasal IPPV delivered by a portable ventilator. With time and advancing muscle weakness, the patient requires increasing periods of noninvasive IPPV to maintain adequate ventilation ($SpO_2 > 94\%$). The patient is taught to use oximetry to gauge the depth of breaths needed without ventilatory assistance, and to decide when assistance is needed. In this manner, an oximeter facilitates optimal daytime use of noninvasive IPPV, as well as helps to reset central ventilatory drive.

16. **When should nocturnal noninvasive ventilation be initiated for patients with hypoventilation (e.g., Duchenne muscular dystrophy)?**

When patients have symptoms of ventilatory insufficiency and some combination of the following:

- Hypercapnia ($EtCO_2 > 50$ mmHg) during sleep with VC $< 50\%$
- Mean $SpO_2 < 95\%$ for longer than 5 min of sleep
- Multiple episodes of oxyhemoglobin desaturation during sleep
- $PaCO_2 > 45$ mmHg when awake

17. **How is SpO_2 useful in managing acute respiratory tract infections?**
Respiratory muscle weakness is exacerbated during acute respiratory infections. This, along with airway mucus encumberment, causes a decrease in the patient's vital capacity. Mucus plugging and hypoventilation can also cause decreases in SpO_2. The patient is instructed to augment ventilation and maintain a normal SpO_2 by taking mouthpiece-assisted insufflations as necessary. When mucus plugging causes a sudden decrease in SpO_2, manually and mechanically assisted coughing are used until the mucus is eliminated and the SpO_2 returns to normal. When the SpO_2 baseline decreases below 95%, despite optimal ventilation and aggressive assisted coughing, at least, microscopic atelectasis is present. This may clear with continued treatment; however, persistent baseline SpO_2 less than 95% may indicate pulmonary infiltration or other complications requiring hospitalization. This justifies hospitalization and intensive care.

18. **What is glossopharyngeal breathing or "frog breathing"?**
The patient is instructed to take a deep breath and then augment it by projecting boluses of air into the lungs by pumping action of the glottis. The glottis closes with each "gulp." One breath usually consists of 6–8 gulps of 60–200 mL each. During training, GPB efficiency is monitored by spirometrically measuring the milliliters of air per gulp, gulps per breath, and breaths per minute. A GPB rate of 12–14 breaths/minute can provide patients with little or no vital capacity with normal tidal volumes, minute ventilation, and hours of ventilator-free breathing ability.

19. **When is GPB useful?**
GPB is most commonly used as a method for providing maximal insufflations and as a noninvasive method for emergent support of ventilation. It is an excellent backup in the event of ventilator failure. Deep GPB is also useful for manually assisted coughing and hyperinflates to prevent microatelectasis. GPB can normalize the volume and rhythm of speech and permits the patient to shout. A tracheostomy virtually precludes use of GPB, because even with the tube plugged, gulped air leaks around the tube and out of the tracheostomy site.

Webber B, Higgens J: Glossopharyngeal breathing—what, when and how? [video] Horsham, UK, Aslan Studios Ltd., 1999.

20. **When is tracheotomy indicated?**
For **chronic ventilatory failure** and:
- SpO_2 persistently less than 95% in ambient air, despite up to continuous noninvasive ventilation and aggressive mechanically assisted coughing
- A mentally incompetent or uncooperative patient, or one who requires ongoing heavy sedation or narcotics
- Severe intrinsic lung disease
- Substance abuse or uncontrollable seizures
- Conditions interfering with the use of IPPV interfaces

Bach JR, Bianchi C, Aufiero E: Oximetry and indications for tracheostomy for amyotrophic lateral sclerosis. Chest 126:1502–1507, 2004.

KEY POINTS: NONINVASIVE PULMONARY REHABILITATION

1. A cardinal rule in respiratory therapy is to always first attempt to normalize oxyhemoglobin saturation (SaO_2) by providing adequate ventilation and assisted coughing before considering oxygen therapy and intubation.

2. Signs of successful noninvasive pulmonary rehabilitation are decreased respiratory rate and accessory respiratory muscle use, increased chest expansion, normalization of end-tidal carbon dioxide and SaO_2, relief of dyspnea, and decreased hospitalization rates.

3. Ventilatory impairment and oxygenation impairment need to be evaluated and managed differently.

4. Respiratory muscle aids can substitute for inspiratory and expiratory muscle function, but not for the function of bulbar-innervated muscles.

5. Nasal ventilation is introduced to treat symptoms of nocturnal hypoventilation; patients increase its use as needed and can use it continuously for full ventilatory support without ever being hospitalized.

6. Polysomnograms diagnose central and obstructive apneas, not symptoms cause by muscle weakness. This is like blaming the brain and throat for what the diaphragm cannot do.

---

21. **Does oxygen therapy ease symptoms of hypoventilation?**
    Although oxygen therapy is routinely given to virtually all ventilator users, whether or not they are hypoxic, for patients with primarily ventilatory impairment, its use is tantamount to putting a bandage on a cancer! Oxygen therapy depresses ventilatory drive, exacerbates hypercapnia, prevents the use of oximetry feedback, increases hypoventilation symptoms (e.g., daytime drowsiness, nightmares, and depression), and can render the nocturnal use of nasal or mouthpiece IPPV ineffective. In addition, hypercapnic patients who are treated with oxygen therapy have a higher incidence of pulmonary complications than patients who are not treated. *A cardinal rule is to always first attempt to normalize SpO_2 by providing adequate ventilation and assisted coughing before considering oxygen therapy and intubation.*

22. **What is the difference between CPAP and BiPAP?**
    - **Continuous positive airway pressure** delivered via a CPAP mask provides a pneumatic splint that maintains airway patency during sleep and allows the patient with obstructive sleep apneas to breathe effectively using his or her own muscles.
    - **Bilevel positive airway pressure** permits independent adjustment of inspiratory (IPAP) and expiratory positive airway pressures (EPAP). The greater the IPAP/EPAP difference (span), the greater the inspiratory muscle support. Spans of approximately 20 cm H_2O are required for effective respiratory muscle rest and for ventilatory support for patients with normal lung compliance.

23. **Are pressure support ventilation, synchronized intermittent mandatory ventilation (SIMV), positive end-expiratory pressure (PEEP), and oxygen administration necessary for ventilator weaning?**
    No. Patients are best managed by clearing the airway of secretions by using MI-E to normalize SpO_2 in ambient air and then extubating/decanulating and letting the patient wean himself or herself by taking fewer and fewer assisted breaths via a mouthpiece/nasal interface until weaned to nocturnal-only noninvasive ventilation.

24. **List five maxims regarding use of intubation and tracheostomy in the rehabilitation of ventilatory failure.**
    1. Intubation and tracheostomy are neither needed nor desired by most patients with primarily ventilatory impairment who require 24-hour-a-day ventilatory support.
    2. Oxygen should never be used as a substitute for assisted ventilation and coughing.
    3. Rehabilitation is not complete for any ventilator user who has not been evaluated for tracheostomy tube removal and had the tube removed when PCFs permit, irrespective of the extent of respiratory muscle failure.
    4. Endotracheal intubation is unnecessary for managing most cases of uncomplicated acute ventilatory failure.
    5. Endotracheal suctioning is often less effective than insufflation-exsufflation via an invasive airway tube (exsufflation creates high expiratory flows to clear both lung fields, whereas suctioning usually only clears the right airways).

    Physical medicine alternatives to the invasive measures of endotracheal intubation, tracheotomy, and airway suctioning are cheaper, safer, more comfortable, and greatly preferred by patients with primarily ventilatory impairment. They deserve wider application.

OBSTRUCTIVE DISEASES (OXYGENATION IMPAIRMENT)

25. **What causes chronic obstructive pulmonary disease (COPD)?**
    Chronic bronchitis, emphysema, asthmatic bronchitis, and cystic fibrosis are the most common causes (Box 66-2).

> **BOX 66-2. CAUSES OF CHRONIC OBSTRUCTIVE PULMONARY DISEASE (COPD)**
>
> Genetic predisposition
> Environmental factors (allergic diseases such as asthma)
> Respiratory infections (e.g., bronchopneumonitis)
> Chemical inflammation (e.g., cigarette smoke, asbestosis)
> Metabolic abnormalities (e.g., α_1-antitrypsin deficiency)
> Cigarette smoking (main cause of chronic bronchitis, emphysema)
> Smokers are 3.5–25 times more likely (depending on the amounts smoked) to die of COPD than nonsmokers

---

26. **What is the difference between emphysema and bronchitis?**
    - **Emphysema** is characterized by distention of air spaces distal to the terminal nonrespiratory bronchiole with destruction of alveolar walls. There is a loss of lung recoil, excessive airway collapse on exhalation, and chronic airflow obstruction.
    - **Chronic bronchitis** and cystic fibrosis are characterized by enlargement of tracheobronchial mucus glands, chronic mucus hypersecretion, and frequent chest infections. Chronic bronchitis is distinguished from asthmatic bronchitis by its irreversibility, lack of bronchial hyperreactivity, lack of responsiveness to bronchodilators, and distinctive abnormalities in ventilation-perfusion.

27. **How can you determine the prognosis for patients with COPD?**
    The extent of pulmonary function abnormalities correlates with prognosis: 30% of COPD patients with forced expiratory volume in 1 second (FEV_1) <750 mL die within 1 one year and

50% within 3 years. However, pulmonary function abnormalities do not predict the extent of the patient's functional impairment.

28. **Who are candidates for pulmonary rehabilitation?**
Any motivated nonsmoker or patient who has quit smoking, whose activities are limited by dyspnea due to COPD, and who has adequate medical, neuromusculoskeletal, financial, and psychosocial resources to permit active participation. Patients who benefit the most usually have a respiratory limitation to exercise at 75% of predicted maximum oxygen consumption and irreversible airway obstruction with an FEV_1 <2000 mL or FEV_1/FVC ratio <60%. Ventilator users should be decanulated and weaned in inpatient programs.

29. **Why use clinical exercise testing?**
Clinical exercise testing, whether done with a treadmill, stationary bicycle, or upper extremity ergometer, includes monitoring of oxygen consumption, CO_2 production, minute ventilation, and metabolic rate. It permits the differentiation of impairment caused by cardiac disease or exercise-induced bronchospasm from pulmonary disease. It indicates the reasons for exercise-related symptoms, and documents the patient's progress during rehabilitation by demonstrating changes in symptom-limited oxygen consumption and other physiologic parameters.

30. **When do you terminate a clinical exercise test?**
The test should continue until oxygen consumption fails to increase, maximum allowable heart rate for age is reached, or electrocardiographic changes, chest pain, severe dyspnea, or fatigue occur. A minute ventilation 35 times the patient's FEV_1 is the goal.

31. **What medical strategies are used to manage patients with lung disease and primarily oxygenation impairment?**
Pulmonary ventilatory function should be optimized medically and by facilitating airway secretion elimination. Hypoxic (PaO_2 < 60 mmHg) patients benefit from oxygen therapy with decreased dyspnea, enhanced performance, and prolonged survival. Medications such as bronchodilators (α_1-adrenergics, anticholinergics, and methylxanthines) and, occasionally, glucocorticoids, expectorants, mucolytics, antibiotics, and mast-cell membrane stabilizers may also be helpful.

32. **Outline a sample rehabilitation prescription for a COPD patient. Name its seven major components.**
    1. **Goals**
        - Improve endurance by exercise training.
        - Optimize medication delivery, oxygen utilization, and airway secretion elimination.
        - Increase walking capabilities and independent functioning.
        - Reduce anxiety and improve self-esteem.
        - Increase community, reintegration, and participation in life activities.
    2. **Precautions**
        - Maintain oxyhemoglobin saturation (SpO_2) > 90%.
        - Discontinue exercise and notify physician if chest pain, severe dyspnea, or ventricular premature beats > 6/min occur during exercise.
        - Maintain heart rate < 120 bpm.
    3. **Respiratory therapy**
        - With oximetry, titrate oxygen flows to maintain SaO_2 > 90% during exercise.
        - Instruct in diaphragmatic and pursed-lip breathing.
        - Instruct in use of incentive spirometer.
        - Instruct in inhaler use to prevent tongue deposition of medications.
        - Evaluate and instruct in methods to eliminate airway secretions.
        - Instruct in home portable oxygen use.
        - Instruct in respiratory muscle resistive exercise training and log use.

4. **Physical therapy**
   - Assess baseline 6- to 12-minute walk, instruct in using log.
   - Supervise incremental exercise program with stationary bicycle or treadmill three times daily, instruct in making log entries.
   - Review body mechanics and coordinate with breathing patterns.
   - Supervise use of diaphragmatic and pursed-lip breathing, and encourage their use during exercise.
5. **Occupational therapy**
   - Assess upper body mobility, strength, and endurance.
   - Develop an upper-extremity exercise program.
   - Evaluate and facilitate activities of daily living (ADLs) and use of adaptive aids as appropriate.
   - Train in energy and work conservation.
   - Evaluate the home, recommend modifications and equipment to improve safety, efficiency, and independence.
   - Train in relaxation exercise.
6. **Nutrition:** Assess nutritional intake, advise modifications as appropriate.
7. **Psychology:** Evaluate cognitive status and adjustment issues; intervene as needed.

33. **What methods can be used to assist the patient in airway secretion elimination?**
   - **Inexpensive methods:** Huffing, chest percussion and postural drainage, autogenic breathing, positive expiratory pressure masks, and use of flutter valves that create positive back pressure and oscillate airflow
   - **Expensive methods:** Vibrating vests, vibrating air under chest shells, and high-frequency oscillations (40–200 times/minute) of the air column delivered via mouthpiece or airway tube; the expensive methods have not been shown to be more effective than the less-expensive approaches

34. **How should the respiratory muscles of COPD patients be rested?**
Diaphragm rest can be achieved by assisting ventilation noninvasively with the use of body ventilators, mouthpiece or nasal IPPV, or tracheostomy IPPV. Although assisting ventilation can exacerbate air trapping in COPD patients, the benefits of resting respiratory muscles and decreasing oxygen consumption may outweigh this in importance. Some studies suggest that use of ventilatory assistance daily, usually delivered overnight, can improve daytime blood gases, vital capacity, dyspnea, 12-minute walking distance, respiratory muscle strength and endurance, functional activities, and quality of life, while decreasing hospitalizations. Patients with some combination of maximal inspiratory force < 50 cm H_2O, $FEV_1 < 25\%$ of predicted normal, $PCO_2 > 45$ mmHg, respiratory rate > 30/min, and chest/abdomen dyssynchrony might be considered for nocturnal ventilatory assistance. If the symptoms improve with its use, the patients are likely to be compliant.

35. **When should supplemental oxygen therapy be used?**
It should be used for patients with $PO_2 < 55$–60 mmHg, whether daytime or nighttime. Home oxygen therapy, when indicated, **decreases reactive pulmonary hypertension,** polycythemia, and perception of effort during exercise and prolongs life. Cognitive function may be improved and hospital needs reduced. It should be given with caution to patients who retain CO_2.

36. **Should supplemental oxygen be used by COPD patients on commercial airlines?**
It should not, unless it is already being used on a regular basis, and then an increase of 0.5 L/min is generally sufficient.

37. **Are nutritional supplements necessary?**

    Yes. As many as 50% of inpatients with COPD are malnourished. Inadequate or inappropriate nutrition (e.g., increased carbohydrate intake can increase PCO_2) can impair lung repair, surfactant synthesis, pulmonary defense mechanisms, control of ventilation and response to hypoxia, respiratory muscle function and lung mechanics, water homeostasis, and the immune system. Patients with significant nutritional impairment have more tracheal bacteria and are more frequently colonized by *Pseudomonas* species. Malnutrition can lead to hypercapnic respiratory failure, difficulty in weaning from mechanical ventilation, and infection. Short-term refeeding of malnourished patients leads to improved respiratory muscle endurance and, in some patients, increases in respiratory muscle strength in the absence of demonstrable changes in peripheral muscle function.

38. **Can respiratory muscles be trained?**

    Maximum sustained ventilation exercises and inspiratory resistive exercises, including inspiratory resistive loading and inspiratory threshold loading, have been shown to improve respiratory muscle endurance. With a few exceptions, studies have not shown improvements in other pulmonary function parameters, and respiratory muscle exercise does not appear to improve general exercise tolerance or ADL capabilities. However, the combination of respiratory muscle exercise and rest, which appears to be especially effective for ventilator weaning, has not been adequately explored for the COPD patient.

    Aldrich T: Respiratory muscle training in COPD. In Bach JR (ed): Pulmonary Rehabilitation: The Obstructive and Paralytic Conditions. Philadelphia, Hanley & Belfus, 1996, pp 123–132.

39. **How should reconditioning exercises be prescribed?**

    The intensity of reconditioning exercises may be guided by clinical exercise testing (e.g., 80–85% of maximum achievable heart rate, or heart rate at ventilation levels of 35 times FEV_1). Walking, stair climbing, calisthenics, bicycling, and pool activities may be used. Upper-extremity reconditioning should also be part of the program. A stationary bicycle should be purchased for the patient's home and used twice a day. In addition, a daily 12-minute walk can be used, as well as several 15-minute sessions daily of inspiratory muscle training. A log should be kept of time and distance bicycled, distance walked, and possibly inspiratory resistance tolerated during 15-minute inspiratory training sessions. Shorter periods of higher-intensity exercise are more effective in increasing exercise tolerance than longer periods of lower-intensity exercise. In general, the pulse should increase at least 20–30% and return to baseline 5–10 minutes after exercise. The program should consist of weekly re-evaluations for several months, after which the patient can continue the home program and maintain the logs.

40. **Should exercise reconditioning be used for advanced patients with marked hypercapnia?**

    There is evidence that even advanced patients with hypercapnia can benefit from an exercise reconditioning program, showing significant improvement in walking distance, ADLs, and, possibly, certain pulmonary parameters.

41. **What are the benefits of pulmonary rehabilitation?**

    1. Reduction in dyspnea and respiratory rate
    2. Increased exercise tolerance, symptom-limited oxygen consumption, work output, and mechanical efficiency
    3. Improvement in ADLs
    4. Decreased anxiety and depression
    5. Increased cognitive function and sense of well-being
    6. Decreased frequency of hospitalizations for respiratory impairment

    Casaburi R, Petty TL (eds): Principles and Practice of Pulmonary Rehabilitation. Philadelphia, W.B. Saunders, 1993.

42. **What is exercise-induced asthma (EIA)?**

EIA is a temporary narrowing of the airways associated with strenuous exercise or activity. EIA may begin during exercise (typically within 15 minutes) and resolves usually within 20–30 minutes of cessation of exercise. EIA can also occur 4–6 hours after completing exercise, usually at night **(a late-phase response).** This is a response to an influx of inflammatory cells in the airways. EIA needs to be differentiated from poorly controlled asthma that develops shortly after beginning exercise. Poorly controlled asthma can make it impossible to complete physical activity. Symptoms of EIA may include coughing, chest tightness, wheezing, and difficulty breathing. Some patients describe feeling winded, tired, or dizzy during or following exercise, and some may complain of stomach pain. EIA occurs in 80–90% of people who have asthma and in almost 50% of people who have allergic rhinitis (i.e., hayfever). Studies have shown that about 5–10% of collegiate athletes have EIA, which is similar to the incidence in the general population. Children are more likely than adults to have EIA.

Stempel DA: The pharmacologic management of childhood asthma. Pediatr Clin North Am 50:609–629, 2003.

43. **What is the management of EIA?**

The administration of an inhaled corticosteroid before exercise is useful to inhibit the late-phase inflammatory response, but it will have no effect on the early-phase response. **Cromolyn sodium** inhibits mast cell degranulation and reduces airway hyperreactivity by an unknown mechanism. Affected patients also should have rescue medication (e.g., albuterol) available when participating in exercise, but sodium cromolyn is the preferred treatment modality because it may prevent symptomatic episodes. Antileukotrienes appear to be more potent than cromolyn sodium.

Bolte RG: Management of pediatric asthma. Clin Ped Emerg Med 5:256–269, 2004.

44. **Are exercise programs beneficial for patients with cystic fibrosis (CF)?**

Aerobic fitness is a strong correlate of 8-year survival, indicating the importance of an active lifestyle. Several studies of CF exercise programs showed results dependent on compliance and intensity of training. Exercise has increased work capacity, improved cardiorespiratory fitness, improved ventilatory muscle endurance, and enhanced immune function. Although increased exercise may not improve pulmonary function, the slowing of progressive pulmonary decline from these other factors suggests an important benefit. No study of individuals with CF has demonstrated harm from exercise. The occasional patient who experiences exercise-related oxygen desaturation can maintain adequate oxygenation through the use of supplemental oxygen during exercise. Exercise might acutely enhance pulmonary function because of its ability to mobilize airway mucus. Adding exercise to standard chest physiotherapy has been shown to result in a clinically important and statistically significant improvement in oxygenation.

Orenstein DM, Hovell MF, Mulvihill M, et al: Strength vs aerobic training in children with cystic fibrosis: A randomized controlled trial. Chest 126:1204–1214, 2004.

45. **What is the best available predictor of survival in patients with CF?**

The FEV_1 is the best predictor of survival. Patients with CF and an FEV_1 less than 30% of predicted value have 50% incidence of 2-year mortality. An FEV_1 of 30% of predicted value is a benchmark for lung transplantation referral.

Yankaskas JR, Marshall BC, Sufian B, et al: Cystic fibrosis adult care: Consensus conference report. Chest 125(1 suppl):1S–39S, 2004.

CHAPTER 67

CANCER REHABILITATION: GENERAL PRINCIPLES

Theresa A. Gillis, MD, Ki Y. Shin, MD, and Fae H. Garden, MD

The truth is, if you asked me to choose between winning the Tour de France and cancer, I would choose cancer. Odd as it sounds, I would rather have the title of cancer survivor than winner of the Tour, because of what it has done for me as a human being, a man, a husband, a son, and a father.

—Lance Armstrong (1971–)

1. **Why is cancer rehabilitation necessary?**
   Advances in early detection and treatment allow more people with cancer to live longer. In the United States an estimated 10 million people are alive today with a diagnosis of cancer, with 1.3 million new cases a year and a relative 5-year survival rate of 65%. *Approximately 7% of the 10 million Americans diagnosed with cancer were longer-term survivors diagnosed more than 27 years earlier.* These cancer survivors frequently are left with physical deficits, cognitive impairments, and psychosocial problems that diminish their quality of life. Rehabilitation professionals have specific experience in minimizing disability, expediting return to "normal" activities, and educating caregivers. Thus caregivers are well trained to assist and direct **cancer survivorship** efforts.

   Many physiatrists have limited experience rehabilitating cancer patients, particularly those with advanced or advancing disease. This may result from a lack of recognition of rehab needs in these patients, training biases, or discomfort in dealing with patients with what is perceived to be a poor or limited prognosis. Cancer rehabilitation can be medically, emotionally, and physically challenging for everyone involved. However, as with most rehabilitation patients, improvements in function and quality of life can be significant and very meaningful among those patients who anticipate a shortened life span.

   Cancer patients with a poor prognosis or very limited life span can still derive significant benefit and improved quality of life from brief, concentrated rehabilitation efforts, including transfer training, bowel and bladder education, skin protection and maintenance skills, and equipment assessments.

   Lehmann JF, DeLisa JA, Warren CG, et al: Cancer rehabilitation: Assessment of need, development and evaluation of a model of care. Arch Phys Med Rehabil 59:410–419, 1978.

   Meyers CA, Abbruzzese JL: Cognitive functioning in cancer patients: Effect of previous treatment. Neurology 42:434–436, 1992.

2. **How might a cancer rehab team differ from other rehab teams?**
   Oncology rehab teams may include the patient's oncologist and, in some settings, may have a chaplain within the team. Head and neck cancer patients may have a prosthodontist involved in their care. Teams are otherwise similar to more typical rehabilitation diagnoses. The rehabilitation team faces typical rehabilitation issues of debility and orthopedic and neurologic impairments. However, patients often have impairments across multiple organ systems and, if facing recurrent cancer or multimodal treatments, may experience repeating cycles of impairments. Because of the nature of cancer treatment, typically involving combinations of surgery, radiation therapy, chemotherapy, or other treatments, often in an outpatient setting over several months, team communications and planning can be challenging.

3. **What are common causes for cancer-related fatigue? How can it be treated?**

   Cancer-related fatigue is a poorly understood but common problem affecting more than 80% of outpatients receiving chemotherapy, and it is reported in 14–96% of different cancer diagnostic groups. This fatigue is not improved by rest, unlike more typical fatigue experiences. Theories for the underlying mechanism include circulating cytokines released by tumor cells, triggering central (e.g., hypothalamic, frontal lobe) and peripheral (neuromuscular junction, neuronal) responses.

   Cancer fatigue is the most common symptom of advanced cancer (90% of patients) but is common throughout the disease continuum. Interventions involving exercise for non–end-stage patients have been studied and have consistently positive outcomes (Table 67-1).

   Gills TA: The role of the physiatrist. In Winningham ML, Barton-Burke M (eds.) Fatigue in Cancer: A Multidisciplinary Approach. Sudbury, MA, Jones & Barlett, 1999, pp 295–301.

TABLE 67-1. CAUSES AND TREATMENT OF CANCER–RELATED FATIGUE	
Causes/Associations of Cancer-Related Fatigue	Treatment
Poor sleep quality	Sleep hygiene, medication
Iatrogenic medications (analgesic, antiepileptic, beta blockers, sedative/hypnotics, antidepressants, etc.)	Medication/dosage reassessment
Pain	Medication, therapy, relaxation
Hormone deficiency	Replacement (if no contraindication)
Distress (anxiety, depression, stress)	Medication, counseling, support
Anemia	Transfusion, erythropoetin
Hypercalcemia	Correction
Inactivity, debility	Exercise
Cognitive failure	Psychostimulants
Malnutrition, dehydration	Supplements, appetite stimulation

4. **Explain some of the nutritional concerns of the cancer patient.**

   Between 40% and 80% of all cancer patients develop clinical **malnutrition**. This is affected by tumor type, stage of disease, and mode of therapy. Clinical effects of malnutrition include poor wound healing, poor skin turgor (which can contribute to skin breakdown and decubiti), wound dehiscence, electrolyte and fluid imbalances, endocrine dysfunction, and compromised immune function. Decreased appetite from nausea and vomiting associated with chemotherapy, as well as endogenous cytokine release, can exacerbate the severity of malnutrition.

5. **What are the potential adverse effects of cancer surgery on nutrition?**

   Surgical procedures such as **radical neck dissection** or **glossectomy** can impair mastication, swallowing, taste, and smell. Patients undergoing esophagectomy, **gastrectomy**, or **bowel resection** can develop gastric stasis, diarrhea, steatorrhea, megaloblastic anemia, malabsorption, and deficiency of vitamins B_{12}, D, and A.

6. **What are the adverse effects of radiation therapy on nutrition?**

   Radiation treatment to the **head and neck area** can produce alterations in taste and saliva. Food texture and sensation alternations can occur from irradiation of the oral mucosa. Ulcerations, stomatitis, or mucositis can also occur. Radiation to the **stomach and intestines** can cause acute nausea, cramps, and diarrhea. Patients with radiation damage to the intestines are usually started on lactose-free, low-residue oral diets. Small, frequent meals and increased fluids are also recommended.

7. **What nutritional deficiencies can occur with chemotherapy?**
Antimetabolite drugs, such as methotrexate, inhibit the metabolism of folic acid, which is necessary for the synthesis of DNA. The resultant **folic acid deficiency** can result in macrocytic anemia, leukopenia, and ulcerative stomatitis. The antimetabolites 5-fluorouracil and 6-mercaptopurine prevent nucleic acid synthesis by interfering with thiamine in DNA synthesis. Clinical **thiamine deficiency** is associated with paresthesias, neuropathy, and heart failure. **Vitamin K deficiency** results from long-term treatment with adjunctive antibiotics, such as moxalactam disodium, leading to a pronounced bleeding tendency.

8. **How does cancer or cancer treatment affect female sexual function?**
Sexual dysfunction can occur at any time during or after treatment. Changes in body image, stress and anxiety related to the diagnosis and treatment, and pain after surgery or other treatments can have a negative impact on sexual response. Fear of partner rejection can lead to the avoidance of sexual intercourse. Women who have undergone pelvic surgery or irradiation need to be counseled about the possible need for vaginal dilators to prevent stenosis, as well as the possibility of bleeding with intercourse. Some women may need to use artificial vaginal lubrication and change from their customary sexual positions. Side effects of chemotherapy and radiation therapy, including nausea, fatigue, hair loss, and weight changes, can produce additional psychological and physical roadblocks to resuming sexual activity.

9. **What are some sexual dysfunctions that occur in male patients undergoing cancer treatment?**
Impotence, retrograde ejaculation, and infertility can result from damage to the vascular or nerve pathways after surgical treatment for prostate cancer. If permanent sterilization is anticipated, preoperative and pretreatment discussion of reproductive concerns, including sperm banking, should be undertaken. Sexual rehabilitation can include the use of oral medications such as sildenafil, tadalafil, and vardenafil, erectile assistive devices, and surgical reconstruction of the phallus. Performance anxiety, fear of rejection or failure, and treatment-induced symptoms previously described can also inhibit sexual function and satisfaction. Couples counseling through knowledgeable trained therapists, psychologists, or social workers may be of help.

10. **What is a paraneoplastic syndrome?**
When tumors produce systemic signs and symptoms at a distance from the tumor or its metastases, it is referred to as a paraneoplastic syndrome. Tumor cells may produce antibodies, hormones or precursors, enzymes, or other physiologically active substances.
   By definition, these syndromes should not be produced as a direct effect of the tumor or its metastases. Paraneoplastic syndromes develop in approximately 10–15% of cancer patients but may be underrecognized and underreported, particularly when associated with cytokine release (*see* "Nonspecific" category in Table 67-2).

11. **An elderly male patient with myeloma is complaining of diffuse abdominal pain and appears confused and dehydrated. What specific metabolic abnormality must be included in your differential diagnosis?**
Hypercalcemia is common in cancer patients, occurring in approximately 10% of patients at some point in their disease (Box 67-1). Most commonly, excessive calcium is released from **osteolytic** bone metastases associated with **breast, lung, renal cell carcinomas,** and **multiple myeloma.** Other tumors such as ovarian, lung, head and neck, esophageal, cervical, multiple endocrine neoplasia, pheochromocytoma, and hepatoma may release a parathyroid hormone-like protein that also leads to increased osteoclastic activity.

TABLE 67-2. PARANEOPLASTIC SYNDROMES

Category	Symptom/Signs	Common Inciting Primary Tumors
Neuromuscular	Lambert-Eaton myasthenic syndrome	Pulmonary, ovarian, renal, breast, lymphoma, thymoma, pancreas
	Motor, sensory, or mixed neuropathies	Lung
Rheumatologic	Polymyalgia rheumatica	Lymphoma, leukemia, colon, pancreas, prostate, CNS
	Polymyositis/dermatomyositis	Lymphoma, lung, gastric, breast, uterus
	Scleroderma	Breast, uterus, lung
	Hypertrophic osteoarthropathy	Lung, mesothelioma
Dermatologic	Pruritus	Many, common in Hodgkin's disease
	Acanthosis nigricans	Melanoma, pancreatic
Endocrine	Cushing's syndrome ($\downarrow K^+$, $\uparrow$ACTH, $\uparrow$cortisol)	Lung (small cell), gonadal, adrenal
	SIADH	Lung (small cell), thymus, pancreas, duodenum, CNS bronchogenic
Gastrointestinal	Diarrhea	Proctosigmoid, medullary thyroid, myeloma, melanoma
Nonspecific	Fever	Lymphoma, leukemia, GI, sarcoma, renal cell, liver
	Cachexia/wasting/anorexia	Common

ACTH = adrenocorticotropic hormone, CNS = central nervous system, GI = gastrointestinal, SIADH = syndrome of inappropriate secretion of antidiuretic hormone.

BOX 67-1. CLINICAL SYMPTOMS/SIGNS OF HYPERCALCEMIA

- Anorexia
- Nausea and vomiting
- Alterations of mental status
- Vague abdominal or flank pain
- Constipation
- Lethargy
- Depression
- Weakness and vague muscle/joint aches
- Polyuria and nocturia
- Headache
- Pruritus

12. **My patient with myeloma has a normal serum calcium level, but his presentation is suggestive of hypercalcemia. Now what?**

Don't forget that the total serum calcium level reflects protein-bound and free biologically active calcium. If the patient's serum albumin level is low, the serum calcium level can appear artificially low, even while the free calcium level may be high. The calcium level must be corrected as follows:

Corrected total calcium (mg/dL) = (measured total calcium [mg/dL]) + 0.8 (4.4 − measured albumin [gm/dL]).

Values greater than 10.5 mg/dL are defined as hypercalcemia. Hydration, loop diuretics, and consultation with a nephrologist and/or oncologist are necessary.

13. **What causes pain in cancer patients?**

Cancer patients may experience a variety of painful conditions, related to both treatment and the tumor processes. The most common treatment-induced pains include **mucositis** from radiation or chemotherapy and **peripheral neuropathies** from chemotherapy, particularly taxanes, vinca alkaloids, and platinum. Both etiologies may produce such severe pains that treatment with opiate analgesics is warranted.

The most common malignant cause of pain is **tumor invasion of bone** from a metastatic lesion.

Compression or **infiltration of peripheral nerves** by tumor is the second most frequent cause. Cancer pain occurs in 51% of all patients and 74% of those with advanced or terminal disease.

14. **How can medications be used in managing cancer pain?**

The World Health Organization recommends the stepwise use of nonopioid analgesics, adjuvant drugs, and opioids, matching the severity of the pain rating to the appropriate potency analgesics. **Aspirin** and nonsteroidal anti-inflammatory drugs **(NSAIDs)** are useful to control the pain of bone metastases because they are potent prostaglandin synthetase inhibitors. However, a therapeutic ceiling prevents significant dose escalation of these medications.

Corticosteroids produce analgesia by preventing the release of prostaglandins and are helpful in reducing pain from tumor infiltration of viscera, bone, peripheral nerves, and spinal cord. Adjuvant therapy includes **tricyclic antidepressants,** which block reuptake of serotonin in the central nervous system (CNS). **Carbamazepine, phenytoin, gabapentin, pregabalin, tramadol, venlafaxine, duloxetine,** and **methadone** can be effective in the treatment of neuropathic pain. Topical medications such as **lidocaine, capsaicin,** and **EMLA** (eutectic mixture of local anesthetics) may be useful for limited areas of deafferentation pain.

Opioid analgesics include **codeine, hydrocodone, oxycodone, morphine, hydromorphone, oxymorphone, methadone,** and **fentanyl**. Preparations may be transdermal or transmucosal (fentanyl), and some are available in sustained-release formulations (12- and 24-hour duration). Methadone has a less predictable half-life, which may vary between 4 and 24 hours among different individuals. There is no ceiling effect for these analgesics. Side effects may necessitate changes in route of delivery or rotation to another agent. Demerol (meperidine) is not recommended for the treatment of cancer pain, because of its short duration of action and its potential for adverse CNS effects on repeated use. Opioid analgesics are often *improperly prescribed* in the treatment of severe cancer pain, and underdosing, improper dose intervals, and failure to manage the expected side-effect of constipation are frequent problems.

Dworkin RH, Backonja M, Rowbotham MC, et al: Advances in neuropathic pain: Diagnosis, mechanisms, and treatment recommendations. Arch Neurol 60:1524–1534, 2003.

Miaskowski C, Clearly J, Burney R, et al: Guideline for the Management of Cancer Pain in Adults and Children. Glenview, IL, American Pain Society, 2005.

15. **When should invasive pain management procedures be considered?**

Studies have shown that approximately 90% of cancer patients can achieve satisfactory relief from oral, rectal, transdermal, or intravenous routes of analgesic administration. However, more invasive measures may be necessary when:

- Pain becomes intractable and not relieved by increasing doses of opiates or rotating to another opiate.
- These medications lead to overwhelming and unmanageable side effects such as extreme nausea, myoclonus, sedation, delirium, or agitation.
- Such massive quantities of opiates are required for comfort that continuation of orally/ transdermally delivered medications becomes impractical and/or prohibitively expensive.
- Pain responds poorly to opiate therapy, and intra-axial (intrathecal) delivery of alternative analgesics, such as clonidine or ziconotide, or anesthetic agents may be beneficial. Options then may include spinal administration of opiate or other analgesic medications, neurolytic blocks, or surgical neuroablative procedures.

16. **Describe some neuroablative procedures used in the treatment of cancer pain.**
Subarachnoid neurolytic blocks involve intrathecal injections of demyelinating agents to cause a chemical posterior rhizotomy. This may be effective for somatic, well-localized pain. Sympathetic plexus blockade can be utilized for visceral pains and do not affect motor or cutaneous sensory functions. Percutaneous cordotomy involves disruption of the lateral spinothalamic tract at the C1–C2 interspace and is more useful for unilateral limb pain. A midline myelotomy may be particularly helpful for visceral lower body pain. Intracranial ablations are more rarely used but may be particularly effective for widespread pain such as diffuse bone metastasis (hypophysectomy, cingulotomy) or specific intractable neuropathic pains (thalamotomy). Nerve block options are summarized in Table 67-3.

TABLE 67-3. NERVE BLOCK OPTIONS

Tumor Pain Location	Possible Ablative Procedures
Cranial/facial structures	Trigeminal radiofrequency ablation/tractotomy Maxillary or mandibular divisions Cervical (superior, middle, or cervicothoracic) ganglion block Glossopharyngeal
Neck/upper extremity	Cervicothoracic (stellate) ganglion
Chest wall	Intercostal nerve
Pericardium, heart, pleura	Cervicothoracic ganglion
Pancreas, distal esophagus, liver	Celiac plexus Splanchnic nerve block (T11–T12)
Lower abdominal viscera	Lumbar sympathetic ganglia
Lower extremity	Lumbar sympathetic ganglia
Pelvic viscera	Hypogastric plexus
Perineum	Ganglion impar

17. **How can psychological interventions be used to manage cancer pain?**
Psychological techniques may enable patients with cancer to regain a much-needed sense of personal control. Mental imagery, hypnosis, relaxation, biofeedback, music therapy, meditation, and other cognitive or behavioral methods can directly relieve pain as well as anxiety, which can enhance analgesia.

18. **What is Pancoast's syndrome?**
Pancoast's syndrome is caused by carcinomas in the superior pulmonary sulcus. Although Pancoast tumor refers specifically to non–small cell carcinoma of the lung, the syndrome can arise from any tumor metastasizing to this area. The tumor produces pain in the distribution of

C7, C8, and T1–T2 nerves, hand weakness, arm edema caused by subclavian vein and/or lymphatic compression, as well as Horner's syndrome (ptosis and miosis). A shadow can sometimes be seen on chest films at the apex of the lung. Patients with Pancoast's syndrome usually complain of severe, unrelenting pain that often begins at the shoulder and vertebral border of the scapula. Radiation and surgery are recommended treatments.

Facial swelling, dilated neck veins, and chest wall pains with headache are presenting symptoms of tumor obstruction of the superior vena cava. The superior vena cava syndrome is most commonly seen in lung cancer, lymphomas, and breast cancer patients and requires urgent antitumor therapy.

19. **What is the most common form of radiation-induced spinal cord damage?**
    Transient myelopathy, or **Lhermitte's syndrome,** is an uncommon complication, occurring more commonly in patients being treated for head and neck tumors or lymphoma. The syndrome typically develops after a latent period of 1–30 months, with the peak incidence for onset of symptoms at 4–6 months after completion of treatment. Symptoms include electrical dysesthesias or paresthesias that radiate from the cervical spine to the extremities. These sensations usually occur in a symmetric fashion. Diagnostic imaging studies are typically normal. The syndrome usually resolves in 1–9 months after onset. **Delayed myelopathy** typically occurs 9–18 months after completion of radiation treatment, is nonpainful in contrast to metastatic disease presentation, and is usually irreversible, although early steroid therapy may lessen its severity.

    Dropcho EJ: Central nervous system injury by therapeutic irradiation. Neurol Clin North Am 9:969–988, 1991.

20. **You are performing an electromyographic (EMG) study for a patient with suspected postradiation brachial plexopathy. What features would help you distinguish this from plexopathy caused by tumor infiltration?**
    Plexopathy caused by tumor invasion is up to 10 times more common than postradiation plexopathy. Horner's syndrome (ptosis, enophthalmos), progressive pain, and lower trunk involvement are more common in neoplastic plexopathies. Upper trunk involvement is more common in radiation plexopathy. Electrodiagnostic findings such as myokymic discharges and abnormal sensory conduction studies are more common in patients with radiation plexopathy.

    Harper CM, Thomas JE: Distinction between neoplastic and radiation-induced brachial plexopathy, with emphasis on the role of EMG. Neurology 39:502–506, 1989.

21. **Many patients undergoing cancer treatment have low platelet counts. Does the presence of thrombocytopenia affect the exercise prescription?**
    Vigorous exercise in the presence of thrombocytopenia may increase the risk of intra-articular bleeding. It is common practice to withhold resistive exercise therapy when platelet levels are $<10,000/mm^3$. In early chemotherapy studies done before the availability of platelet transfusions, the risk of intracerebral bleeding became more significant below this level, especially when accompanied by fever or sepsis.

22. **How do cancer amputees differ from dysvascular or traumatic amputees?**
    Patients with cancer often face functional declines associated with chemotherapy or recurrent disease. Many sarcoma patients are treated with preoperative and postoperative chemotherapy protocols, with the attendant risks of anemia, fatigue, anorexia and nutritional depletion, nausea, and cardiovascular toxicity while recovering from the amputation. Prosthesis fitting can also be complicated in patients who are receiving chemotherapy due to weight fluctuations caused by poor nutrition and/or edema. Irradiated skin is often less tolerant to prosthesis contact. All patients should be considered for prosthetic prescription, but special attention must be given to the cancer treatment protocol when planning fabrication, fitting, and training.

The energy costs of prosthetic gait may be particularly unrealistic in severely compromised patients; avoidance of immobility and deconditioning should be a primary concern for these patients *prior to* amputation. Cosmetic prosthesis should be offered to patients unable to use a functional limb.

23. **What is meant by "limb salvage"? What procedures does it entail?**
Limb salvage describes efforts toward maintaining a functional extremity and avoiding amputation in the treatment of sarcomas and bone metastases from other tumors. The plan may employ the use of reconstruction techniques with custom or modular segmental prostheses and/or allograft or autograft transfer of bony or muscular tissues. Limited resections of muscle groups, compartments, or partial bones may be necessary. Partial resections of the sacrum, pelvis, scapulae, and femur, such as the Girdlestone procedure and internal hemipelvectomy, are frequently seen. Cemented prosthetic hip and knee components and intramedullary rods of the humerus and femur are very common. Rehabilitation must be tailored to address intact and unstable structures.

24. **What are the most common malignant bone tumors?**
Carcinomas **metastatic to bone** account for >40 times more cases than all primary bone tumors combined. Breast cancer accounts for most bone metastases, with an incidence of bone metastases in this disease of 50–85%. Prostate carcinoma is the most common primary tumor for metastatic lesions in men, with bone metastases occurring in >90% of patients with advanced disease. Lung, renal, bladder, thyroid, and bowel primaries each have an incidence of bone metastases of 20–40% at autopsy. Most bone metastases are asymptomatic.
Myeloma is the most common primary malignant tumor of bone in adults, arising within the bone marrow from plasma cells. Osteosarcomas, Ewing's sarcoma, and chondrosarcoma are the most common tumors arising from bone tissue itself. In children, osteosarcoma, Ewing's sarcoma, and primitive neuroectodermal tumors (in descending order) are the most predominant primary malignant bone tumors.

25. **When is a bone susceptible to pathologic fracture?**
Pathologic fractures occur in 10–30% of patients with metastases and are seen most frequently in the long bones, particularly the femur and humerus. Bone strength is determined by the cortical and trabecular structure. Cortical destruction increases susceptibility of bone to torsional/rotational forces. The guidelines most frequently cited for increased risk of fracture are as follows:
- Cortical bone destruction affecting ≥50% of the circumference as seen on anteroposterior and lateral radiographs or cross-sectional computed tomography
- Lytic lesions ≥2.5 cm in the proximal femur
- Pathologic avulsion fracture of the lesser trochanter of the femur
- Persisting or increasing pain with weight-bearing despite completion of radiotherapy
These estimates of fracture risk are used synonymously as indications for prophylactic fixation; an inherent limitation to this list is that tumor extent can be greatly underestimated by radiographs.

Mandi A, Szepesi K, Morocz I: Surgical treatment of pathologic fractures from metastatic tumors of long bones. Orthopedics 14:43–50, 1991.

26. **What rehabilitation methods may be used in managing bone metastases?**
Some patients receive prophylactic fixation of metastatic lesions, employing internal fixation, methylmethacrylate and modular prosthesis, or other hardware. After operative management, restoration of mobility and self-care through a rehabilitation approach is essential.
Painful bone metastases are often treated with radiotherapy. During radiation, bone is placed at increased risk of fracture as a result of hyperemic softening of bone and necrosis of tumor cells, and complete reossification may not occur until 6 months or more after treatment.

In theory, therefore, precautions and reduced load-bearing may be indicated for many months. During periods of greatest risk, and for nonsurgical candidates, unloading affected bones with assistive devices, braces, or immobilizers is recommended. Mobility issues with activity restrictions and adaptive equipment for activities of daily living (ADLs) should be addressed by physiatrists.

27. **What are the most common initial symptoms caused by metastases to the spine?**
Four symptoms characterize the clinical picture of spinal cord compression: pain, weakness, autonomic dysfunction, and sensory loss (including ataxia). Pain is usually the initial symptom and can manifest as central back pain with or without radicular pain.

28. **Does the pain of spinal cord tumor differ from the pain caused by a herniated intervertebral disc?**
The pain caused by an epidural tumor is described as being worse when the patient is lying down. Patients may complain of being awakened from sleep several times during the night, and some may describe a need to sleep in a sitting position.

29. **When should one consider epidural spinal cord compression in a cancer patient with back pain?**
Always! The spine is the most common site for skeletal metastases, regardless of the primary tumor. Early diagnosis is essential, because the outcome is related to patient function at diagnosis—that is, if a patient is paraplegic at diagnosis, he or she will nearly always remain so after treatment. Epidural spinal cord compression from metastasis occurs in 10–33% of cancer patients, and in 10% of these patients, cord compression is the presenting manifestation of malignancy.

The most common presenting symptom of spinal cord compression by epidural tumor is **pain,** which often precedes neurologic signs by weeks or months. Early recognition is essential for effective treatment, as the majority of patients who present with paraplegia will remain thus despite treatment, whereas 75% of patients who begin treatment while ambulatory will not develop further neurologic impairment

30. **When evaluating for spinal metastases, what radiologic studies are indicated?**
In patients with cancer or high suspicion for malignancy or epidural spinal cord compression, magnetic resonance imaging (MRI) is often the first diagnostic test. Plain films and bone scan are of additional help in planning for surgical intervention and radiation therapy. Remember that metastatic disease can also arise in the epidural space or paraspinal tissues, and plain film and bone scan will not reveal tumors in these areas. In patients with back pain but without cancer or a high suspicion for malignancy, radiographs are often obtained when a patient does not respond to therapy. Although the vertebral body is usually the site first affected by metastases, 30–50% of cancellous bone here must be destroyed before change is seen on plain film. Destruction of the pedicle is usually discovered first on anteroposterior films. If back pain persists and radiographs are normal, bone scintigraphy or MRI is indicated. The sensitivity of bone scans for metastases is high. A gadolinium-enhanced MRI will clearly delineate epidural disease and tumors arising in the paraspinal soft tissues.

31. **What interventions are most appropriate for metastatic spinal disease?**
When epidural spinal cord compression is present, all patients require urgent intravenous steroid therapy. Studies show better functional outcomes and reduced pain with surgical resection and stabilization, followed by radiation. A posterolateral surgical approach allows access to the vertebral body, where most metastases occur. Laminectomies alone do not resect tumor and may further destabilize the spine. For patients who are not surgical candidates, radiation alone can be offered, but it does not address concerns of spinal bony stability.

When tumor does not invade beyond the cortex, fluoroscopically guided injections of methylmethacrylate may be used to increase stability and reduce pain. Radiation therapy is the standard treatment for most bone-only spinal metastases.

32. **What are some primary spinal cord tumors?**
Ependymomas and astrocytomas are common intramedullary (located in the substance of the cord) tumors. Extramedullary tumors include neurofibromas and meningiomas. The most common malignant lesions affecting the spinal cord are metastases from various primary tumors. Extradural spinal cord compression is a common neurologic complication of systemic malignancy.

33. **Your office has been following up with a 50-year-old woman with a history of breast cancer 2 years previously for chronic stable lymphedema in the right arm. She presents with a sudden onset of severe headache, diplopia, right hemifacial numbness, left-arm radicular pains, bilateral quadricep weakness, and patchy sensory loss in her legs. What diagnosis must be included in your differential?**
The CNS dysfunction in more than one level of the neuraxis seen in this patient should trigger a search for leptomeningeal carcinomatosis (LC) (or carcinomatous meningitis). LC is an underdiagnosed complication affecting 1–8% of patients with cancer. It is most commonly encountered in patients with lung, breast, or gastrointestinal malignancies and melanoma, and may also occur with primary brain tumors and acute lymphocytic leukemias. LC is often seen in late stages of disease but may be present at the time of diagnosis, or can be a presenting feature of sudden relapse. The median survival without treatment is 4–6 weeks due to progressive neurologic compromise. Treated patients usually will ultimately succumb later due to systemic cancer complications, whereas leukemia or lymphoma patients may still achieve a cure.

34. **What diagnostic steps should be taken when evaluating leptomeningeal carcinomatosis?**
A high index of suspicion should be present when neurologic symptoms arise in a cancer patient, particularly pain (headache, radicular, meningeal) or seizures. Diagnostic studies are required when neurologic signs and symptoms occur at more than one level of the CNS, or signs/symptoms are consistent with a single lesion but without evident lesions on imaging studies, or when imaging suggests flow obstruction of cerebrospinal fluid.
An MRI with gadolinium enhancement of the symptomatic areas—often the entire CNS—is performed. Enhancement of tissues, or enlargement of nerve roots or spinal cord, nodularity of the subarachnoid space, or epidural tumor, are common findings, as are hydrocephalus, gyral effacement, or periventricular edema If no evidence of elevated intracranial pressure is found, then lumbar punctures (LPs) for opening pressure determination, and cerebrospinal fluid cell counts, and chemical and cytologic exams are needed. The incidence of false-negative cytology studies drops to approximately 15% with the third LP.
Treatment typically entails radiation to the neuraxis and intrathecal chemotherapy.

35. **What disability results after neck dissection? How is it best managed?**
The spinal accessory nerve is typically sacrificed during radical neck dissection, causing loss of trapezius function. In modified radical dissections the spinal accessory nerve is preserved but may still experience operative manipulation or blood flow changes, which may lead to postoperative demyelination and/or neurapraxia. The medial border of the scapula rotates upward, the scapula deviates laterally and wings medially, despite intact serratus function. Abduction is limited to only 60–80 degrees in nearly all patients. Shoulder pain frequently results, and lifting and overhead activities may become impossible.
Strengthening the levator scapulae, rhomboideus, and serratus anterior muscles may help stabilize the scapula, allow improved shoulder elevation, and reduce pain. Attempts to

strengthen the deltoids, supraspinatus, or infraspinatus should be discouraged, because this only increases pain and further overworks the disadvantaged muscles. Pectoralis muscle contracture aggravates the protracted shoulder and results from lack of pull from the opposing trapezius. Therefore, pectoral stretches and maintenance of good scapular positioning is crucial. Some patients reduce their discomfort through use of a figure-of-eight orthosis, sling, or other orthoses to provide support against gravity, or by habitually resting their hand in a pants pocket or waistband.

36. **How do brain tumor patients differ from brain injury patients?**
Most patients with primary brain tumors experience rapid improvement in function after tumor excision. Normal brain tissue has been compressed by tumor, so with pressure relief, recovery can be dramatic and the patient may return to normal function. However, many tumors recur, and with repeated excisions and invasion of normal tissue by tumor, further functions are lost. Radiation and chemotherapy can further limit recovery through lost plasticity and cognitive effects. Despite advances in treatment, most patients with glioblastoma multiforme or high-grade astrocytomas survive 2 years or less; therefore, rehabilitation goals should be congruent with this pattern of decline.

Gillis TA, Yadav R, Guo Y: Rehabilitation of patients with neurologic tumors and cancer-related central nervous system disabilities. In Levin VA (ed): Cancer in the Nervous System, 2nd ed. New York, Oxford University Press, 2002, pp 470–492.

37. **What is the most common primary brain tumor? Metastatic tumor?**
Gliomas comprise approximately 60% of all primary CNS tumors. The most common tumors that metastasize to the brain are **carcinomas of the lung and breast**. Most brain metastases involve the cerebrum, with the frontal lobe being the most common site. Metastases to the cerebellum are less frequent, and those to the brain stem are the least frequent.

38. **What rehabilitation needs are greatest among brain tumor patients?**
Deficits experienced by brain tumor patients are clearly related to the involved structures. Cognitive deficits are quite prevalent and also related to the site of lesions. Neurobehavioral changes may be the most prominent problems faced by patients with tumors. Memory losses, impaired reasoning and problem-solving skills, decreased energy or initiative, and inability to return to work are problems cited more frequently by family members as problems than difficulty with ambulation, bowel or bladder dysfunction, ADLs, or aphasia.

39. **Describe the neuropsychological abnormalities found in patients with brain tumors.**
The scope of cognitive effects ranges from subtle attention and motivational problems to frank delirium and clouding of consciousness. These deficits can be caused by the primary effects of tumor or secondary effects of treatment. Patients with rapid-growing tumors, such as glioblastoma multiforme, exhibit behavioral and cognitive deficits secondary to rapid destruction of white matter tracts, increased intracranial pressure, and metabolic deficits. Patients with slow-growing tumors often do not demonstrate neuropsychological deficits, possibly due to a reorganization of cognitive functions to other brain regions.

Following radiotherapy to the brain, 14% of patients show subacute cognitive effects occurring 1–4 months after treatment; this effect results from a reversible demyelination, and gradual improvement in functional status over the next 2–3 months distinguishes this condition from signs of early tumor recurrence.

40. **Define postmastectomy lymphedema.**
Postmastectomy lymphedema is a collection of lymph in the interstitial tissues, resulting in a functional overload of the lymphatic system. The edema is usually confined to subcutaneous fat and skin. Lymphedema can follow any breast resection but is more likely if lymph node

dissection or irradiation is given. Its etiology is likely multifactorial, caused by a combination of excision of lymph channels, inflammation of involved tissues, and coagulation of lymph. Fibrosis of breast tissue by radiation and local infection can also increase the risk of developing lymphedema. Some studies report that lymphedema affects between 25.5% and 38.3% of patients having axillary node dissection and radiation therapy.

41. **Explain the conservative management techniques used for lymphedema.**
Elevation, compression wrapping, manual lymph drainage massage techniques, and low-resistance exercise of the distal musculature have been advocated. Compression of the affected extremity with low stretch bandages or a garment may be sufficient, but refractory edema may require a combination of compressive wrapping, manual lymph massage, and activity restrictions to control swelling. Some centers and therapists continue to use sequential compression pumps for lymphedema management with good results. Lymphedema treatments should be monitored closely for patient complaints of shortness of breath and significant pain. Ideally with either treatment, when limb circumference becomes stable without further improvements, the patient should be fitted for a custom support sleeve to be worn daily.

Once lymphedema occurs, it needs to be treated, and a lifelong maintenance program will be necessary, including intermittent aggressive treatment of exacerbations. Complications from chronic lymphedema cause significant morbidity, including chronic cellulitis, chronic shoulder dysfunction, or even a malignant cutaneous hemangiosarcoma (Stewart-Treves syndrome).

KEY POINTS: CANCER REHABILITATION

1. The most common presenting symptom of spinal cord compression by epidural tumor is pain, which often precedes neurologic signs by weeks or months. Early recognition is essential for effective treatment, because the majority of patients who present with paraplegia will remain thus despite treatment, whereas 75% of patients who begin treatment while ambulatory will not develop further neurologic impairment.

2. Facial swelling, dilated neck veins, and chest wall pains with headache are presenting symptoms of tumor obstruction of the superior vena cava. This syndrome is most commonly seen in lung cancer, lymphomas, and breast cancer and requires urgent antitumor therapy.

3. Cancer patients with a poor prognosis or very limited life span can still derive significant benefit and improved quality of life from brief concentrated rehabilitation efforts, including transfer training, bowel and bladder education, skin protection and maintenance skills, and equipment assessments.

4. Once lymphedema occurs, it needs to be treated, and a lifelong maintenance program will be necessary, including intermittent aggressive treatment of exacerbations. Complications from chronic lymphedema cause significant morbidity, including chronic cellulitis, chronic shoulder dysfunction, or even a malignant cutaneous hemangiosarcoma (Stewart-Treves syndrome).

5. Cancer fatigue is the most common symptom of advanced cancer (90% of patients) but is common throughout the disease continuum. Interventions involving exercise for non–end-stage patients have been studied and have consistently positive outcomes.

42. **What concerns should be raised when examining a patient with postmastectomy lymphedema?**
Recurrent disease, upper extremity deep venous thrombosis, and cellulitis can all precipitate and/or exacerbate lymphedema. A proper evaluation and work-up should precede any conservative treatment program. These same concerns should arise when patients with a history of pelvic, groin, or lower extremity tumors develop lower extremity edema.

WEBSITES

1. The National Cancer Institute Comprehensive Database provides information regarding specific cancer diagnoses and treatments, as well as supportive care and symptom management.
www.cancer.gov and www.cancer.gov/cancertopics/paq

2. Similar information can be found at the following address.
www.oncolink.upenn.edu

3. The National Lymphedema Network has disease information and treatment provider listings.
www.lymphnet.org

CHAPTER 68

RHEUMATIC DISEASES: DIAGNOSIS, TREATMENT, AND REHABILITATION

Galen O. Joe, MD, Jay P. Shah, MD, and Jeanne E. Hicks, MD

The grand aim of all science is to cover the greatest number of empirical facts by logical deduction from the smallest number of hypotheses or axioms.

—Albert Einstein (1879–1955)

1. **Is there a difference between noninflammatory and inflammatory arthritis?**
   See Table 68-1.

TABLE 68-1. NONINFLAMMATORY VERSUS INFLAMMATORY ARTHRITIS*				
Type	Onset	Clinical Findings	Joint Fluid/ Serum Labs	Radiographic Findings
Noninflammatory (most common: osteoarthritis)	Slow	Joint pain	High viscosity	Articular
	Progressive	Tenderness with palpation	WBC < 2000 cells/mm^3	Joint space loss
	Degenerative	Some swelling	<25% PMN	Cartilage loss
		Crepitus on passive range of motion	Serum—ESR and others—usually normal	Subchondral sclerosis
				Bony spurs at joint margin
Inflammatory (most common: rheumatoid arthritis)	Usually acute onset	Pain	Lower viscosity	Articular and extra-articular
		Fever	WBC > 3000 cells/mm^3	Soft tissue swelling
		Erythema over joints	>70% PMN	Periositis
		Warmth over joints		
		Inflammation	Serum—ESR elevated	Bony erosion
		Tenderness to palpation	Elevated WBC with elevated PMN (left shift)	Uniform cartilage loss

ESR = erythrocyte sedimentation rate, PMN = polymorphonuclear leukocytes, WBC = white blood cells.
*Inflammatory and noninflammatory arthritis can involve single or multiple joints and can be symmetric or asymmetric.

2. **What are the distinct groups of inflammatory arthritis?**
   See Table 68-2.

TABLE 68-2. DISTINCT GROUPS OF INFLAMMATORY ARTHRITIS	
Group	Examples
Inflammatory connective tissue disease	Rheumatoid arthritis, juvenile rheumatoid arthritis, systemic lupus erythematosus, polymyositis, dermatomyositis, polyarteritis nodosa, mixed connective tissue disorders
Inflammatory crystal-induced disease	Gout, pseudogout
Inflammation induced by infectious agents	Bacterial, viral, tuberculous, and fungal arthritis
Seronegative spondyloarthropathies	Ankylosing spondylitis, psoriatic arthritis, Reiter's disease, inflammatory bowel disease

3. **What is the role of ultrasound in physiatric musculoskeletal assessment?**
   High-resolution ultrasound has shown good results in aiding the diagnosis and localization of joint and bursal fluid. It is also reported to be more sensitive than plain radiographs in detecting early erosions. Imaging of muscle, peripheral nerve, and cartilage pathology have also been demonstrated on musculoskeletal ultrasound.

   Kane D, Balint PV, Sturrock R, Grassi W: Musculoskeletal ultrasound—a state of the art review in rheumatology. Part 2: Clinical indications for musculoskeletal ultrasound in rheumatology. Rheumatology 43:829–838, 2004.

REHABILITATIVE TREATMENTS

4. **What is the mechanism of action of aspirin?**
   - Blocks the synthesis of prostaglandins in the anterior hypothalamus **(antipyretic effect)**
   - Inhibits prostaglandin synthesis **(anti-inflammatory and analgesic effects)**

5. **What are the mechanisms of action of nonsteroidal anti-inflammatory drugs (NSAIDs)? What are their common toxicities?**
   Mechanisms of action
   - Suppress inflammation through prostaglandin synthesis inhibition
   - Inhibit leukocyte migration
   - Inhibit cyclo-oxygenase and lipoxygenase
   Toxicities
   - Gastrointestinal (GI) bleeding
   - Pancreatitis
   - Hepatotoxicity
   - Decreased renal blood flow
   - Allergic interstitial nephritis

6. **What are the COX-2 inhibitors?**
   These are a class of NSAIDs that selectively inhibit cyclo-oxygenase 2 and reduce prostaglandin synthesis. They were believed to have less GI toxicity than original nonselective NSAIDs.

Examples include rofecoxib, celecoxib, and valdecoxib. Recent studies showed increased cardiovascular risk with rofecoxib, and as a result it is no longer FDA approved. Higher doses of the latter two also can increase this risk. Doses of celecoxib at 200 mg have proved safer than some of the nonselective agents at higher doses. Meloxicam is considered a COX-2 inhibitor in Europe.

Kaplan RJ: Current status of nonsteroidal anti-inflammatory drugs in physiatry: Balancing risks and benefits in pain management. Am J Phys Rehabil 84:885–894, 2005.

7. What are the DMARDS? What are SAARDS?

Disease-modifying antirheumatic drugs (DMARDs) have been shown to produce sustained improvement in the course of rheumatoid arthritis (RA) for at least 1 year, as supported by a reduction in synovitis and structural joint disease shown on x-rays and enhanced physical function. Slow-acting antirheumatic drugs (SAARDS), a subset of DMARDS, are classified according to their presumed mechanism of action (antimetabolite, cytotoxic, or immunosuppressor), benefit, or clinical effect. It usually takes several weeks or more of use to see clinical improvement. Examples include methotrexate, leflunomide, and cyclosporine.

Wolf F, Rehman V, Lane NE, et al: Starting a disease-modifying antirheumatic drug or biologic agent in rheumatoid arthritis: Standards of practice for RA treatment. J Rheumatol 28:1701–1711, 2001.

8. What are the adverse effects associated with long-term methotrexate use?

GI toxicities such as stomatitis and dyspepsia are most common. Pulmonary and hepatic toxicity are the main concerns. Pulmonary hypersensitivity can occur in 2–6% and be life threatening, but it is usually reversible. Transaminitis occurs in 50%, but cirrhosis is rare. Teratogenicity is a known side effect. Pretreatment liver biopsy is recommended in patients with a history of alcohol abuse.

9. Do low-dose steroids cause muscle atrophy?

Muscle atrophy has been shown both in patients on high-dose steroids (prednisone > 15 mg/day) used in systemic lupus erythematosus (SLE) and stable, active polymyositis, and on low doses (5–12.5 mg/day) used in these and RA. All of these diseases cause muscle atrophy from the systemic disease and decreased patient activity.

10. What are the TNF-blocking agents?

The tumor necrosis factor (TNF) inhibitors, etanercept and infliximab, have been approved to treat several of the rheumatic diseases. These drugs bind and inhibit TNF-alpha, reducing inflammation and altering immune response. Common side effects include injection site pain and erythema, increased risk of infection, headache, and autoantibody production.

11. What effect does application of superficial heat have on soft tissue and joint temperature in arthritis?

Superficial moist heat applied for 3 minutes causes elevation of the soft tissue temperature by 3°C, to a depth of 1 cm, and significantly increases the temperature of hand and knee joints. Superficial heat causes decreased soft tissue pain by acting on pain receptors and by relieving muscle spasm. It also increases collagen extensibility, allowing for more effective stretching programs. However, it is associated with increased collagenase enzyme in the rheumatoid joint, an enzyme that causes joint destruction. Therefore, it is best if cold is used on acutely inflamed joints, and heat reserved for subacute or chronic joints.

Hicks JE: Modalities and devices for rheumatoid arthritis. J Musculoskeletal Med 17:385–398, 2000.

12. **What are the indications, benefits, and contraindications of hot and cold modalities in the treatment of inflammatory joint diseases?**
See Table 68-3.

TABLE 68-3. USE OF HOT AND COLD MODALITIES IN THE TREATMENT OF INFLAMMATORY JOINT DISEASES

Modality	Indication	Benefits	Contraindications
Heat (superficial and/or deep)	Subacute or chronic stages	Increases range of motion Increases tendon extensibility Relaxes spastic muscles Decreases pain	Acute inflamed joint or tissue Impaired sensation Malignancy Infection Impaired circulation Atrophic skin
Cold	Acutely inflamed stage	Relieves pain Relaxes surrounding spastic muscles Decreases inflammation	Cryopathies Raynaud's phenomenon Cold hypersensitivity cryoglobulinemia Paroxysmal cold hemoglobinuria Arterial insufficiency Neurapraxia or other injury to superficial nerves Cognitive impairment or impaired sensation that would limit the ability to report pain or discomfort Cardiovascular disease

13. **Discuss the detrimental effects of prolonged rest.**
Rest is an accepted treatment for inflammatory rheumatic disease. However, prolonged rest can have detrimental effects. Decreased mobility may promote stiffening of periarticular structures, reduction of cartilage integrity, and decreased cardiovascular fitness, muscle mass and strength, bone density, and coordination.

14. **List the factors to be considered in designing an exercise program for patients with inflammatory arthritis.**
- Assessment of local or systemic involvement
- Stage of joint involvement
- Type of pain
- Age of patient
- Comorbid medical conditions
- Compliance
- Preparation for exercise and exercise sequence

15. **List the beneficial effects of exercise programs for patients with rheumatic diseases.**
- Increases and maintains joint motion
- Re-educates and strengthens muscles

- Increases static muscle endurance
- Increases aerobic capacity
- Decreases the number of swollen joints
- Enables joints to function better biomechanically
- Increases bone density
- Increases overall patient function and well-being

16. **What are the signs of excessive exercise in patients with rheumatic diseases?**
Postexercise pain of >2 hours, undue fatigue, transient increased weakness, and increased joint swelling. If any or all of these problems occur, the program should be reassessed and appropriate adjustments made. The type of exercise, duration, and intensity need to be reevaluated periodically in light of the disease stage and the condition of various joints.

17. **Compare the indications and contraindications of passive and active range-of-motion (ROM) exercise in patients with rheumatic disease. When should forceful stretching of a tendon or joint be avoided?**
Passive ROM exercise is beneficial for patients with severe weakness caused by polymyositis or neuropathic disease, stroke, peripheral neuropathy, and vasculitis. Patients with acute joints may passively put their joints through an arc of motion once daily to prevent the development of joint contracture, but passive motion with many repetitions increases joint inflammation. Active ROM can exacerbate inflammation in acute joints. It is used for subacute or chronic joints to enhance ROM.
Forceful **tendon stretching** should be avoided when the tendon is inflamed, very tight, or lax, because this can increase inflammation and tendon sheath fluid accumulation. Forceful stretching of a very tight tendon can be very painful, and rupture might occur at the musculotendinous junction. Stretching of lax tendons as in SLE (particularly of the patellar and Achilles tendons) may cause rupture. For a tight, noninflamed tendon, prolonged periods of stretch are more effective in lengthening the tendon without causing undue pain.
Forceful **joint stretching** should also be avoided if there is a moderate or large effusion, joint inflammation, or joint laxity, because this can cause a capsular rupture. Forceful stretching of joints with much ligamentous and capsular laxity can cause joint subluxation (common in RA, juvenile RA, and SLE).

18. **Which type of exercise is least likely to increase inflammation in an inflamed joint: isotonic, isokinetic, or isometric?**
Isometric exercise is associated with the least joint inflammation and juxta-articular bone destruction.

19. **What type of strengthening exercise can be used in rheumatic diseases?**
For nonacute arthritis, strengthening begins with an isometric exercise program of key large muscles around joints. This is followed by an isotonic program with low weights and joint motion. Isokinetic exercise (particularly) at low speeds places high forces across joints, is expensive and used only in the clinic, and thus has limited use for arthritis patients.

Hicks JE: Exercise in patients with inflammatory arthritis and connective tissue disease. Rheum Dis Clin North Am 16:845–870, 1990.

20. **What type of aerobic exercise is used in rheumatic disease?**
Both the bike ergometer and pool are used for aerobic exercise. Because rheumatic disease (RD) patients are often much deconditioned, low-intensity exercise for 15–20 minutes two to three times a week can increase aerobic capacity.

21. **How do knee and hip effusions affect the surrounding muscle?**
Hip effusions in RA patients have an inhibiting effect on contraction of the gluteus medius muscle, and knee effusions inhibit contraction of the quadriceps mechanism. This diminishes

the effect of muscle-strengthening programs in the knee. It also allows for overpull by the stronger, less atrophied hamstring muscles and makes the knee prone to flexion contracture.

It is recommended that moderate to large knee joint effusions, easily detected by clinical exam, be removed in rheumatic disease patients before initiating a quadriceps-strengthening program. It is harder to detect hip effusion clinically. However, if the patient is unable to strengthen the gluteus medius muscle and has pain with exercise, you may wish to check the hip by plain film or ultrasound to see if significant effusion is present.

22. **What factors contribute to fatigue in patients with RD?**
Medication, chronic inflammation, anemia of chronic disease, abnormal posture and gait, decreased aerobic capacity, abnormalities of the sleep cycle, atrophy of muscle secondary to disease or chronic pain, and cardiovascular and pulmonary problems may contribute to fatigue. Fatigue is difficult to quantify because a decrease in overall stamina, true muscle fatigue, and lack of motivation all result in an inability to complete tasks.

23. **You are asked to educate the RD patient about energy conservation. What would your recommendations to the patient be?**
   - Maximize biomechanical function of joints by using proper orthotics and assistive devices to maintain energy-efficient ambulation and hand function.
   - Use appropriate clothing and adaptive devices; prepare proper environmental designs; maintain strength, ROM, and posture; take short rest periods during the day.

24. **Name some appropriate techniques for joint protection.**
   - **Avoid prolonged periods in the same position:** To minimize joint stress
   - **Maintain ROM:** To maintain strength
   - **Maintain good joint alignment:** To reduce joint pain
   - **Avoid joint overuse during acute flare:** To unload painful joint
   - **Use adaptive equipment and splints as indicated:** To modify tasks

25. **What is the purpose of prescribing orthotics for the RD patient?**
To decrease pain and inflammation and improve joint alignment and function. Prevention of progression of joint deformity has not yet been clinically proven.

26. **Discuss the key reasons for referring rheumatoid patients for surgery.**
Pain caused by joint destruction by inflammation (JRA, RA) or mechanical degeneration (osteoarthritis) unresponsive to adequate medical and rehabilitation management and decreased overall function are the two most common indications for joint replacement. Suspicion of a **pending extensor tendon rupture,** particularly in the RA hand, or actual **tendon rupture** is another valid reason for surgery. Elective tendon realignment and metacarpophalangeal (MCP) replacement in RA should be carefully considered only if function will clearly be increased. **Deformity alone,** fixed or not, is usually not a reason for surgery, because significant deformity can be present and fairly good function maintained. Arthrodesis of unstable joints in a functional position, particularly the thumb or hindfoot, is also useful.

Gerber L, Hicks JE: Surgical and rehabilitation options in the treatment of the rheumatoid arthritis patient resistant to pharmacologic agents. Rheum Dis Clin North Am 21(1):19–39, 1995.

RHEUMATOID ARTHRITIS

27. **Name the seven criteria used to establish the diagnosis of RA.**
See Table 68-4.

28. **What are the most common extra-articular manifestations of rheumatoid arthritis?**
See Table 68-5.

TABLE 68-4. 1987 AMERICAN COLLEGE OF RHEUMATOLOGY (ACR) REVISED CRITERIA FOR THE CLASSIFICATION OF RHEUMATOID ARTHRITIS*

Criterion	Definition
Morning stiffness	Morning stiffness in and around the joints, lasting at least 1 hour before maximal improvement
Arthritis involving 3 or more joints	At least 3 joint areas simultaneously have had soft-tissue swelling or fluid observed by a physician; 14 possible areas are right or left PIP, MCP, wrist, elbow, knee, ankle, and MTP joints
Arthritis of hand joints	At least 1 area swollen (as defined above) in a wrist, MCP, or PIP joint
Symmetric arthritis	Simultaneous involvement of the same joint areas (as defined in criterion 2) on both sides of the body (bilateral involvement of PIPs, MCPs, or MTPs is acceptable without absolute symmetry)
Rheumatoid nodules	Subcutaneous nodules over bony prominences, or extensor surfaces, or in juxta-articular regions, observed by a physician
Serum rheumatoid factor	Abnormal amounts of serum RF demonstrated by any method for which the result has been positive in < 5% of normal control subjects
Radiographic changes	Radiographic changes typical of RA on posteroanterior hand and wrist radiographs, which must include erosions or unequivocal bony decalcification localized in or, most marked, adjacent to the involved joints (osteoarthritis changes alone do not qualify)

MCP = metacarpophalangeal joint, MTP = metatarsophalangeal joint, PIP = proximal interphalangeal joint, RA = rheumatoid arthritis, RF = rheumatoid factor.
Adapted from Arnett FC, Edworthy SM, Bloch DA, et al: The American Rheumatism Association's 1987 revised criteria for the classification of rheumatoid arthritis. Arthritis Rheum 31:315–324, 1987.
*For classification purposes, a patient is considered to have RA if he or she satisfies at least four of these seven criteria. Criteria 1–4 must have been present for at least 6 weeks. Patients with two clinical diagnoses are not excluded. Designation as classic, definite, or probable rheumatoid arthritis is not to be made.

TABLE 68-5. COMMON EXTRA-ARTICULAR MANIFESTATIONS OF RHEUMATOID ARTHTITIS

System	Manifestations
Dermatologic	Rheumatoid nodules in 25–35% of patients (most often on extensor surfaces), vasculitic lesions
Neurologic	Entrapment neuropathies, myelopathies related to cervical spine instability
Cardiovascular	Inflammatory pericarditis, valvular dysfunction, vasculitis
Pulmonary	Inflammation of the cricoarytenoid joint, interstitial lung disease
Hematologic	Normocytic hypochromic anemia, Felty's syndrome
Systemic	Fatigue, malaise, fever
Renal	Renal vasculitis, glomerulonephritis
Ocular	Scleritis

29. **What is a rheumatoid factor? Is it pathognomonic for RA?**
Rheumatoid factors (RFs) are immunoglobulins (e.g., IgM) that react with the Fc portion of IgG molecules. They are found in the serum of 85% of patients with RA but are not pathognomonic of this disease. RFs are also found in some patients with Reiter's syndrome, psoriatic arthritis, sarcoidosis, the elderly population, bacterial endocarditis, and in 3% of apparently healthy people. RFs are of clinical value because their presence in high titer tends to correlate with severe and unremitting disease, RA nodules, and extra-articular manifestations of RA.

30. **What are the x-ray hallmarks of RA?**
The early x-ray abnormalities seen in RA are soft-tissue swelling and juxta-articular osteoporosis. Later changes include bilaterally symmetric joint-space narrowing and cartilage and bony erosions.

31. **What are "swan neck," boutonnière, and mallet digit deformities?**
The "swan neck" deformity results from contracture of the interosseous and flexor muscles and tendons of the fingers, resulting in a flexion contracture of the MCP joint, hyperextension of the proximal interphalangeal (PIP) joint, and flexion of the distal interphalangeal (DIP) joint. It commonly occurs in RA. However, it may be seen due to ligamentous laxity in SLE and polymyositis. The **boutonnière** deformity consists of hyperflexion of the DIP and hyperextension of the PIP joints when the extensor hood of the PIP is stretched. The **mallet** deformity is hyperflexion at the PIP. These deformities, when reducible, can be corrected with custom-made orthoplast or Silver Ring splints.

32. **A patient with a long history of RA presents with sudden onset of unsteady gait, paresthesias, and neck pain. A lateral x-ray of the cervical spine should be obtained to rule out what condition?**
Atlantoaxial subluxation is common in RA. It may occur with up to 9–10 mm of subluxation with no neurologic findings. However, neurologic findings may occur early, and whenever they do occur, it is important to repeat the cervical spine x-ray and compare it to previous ones. High-resolution computed tomography (CT) or magnetic resonance imaging (MRI) may show anatomic abnormalities in the presence of neurologic findings; surgery to reduce the deformity may be indicated.

33. **What are the most common foot abnormalities in patients with RA?**
See Table 68-6.

34. **Name some typical gait characteristics observed in patients with RA involvement of the feet.**
The typical gait pattern is a nonpropulsive gait with decreased velocity, stride length, short single-limb stance, prolonged heel contact, and longer double-limb support phase.

35. **What key muscles should be strengthened and stretched in RA?**

Strengthened	**Stretched**
Foot intrinsics	Toe extensors, peroneus, gastrocnemius
Quadriceps	Hamstrings, hip flexors, iliotibial band
Finger, wrist extensors	Hand intrinsics

Strengthening and stretching of these key muscles is particularly important to encourage muscle balance. Certain muscles become weaker than others, and an overpull of the stronger muscles around an RA joint may lead to joint contractures. For example, a weak, atrophied quadriceps with overpull by the stronger hamstrings can create a flexion contracture of the knee.

Hicks JE: Exercise in rheumatoid arthritis. Phys Med Rehabil Clin North Am 5(4):701–728, 1994.

TABLE 68-6.   COMMON FOOT ABNORMALITIES IN PATIENTS WITH RHEUMATOID ARTHRITIS

Region of Foot	Most Common Abnormalities	Treatment
Forefoot	Widening of the metatarsal area Metatarsalgia Hammertoe Hallux valgus	Wide and extra-depth footwear, soft-lined; custom-molded orthosis with MTP relief
Midfoot	Decreased medial longitudinal arch Posterior tibialis tendon (PTT) tendinitis	Footwear crepe wedge or conventional heel–sole combination with a shank support system Custom orthosis with corrective medial column support to prevent excessive pronation and PTT strain
Hindfoot	Pronation with subtalar joint and ankle disease PTT tendinitis Ligamentous laxity	Footwear with a firm heel counter Custom orthosis with full medial column support, hind foot post, and midfoot post

MTP = metatarsophalangeal.

SPONDYLOARTHROPATHIES

36. **Which joint must be affected before establishing a diagnosis of one of the spondyloarthropathies?**
    The sine qua non of spondyloarthropathies is **sacroiliitis**. Early SI joint changes include superficial bony erosions and eburnation, which may enlarge, and are followed by progressive sclerosis and focal narrowing of the articular space. At more advanced stages, extensive sclerosis and focal ankylosis complete ankylosis of the synovial and ligamentous portions of the SI joint.

37. **What are the spondyloarthropathies?**
    This group of disorders includes ankylosing spondylitis, psoriatic arthritis, reactive arthritis, and inflammatory bowel disease. They involve the axial skeleton and are accompanied by enthesopathy (inflammation at the site of a tendon or ligament attachment to bone). Extra-articular manifestations may include skin rashes, psoriasis, uveitis, and aortitis.

38. **What are the diagnostic signs and symptoms for the spondyloarthropathies?**
    Inflammatory spinal pain should be present, or synovitis, which is asymmetric or predominantly involves the lower limbs. Either of these in combination with one or more of the following supports the diagnosis of a spondyloarthropathy:
    - Positive family history
    - Psoriasis
    - Inflammatory bowel disease
    - Urethritis, cervicitis, or acute diarrhea within 1 month before arthritis

- Buttock pain alternating between right and left gluteal areas
- Enthesopathy
- Sacroiliitis

Dougados M, Van Der Linden S, Juhlin R, et al: The European Spondyloarthropathy Study Group preliminary criteria for the classification of spondyloarthropathy. Arthritis Rheum 34:1218–1227, 1991.

39. **What triad of disorders make up Reiter's syndrome?**
Urethritis, conjunctivitis, and **arthritis.** Reiter's syndrome, or reactive arthritis, typically follows a bout of urethritis or diarrhea 2–4 weeks previously (the urethritis may persist) and is presumed to involve the migration of bacterial antigens into these sites, where an inflammatory response ensues.

40. **Which clinical test is used to measure the progression of spinal involvement in ankylosing spondylitis?**
The **Wright-Schöber test** can be used to measure the progression of motion limitation in ankylosing spondylitis. This test measures the distraction on anterior spinal flexion measured vertically above the level of the posterior iliac spines. On anterior flexion, a reading of 5–10 cm is considered normal.

41. **Describe an appropriate exercise program for a patient with ankylosing spondylitis.**
The joint and spinal motion loss, muscle weakness, and decreased endurance seen in this disorder are less severe in patients who participate in an active and consistent ROM, stretching, strengthening, and aerobic exercise program, as well as maintain good posture:
- **Posture** advice includes sleeping on a firm mattress with no pillow or a very thin pillow; lying prone for 15–20 minutes twice a day; sitting upright in a chair that reaches to the thoracic level; having an eye-level computer; and placing reading materials on an eye-level stand.
- A twice-daily **ROM stretching program** should be done for the large peripheral joints (shoulder and hips).
- **Spinal extension exercises** should be done using the corner-pushup exercise.
- **Strengthening** of the shoulder, hip, and spinal extensor muscles should be included as well.
- **Aerobic exercise** in the pool (laps using a snorkel) encourages spinal extension.
- **Sports** or activities that involve heavy contact or encourage spinal flexion should be discouraged (golf, bicycling, bowling, crochet), and those encouraging spinal extension should be recommended (archery, table tennis, badminton).
To be effective, the program must be done for the entire course of this chronic disease.

Vitanen JV, Heikkila S: Functional changes in patients with spondyloarthropathy. A controlled trial of the effects of short term rehabilitation and a 3 year follow-up. Rheumatol Int 20:21–25, 2001.

OSTEOARTHRITIS

42. **What is the pathophysiology of osteoarthritis (OA)?**
The normal joint provides an extremely smooth bearing surface, permitting virtually frictionless movement of one bone over another within the weight-bearing joint; second, it distributes load, preventing concentration of stress within the joint. Although cartilage degeneration is the hallmark of OA, it does not represent the failure of a single tissue but of an organ—the diarthrodial joint. The primary abnormality in OA may reside in the articular cartilage, synovium, subchondral bone, ligaments, or neuromuscular apparatus.
Nonetheless, the marked changes that occur in osteoarthritic cartilage and bone are cartilage wear and tear, decreased joint space, and osteophyte formation.

Stitik TP (ed): Osteoarthritis. Physical Medicine and Rehabilitation: State of the Art Reviews, Vol 15, No 1. Philadelphia, Hanley & Belfus, 2001.

43. **What types of sports activities typically increase the likelihood for OA?**
See Table 68-7.

TABLE 68-7. TYPES OF ACTIVITIES THAT INCREASE THE LIKELIHOOD OF OSTEOARTHRITIS

Incidence of Osteoarthritis	Sports Activity
High	Ballet (talus, ankle, MTP joint, hip)
	Soccer (ankle, talus, knee)
	Baseball (elbow, shoulder)
Low	Running (hip)
Possible	Running (knee)
	Gymnastics (shoulder, elbow, wrist)

MTP = metatarsophalangeal.

44. **Which joints does OA typically involve? In which joints is it most likely to lead to disability?**
In primary or idiopathic OA, the joints that develop OA (in order of decreasing frequency) are the knees, first MTP joints, DIP joints, carpometacarpal (CMC) joints, hips, cervical spine, and lumbar spine. It spares the elbows and shoulders, unless it is truly primary OA caused by an injury, fracture, or an occupation-related task. Significant disability in OA is caused by involvement of the large weight-bearing joints of the hip and knee. CMC joint involvement in the hand causes pain and limitation in functional activities, particularly those of a repetitive nature. However, splinting of the CMC joint reduces pain and allows for a very functional thumb.

45. **What are the most commonly encountered problems in a foot with OA?**
Hallux valgus, with or without bunions; hallux rigidus with cocked toes; metatarsal head calluses; and abrasions on the dorsum of the toes.

46. **What exercises should patients with OA perform?**
Patients can improve ROM, local muscle endurance, aerobic capacity, gait characteristics, balance, and overall function and decrease pain and disability with a combined strengthening and aerobic exercise program. Both isometric and isotonic exercise are indicated. Aerobic exercise can be done by mall walking, bike ergometer, treadmill, or pool. Those patients with significant hip and knee disease should use the pool for exercises.

Hicks JE, Perry M, Gerber LH: Rehabilitation in the management of patients with osteoarthritis. In Moskowitz RW, Howell DS, Goldberg VM, Mankin HJ (eds): Osteoarthritis: Diagnosis and Medical/Surgical Management, 2nd ed. Philadelphia, W.B. Saunders, 2000, pp 413–446.

47. **Is there a role for acupuncture in the management of osteoarthritis?**
Yes. A recent study by Berman et al. demonstrated that acupuncture provides both pain relief and functional improvement for people with osteoarthritis of the knee and serves as an effective complement to standard medical management. This multisite study, the longest and largest randomized, controlled phase III clinical trial of acupuncture yet conducted, enrolled 570 patients, aged 50 or older with knee pain secondary to OA. Participants were randomly

assigned to one of three treatment groups: acupuncture, sham acupuncture, or participation in a control group that followed the Arthritis Foundation's self-help course for managing the condition. Participants continued to receive standard medical care from their primary physicians, including anti-inflammatory medications, NSAIDs, and opioid pain relievers.

Primary outcome measures were changes in the Western Ontario and McMaster Universities Osteoarthritis Index (WOMAC) pain and function scores at 8 and 26 weeks. Secondary outcome measures included patient global assessment, 6-minute walk distance, and physical health scores of the 36-item Short-Form Health Survey (SF-36). Subjects in the true acupuncture group experienced greater improvement in WOMAC function scores than the sham acupuncture group at 8 weeks but not in WOMAC pain score or the patient global assessment. At 26 weeks, the true acupuncture group experienced significantly greater improvement than the sham group in the WOMAC pain score, WOMAC function score, and patient global assessment.

Berman BM, Lao L, Langenberg P, et al: Effectiveness of acupuncture as adjunctive therapy in osteoarthritis of the knee: A randomized, controlled trial. Ann Intern Med 141(12):901–910, 2004.

POLYMYOSITIS

48. **List the five criteria for diagnosis and typing of polymyositis.**
    See Table 68-8.

TABLE 68-8. FIVE DIAGNOSTIC CRITERIA FOR AND TYPES OF POLYMYOSITIS	
Diagnostic Criteria	**Types**
1. Symmetrical muscle weakness	1. PM
2. EMG with myopathic pattern	2. Adult DM
3. Elevated CPK/aldose	3. Polymyositis–dermatomyositis associated with other connective tissue diseases (Sjögren's, RA, SLE, PSS, MCTD)
4. Muscle biopsy with inflammation of muscle	4. PM–DM of childhood
5. Dermatologic features (dermatomyositis)	5. PM–DM with malignancy
	6. Inclusion body myositis

CPK = creatine phosphokinase, DM = dermatomyositis, EMG = electromyography, MCTD = mixed connective tissue disease, PM = polymyositis, PSS = progressive systemic sclerosis, RA = rheumatoid arthritis, SLE = systemic lupus erythematosus.
Adapted from Wortman RL: Inflammatory diseases of muscle and other myopathies. In Ruddy S, Harris ED, Sledge CB, et al (eds): Kelly's Textbook of Rheumatology, 6th ed. Philadelphia, W.B. Saunders, 2001, pp 1339–1376.

49. **Describe an appropriate exercise program for patients with polymyositis.**
    In the past, exercise for patients with polymyositis was not recommended because of fear it would cause muscle inflammation. Currently, it has been shown that a 1-month isometric exercise program can increase strength in patients with inactive or stable active myositis without causing sustained creatine phosphokinase (CPK) elevations. Patients with significant muscle atrophy and very weak muscles do not respond as well.

It is reasonable to place polymyositis patients with chronic or stable active disease on a three-times-a-week or even daily **isometric program** consisting of 6–10 isometric contractions, each held for 6 sec, with a 20-sec recovery time between contractions. The main muscles to exercise are the deltoids, biceps, hip abductors, extensors, and quadriceps muscles. Those patients who also have some distal weakness (20–40%) may wish to exercise wrist and hand muscles and ankle dorsiflexors/plantar flexors. A significant proportion of patients with inclusion body myositis have both proximal and distal weakness. A few studies support isotonic resistive exercise for myositis with low 1–2 lb weight two to three times a week.

Studies reveal adults and children with myositis also have decreased aerobic capacity. **Aerobic training** in stable, nonactive adult patients with myositis has revealed an increase in aerobic capacity without a disease flare. Low-level aerobic program on a cycle or in a pool can be done. Exercise programs should be reassessed if there is increased muscle weakness and soreness along with significant rises in CPK.

Stretching exercises may be performed to maintain ROM chronic and stable, active disease. Adult patients frequently lose significant shoulder motion, and children lose motion quickly in shoulders, elbows, hips, and knees, and sometimes wrist and ankles. Calcium deposits in the soft tissues around joints in childhood dermatomyositis make them particularly prone to loss of joint motion.

Alexanderson H, Lundberg IE: The role of exercise in rehabilitation of idiopathic inflammatory myopathies. Current Opin Rheumatol 17(2):164–171, 2005.

KEY POINTS: RHEUMATIC DISEASE

1. Early diagnosis of rheumatic disease is often associated with better disease control and functional outcome.

2. Some rheumatoid arthritis medications slow the progression of disease damage and are associated with improved functional outcome.

3. Exercise has been proven to have a number of benefits for persons with rheumatic diseases.

4. Acupuncture, a type of complementary and alternative medicine, has been proven to reduce the pain of knee osteoarthritis.

5. Referral for surgical interventions such as joint replacement is indicated if there is persistent pain and decreased function despite appropriate medical and rehabilitation treatment.

50. **How can you stabilize the knee in the presence of a very weak quadriceps mechanism?**

Patients with polymyositis often develop very weak quadriceps muscles and begin to fall when their strength is 3 out of 5 or below. Although weakness is generally symmetrical in a proximal distribution, one quadriceps may be weaker than the opposite one, and bracing the weaker limb may dramatically decrease the incidence of falling. The brace used is a short-leg metal or plastic one locked in 5 degrees of plantar flexion to create a stabilizing extension moment at the knee. This brace may also be used if there is concomitant plantar flexor weakness, because the locked position at 5 degrees will prevent tripping on the toes.

Do not put a dorsiflexion assist on a brace when the quadriceps is weak. A flexion moment will be created at the knee and make it less stable. If the hip flexors are very weak, use the lighter plastic brace fixed in plantar flexion. Braces that create a hyperextension moment at the knee should be used with caution in patients with joint involvement from arthritis because knee pain can be increased as a result of the hyperextension force.

SYSTEMIC LUPUS ERYTHEMATOSUS

51. **What are the signs and symptoms for the diagnosis of systemic lupus erythematosus (SLE)?**
    - Malar rash
    - Discoid rash
    - Photosensitivity
    - Oral or nasopharyngeal ulceration
    - Nonerosive arthritis
    - Serositis
    - Pleuritis or pericarditis
    - Renal disorder
    - Neurologic disorder (seizures) or psychosis
    - Hemolytic anemia—with reticulocytosis, leukopenia, lymphopenia, or thrombocytopenia
    - Immunologic disorder (positive LE cell preparation; anti-DNA: antibody to native DNA in abnormal titer; or anti-Sm: presence of antibody to Sm nuclear antigen; or false-positive serologic test for syphilis known to be positive for at least 6 months and confirmed by *Treponema pallidum* immobilization or fluorescent treponemal antibody absorption test) Antinuclear antibody must be present. The proposed classification is based on 11 criteria. A person is said to have SLE if any 4 or more of the 11 criteria are present, serially or simultaneously, during any interval of observation.

    Tan EM, Cohen AS, Fries JF, et al: The 1982 revised criteria for the classification of systemic lupus erythematosus (SLE). Arthritis Rheum 25:1271–1277, 1982.

52. **Which sex is overwhelmingly affected by SLE?**
    SLE is primarily a disease of young women. Its peak incidence occurs between the ages of 15 and 40, with a female-to-male ratio of approximately 5:1.

53. **What are the typical musculoskeletal and systemic manifestations of SLE?**
    Arthralgias are the most common presenting manifestations of SLE. These patients may develop arthritis with joint deformities (Jaccouds arthritis) and complain of muscle pain and weakness. They often have significant **ligamentous** laxity, leading to dislocation of the shoulder, significant knee instability, and swan-neck deformities of the hands. The laxity makes them prone to tendon rupture during sports activities, particularly of the Achilles and patellar tendons. **Fatigue** and **psychological and neurologic disorders** may also be complications of SLE.

54. **Describe an appropriate exercise program and its rationale for a patient with SLE.**
    Patients with SLE have prominent fatigue, and significant decreased aerobic capacity has been shown in patients with mild SLE. These patients should be on an aerobic exercise program. Aseptic necrosis of the knee and hips often occurs as a result of the disease itself or steroids. An isometric and isotonic strengthening program for the quadriceps and hip musculature is important to help maintain biomechanical integrity.

JUVENILE RA (JRA)

55. **List the types of JRA. What are some common problems seen in these patients?**
    Types of JRA
    - Pauciarticular: Involvement of ≤3 joints
    - Polyarticular: Involvement of >3 joints

- Systemic: Associated with a systemic onset of high fever, rash, and acute joint pain
  Common problems with JRA are decreased joint motion and strength, limb-length discrepancies, and gait abnormalities.

56. **You are asked to evaluate and recommend a treatment plan for a 5-year-old boy with pauciarticular JRA. Describe an appropriate exercise program and its rationale.**

   Children with JRA quickly lose strength around inflamed joints, and motion of the joint is compromised at an early stage. ROM and a few isometric exercises are done even when the joint is acute. Incorporating exercise into play routines is important. Use of a tricycle can increase motion strength and conditioning. Pool programs are very helpful. The parent should be instructed in the importance of exercise and incorporate this into the child's daily routines.

ACKNOWLEDGMENT

Special thanks are extended to Frances Stevens, who was responsible for typing the revisions for this manuscript.

WEBSITES

1. American College of Rheumatology
   www.rheumatology.org

2. Arthritis Foundation
   www.arthritis.org

3. Myositis Association
   www.myositis.org

BIBLIOGRAPHY

1. Hicks JE, Joe GO, Gerber L: Rehabilitation of the patient with inflammatory arthritis and connective tissue disorders. In DeLisa J (ed): Physical Medicine and Rehabilitation: Principles and Practice. Philadelphia, J.B. Lippincott Williams & Wilkins, 2004, pp 1047–1081.

2. Hicks J, Nicholas J, Swezey R (eds): Handbook of Rehabilitative Rheumatology. Bayville, NY, Contact Associates, 1988.

3. Munster T, Furst DE: Pharmacotherapeutic strategies for disease modifying anti-rheumatic drug (DMARD) combinations to treat rheumatoid arthritis (RA). Exper Rheumatol 17(Suppl 18):S29–S36, 1999.

4. Ruddy S, Harris ED, Sledge CB, et al (eds): Kelly's Textbook of Rheumatology, 6th ed. Philadelphia, W.B. Saunders, 2001, pp 1339–1376.

5. Schumacher HR Jr: Primer on the Rheumatic Diseases, 12th ed. Atlanta, Arthritis Foundation, 2001.

CHAPTER 69

BURN INJURIES: EPIDEMIOLOGY, TREATMENT, AND REHABILITATION

Peter C. Esselman, MD, Vincent Gabriel, MD, Arieh Eldad, MD, and Karen J. Kowalske, MD

> *Healing is a matter of time, but it is sometimes also a matter of opportunity.*
> —Hippocrates (460–377 BC), *Precepts*

1. **Describe the type of injury occurring in a burn wound.**
   A burn wound can be divided into three zones:
   - In the **zone of coagulation,** the protein destruction is most severe and cellular necrosis is complete, forming eschar.
   - In the **zone of stasis,** the majority of cells are initially intact, but inflammation can lead to ischemia and necrosis.
   - The most peripheral is the **zone of hyperemia** with increased blood flow and negligible cellular injury.

   Willams Geoff W: Pathophysiology of the burn wound. In Herndon DN (ed): Total Burn Care, 2nd ed. Philadelphia, W.B. Saunders, 2002, pp 514–521.

2. **What different agents can cause a burn?**
   Burns are caused by thermal, electrical, chemical, and radiation agents. Scalds are the most common overall cause, whereas flame is the predominant cause in patients requiring burn center admission. Radiation burns are rare.

3. **How common are burns?**
   In the United States, more than 1 million burn injuries occur each year. There are approximately 700,000 emergency department visits per year and approximately 45,000 patients admitted to the hospital.

   Burn Incidence and Treatment in the US: 2000 Fact sheet. Available from the American Burn Association: www.ameriburn.org/resources_factsheet.php

4. **What factors determine burn injury survival?**
   Burn depth, percentage of total body surface area (TBSA) burned, inhalation injury, patient age, associated trauma, and premorbid health determine survival after a burn injury. Survival has increased over time due to improved acute care, as well as early excision, and grafting of severe burns. The LD_{50} or burn size lethal to 50% of the population increased from 65% TBSA in the 1980s to more than 80% TBSA in the 1990s.

5. **What is the "rule of nines"?**
   The rule of nines is a convenient and fairly accurate way of estimating adult percentage TBSA burned (Fig. 69-1). The rule of nines is not accurate for children who have different proportions, especially the head, which is 19% of the TBSA in an infant.

6. **How are burns classified?**
   Burns are classified by the depth of injury.
   1. **Superficial (first degree):** Involves only the epidermis. Skin is erythematous, painful, but not blistered. Heals in 3–7 days.

2. **Partial thickness (second degree):**
   - Superficial partial thickness: Includes the epidermis and superficial dermis. Burn may blister, is red and painful, will blanch with pressure, and will heal in 7–21 days.
   - Deep partial thickness: Extends into deeper dermis. Wound is mottled pink to white with poor capillary refill. May heal with hypertrophic scarring but usually needs grafting.
3. **Full thickness (third degree):** Involves entire epidermis and dermis. Eschar is present. Wound is not painful because of destruction of sensory nerve endings. Requires grafting.

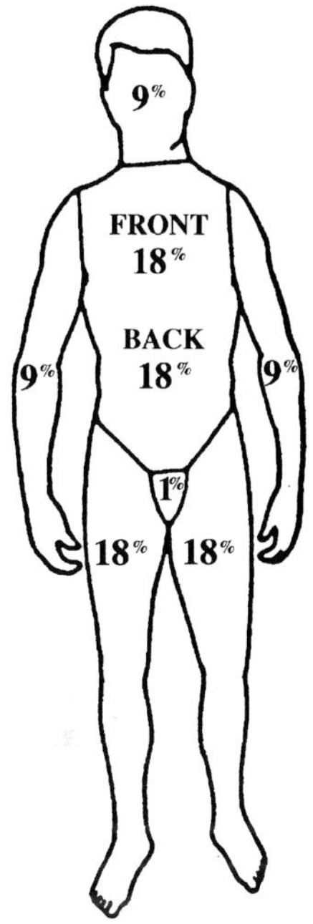

7. **How do partial-thickness burns heal?**
   The epidermis is destroyed, so healing can occur only from the edges of the wound or from epidermal cells in the dermal appendages (hair follicles, sweat glands).

8. **When are grafts necessary?**
   Any full-thickness burn or deep partial-thickness burn that will not heal within 28 days benefits from skin grafting. Early excision of nonviable tissue and grafting reduce pain, length of hospital stay, wound infection, risk of hypertrophic scarring, and medical complications.

9. **What types of grafts are available?**
   - An **autograft** is taken from a donor site on the patient's body. Split-thickness skin grafts (STSG) include the epidermis and superficial dermis. An autograft can be used intact as a sheet graft on the face, hands, and joints or as a mesh graft to cover larger areas. A full-thickness skin graft (FTSG) includes the epidermis and entire dermis and is used to graft very small areas such as the eyelid or tip of the nose. An FTSG donor site usually requires primary closure for healing.
   - A **xenograft** is skin from a pig and provides a biologic dressing to promote healing and prevent infection.
   - An **allograft** is taken from cadavers and also provides a temporary covering that will be rejected by the immune system in several weeks. If an allograft remains intact before rejection, an autograft placed on the wound can be expected to survive.
   - **Integra** is a dermal replacement product consisting of bovine collagen in a matrix of shark cartilage covered by silicone. The collagen is vascularized over 2–3 weeks, at which time the silicone is removed and a thin autograft is placed on the wound.

   Heimbach DM, Warden GD, Luterman A, et al: Multicenter postapproval clinical trial of Integra dermal regeneration template for burn treatment. J Burn Care Rehabil 24:42–48, 2003.

Figure 69-1. The "rule of nines" is used to estimate total body surface area (TBSA).

10. **How do electrical injuries cause burns?**
    Tissue damage is caused by electrical conduction. In the distal extremities, current density increases as cross-sectional area decreases, resulting in greater tissue damage. The surface wound may look minor, but the damage to deep structures can be severe, resulting in compartment syndrome and neuropathy. Injuries include amputations, seen in up to 40% of individuals with high-voltage injuries (>1000 volts), muscle damage with myoglobinuria and renal injury, and neurologic injury (peripheral nerves, spinal cord). There is a high prevalence of

neuropsychological problems, post-traumatic stress disorder, and depression after electrical injury.

Kelley KM, Tkachenko TA, Pliskin NH, et al: Life after electrical injury. Risk factors for psychiatric sequelae. Ann NY Acad Sci 888:356–363, 1999.

11. **Describe the clinical features of hypertrophic scars.**
Hypertrophic scars are raised, red, rigid, and itchy, and can result in joint contractures and deformities. The epidermis and dermis are thicker, with fewer epithelial ridges, indistinct collagen fibers, increased water content, and mast cells. Burns that take more than 21 days to heal and individuals with greater skin pigmentation are at increased risk.

12. **How does applying pressure help in treating a hypertrophic scar?**
Pressure applied with pressure garments or facial masks may be used to reduce and remodel scar tissue in burns that take more than 21 days to heal. Hypertrophic scars that have been treated with pressure tend to have fewer mast cells and fewer nodules; they also show decreased space between collagen fibrils and better organization of collagen. However, the mechanism is unclear; there are limited controlled trials evaluating the benefits of pressure garments.

KEY POINTS: HYPERTROPHIC SCARRING

1. A hypertrophic scar is red, raised, and rigid.

2. Patients with increased skin pigment are at greater risk.

3. Burns that do not heal within 3 weeks are at higher risk.

4. A hypertrophic scar causes contractures and facial and joint deformities.

5. It can be treated with pressure, using pressure garments and facial masks.

13. **How should the patient be positioned to avoid contracture formation?**
   - Neck extension
   - Shoulder abduction at 80 degrees and flexed at 15 degrees
   - Elbows extended and supinated
   - Wrists and hands in the intrinsic plus position
   - Hips extended, abducted at 10 degrees with no external rotation
   - Knees extended
   - Ankles in neutral dorsiflexion
      Remember not to leave your patient in this position. Patients need stretching and active exercise!

   Esselman PC, Nakamura DY, Patterson DR: Burns. In Robinson LR (ed): Trauma Rehabilitation. Philadelphia, Lippincott Williams & Wilkins, 2006, pp 181–204.

14. **How should a burned hand be splinted?**
The most common hand deformity is a **claw hand,** with metacarpophalangeal (MCP) extension, proximal interphalangeal (PIP) flexion, and distal interphalangeal (DIP) flexion, and thumb adduction. General splinting guidelines to prevent the claw hand are as follows:
   - Wrist in 15–30 degrees of extension
   - MCP flexion in 60–90 degrees
   - Proximal and distal IP joints in full extension
   - Thumb in radial or palmar abduction

   Tilley W, McMahon S, Shukalak B: Rehabilitation of the burned upper extremity. Hand Clin 16(2):303–318, 2000.

15. **How should a hand with exposed tendons be splinted?**
Tendons that are exposed should be covered with a moist dressing and maintained in a slack position. Disruption of the extensor tendon at the PIP joint can result in a **boutonnière deformity** (PIP flexion and DIP hyperextension). Damage to the extensor tendon at the DIP joint can result in a **mallet deformity** with DIP flexion. Contractures of the dorsal hand structures can result in a **swan-neck deformity** (PIP hyperextension, DIP flexion).

16. **What are five common disfiguring complications of deep facial burns?**
Deep facial burns may result in:
- Hypertrophic scarring
- Eyelid ectropion (when the lower eyelid is everted and pulled downward)
- Microstomia with decreased mouth opening
- Nasal deformities with retraction of the alar margin and nostril stenosis
- Alopecia

Klein M, Moore M, Costa B, Engrav L: Primer on the management of face burns at the University of Washington. J Burn Care Rehabil 26(1):2–6, 2005.

17. **What happens to the skeletal muscles in a patient with a large burn?**
Lots! A large burn results in a catabolic state throughout the body. Treatment with anabolic agents, such as oxandrolone, has demonstrated decreased nitrogen loss, increased muscle protein synthesis, increased weight gain, and increased lean body mass.

Murphy KD, Thomas S, Mlcak RP, et al: Effects of long-term oxandrolone administration in severely burned children. Surgery 136:219–224, 2004.

18. **What is the risk of developing heterotopic ossification?**
The incidence of heterotopic ossification (HO) after burn injury is reported to be between 1% and 3%. It is difficult to predict, but it is more common in larger burns and in joints with an overlying deep burn. HO after burn injury most commonly develops around the elbows. Treatment includes early recognition with modification of therapy to use only active or passive range of motion (ROM) within the pain-free arc. Some patients may need surgical resection, especially if there is ulnar nerve compression.

19. **Can neuropathies be prevented?**
Many neuropathies cannot be prevented and may be caused by ischemia or some other factor. The incidence of peripheral neuropathy is estimated at 15–30% in burn patients. Neuropathies are more commonly seen in patients with >20% TBSA and electrical burns. Iatrogenic causes include stretch and pressure from improper positioning or tight, bulky dressings.

20. **What is the best approach for the management of pain?**
Adequate pain control is essential. Background pain or pain that is present when the patient is at rest is best treated with a continuous infusion of opiates in the intensive care unit or with long-acting opiate medications. Procedural pain such as that experienced during wound care and therapy sessions can be treated with short-acting opiate pain medications given before and during the treatment. Studies have shown that the use of hypnosis and immersive virtual reality distraction can assist in decreasing procedural pain.

Hoffman HG, Patterson DR, Magula J, et al: Water-friendly virtual reality pain control during wound care. J Clin Psychol 60:189–195, 2004.

21. **What psychological problems are seen in burn patients?**
Anxiety, depression, and post-traumatic stress disorder are common in burn patients. Research has demonstrated that the size of the burn does not correlate with psychological outcome.

Ehde DM, Patterson DR, Wiechman SA, Wilson LG: Post-traumatic stress symptoms and distress 1 year after burn injury. J Burn Care Rehabil 21:105–111, 2000.

22. **What causes problems with self-image and appearance in burn patients?**
Paradoxically, the severity of the initial burn injury is not a good predictor of problems with body esteem and self-image. The visibility of the burn scar and variables such as social adjustment, depression, and family support are better predictors of difficulties in this area.

   Lawrence JW, Fauerbach JA, Heinberg L, Doctor M: Visible vs hidden scars and their relation to body esteem. J Burn Care Rehabil 25:25–32, 2004.

23. **When should children return to school after a burn injury?**
After an injury, a child should go back to school as quickly as possible despite splints, scars, and ongoing therapies. Early reintegration promotes a positive body image and prevents disruptive and maladaptive behavior. Many burn centers have school reentry programs involving on-site visits to the school.

24. **What three factors reduce the likelihood of a burned patient returning to work?**
One study demonstrated that the average time off work after a burn injury is 17 weeks, with 66% of individuals with burn injuries having returned to work within 6 months. Predictors of not returning to work are as follows:
   - Larger percentage TBSA burned
   - Psychiatric history
   - Extremity burns

   Brych SB, Engrav LH, Rivara FP, et al: Time off work and return to work rates after burns: Systematic review of the literature and a large two-center series. J Burn Care Rehabil 22(6):401–405, 2001.

XIV. CHRONIC PAIN

CHRONIC PAIN: ASSESSMENT AND MANAGEMENT

David A.N. Siegel, MD, Charles Kim, MD, CAc,
Russell K. Portenoy, MD, and Robert J. Gatchel, PhD, ABPP

CHAPTER 70

Pain is inevitable; suffering is optional.

—Anonymous

1. **What is "pain"?**
   The most widely cited definition of pain comes from the International Association for the Study of Pain (IASP): Pain is "an unpleasant sensory and emotional experience associated with actual or potential tissue damage or described in terms of such damage." This definition emphasizes that pain is a subjective, multidimensional experience that may or may not be linked to identifiable tissue injury.

   Merskey H, Bogduk N (eds), for the IASP Task Force on Taxonomy: Classification of Chronic Pain, 2nd ed. Seattle, IASP Press, 1994, pp 209–214.

2. **What is meant by "acute" versus "chronic" pain?**
   - **Acute pain** is, or is expected to be, transient, typically disappearing with the resolution of the initial insult or event (generally 3–6 months). It usually reflects a predictable response to noxious events (e.g., trauma, surgery, acute illnesses).
   - **Chronic pain** has been defined in temporal terms, typically either as pain that persists for a period beyond either 3–6 months, or in a more nuanced manner, as pain that persists for more than a month beyond the healing of an acute injury, recurring frequently over a period of time, or associated with a lesion that is not expected to heal. The significant interplay of the emotional, cognitive-behavioral, and physiologic adaptations to the pain can be highly apparent in the patient's clinical course. For most patients, chronic pain is best perceived to be an illness in its own right. The goal is to "manage" the pain to enable the patients to function better in their daily life activities and vocations.

3. **What is the "vicious cycle" of pain?**
   The vicious cycle of pain is a concept that relates to the maladaptive and downward functional spiraling of many patients in the chronic pain state. The pain becomes associated with deconditioning, psychological disorders (such as mood disturbance and catastrophization), and progressive functional impairments—a cycle of worsening pain and progressive disability.

4. **Why is it important for the physiatrist to understand and treat pain?**
   The top two causes of disability in the United States are osteoarthritis and back pain (Centers for Disease Control and Prevention). The disability produced by these conditions exceeds that caused by heart disease. Physiatrists are often on the front lines in managing their adverse effects. The prevalence of these problems, and other common sources of chronic pain (e.g., neck pain, myofascial pain) are likely to increase with the aging of the population. The adverse financial and societal impact of this chronic pain is astronomical, and the discipline of physiatry should be positioned to assist in its management.

   Pain is also one of the leading reasons for a patient not to continue with physical therapy programs or in performing the exercises correctly. In a group of 544 subjects, Snih et al. found that the presence of pain was associated with decreased muscle strength and physical function. The physiatric goal for patients with chronic pain is to break the "vicious cycle" of pain and disability, thereby reducing the individual and societal impacts of these disorders. For patients, this approach is essential to develop better adaptive behaviors, engage in a more effective participation in a functional restorative program, and, ultimately, lead more fulfilling lives.

CDC: Prevalence of disability and associated health conditions—United States, 1991–1992. MMWR 43(40):730–731, 737–739, 1994.

Snih SA, Raji MA, Peek MK: Pain, lower extremity muscle strength, and physical function among older Mexican Americans. Arch Phys Med Rehabil 86:1394–1400, 2005.

KEY POINTS: ESSENTIAL PRINCIPLES

1. Pain is a subjective, multidimensional experience that may or may not be linked to identifiable tissue injury.

2. The "vicious cycle" of pain is a concept that relates to the maladaptive and downward functional spiraling of many patients in the "chronic pain state."

5. **What role does "self-efficacy" have in chronic pain conditions?**
It is imperative for patients to obtain a sense of control over their pain. High self-efficacy decreases the risk that a patient will tumble down the spiral of the "vicious cycle." A study by Turner et al. showed that among retirement community residents, higher self-efficacy measures for the management of their pains were associated with less disability, less depression, and better pain coping strategies.

Turner JA, Ersek M, Kemp C: Self-efficacy for managing pain is associated with disability, depression, and pain coping among retirement community residents with chronic pain. Pain 6(7):471–479, 2005.

6. **What is the approach to assessing pain complaints?**
Because pain is a purely subjective experience, the person experiencing it can be the only one who can truly describe it. The first and most important rule of pain medicine is to believe that the patient's pain complaint is real. Although dissembling is possible, there is no way for a clinician to know and it is far better to simply believe that the patient is truly experiencing what is described. The clinical challenge is then to understand the nature of this experience and determine the best course of pain-modulating and rehabilitative therapy. Besides the standard medical history and physical examination, more specific characteristics of the pain must be ascertained and documented, including:

- **Location** (e.g., low back, neck). Any radiating pains?
- **Descriptors** of the pain (e.g., shooting, throbbing, burning, lancinating, aching)
- Pain **intensity** rating (e.g., rate the pain "on average" and "at its worst" on a scale of 0–10, where 0 is "no pain" and 10 is "the worst pain imaginable")
- **Temporal features** (e.g., duration, course over time, daily fluctuations)
- **Modifying factors** (e.g., Does sitting, walking, bowel movements/coughing, or laying down worsen or improve the pain?)
- **Impact of the pain** (e.g., Does the pain affect activities of daily living (ADLs)? Does the pain awaken them from sleep? How does the pain affect daily life-functions, such as work, leisure, and sexual activities?)
- **Past pain treatments** and **responses** (e.g., past pain medication use, injections, surgeries, physical therapy, acupuncture, chiropractic treatments)

7. **Why are such descriptors important in pain treatments?**

The **descriptions** that patients use to communicate their pain can help clinicians infer a potential etiology and pathophysiology for the pain and point toward more effective treatments. Inferred pathophysiologies are denoted as "nociceptive" (either somatic or visceral), "neuropathic," "mixed," or "psychogenic." A report of "burning," "pins/needles," or "lancinating" pain often suggests a neuropathic origin. "Crampy, dull, achy" pain is more indicative of nociceptive pain. These determinations may suggest specific treatment strategies.

In a similar way, the **temporal characteristics** of pain may suggest the value of different types of medications. If an opioid is indicated, for example, a long-acting drug typically is preferred for continuous or nearly continuous pain, whereas a short-acting drug may be appropriate for episodic pain or pain known as "breakthrough" pain.

8. **What is meant by "breakthrough" pain?**

Breakthrough pain is a type of episodic pain that is usually defined as a transitory flare of severe pain that occurs in the context of a chronic baseline, generally controlled with drug therapy. Originally described in populations with cancer pain, the term is now used in all chronic pain settings.

Incidental pain is a subtype of breakthrough pain, which is precipitated by a voluntary activity, such as walking. Some breakthrough pains occur at the end of an analgesic dosing cycle and may be described as **end-of-dose failure**. In opioid-treated patients with breakthrough pain, the use of a short-acting opioid (known as a **rescue** medication) combined with a fixed schedule regimen of a long-acting opioid for the baseline pain is a common approach to management. This approach has become a standard of care in cancer pain management and should be considered on a case-by-case basis during the management of chronic noncancer pain with opioid drugs. Because rescue medications have a faster onset of action and shorter half-life compared to the drugs used for the baseline pain, this theoretically allows for a "tighter" and more effective analgesic regimen.

9. **Describe the ways that pain intensity can be measured.**

The measurement of pain intensity is an essential element in the broader assessment of the pain. Besides the utility of such scales in the research world, the most effective applicability of such scales is in the temporal measure of effectiveness, or lack thereof, of the ongoing treatments. The specific tool used to quantitate the pain is less important than its regular and consistent use over time. Some of the common pain intensity tools include:

- **Visual analog scale (VAS):** A patient is asked to mark his or her level of pain (clearly described, e.g., "pain on average during the past day") on a 10-cm line anchored at one end by "no pain" and at the other end by "pain at its worst imaginable." The number of millimeters measured from the "no pain" end to the patient's marked level of the pain is the VAS pain score.
- **0–10 scale:** Probably the most popular scale used in typical pain practices. The patient is asked to verbally rate his or her pain (again, clearly described) on a scale from 0–10, with 0 being no pain and 10 being the worst pain imaginable.
- **FACES Diagram** (e.g., Wong and Baker): A scale comprising a series of pictures from a smiling face to a crying face, with gradations of distress in between. These types of scales have been studied and modified and have also been used in the "Oucher Scale," a scale for pediatric patients with pain, with varying successes.

Belville RG, Seupaul RA: Pain measurement in pediatric emergency care: A review of the faces pain scale—revised. Pediatr Emerg Care 21(2):90–93, 2005.

Wong DL, Hockenberry-Eaton M, Wilson D, et al: Wongs Essentials of Pediatric Nursing, 6th ed. St. Louis, Mosby, 2001.

10. **What terms can be used to describe the pain or abnormal sensations?**
    - **Hyperesthesia/hypesthesia:** Increased/decreased sensitivity to nonnoxious stimulation, excluding the special senses.
    - **Hyperalgesia/hypalgesia:** Increased/decreased response to a stimulus that is normally painful.
    - **Paresthesia:** Nonpainful, abnormal sensation (e.g., "pins and needles"), either evoked or spontaneous.
    - **Dysesthesia:** Unpleasant abnormal sensation (e.g., pain that "burns" or is "electric-like"), either evoked or spontaneous.
    - **Allodynia:** Pain induced by a nonnoxious stimulus, specifically light touch.
    - **Hyperpathia:** Exaggerated pain response to a stimulus, which may be characterized by very intense pain out of proportion to the stimulus, after-sensation, and emotional overreaction.

    Turk DC, Okifuji A: Pain terms and taxonomies of pain. In Loesser JD, Butler SH, Chapman CR, Turk D (eds): Bonica's Management of Pain, 3rd ed. Philadelphia, Lippincott Williams & Wilkins, 2001, pp 17–19.

11. **What are the goals of treating pain with medications?**
    - **Decrease** the pain levels, as subjectively described by the patient.
    - Follow the patient's pain scales and breakthrough medication use.
    - Improve the patient's **functional** status.
    - Ask about any changes to ADLs, psychosocial status, and work activities.
    - Monitor and control the potential **side effects** of the medications. The most commonly seen are sedation, nausea, and constipation. Warn patients about driving and operating heavy machinery.
    - Monitor and observe for the **improper use** or **abuse** of medications.

    Hendler NH: Pharmacological management of pain. In Raj PP, Abrams BM, Benzon HT, et al (eds): Practical Management of Pain, 3rd ed. St. Louis, Mosby, 2000, pp 145–155.

12. **What is an adjuvant pain medication?**
    Adjuvant pain medications have been defined as drugs with primary indications other than pain, which are analgesic in specific circumstances. The term has become a misnomer with the appearance on the market of antidepressants and anticonvulsants specifically approved for pain. The adjuvant analgesics are distinguished from the opioids and the nonopioid analgesics, acetaminophen, and nonsteroidal anti-inflammatory drugs (NSAIDs). The category of adjuvant pain medication includes many specific drug classes, such as antidepressants, anticonvulsants, central-acting adrenergic agents, muscle relaxants, and others.

13. **What is the role of antidepressants in pain management?**
    There are so many randomized controlled trials demonstrating the effectiveness of antidepressant medications on different types of chronic pain that these drugs are best considered multipurpose analgesics, potentially useful for any patient with pain. They have primary analgesic effects, and although they may be particularly helpful for patients with comorbid major depression, they should be considered for those patients with pain unassociated with a mood disorder.

    The best-studied drugs are tricyclic antidepressants **(TCAs)**. The tertiary amine drugs, particularly amitriptyline, are more likely to be efficacious than the secondary amine drugs, such as desipramine and nortriptyline. The latter have fewer side effects. Overall, TCAs are probably more effective than newer antidepressants, but the latter are better tolerated than the secondary amine group. Among the newer drugs, evidence is best for the serotonin-norepinephrine selective reuptake inhibitors (SNRIs), specifically duloxetine (approved for the management of pain in diabetic neuropathy) and venlafaxine. Evidence is less supportive for serotonin selective reuptake inhibitors (SSRIs), but paroxetine and citalopram have had some favorable studies. Selective norepinephrine reuptake inhibitors, specifically bupropion, also are analgesic and may be well tolerated by some patients.

14. **How about the role of anticonvulsant medications?**
Historically developed for the treatment of seizures, these agents have been found to be effective analgesics in a variety of conditions. They are now widely used in the management of neuropathic pains and headaches. Gabapentin is the most widely prescribed. Pregabalin, which has the same mechanism of action as gabapentin, was recently approved for both painful diabetic polyneuropathy and postherpetic neuralgia. Older drugs that have been used for this indication include carbamazepine, phenytoin, and valproate. Newer drugs have lower side-effect profiles. Evidence is best that lamotrigine is analgesic, but many other anticonvulsants, including topiramate, levetiracetam, tiagabine, oxcarbazepine, and zonisamide, are sometimes utilized for more refractory cases.

15. **Do antianxiety or hypnotic medications also play a role in chronic pain?**
Anxiety and sleep disturbances are quite commonly seen in patients with chronic pain. The use of benzodiazepines (e.g., diazepam) may help ease the anxiety associated with chronic pain, as well as help with muscle spasms. Clonazepam is a benzodiazepine that has been used empirically for neuropathic pain. In general, none of the benzodiazepines are preferred for pain-related sleep disturbances, as they do not provide a favorable restoration of sleep architecture (mainly stage IV sleep). The newer nonbenzodiazepine hypnotics (e.g., zolpidem, zaleplon) may be better choices for sleep, as they have more favorable effects on sleep architecture.

16. **What are nonopioid analgesics?**
In the United States, the nonopioid analgesics include acetaminophen and NSAIDs. These drugs produce analgesia through both peripheral and central mechanisms. Unlike opioids, the analgesia produced by these agents is characterized by a **ceiling effect** (a dose level above which additional amounts provide no added analgesia). None of these drugs are subject to abuse. NSAIDs are anti-inflammatory as well as analgesic. Aspirin and NSAIDs (e.g., ibuprofen) inhibit the synthesis of prostaglandins by different mechanisms. Aspirin is unique in that it irreversibly inactivates cyclooxygenase (COX). Acetaminophen inhibits prostaglandin synthesis in the central nervous system and is antipyretic but not anti-inflammatory.

A major toxicity of NSAIDs is gastroduodenopathy, with effects ranging from abdominal pain and bloating, to massive gastrointestinal hemorrhage. The COX-2 selective NSAIDs (e.g., celecoxib) are less likely to produce these outcomes. It is not known whether this risk reduction is greater or less than that achieved by the administration of concomitant gastroprotective therapy, specifically the addition of a proton pump inhibitor (e.g., omeprazole), misoprostol, or a high dose of a H2 blocker (e.g., famotidine). All NSAIDs can impair renal function, with effects that vary from peripheral edema to either acute or chronic renal failure. COX-2 drugs are not renal sparing.

Recently, rofecoxib was withdrawn by its manufacturer from the U.S. market, and valdecoxib was withdrawn on request from the U.S. Food and Drug Administration (FDA) because of concerns of increased risk of cardiovascular events (transient ischemic attack/stroke, myocardial infarction, and peripheral vascular disease) from these drugs. The data are still very limited. There is one study suggesting that this risk may exist for the nonselective COX-1/COX-2 inhibitors, too, and the FDA has therefore requested that a warning be included in the package inserts of all NSAIDs. The existing data, however, suggest that the risk varies by drug (there is much more evidence that rofecoxib increases these risks, more so than celecoxib), although these risks are relatively small. For example, in the key rofecoxib study, the risk of a cardiovascular event after three years of treatment was 3% in the drug-treated group and 1.5% in the placebo-treated group, but the risks may increase with higher doses and may increase over time of use.

The potential for renal and cardiovascular toxicity must be considered when decisions are made about selecting an NSAID for long-term pain therapy. A recent study also demonstrated a relationship between acetaminophen and NSAID treatments, with elevated blood pressures. Poorly controlled hypertension is another relative contraindication, and thus blood pressure must be monitored if therapy is undertaken.

Forman JP, Stampfer MJ, Curhan GC: Non-narcotic analgesic dose and risk of incident hypertension in US women. Hypertension 46(3):500–507, 2005.

17. What is the role of muscle relaxants in chronic pain control?

Drugs such as cyclobenzaprine, metaxalone, methocarbamol, and carisoprodol are centrally acting analgesics and do not relax skeletal muscle. Diazepam and tizanidine affect muscle directly (note that tizanidine, an alpha 2-adrenergic agonist, is also a centrally acting analgesic). Baclofen can relax hypertonic muscle affected by a pyramidal tract lesion. Dantrolene acts directly on skeletal muscle but is rarely used because of potential liver toxicity.

All of these drugs are used to treat musculoskeletal pains, and tizanidine and baclofen also have been used in the treatment of other chronic pain disorders. There are no comparative data by which to judge relative efficacy against each other, NSAIDs, or opioids. Drug selection is empirical. Use is usually, but not always, short-term and the most troubling side effects are sedation and mental clouding.

18. Are topical agents also effective in pain management?

Topical agents can be applied directly over the painful areas involved. The lidocaine 5% patch is an adhesive preparation with the local anesthetic impregnated in the adhesive. It is approved for postherpetic neuralgia, but now pain specialists commonly utilize it for virtually all types of regional pains. If the patient does not report improvement by 1 week, discontinue use. Capsaicin cream (0.025–0.075%) is sometimes used for patients with painful neuropathies, as well as other musculoskeletal conditions such as arthritis. It is derived from the active ingredient in hot chili peppers and depletes the levels of substance-P at the periphery. Other topical agents (e.g., antidepressants, NSAIDs) can be compounded and mixed in cream and ointment preparations and are supported by trials that demonstrate their efficacy.

19. What is the difference between an opiate and an opioid?

- An **opiate** is a drug that is derived from the poppy plant *Papaver somniferum*. Morphine and codeine, in this respect, are defined as opiates and exist in nature.
- An **opioid** is defined as having "morphine-like" properties. An opioid can be an opiate or be synthetic (e.g., fentanyl, methadone, meperidine) or semi-synthetic (e.g., hydromorphone, oxycodone, hydrocodone, heroin). Endogenous opioids are a class of peptides produced by, and distributed widely in, the body. They include subclasses of compounds—endorphins, enkephalins, and dynorphins—that are widely distributed and involved in numerous physiologic functions, including the modulation of nociception.

Uppington J: Opioids. In Ballantyne J: The Massachusetts General Hospital Handbook of Pain Management, 2nd ed. Philadelphia, Lippincott Williams & Wilkins, 2002, pp 103–124.

20. Where do the opioids act to produce their analgesic effects?

Opioids act at the **opioid receptors** (*mu, kappa, delta,* and *sigma*), which are located in the central and peripheral nervous systems and at other sites, such as the immune cells. Receptors involved in nociceptive processing are found mainly in the brain stem, medial thalamus, substantia gelatinosa of the spinal cord, hypothalamus, limbic system, and the peripheral sensory nerve fibers and terminal branches. The potency of an opioid is defined as the milligram amount needed to produce a defined effect; it is related to a number of factors, including the affinity for these receptors.

Mycek MJ, Harvey RA, Champe PC (eds): Opioid analgesics and antagonists. In Pharmacology, 2nd ed. Philadelphia, Lippincott-Raven, 1997, pp 133–142.

21. **What are the most important opioid side effects?**
See Table 70-1.

TABLE 70-1. SIDE EFFECTS OF OPIOIDS	
Side Effects	**Comments**
Euphoria/ contentment	A powerful sense of contentment and well-being due to central effects in the ventral tegmentum. Although a sense of contentment is sometimes seen during acute administration of an opioid in the setting of acute pain, positive mood effects appear to be rare during chronic administration in the population without a history of addiction. Opioid-induced euphoria in the clinical setting is rarely encountered.
Sedation/ mental clouding/ dysphoria	The physiology of these effects is presumably complex and involves multiple brain areas. Sedation and mental clouding are usually transitory effects that occur when therapy is initiated or the dose is increased. Some patients have persistent symptoms of this type, however.
Nausea and vomiting	Opioids directly stimulate the chemoreceptor trigger zones in the area postrema.
Constipation	Opioids decrease peristalsis by acting on receptors in both the bowel and central nervous system.
Pruritus	Opioids stimulate mast cells to secrete histamine. Morphine tends to produce this effect more than the others. Care must be taken in prescribing opioids to asthmatics.
Respiratory depression	A central effect on the respiratory drive centers that decrease the sensitivity to carbon dioxide. This effect is extremely rare when dosing is done according to appropriate clinical guidelines. Respiratory depression is usually preceded by slowed respirations and somnolence. The patient who presents with anxiety and dyspnea or tachypnea is not experiencing an opioid-related adverse respiratory effect. If a patient who has been stable while receiving an opioid regimen develops respiratory problems, another source should be investigated, even if there is transitory improvement following administration of *naloxone*. The latter effect means the opioid is contributing a reversible component to the problem; it does not imply that the opioid is the cause. Respiratory failure is the most common cause of death due to opioid intoxication.

22. **What is tramadol?**
Tramadol is a unique compound that acts as a weak opioid receptor agonist (mainly at the *mu* receptor) and is also a reuptake inhibitor at both norepinephrine and serotonin receptors. It is an effective analgesic but carries a risk of seizures that is partially idiosyncratic and partially dose-related. Care must be used to avoid this medication in patients with a seizure history and who are also on norepinephrine and serotonin reuptake inhibitors. It is seldom abused by opioid addicts and is not scheduled under the Controlled Substance Act in the United States. Overall, it is a good choice for mild to moderate pain conditions.

KEY POINTS: PAIN MEDICATIONS

1. The goals of treating pain with medications are to decrease the subjective pain levels, improve the patient's functional status, monitor and control for potential treatment side effects, and monitor and observe for the proper use or abuse of the medications.

2. Unlike most other medications used to treat pain, opioids do not have a pharmacologic "ceiling effect" and should be titrated to therapeutic efficacy while monitoring side effects.

3. Many pain conditions can be effectively treated with nonopioid adjuvant medications.

23. **Is methadone used for drug addicts?**
Many patients perceive methadone very negatively because of its use as a treatment for heroin addiction. It is an effective analgesic, however, and its clinical use for chronic pain has been growing recently. The formulation available in the United States is a racemic mixture of two isomers. *L-methadone* is an opioid, and *d-methadone* is an NMDA (N-methyl-D-aspartate) receptor antagonist. The latter activity may produce independent, nonopioid analgesia and reduce whatever analgesic tolerance exists. The NMDA receptor is thought to be involved in the **"wind-up" phenomenon** of central sensitization in the dorsal horn of the spinal cord and appears to be key in the development of some types of neuropathic pains.
   Methadone may be more potent than expected or calculated when a patient is switched from another opioid. This may reflect the impact of the d-isomer. This variable potency and an equally variable half-life, which is typically about 24 hours but varies from less than 12 hours to more than 150 hours, mean that the effects of this drug require close monitoring in the clinical setting. It can take many days or even weeks for the plasma concentration to gradually ascend to steady state levels; close monitoring is imperative during this time. It also must be noted that higher doses of methadone (some data suggest doses >300 mg/day, but the information available is limited) have been associated with QT prolongation, which may predispose to torsades de pointe, a life-threatening arrhythmia. Methadone can be used safely and very effectively for pain, but the unique characteristics of the drug must be appreciated to ensure appropriate use. The risks of the drug are greater in the elderly.

   Martell BA, Arnsten JH, Ray B, Gourevitch MN: The impact of methadone induction on cardiac conduction in opiate users. Ann Intern Med 139(2):154–155, 2003.

24. **Is it true that meperidine is "falling out of favor" in the pain circles?**
Meperidine is the only opioid that can produce tachycardia. But of more concern is that its active metabolite, normeperidine, has been found to be significantly neurotoxic and increases the risk of tremors, convulsions, and seizures.

25. **What is unique about fentanyl?**
Fentanyl is a highly lipid-soluble opioid that is 50–80 times more potent than morphine. It is typically used in pain practice in the transdermal modified-release and quick-acting transmucosal lozenge preparations of administration.

26. **Is the term *narcotic* exclusive to opiates and opioids?**
The term *narcotic* is mainly a regulatory and legal definition that can include opioids and opiates, but it can include virtually any other agent that can be abused, diverted, and used illegally. The term should not be used in clinical practice.

27. **Outline a good 8-step approach to managing a patient with chronic benign pain.**
   1. As a physician, one must **accept that the patient's pain is real**. Find out why the patient experiences so much discomfort. Try to analyze to what degree the different dimensions of pain are contributing to the patient's total pain experience.
   2. **Avoid excessive, unnecessary, invasive procedures and tests** that do not help in the management of the patient's pain and only fuel the fires of the chronic pain process.

3. **Set realistic goals**. Make it clear to the patient that you are not trying to cure the pain, but rather to manage it and help the patient to be as functional as possible despite the pain.

4. **Evaluate the patient's level of function**. Make realistic goals to increase his or her function gradually in terms of different physical tolerances, such as walking, sitting, and standing. The patient should be taught how to pace himself or herself and how to organize work activities so that he or she can carry out the needed or wanted tasks despite the pain. In other words, the patient has to learn to work his or her life around the obstacle of pain rather than let pain restrict the quality of life.

5. If the patient is on medication for pain, he or she should take **medication on a standing basis** rather than on an as-needed basis. Taking the medication as needed may reinforce pain behavior and may not be the best way to approach chronic pain. Also, very gradually reduce the amount of pain medication that the patient is taking.

6. **Prescribe an exercise program** for the patient, including a physical activity program, that should be very gradually increased over time. Many patients with chronic pain are deconditioned because of lack of activity due to the fear of pain in the past. These patients need a reconditioning exercise program.

7. **Educate the patient and family** regarding the chronic pain process. If the patient and family understand the problem well, it then becomes easier to deal with it. The patient's focus should be directed toward becoming more functional and active in society despite the discomfort and pain.

8. **Help the patient to get involved in recreational and pleasurable activities** to keep himself or herself physically as well as mentally busy. People who have something better to do don't hurt as much.

Patil J: Pain management. In O'Young BJ, Young MA, Stiens SA (eds): Physical Medicine and Rehabilitation Secrets, 2nd ed. Philadelphia, Hanley & Belfus, 2002, pp 363–369.

28. **So with all this knowledge about pain management, how can we break the "vicious cycle" of the patient with chronic pain?**

The field of pain medicine has grown rapidly over the past several years and will continue to grow in leaps and bounds. There was a time not long ago when the number of medications that pain practitioners utilized could be counted on one hand. Now the numbers of pain-related medications are in the several hundreds, with new ones being approved by the FDA every year.

In addition, the growing subfield of pain medicine—interventional pain medicine—brings to the treatment table countless pain-modulating procedures that are minimally invasive and potentially effective alternatives or complements to traditional surgeries and chronic medication therapies. With the effectiveness of structured physical therapeutics, psychological supports, and a better understanding of pain, the future of millions of pain sufferers looks more promising.

WEBSITES

Pain Medicine Forums and Clinical Information

1. www.painphysicians.org

2. www.painrounds.com

Pain Medicine Organizations

1. www.ampainsoc.org

2. www.asra.com

3. www.painmed.org

CHAPTER 71

SPINAL SEGMENTAL SENSITIZATION: DIAGNOSIS AND TREATMENT

Andrew A. Fischer, MD, PhD, Marta Imamura, MD, PhD, Hy Dubo, MD, Bryan J. O'Young, MD, and David A. Cassius, MD

> *Spinal neuronal plasticity is shown to be a key contributor to pathologic pain hypersensitivity. We need to treat both the disease/injury process in the periphery and the changes it induces or triggers in the CNS. Prevention of central sensitization will substantially eliminate the hyperalgesia and allodynia that patients find so distressing.*
>
> —Clifford J. Woolf, MD

From Woolf CJ: A new strategy for treatment of inflammatory pain prevention or elimination of central sensitization. Drugs 47(Suppl):1–9; discussion, 46–47, 1999.

Dr. Woolf founded and leads the Neural Plasticity Research Group of the Department of Anesthesia and Critical Care, Massachusetts General Hospital and Harvard Medical School. Modern understanding of pain and its underlying mechanisms, as well as many specific treatments, is based mainly on Dr. Woolf's pioneering research. He developed the concept of central sensitization and contributed essentially to the understanding of the role of neuroplasticity.

1. **What are the goals of future pain management?**
   According to Dr. Woolf, "Future steps [in pain management] require the development of diagnostic tools that will allow us to identify the mechanisms of pain in an individual patient and pharmacologic tools that act specifically on these mechanisms." The present chapter is a step in this direction, describing the diagnosis of some pain mechanisms and specific nonpharmacologic treatment of pain in individual patients.

2. **What are the four primary types of pain, according to Woolf?**
   - **Nociceptive pain:** Noxious peripheral stimulus to sensory neuron ("early warning")
   - **Inflammatory pain:** Inflammation, tissue damage, sensitizing the nociceptor sensory neuron
   - **Neuropathic pain:** Peripheral nerve damage
   - **Functional pain:** Abnormal central processing with normal peripheral tissues and nerves

   Woolf CJ: Pain: Moving from symptom control toward mechanism: Specific pharmacologic management. Ann Intern Med 140:441–451, 2004.

3. **How is peripheral sensitization (PS) defined?**
   PS is characterized by **hyperexcitability (i.e., hyperreactivity)** of sensory nerve fibers to stimuli. The clinical manifestations of nerve fiber sensitization consist of **hyperalgesia** (increased reaction to painful stimuli, such as scratching or pinprick) and **allodynia** (stimuli that normally fail to cause pain, such as pressure or compression, become painful). The usual mechanism of sensitization consists of local tissue damage that produces sensitizing, inflammatory, irritating substances, such as prostaglandins and bradykinin. A vicious cycle develops between spinal segmental sensitization (SSS) and irritative foci (i.e., tender spots/trigger points [TS/TrPs]), each increasing the sensitization of the corresponding component. Increased sympathetic outflow potentiates the sensitization of peripheral nerves in the acute state. **Edema** around the tissue damage entraps inflammatory substances along with nerve endings (Fig. 71-1).

   Abram SE: Pain management. In Abram SE (ed): Atlas of Anesthesia, Vol. VI. New York, Churchill Livingstone, 1998, pp 1.2–1.9.

   Mense S, Simons DG: Muscle Pain. Philadelphia, Lippincott Williams & Wilkins, 2000, pp 158–205.

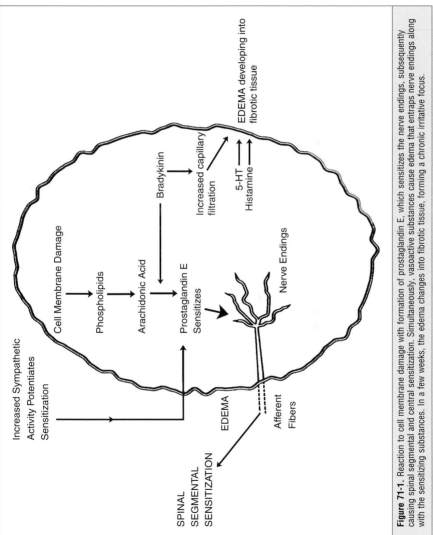

Figure 71-1. Reaction to cell membrane damage with formation of prostaglandin E, which sensitizes the nerve endings, subsequently causing spinal segmental and central sensitization. Simultaneously, vasoactive substances cause edema that entraps nerve endings along with the sensitizing substances. In a few weeks, the edema changes into fibrotic tissue, forming a chronic irritative focus.

4. **Define SSS and central sensitization (CS).**

   SSS is a condition characterized by hyperactivity, facilitation, and hyperexcitability of a spinal segment that develops in reaction to an irritative focus, which constantly bombards the sensory ganglion by nociceptive stimuli. The irritative focus usually consists of a small area of damaged or dysfunctional tissue where peripheral sensitization or irritation of the nerve fibers generates the continuous nociceptive stimuli, causing sensitization of the central nervous system (CNS). The sensitization and hyperexcitability spread from sensory to motor components of the segment, inducing hypertonicity and tenderness (muscle spasm), and activate TS/TrPs within the myotome. This **CS** starts with the spinal segment (i.e., SSS is the initial step in CS). The most frequently affected segments are C5 and C6 as well as L5 and S1.

   Fischer AA: Functional diagnosis of musculoskeletal pain by quantitative and objective methods. In Rachlin ES, Rachlin IS (eds): Myofascial Pain and Fibromyalgia. Trigger Point Management, 2nd ed. St. Louis, Mosby, 2002, pp 145–173.

5. **What is the anatomic basis of SSS?**

   Each spinal segment is a switchboard for several nerve fiber connections: horizontal structures connect the spinal segment with afferent and impulses from and efferent signals to different peripheral tissues. Both incoming afferent and outgoing efferent pathways connect the spinal segment with different organs. The afferent pathways, which carry information sensation from different tissues, connect with ascending spinothalamic and thalamocortical tracts, which relate sensory information to the cortex. Descending tracts such as cortico-spinal connect with efferent segmental structures, including somatic, and with visceral motor neurons. Unlike a telephone switchboard, the spinal segmental connections are dynamic (i.e., every second their activity and function depend on balance between the excitatory and inhibitory impulses coming from the periphery, as well as their modulation by higher nerve centers). The hyperexcitability connected with sensitization is increased by sensitized peripheral tissues as well as by descending tract control. The steps in peripheral and central sensitization are summarized in Figure 71-2.

   Woolf CJ: Dissecting out mechanisms responsible for peripheral neuropathic pain: Implications for diagnosis and therapy. Life Sci 74:2605–2610, 2004.

6. **What is the innervation area of a myotome?**

   A myotome consists of a group of muscles, the motor innervation of which originates in the identical spinal segment. Each muscle receives motor and sensory nerve supplies from at least two spinal segments. This information unfortunately leads to the *incorrect* concept that each and every part of the muscle is supplied by both spinal segments. Improved examination methods for both motor and sensory functions reveal that *each spinal segment supplies the motor innervation only to part of a muscle belonging to the myotome*. This conclusion is based on findings of sensitization, which is limited to the part of the muscle lying under the corresponding sensitized dermatome. For example, typically the gastrocnemius muscle is known to be innervated by S1 and S2 segments. However, findings indicating sensitization of the muscle, such as spasm as well as taut bands with TS/TrPs, suggest that in case of S1 sensitization, only the lateral part of the gastrocnemius muscle is sensitized. On the contrary, when solely S2 sensitization was detected by sensitized S2 dermatome, the typical findings of muscle sensitization were present only in the medial head of the gastrocnemius muscle. *Therefore, each myotome consists only of a part of the muscle innervated by a spinal segment.*

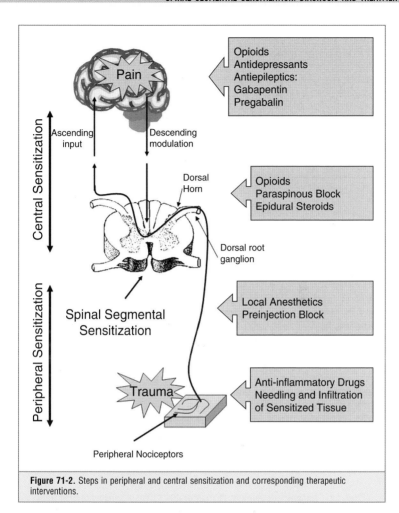

Figure 71-2. Steps in peripheral and central sensitization and corresponding therapeutic interventions.

KEY POINTS: SEGMENTAL NEUROMYOTHERAPY

1. The system of diagnosis and treatment is based on spinal segmental sensitization (SSS).

2. SSS can be diagnosed only by improved, more sensitive, and precise examination methods.

3. Specific treatments, including special injection techniques, are combined with physical therapy and exercises concentrated on the involved spinal segment.

7. **What is the role of neuroplasticity in sensitization?**
   According to Mannion and Woolf, "The afferent input generated by injury and intense noxious stimuli triggers an increased excitability of nociceptive neurons in the spinal cord." There is

a "specific role of dorsal horn of the spinal cord in the mechanism of nociceptive pain and spinal plasticity that occurs after nerve and tissue injury. The spinal neuronal plasticity is shown to be a key contributor to pathologic pain hypersensitivity."

Mannion RJ, Woolf CJ: Pain mechanisms and management: Central perspective. Clin J Pain 16(3 suppl): S144–S156, 2000.

8. **What are the physical findings indicating sensitization?**
See Table 71-1.

KEY POINTS: SIGNIFICANCE OF SENSITIZED SPINAL SEGMENT

1. This step indicates that the sensitizing process, which starts at the periphery, has reached the central nervous system.

2. Effective management requires treatment of both peripheral and central sensitization.

3. Its presence, along with peripheral tissue sensitization, may escape diagnosis when conventional examination techniques are employed.

4. This condition can be successfully diagnosed by quantitative objective methods with high sensitivity and precision (e.g., algometry, electric skin conductance, tissue compliance measurement).

9. **How is SSS diagnosed in clinical practice?**
SSS is diagnosed by **hyperalgesia** and **pressure pain sensitivity** that extends over the sensory, motor, and skeletal areas as well as viscera supplied by the involved spinal segment (i.e., its dermatome, myotome, sclerotome, and viscerotome).

Dermatomal hyperalgesia is diagnosed by the following methods:

- **Sensory testing for diagnosis of SSS: Scratching the skin** with the tip of an opened paper clip tests sensitivity to painful stimuli more precisely than a pinprick. The sharp object is slowly dragged across the dermatomal borders. Patients are asked to indicate if the sensation of the paper clip changes and gets sharper or duller. Use of **sensory testing tracks** allows more accurate diagnosis and requires only a fraction of the time as compared to the conventional pinprick method (Fig. 71-3).

- **Sensitivity of subcutaneous tissue** is tested by the **pinch and roll method**. This test is performed by picking up the skin between the thumb and forefinger and rolling the tissue beneath. It is the most sensitive test for the diagnosis of sensitization.

- **Electric skin conductance (ESC)** is an objective test of sympathetic dysfunction and can be measured by a microampere meter.

Head H: On disturbances of sensation with especial reference to the pain of visceral disease (Parts I and II). Brain 16:1–130, 1893.

Keegan JJ, Garrett FD: The segmental distribution of the cutaneous nerves in the limbs of man. Anat Rec 102–409, 1948.

TABLE 71-1. DIAGNOSIS OF PERIPHERAL AND SEGMENTAL (CENTRAL) SENSITIZATION

Findings	Quantification Methods
A. Peripheral sensitization	
1. Hyperalgesia of skin: sharper feeling on scratch and pinch and roll	
2. Tenderness: decreased pressure pain threshold	Algometer
a. Skin	
b. Subcutaneous	
c. Deep tissues, muscles	
3. Micro-tropho edema: indentation by nail persists	Algometer
4. Subcutaneous edema: thicker skin fold	Caliper, ultrasound
5. Electric skin conductance: Increased	Micro Amp meter
B. Segmental (central) sensitization	
1. Dermatomal distribution of peripheral sensitization findings	See Part A
2. Temporal summation of repetitive stimuli; pinprick or electric stimuli repeated 1 per second causes gradually increasing pain reaction	Pinprick or electrical stimulation
3. Myotomal distribution of muscle sensitization	
a. Tender spots/trigger points	Algometer
b. Taut bands	Tissue compliance meter
c. Muscle spasm (tender hypertonicity)	Tissue compliance meter
4. Sclerotomal inflammation	
a. Enthesopathy at insertions of taut bands	Algometer
b. Tendinitis, bursitis, epicondylitis	
c. Joint changes, capsulitis	
d. Ligament tenderness	
5. Viscerotome: Segmental organ irritation and dysfunction (*see* Table 71-2)	Palpation/auscultation of target organs
6. Spatial irradiation: spreading of segmental sensitization proximally and distally	All of the above tools are used to identify spinal segmental sensitization.

From Fischer AA: Algometry in diagnosis of musculoskeletal pain and evaluation of treatment outcome: An update. Fischer AA (ed): Muscle Pain Syndromes and Fibromyalgia. New York, Haworth Press 1998, pp 5–32.

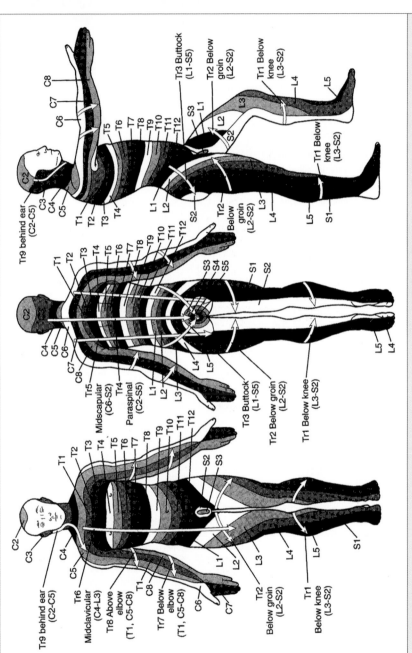

Figure 71-3. The correct dermatomes and superimposed sensory testing tracts for fast and precise diagnosis of sensory dysfunction.

KEY POINTS: ACCURATE DIAGNOSIS OF PAIN DISTRIBUTION

1. An accurate diagnosis requires identification of sensitized spinal segment.

2. This diagnosis can be achieved only if based on the correct dermatomes described by Keegan and Garret (1948).

3. Sensitization of myotomes can be detected only if the correct innervation pattern is kept in mind.

4. Each myotome innervates only part of a muscle, which is covered by the corresponding dermatome.

10. **What are the manifestations of SSS in viscerotome and other segmental components?**
    - **Viscerotome:** Pain, local and referred, with symptoms specific to each organ (i.e., for gastrointestinal: gastroesophageal reflux disease, nausea, vomiting, irritable bowel syndrome) (*see* Table 71-2)
    - **Myotome:** Tender spots/trigger points, taut bands, spasm. Myotomal deep tissue (muscle) tenderness is assessed by digital pressure and quantified with a pressure algometer. Pressure pain threshold, which is the minimum pressure that induces pain, is considered abnormal if it is lower than 2 kg/cm^2 compared to a normosensitive control point.
    - **Dermatome:** Skin and subcutaneous tissue tender on pinch and roll and scratch tests, increased electric skin conductance
    - **Sclerotome:** Tenderness over sclerotomal tissues (i.e., ligaments, bursa, enthesopathy, joints) within the involved segment
    - **Sympathetic:** Segmental sweating, skin cooling and discoloration, microedema, and increased electric skin conductance over the involved segment (dermatome)

    Head H: On disturbances of sensation with especial reference to the pain of visceral disease (Parts I and II). Brain 16:1–130, 1893.
    Loeser J, Butler S, Chapman C, Turk D: Bonica's Management of Pain, 3rd ed. Philadelphia, Lippincott Williams & Wilkins, 2001.

11. **What are the diagnostic criteria indicating that central sensitization (CS) has occurred?**
    See Table 71-1. Also note the following characteristics of CS:
    - **Temporal summation** is characteristic for CS and consists of increased pain intensity on repeated stimuli such as pinprick or electric stimulation, one per second. Such "wind-up" can be explained by abnormal continuous electrical activity of the sensitized hyperexcitable nerve. Local anesthetic reverses the hyperexcitability and interrupts the continuous activity, which is the basis of sensitization. Once the normal sensitivity and reactivity of the nerve have been restored, the condition is *maintained until an irritative focus causes its sensitization again*.
    - **Spatial irradiation** is another characteristic of CS and consists of spreading the hyperexcitability to the adjacent areas and tissues, as well as to the entire spinal segment. In addition, the spreading of the spinal sensitization proceeds also vertically to the adjacent cranial and caudal segments.
    - The more intense the peripheral sensitization is in the irritative focus, manifested by a lower pressure pain threshold, the more intense the local and central sensitization. The signs

TABLE 71-2. SYMPTOMS AND SIGNS OF SPINAL SEGMENTAL SENSITIZATION RELATED TO VISCEROTOMES AND OTHER SEGMENTAL STRUCTURES

Visceral Organ	Innervating Spinal Segments	Symptoms	Components of Sensitized Spinal Segment
Lungs	T2–T6	Chest pain	T2–T6 innervated myotomes, including paraspinal and intercostal muscles T2–T6 innervated sclerotomes T2–T6 innervated dermatomes
Heart	T1–T4 C5–C6 C7–C8	Chest pain and tightness Referred pain to upper limb Referred pain to neck and interscapular regions	T1–T4 and C5–C8 innervated myotomes, including paraspinals, intercostals, pectoralis major/minor, and sternalis T1–T4 and C5–8 innervated sclerotomes T1–T4 and C5–C8 innervated dermatomes
Upper gastrointestinal (esophagus, stomach, duodenum, small intestine, gallbladder, liver)	T5–T9	Substernal pain, epigastric pain, rib cage pain, mid-thoracic pain, abdominal pain, nausea, emesis, dyspepsia, heartburn	T5–T9, T10–L1 innervated myotomes, including rectus abdominis, abdominal obliques, and iliocostalis T5–T9, T10–L1 innervated sclerotomes, including supra/interspinous ligaments and muscle attachment site on ribs, sternum
Lower gastrointestinal (large intestine, appendix)	T10–L1	Lower abdominal pain, diarrhea, constipation, flatulence (irritable bowel syndrome–like symptoms)	T5–T9, T10–L1 innervated dermatomes

Genitourinary (kidneys, ureters)	T10–L1	Abdominal/pelvic pain, flank pain, groin/scrotal pain	T10–L2 innervated myotomes, including paraspinals, quadratus lumborum, abdominal obliques
Bladder, urethra, prostate, epididymis, testes	T12–L2	Bladder pain, pelvic pain, urinary frequency (e.g., interstitial cystitis)	T10–L2 innervated sclerotomes T10–L2 innervated dermatomes
Pelvic (gynecologic)		Pelvic pain, dysmenorrhea (e.g., chronic inflammatory pelvic disease, chronic endometriosis)	T10–L1 innervated myotomes, including pelvic floor muscles, lower abdominal muscles, and paraspinals
Ovaries	T10		
Uterus	T10–L2		T10–L1 innervated sclerotomes T10–L1 innervated dermatomes

and symptoms of sensitization, hyperalgesia, allodynia, and augmented ESC increase **exponentially** in relation to the progressive sensitization of the irritative focus.

Curatolo M, Arendt-Nielsen L, Petersen S: Evidence, mechanisms, and clinical implications of central hypersensitivity in chronic pain after whiplash injury. Clin J Pain 20:469–476, 2004.

12. **How do you treat peripheral sensitization?**
The elimination of the irritative foci within the somatic components of the SSS is necessary for the effective treatment of pain and dysfunction originating in the periphery or in the viscerotome (*see* Box 71-1). Early effective treatment of peripheral sensitization can prevent the onset of central sensitization and chronicity.

Kraus H: Clinical Treatment of Back and Neck Pain. New York, McGraw-Hill, 1970, pp 1–17.

BOX 71-1. MANAGEMENT OF PERIPHERAL SENSITIZATION AND PREVENTION OF CENTRAL SENSITIZATION

A. Noninvasive methods
1. Start treatment as soon as possible.
2. Do **not** use RICE (rest, ice, compression, and elevation). Do **not** rest injured part! Use **MECE** (move, ethylchloride spray, compression, and elevation).
   - Use vapocoolant spray to deactivate trigger points, which limit movement. The spray inactivates the trigger points' tender spots and makes relaxation exercises and passive stretching of the involved muscle more effective.
   - No weight-bearing; only use crutches until normal ambulation is possible.
   - Return to activities only when scale test (knee bend, standing on two scales) shows equal distribution of weight on both lower extremities.
   - Relaxation and stretching: relax by deep exhalation, eye movement, and activation of antagonist. Stretch passively by gravity.
3. Medications
   - Take anti-inflammatory drugs, but steroids only as an exception.
   - Use short-acting opiates on a regular basis to desensitize and prevent pain.
   - Do not use medications for early return to activity.

B. Injections: most effective treatment with dramatic, instantaneous pain relief and restoration of function
1. Preinjection block pre-empts the pain and irritation caused by injections of tender areas.
2. Needling and infiltration break through and eradicates edema, which later becomes fibrotic tissue entrapping nerve endings along with sensitizing substances; eliminate irritative foci.

---

13. **What are the new, more effective injection techniques for treatment of peripheral sensitization, irritative foci, and tissue damage?**
   - **Needling and infiltration (N&I) of the damaged tissue** eradicate the TS/TrPs. Such outcomes are confirmed by improved pressure sensitivity quantified by algometry along with pain relief.
   - **Preinjection block** interrupts the sensory impulses from the irritative focus, TS/TrPs so that needling and infiltration, which follow, can be carried out relatively pain-free. Preinjection

block consists of spreading 1% lidocaine on the side of nerve entry to the treated tissue (*see* Chapter 73). Other advantages of preinjection block include prevention of central sensitization caused by needling or injecting a sensitized area. In addition, preinjection block relieves the neurogenic component of the taut band, shrinking it to about 20% of its original size. A "fibrotic core" located within the taut band is uncovered, which is the sole target for N&I. By shrinking the taut band, preinjection block allows the practitioner to concentrate the N&I on the fibrotic core, which makes the procedure more efficient and renders substantially better results.

Fischer AA (ed): Myofascial pain: Update in diagnosis and treatment. Phys Med Rehabil Clin North Am 8:153–169, 1997.

14. **What are the basic principles of segmental neuromyotherapy (SNMT) developed as a system for diagnosis and pain management based on spinal segmental sensitization?**
Segmental neuromyotherapy consists of a system of diagnosis based upon quantified and objective assessment methods that are distinguished by a higher degree of sensitivity in the detection of abnormal neurologic and other tissue dysfunction, as compared to the conventional examination methods. Employing the improved sensory and motor techniques, as well as other tissue evaluation, two clinical pain syndromes have been described: **SSS** and **the pentad of vertebrogenic dysfunction (PVD)**. The significance of the new pain syndromes lies in the fact that they are consistently associated with pain of different etiologies. In addition, specific injection techniques promptly relieve pain by rectifying the abnormalities.

The therapeutic approaches employed in SNMT are focused on desensitization of the sensitized segment. In the first step, this is achieved by special blocks, such as paraspinous block and application of physical modalities (relaxation, limbering exercises), which decrease sensitization and hyperexcitability of the myotome, dermatome, and other components of the spinal segment.

15. **What are the components of the pentad of vertebrogenic dysfunction (PVD)?**
    1. Sensitized supraspinous and interspinous ligaments, which are pressure-sensitive and show microedema (impression of fingernail fails to recover for a few minutes). The sensitized ligament acts as an irritative focus causing SSS or contributing to the SSS.
    2. Paraspinal spasm, which is part of SSS and causes.
    3. Narrowed neural foramina.
    4. Root compression.
    5. Narrowed disc space.
    These latter two are manifested clinically by narrowed space between the spinous processes. Specific treatment of PVD is N&I of the interspinous/supraspinous ligaments, usually performed in conjunction with paraspinous block with 1% lidocaine at the identical level.

16. **What are the basic principles of treatments according to the concept of segmental neuromyotherapy?**
The first principle is to alleviate pain immediately by desensitization of the spinal segment. Segmental desensitization is achieved by four components:
    - **Injections:** Paraspinous block (PSB) with 1% lidocaine alleviates pain instantaneously by reversing SSS to normal sensitivity; N&I with 1% lidocaine of the supraspinous/interspinous ligament and then N&I of muscle TrPs eradicate the irritative foci. This is a prerequisite for long-term relief. Preinjection blocks pre-empt the pain and irritation caused by injections of TrPs and tender areas.
    - **Specific physical therapy:** The healing of the needling is supported by electric stimulation, hot packs, and relaxation exercises. The **relaxation exercises** should concentrate on all

the muscles of the involved myotome. The exercises should be limited to relaxation and limbering, which decrease sensitization and prevent its recurrence. Strengthening exercises in the early stage after injection has the opposite effect, causing aggravation of the existing sensitization.

- **Removal of conditions causing irritative foci** (TrPs, TS, inflammation).
- **Medications** that induce or support peripheral and central desensitization.

Fischer AA: New injection techniques for treatment of musculoskeletal pain. In Rachlin ES, Rachlin IS (eds): Myofascial Pain and Fibromyalgia: Trigger Point Management, 2nd ed. St. Louis, Mosby, 2002, pp 403–419.

Kidd RF: Neural Therapy. Renfrew, Canada, Custom Printers of Renfrew, 2005, pp 24–66.

Maigne R: Segmental vertebral cellulotenoperiosteomyalgic syndrome. In Maigne R: Diagnosis and Treatment of Pain of Vertebral Origin: A Manual Medicine Approach, 2nd ed. New York, Taylor & Francis, 2006, pp 103–112.

17. **Describe the technique of paraspinous block (PSB) and its effects.**
    PSB (Fig. 71-4) is a special injection technique that effectively desensitizes the SSS and alleviates the pain in the segment. PSB consists of spreading local anesthetic (1% lidocaine)

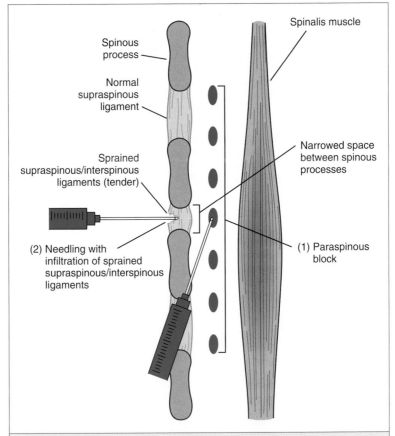

Figure 71-4. Technique of paraspinous block combined with needling and infiltration of sprained supra-spinous/interspinous ligaments.

along the spinous processes and their connection in the form of the supraspinous/interspinous ligaments. PSBs are effective in specifically desensitizing (reversing to normal sensitivity) the sensitized segment and so relieving the segmental pain. This is manifested by normalization of the hyperalgesic dermatome on scratch, electric skin conductance, and pinch and roll; on motor testing, the TS/TrPs become less tender, and the spasm within the corresponding myotome is relieved. PSB achieves this effect by blocking the nociceptive impulses from the sprained interspinous ligament(s), which acts as an irritative focus, mediating the SSS.

18. **What are the roles of medications and exercises in management of SSS?**
    - **Medications** should be used as an adjunct to therapy and consist of anti-inflammatory medications, as well as drugs for reduction of central sensitization (antidepressants, anticonvulsants, opiates).
    - **Exercises** are prescribed to reduce risk factors for recurrence, such as postural correction restoring cervical and lumbar lordosis, and to relax key postural muscles that lack flexibility. Endurance of the weak key postural muscles should be enhanced, but strengthening against high resistance should be employed only in the final stage of rehabilitation. Most relaxation exercises are active, slow through range of motion without resistance, combined with eye movement, deep exhalation, as well as mild activation of the antagonist muscle(s). This can be followed with passive stretching, preferably by gravity.

    Fischer AA: Myofascial pain: Update in diagnosis and treatment. Phys Med Rehabil Clin North Am 8:153–169, 1997.

KEY POINTS: EFFECTIVE TREATMENT OF PAIN

1. Treatment cannot be limited to the alleviation of pain.

2. Identify and remove the causes of pain and address the mechanisms underlying the sensitization.

3. Treatment of spinal segmental sensitization should involve all of its affected components.

4. Treatment consists of desensitization of the involved segment.

5. Long-term results require eradication of irritative foci, which induce the sensitization.

19. **How do you prevent recurrence of SSS?**
    Remove factors that cause recurrence of SSS, such as TrPs, TSs, muscle spasm, and inflammation, all of which cause peripheral sensitization that spreads to the CNS, causing SSS. For this purpose, special injection techniques include N&I of the entire sensitized abnormal tissues to eradicate the underlying pathologic, particularly fibrotic, tissue. Prior to N&I, a preinjection block is performed, which prevents nociceptive and irritative impulses from reaching the CNS and decreases the sensitization at the spinal level.

20. **Outline an algorithm for diagnosis and management of musculoskeletal pain based on SSS.**
    See Box 71-2.

BOX 71-2. ALGORITHM FOR DIAGNOSIS AND MANAGEMENT OF MUSCULOSKELETAL PAIN BASED ON SENSITIZED SPINAL SEGMENTS

Goals

- **Short-term:** to alleviate pain before patient leaves the office. This is achieved by treating the immediate cause of pain, which most frequently consists of tender spots (TSs), trigger points (TrPs), muscle spasm (MSp), or inflammation.
- **Long-term:** to remove perpetuating and etiologic factors responsible for the immediate cause(s) of pain in order to prevent recurrence of the condition.

Phase I: Identify the immediate cause of pain: TrPs/TSs, MSp, inflammation

1. Ask the patient to point with one finger to the spot of the most intensive pain.
2. Find the point of maximum tenderness or TrP.
3. Quantify the tenderness (degree of sensitization) with an algometer.
4. Reproduction (recognition) of pain: Press over the maximum tender point and ask, "Is this the pain you are complaining about?"

Phase II: Diagnose the SSS and specify the segment corresponding to the TrP/Ts spot.

Diagnoses of SSS:

1. **Sensory.** Diagnose the hyperalgesic dermatomes.
   - Scratching along the sensory diagnostic tracks
   - Electric skin conductance, which objectively documents nerve fiber dysfunction
   - Pinch and roll, which tests sensitization of subcutaneous tissue; can be quantified by pressure algometer
2. **Motor.** Diagnose the affected myotome.
   - TrP/TSs by palpation and algometry
   - Taut bands (TBs) by palpation and tissue compliance meter
   - Muscle spasm, by palpation and tissue compliance meter
3. **Sclerotome.** Bursitis, tendinitis, epicondylitis, enthesopathy

Phase III: Treatment. Concentrate on the SSS corresponding to the immediate cause of pain (TrPs/TSs, MSp, neurogenic inflammation), the associated supraspinous ligament sprain, and pentad.

1. **Injections:** for immediate and long-term relief of pain
   - Paraspinous block to desensitize the SSS
   - Preinjection block to anesthetize the painful sensitive area to be infiltrated
   - Needling and infiltration of the TB to break up the entire underlying pathology around the TrPs/TSs
2. **Physical therapy:** to promote healing after injections, restore function, and prevent recurrence
   - Modalities: Heat or cold; electric stimulation (sinusoid surging and tetanizing currents)
   - Exercises: Relaxation exercises and stretching: general and specific for the involved myotome, in which the pain-generating TrPs/TSs, MSp are located. Relaxation by activation of antagonist muscle(s)
   - Postural correction: **Kraus-Weber test** to specifically diagnose dysfunction (weakness or loss of flexibility) in key postural muscles and **Robin McKenzie test:** flexion deficiency of the lumbosacral spine is indicated by knee-chest over 5 cm. Extension deficiency is considered if on push-up, pelvis-floor distance is over 2.5 cm. On lateral bending, shoulder should pass midline. Induce corresponding correction by specific postural exercises (Robin McKenzie, Hans Kraus).

continued

BOX 71-2. ALGORITHM FOR DIAGNOSIS AND MANAGEMENT OF MUSCULOSKELETAL PAIN BASED ON SENSITIZED SPINAL SEGMENTS – CON'T

Phase IV: Diagnosis and removal of perpetuating and etiologic factors
1. **Mechanical:** overuse, sport injuries, cumulative trauma disorder
2. **Postural deficiencies:** muscle deficiencies (loss of strength or flexibility)
3. **Lab results:** endocrine and metabolic tests, electrolytes, vitamins, disorders

---

Kraus H: Diagnosis and Treatment of Muscle Pain. Chicago, Quintessence Publishing, 1998, 9–54.

McKenzie: 7 Steps to a Pain-Free Life. New York, Dutton, 2000, 65–105.

Editors' note: Andrew A. Fischer, MD, PhD is credited with several original scientific discoveries that have revolutionized the practice of pain management and enhanced functional outcomes of pain sufferers throughout the world. One important basic contribution has been the discovery of the syndrome called Spinal Segmental Sensitization (SSS). The significance of SSS lies in the awareness that it is a consistent component of all painful conditions. Furthermore, it can be diagnosed and treated successfully in daily clinical practice if the special examination and treatment methods developed by Dr. Fischer are being employed. This groundbreaking, seminal scientific observation by Dr. Fischer has led to the development of the Segmental Neuromyotherapeutic (SNMT) model. The SNMT consists of a unique system of objective and quantitative examination methods that detect the basic pathophysiological components of pain. It provides not only a scientifically valid and reproducible diagnosis, but also an assessment of the efficacy of various treatment methods. Only the exceptional sensitivity of these methods, as compared with conventional techniques, makes the diagnosis of SSS in clinical practice possible.

Based on the diagnosis of SSS, a more efficacious treatment plan can be formulated. In therapeutic terms, Dr. Fischer has poineered a novel system of safe and efficacious injection techniques, including Paraspinous Blocks (designed to control pain by reversing the SSS to normal), Preinjection Blocks, and Needling and Infiltration of taut bands, which eradicates the pain generator. Dr. Fischer's model of diagnosing spinal segmental sensitization and his new injection techniques have been successfully employed and are gaining increasing acceptance on a national and international level.

ACKNOWLEDGMENT

The authors thank Ruth Frischer, PhD, for preparation of figures.

CHAPTER 72

CENTRAL PAIN: PATHOPHYSIOLOGY, DIAGNOSIS, AND TREATMENT

Charles E. Argoff, MD

> *The lesion is in the area of my brain that is responsible for motor function, so I have continual chronic pain in my left arm from elbow to fingertips and the right side of my body from my ear to my breast area.*
>
> —Karen Duffy, model and actress who suffers from neurosarcoidosis

1. **What is central pain?**
   Central pain is defined as pain associated with lesions of the central nervous system. Most experts agree that central pain syndromes are among the most difficult and intractable pain syndromes to evaluate and treat successfully. The most commonly cited central pain syndromes are central post-stroke pain (CPSP) and spinal cord injury (SCI) pain; however, one should not overlook the potential for central pain in patients with multiple sclerosis, syringomyelia, Chiari malformation, neoplasms, or other lesions of the spinal cord or brain. Identifying and treating central pain is extremely important, especially in the rehabilitation setting, since impaired pain control may lead to difficulty with rehabilitation program participation.

   Merskey H: Classification of chronic pain: Description of chronic pain syndromes and definitions of pain terms. Pain 3(Suppl):S1–S25, 1986.

2. **What are the causes of spinal cord injury pain?**
   The most common cause of SCI-related pain is trauma (60–70% of SCI patients). Other causes of SCI include postsurgical, neoplastic, inflammatory, and vascular conditions, as well as demyelination and congenital abnormalities. SCI-related pain occurs in 60–70% of central pain-affected patients. There is often a significant delay of months following the injury before the onset of the SCI-related pain. Almost one-third of patients with SCI-related pain rate their pain as severe. Almost two-thirds of these patients continue to complain of pain for over 1 year. SCI pain may be associated with a number of different patterns, including the following.
   - Diffuse pain below the level of the injury
   - Band-like or dermatomal region of pain
   - Development of a cystic lesion in the spinal cord following the injury, which ultimately results in a syringomyelia

   The onset is most delayed in the third pattern. One should keep in mind that non-SCI pain syndromes may coexist, including radiculopathies, secondary overuse syndromes, and spasticity, to name a few.

   National Spinal Cord Injury Statistical Center: Spinal Cord injury—Facts and Figures at a Glance. Birmingham, AL, 2001: www.spinalcord.uab.edu

3. **What are the causes of central pain induced by brain lesions?**
   The most common central pain syndrome associated with brain injury is that which may occur following a stroke. CPSP was first described in 1906 and is thought to occur in approximately 8% of patients with strokes. The onset of pain following a stroke can be as early as 1–2 months or as long as 1–6 years. Patients often describe their pain in vague terms, sometimes delaying diagnosis.

   Andersen G, Vestergaard K, Ingemann-Nielsen M, et al: Incidence of central poststroke pain. Pain 61:161–164, 1995.

4. **Discuss the pathophysiology of central pain syndromes.**

Nociceptor hyperexcitability has been postulated as one of the mechanisms of SCI-related pain. This can lead to both spontaneous and evoked pain. When both types of pain are present, both spinal and supraspinal pathways are assumed to be affected. Some experts have postulated that the spontaneous pain associated with SCI occurs most commonly in individuals with lesions of the dorsal or dorsolateral aspects of the spinal cord, with resulting abnormalities of descending pain inhibitory input to the spinal cord.

CPSP has frequently been termed "thalamic" pain, in part, because early research pointed toward the thalamus as a source of the pain. Cortical processing has now been shown to be important as well in the development of CPSP, in addition to any role that the thalamus might play. Spinal thalamic cortical pathways may be injured following an ischemic or hemorrhagic infarct. Thalamic areas most commonly involved include the ventroposterior inferior and ventromedial nuclei of the thalamus. Alternations in thalamic and cortical processing of "normal" nociceptive pathways may lead to sensitization and loss of inhibition, resulting in a subnormal threshold activation of pain pathways.

Eide PK: Pathophysiological mechanisms of central neuropathic pain after spinal cord injury. Spinal Cord 36:601–612, 1998.

Jensen TS, Lenz FA: Central post-stroke pain: A challenge for the scientist and the clinician. Pain 61:161–164, 1995.

5. **What are the clinical features of central pain syndromes?**

Very often, the terms that patients use to explain their experience of central pain syndrome may be vague and strange. Their complaints may vary considerably from day to day and may sometimes confuse clinicians. SCI-related pain may be associated with nerve root lesions, partial or segmental cord damage, more complete cord injury, secondary visceral involvement through connections via the sympathetic nervous system, and injury to the cauda equina. Patients with SCI pain may complain of band-like muscle pain, described at times as a crushing or aching sensation. Any patient with central pain may complain of abnormal sensations, which are often poorly localized and quite upsetting to the patient. Allodynia (pain from a normally nonpainful stimulus) and hyperalgesia (more pain than normal following a normal painful stimulus) are common in central pain. Patients will also commonly complain of lancinating as well as shooting pain, "pins and needles," and sensations of bloating or bladder fullness. Painful micturition is also common.

McHenry KW, International Association for the Study of Pain: Lessons from my central pain. Pain 10(3):1–6, 2002.

KEY POINTS: CENTRAL PAIN

1. There are multiple etiologies of central pain; the most commonly cited central pain syndromes are SCI pain and CPSP.

2. Central disinhibition of various sensory systems is a likely mechanism of central pain.

3. Although central pain is one of the most difficult pain types to treat, various medical and nonmedical treatments are available for properly selected patients.

6. **What are the medical treatments for central pain?**

Surprisingly, few controlled studies have been completed for patients with central pain. Evidence for pain relief in patients with CPSP has been noted with the use of the tricyclic antidepressant, amitriptyline. At doses of 50–75 mg/day, significant pain relief compared with placebo was noted in 10 of 15 patients. One might also consider similar agents with fewer side effects.

As might be expected, anticonvulsant medications have been studied in central pain syndromes as well. Lamotrigine has been shown to be effective in the treatment of both CPSP as well as SCI-related pain in separate studies. Gabapentin has been shown to be effective in the treatment of SCI-related pain. Both topiramate and carbamazepine have been shown to be ineffective in the management of central pain states.

The use of opioids, especially intravenously administered morphine, has been shown to be effective in the management of spontaneous and certain types of evoked pain in patients with CPSP or SCI-related pain. When patients in this trial were switched to oral morphine, however, 6 of 15 could not tolerate the oral regimen and discontinued use of the morphine.

Nicholson BD: Evaluation and treatment of central pain syndromes. Neurology 62:S30–S36, 2004.

7. **What are some of the available interventional treatments for central pain?**
Intravenous lidocaine has been shown to be quite effective in the management of central pain; however, doses need to be repeated in order to maintain its effect. In a randomized controlled study, the intensity of spontaneous, burning pain as well as brush allodynia was reduced compared to placebo. Overall, in the same study, 69% of patients receiving intravenous lidocaine, compared with 38% of patients receiving placebo, experienced moderate or complete relief. Unfortunately, patients subsequently treated with the oral antiarrhythmic agent, mexiletine, after the use of intravenous lidocaine were, in general, not effectively treated.

Direct lesioning of either the brain or the spinal cord, except in selected cancer pain syndromes, has not been shown to be particularly effective in the management of central pain. When these treatments have been utilized in noncancer pain, there is a 60–80% recurrence of pain within 2 years.

Both spinal stimulation and deep brain stimulation have been shown to be effective in central pain syndromes such as phantom limb pain and CPSP. A recent report suggests the potential benefit of botulinum toxin injected subcutaneously for the treatment of SCI pain. The use of intrathecal analgesics, including both opioid and nonopioid analgesics, can also be considered in refractory situations.

Attal N, Gaude V, Brasseur L, et al: Intravenous lidocaine in central pain: A double-blind, placebo-controlled, psychophysical study. Neurology 54:564–574, 2000.

Katayama Y, Yamamoto T, Kobayashi K, et al: Motor cortex stimulation for post-stroke pain: Comparison of spinal cord and thalamic stimulation. Sterotact Funct Neurosurg 77:183–186, 2001.

WEBSITES

1. www.hmcnet.harvard.edu/brighampain/therapy/centralpain.html

2. www.ninds.nih.gov/disorders/central_pain/central_pain.htm

3. www.painonline.org/intro.htm

BIBLIOGRAPHY

1. Garcia-Nicas E, Laird JMA, Cervero F: What the brain tells the spinal cord: Lamina I/III NK1-expressing neurons control spinal activity via descending pathways. Proceedings of the 10th World Congress on Pain, San Diego, CA, 2002.
2. Yezierski RP: Spinal cord injury: A model of central neuropathic pain. Neurosignals 14:182–193, 2005.

CHAPTER 73

PERIPHERAL NEUROPATHIC PAIN: USING MECHANISMS TO DESIGN TARGETED, MULTIMODAL TREATMENT

Steven A. Stiens, MD, MS, Mark A. Young, MD, MBA, and Bryan J. O'Young, MD

Pain is temporary. It may last a minute, or an hour, or a day or a year, but eventually it will subside and something else will take its place. If I quit, however, it lasts forever.

—Lance Armstrong (1971–)

1. **What is neuropathic pain (NP)?**
   According to the International Association for the Study of Pain (IASP) Task Force on Pain Taxonomy:
   - **Neuropathic pain** is initiated or caused by a primary lesion or dysfunction anywhere in the nervous system.
   - **Central pain** is initiated or caused by a primary lesion or dysfunctions in the central nervous system.
   - **Peripheral neuropathic pain** is initiated or caused by a primary lesion or dysfunction in the peripheral nervous system.
     This chapter addresses the variety of presentations of neuropathic pain resulting from insults to the peripheral nerves.

   Merskey H, Bogduk N: Classification of Chronic Pain, 2nd ed. In Merskey H, Bogduk N (eds): IASP Task Force on Taxonomy. Seattle, IASP Press, pp 209–214, 1994.
   www.iasp-pain.org/AM/Template.cfm?Section=Pain_Definitions&Template=/CM/HTMLDisplay.cfm&ContentID=1728#Peripheral%20Neurogenic%20Pain

2. **How does neuropathic pain differ from nociceptive pain?**
   - **Nociceptive pain** originates from stimuli to somatic and/or visceral nociceptors.
   - **Neuropathic pain** originates from an insult to the nervous system that results in a subsequent nervous system dysfunction, resulting in the perception of pain without a normal nociceptive stimulus.

   Chen H, Lamer T, Rho R, et al: Contemporary management of neuropathic pain for the primary care physician. Mayo Clin Proc 79(12):1522–1545, 2004.

3. **What are the positive and negative symptoms of neuropathic pain?**
   Positive symptoms:
   - Paresthesia (spontaneous or evoked abnormal sensation such as pins and needles and/or a burning-like sensation)
   - Dysesthesia (spontaneous or evoked unpleasant abnormal sensation, including unpleasant pins and needles and/or a burning-like sensation)
   - Allodynia (pain from a stimulus that is normally nonpainful)
   - Hyperalgesia (increased pain from a stimulus that is normally less painful)
   - Hyperpathia (prolonged sensation of pain that persists after repetitive stimulation)
   Negative symptoms:
   - Reduced perception of light touch
   - Reduced perception of pinprick
   - Reduced perception of temperature

The variety and severity of these symptom patterns may suggest separate mechanisms that theoretically may be amenable to specific targeted therapy.

Mersky H, Bogduk N: Classification of Chronic Pain, 2nd ed. In Mersky H, Bogduk N (eds): IASP Task Force on Taxonomy. Seattle, IASP Press, pp. 209–214, 1994.

4. **What are the hallmark features of peripheral neuropathic pain?**
Neuropathic pain is often worse at night and leads to sleep disruption. Reduced pain or temperature perception may occur with damage to smaller sensory fibers without myelin sheaths. Also, the patient may experience allodynia over sensitized skin (e.g., pain from bed sheets in contact with the body). The loss or absence of protective pain sensation among diabetics can contribute to amputations.

5. **Why is the distribution of pain important? How can this information be used to confirm the diagnosis and record a baseline?**
A distribution of symptoms and findings that relate directly to the receptive fields of particular peripheral nerves or stocking and glove patterns implicate peripheral nerves as pain generators. A clinical baseline can be recorded by diagramming the areas of the body affected, characteristics of the perceptions, and intensity.

Dworkin RH, Backonja M, Rowbotham MC, et al: Advances in neuropathic pain: Diagnosis, mechanisms, and treatment recommendations. Arch Neurol 60:1524–1534, 2003.

6. **What are the causes of peripheral neuropathic pain?**
Toxic/metabolic
- Endocrine: diabetic polyneuropathy
- Chemotherapy: isoniazid
- Nutritional: deficiency of vitamins B_6 and B_{12}

Post-traumatic
- Complex regional syndrome, types I and II

Compression/injury
- Entrapment neuropathy
- Amputation

Irradiation
- Gradually progressive weakness and sensory symptoms months after radiation therapy

Infections
- Viral (e.g., HIV)
- Spirochetal (Lyme disease)

Autoimmune
- Demyelination
- Paraneoplastic syndrome
- Postinfectious (e.g., postherpetic neuralgia)

Hereditary
- Fabry's disease
- Amyloidosis

Sommer C: Painful neuropathies. Curr Opin Neurol 16:623–628, 2003.

7. **How common is peripheral neuropathy?**
Peripheral nerve disorders affect 2.4% of the population, and prevalence may increase to 8.0% with advancing age. In the United States, there are over 3 million people with painful diabetic neuropathy and 1 million with postherpetic neuralgia.

Duby J, Campbell R, Setter S, et al: Diabetic neuropathy: an intensive review. Am J Health-Syst Pharm 61:160–173, 2004.
Lycka BAS: Dermatological aspects of herpes Zoster. In Watson CPN (ed): Herpes Zoster and Postherpetic Neuralgia New York, Elsevier, pp 59–72, 1993.

8. **What is the most common cause of peripheral neuropathic pain?**
The most common generalized polyneuropathy is **diabetic sensorimotor polyneuropathy,** which may be present in up to 66% of type 1 diabetic patients and in nearly 59% of type 2 diabetic patients. Clinicians need to ask about the condition, quantify a baseline, and initiate trial treatment.

Barbano RL, Herrmann DN, Hart-Gouleau S, et al: Effectiveness, tolerability, and impact on quality of life of the 5% lidocaine patch in diabetic polyneuropathy. Arch Neurol 61:914–918, 2004.

Vinik A: Use of antiepileptic drugs in the treatment of chronic painful diabetic neuropathy. J Clin Endocrinol 90:2067–2072, 2005.

9. **What pathophysiologic mechanisms have been proposed to explain peripheral neuropathic pain?**
Damage to the peripheral nerve, due to toxic insult, ischemia, or pressure, starts intraneural inflammation. Reparatory processes and inflammation in adjacent tissues make primary afferent nociceptors hyperexcitable, a condition called **peripheral sensitization.** Thereafter, central neurons responding to such nociceptors functionally transform to become hyperexcitable; a process termed **central sensitization.** See Table 73-1 for a list of proposed neuropathic pain mechanisms.

Backonja MM: Painful neuropathies. In Loesser J, Butler S, Chapman C, et al (eds): Bonica's Management of Pain, 3rd ed. Philadelphia, Lippincott Williams & Wilkins, pp 371–387, 2001.

Dworkin R, Backonja M, Rowbotham M, et al: Advances in neuropathic pain. Arch Neurol 60:1524–1534, 2003.

10. **How can the proposed mechanisms be related to symptoms and physical findings?**
Constant burning and tingling may be clues to increased spontaneous peripheral afferent firing due to sodium and other membrane channel abnormalities. Sudden shooting pains from ectopic impulses or ephaptic transmissions may be generated from damaged peripheral nerve fibers spontaneously depolarizing. Decreased inhibition of pain messages at the dorsal horn entry zone may transmit otherwise insignificant sensory messages to the thalamus and onto conscious perception. Altered sensory processing at the spinal cord and beyond (central sensitization) may further amplify pain.

Rothbotham M: Mechanisms of neuropathic pain and their implications for the design of clinical trials. Neurology 65:S66–S73, 2005.

KEY POINTS: PERIPHERAL NEUROPATHIC PAIN

1. Peripheral neuropathic pain is initiated by a primary lesion or dysfunction in the peripheral nervous system.

2. Nociceptive pain originates from injury, disease, or a noxious stimulus to soft tissue or somatic or visceral nociceptors.

3. Mechanisms that maintain pathologic pain perception may operate within the central or peripheral nervous system.

4. Peripheral nerve disorders affect 2.4% of the population; prevalence may increase to 8.0% with advancing age.

5. Transdermal patch containing 5% lidocaine (Lidoderm) has been demonstrated to be effective for post-herpetic neuralgia and other forms of peripheral neuropathic pain states.

6. Effective control of peripheral neuropathic pain may require targeting more than one treatment (pharmacologic and/or nonpharmacologic) at various pain mechanisms suggested by symptoms and signs.

TABLE 73-1. VARIOUS PAIN MECHANISMS, ASSOCIATED SYMPTOMS, AND MEDICATIONS

Pain Mechanisms	Associated Symptoms	Medications
Receptor sensitization	Allodynia, pain perception in response to touch	Topicals, including emollient cream and capsaicin cream
Upregulation of sodium channels	Constant burning, tingling associated with allodynia, which exacerbates all symptoms Sensory examination reveals mild deficits	Sodium channel blocker: lidocaine patch Sodium channel modulators: carbamazepine, oxcarbazepine, lidocaine, tricyclic antidepressants
Spontaneous afferent activation	Sudden shooting pains unprovoked by stimuli	Carbamazepine, gabapentin
Ephaptic transmission	Shooting pain that varies in frequency and severity	Carbamazepine, gabapentin
Ectopic discharge at dorsal root ganglion	Pain perceived as shooting out into the affected area	Activation of descending pain inhibition pathways: tricyclic antidepressants; voltage-gated calcium channel blockers Inhibition of glutamate in the spinal cord dorsal horn: gabapentin, pregabalin; opioids
Sensitized adrenergic receptors	Burning, exaggerated pain response	Alpha blockers: clonidine
Central sensitization	Burning or diffuse pain not seemingly confined to a peripheral nerve pattern Unaffected by sensory stimulation in distribution	Centrally active agents: anticonvulsants (gabapentin), antidepressants (selective serotonin reuptake inhibitors, selective norepinephrine reuptake inhibitors), opioids

Data from Gallagher R: Management of neuropathic pain: translating mechanistic advances and evidence-based research into clinical practice. Clin J Pain 22:S2–S8, 2006; and White W, Patel N, Drass M, Nalamachu S: Lidocaine patch 5% with systemic analgesics such as gabapentin: A rational polypharmacy approach for the treatment of chronic pain. Pain Medicine 4(4):321–330, 2003.

11. **What components of treatment should be considered in designing a treatment program for a patient with peripheral neuropathic pain?**

Treatment is simultaneously directed toward at least two objectives: halting and reversing the disease process (primary objective) and reducing symptom severity (secondary objective).

All factors contributing to the problem must be considered from a biopsychosocial perspective, including biologic, psychological, and social contributions. Protection of the painful region from nociceptive stimulants with topical emollients and avoidance of restrictive clothing is helpful. The clinician must consider predisposing factors, precipitating factors, the patient's illness pattern factors, and perpetuating factors. Early implementation may reduce overall severity and improve outcomes by teaching patients to be observant of symptoms and to actively engage in self management.

Gallagher RM: Rational integration of pharmacologic, behavioral, and rehabilitation strategies in the treatment of chronic pain. Am J Phys Med Rehabil 84(Suppl):S64–S76, 2005.

12. **How can the various therapeutic modalities be used in the initial treatment of neuropathic pain?**
    - **Desensitization** of the sensitized denervated structures (peripheral desensitization). When a nerve is dysfunctional and/or injured, the denervated regions (e.g., skin, muscles, tendons) become irritable or supersensitive to the surrounding stimuli. Patients are taught to survey the hypersensitive areas using their hands as stimulators and then use creams and cloths to rub the areas to increase their tolerance and reduce the perceived discomfort over time.
    - **Shielding from stimulus.** Many triggers for hyperpathia and allodynia can be prevented. Patients are taught to desensitize the areas during bathing. Afterward, they can apply thick emollients with massage to keep skin from drying and prevent stimulation of the C fibers. Patients don garments such as cotton socks and use protective footware.
    - **Transcutaneous electrical stimulation (TENS).** One of the physiologic effects of TENS is to desensitize supersensitized regions. One proposed mechanism introduced by Melzack and Wall is the gate theory (i.e., stimulation of large myelinated fibers stimulates interneurons in the substantia gelatinosa of the dorsal horn, which, in turn, exerts an inhibitory influence on lamina V of the dorsal horn, where the small unmyelinated pain fibers synapse with the spinal neurons). The desensitization of the dorsal horn is a central desensitization process.
    - **Stimulating the peripheral sensory receptors.** This can be achieved by different means; for example, heat and cold activate the thermal receptors; exercise, manipulation, and dry needling stimulate the muscle spindles and Golgi organs; and massage triggers the tactile and pressure receptors. These stimuli are detected by the specific receptors that trigger nerve impulses relayed to the dorsal horn. The dorsal horn stimulus can lead to the inhibition of the supersensitized dorsal horn (central desensitization), resulting in decreased pain. The various forms of treatment, including dry needling, are effective only when the nerve to the painful region is still intact.
    - **Desensitization of central and peripheral sensitization by the segmental neuromyotherapy** approach to diagnosis and treatment of neuromusculoskeletal pain. (See Chapter 71, Spinal Segmental Sensitization: Diagnosis and Treatment.)
    - **Direct stimulation of the spinal cord.** Spinal cord stimulation attenuates the augmented dorsal horn release of excitatory amino acids in neuropathy via a GABAergic mechanism. This leads to inhibition of the dorsal horn (central desensitization), resulting in pain reduction.

Gunn C: Neuropathic myofascial pain syndromes. In Loesser J, Butler S, Chapman C, et al (eds): Bonica's Management of Pain, 3rd ed. Philadelphia, Lippincott Williams & Wilkins, p 527, 2001.
Melzack R, Wall PD: Pain mechanisms: a new theory. Science 150:171–179, 1965.
Meyerson BA, Linderoth R: Spinal cord stimulation. In Loesser J, Butler S, Chapman C, et al (eds): Bonica's Management of Pain, 3rd ed. Philadelphia, Lippincott Williams & Wilkins, pp 1857–1876, 2001.

13. **Knowing symptoms, signs, and proposed mechanisms, how can a systematic method for pharmacologic intervention be designed to get the best symptom control?**
    The following medications have been demonstrated to be independently efficacious in treating neuropathic pain in randomized controlled studies. The most commonly recruited subjects had diabetic neuropathy or postherpetic neuralgia. Reviewing the medication options and selection for safety and consistent efficacy in randomized controlled trials produces a group of medications that can be utilized to alleviate particular symptoms and find combinations in treatment of neuropathic pain.
    - **Topicals:** These are locally administered treatments such as lidocaine 5% patch, capsaicin, EMLA (eutectic mixture of local anesthetics) cream, lidocaine 2.5%, and prilocaine 2.5%

creams. These should undergo trial in the range of 2–3 weeks for lidocaine and for 4 weeks with capsaicin.

- **Sodium channel blocker:** Lidocaine
- **Tricyclic antidepressants:** Nortriptyline, desipramine. These should be avoided in the elderly and in patients with cardiac symptoms.
- **Selective norepinephrine reuptake inhibitors:** Venlafaxine, duloxetine
- **Alpha adrenergic antagonist:** Clonidine
- **Anticonvulsants:** Gabapentin, pregabalin, valproate, carbamazepine
- **NMDA antagonist:** Dextromethorphan
- **Opioids:** Oxycodone, methadone, tramadol

Meier T, Wasner G, Faust M: Efficacy of lidocaine patch 5% in the treatment of focal peripheral neuropathic pain syndromes: A randomized, double-blind, placebo-controlled study. Pain 106:151–158, 2003.

14. **How can these medications be categorized differently based on mechanisms for treatment of neuropathic pain?**
Medications that may be considered based on pain mechanisms and associated symptoms are included in Table 73-1.

15. **How are various agents trialed and clinically followed to assess efficacy for symptom improvement in individual patients?**
New medications are introduced when the patient is in a stable condition with well-quantified pain quality, intensity, distribution, and duration.

- One medication at a time is started and adjusted.
- The trial medication is started at the **lowest effective dose**.
- Medication dosing increases are made in increments that are expected to make a change in symptomatic response but avoid adverse consequences. The trial interval is 3–7 days or 5 half-lives.
- Increases are continued until the pain symptom is adequately controlled, intolerable side effects develop, toxic serum levels are measured, or maximal recommended doses are reached.

Argoff CE, Galer BS, Jensen MP, et al: Effectiveness of the lidocaine patch 5% on pain qualities in three chronic pain states: Assessment with the Neuropathic Pain Scale. Curr Med Res Opin 20(Suppl 2):S21–S28, 2004.

Hughes RAC: Peripheral neuropathy. Assessment of pain quality in chronic neuropathic and nociceptive pain clinical trials with the Neuropathic Pain Scale. BMJ 324:466–469, 2002.

WEBSITES

1. www.ahrq.gov/clinic/epcsums/neurosum.htm

2. www.clevelandclinicmeded.com/diseasemanagement/neurology/pneuro/pneuro.httm

3. www.en.wikipedia.org/wiki/Neuropathy

4. www.ninds.nih.gov/disorders/peripheralneuropathy/peripheralneuropathy.htm

CHAPTER 74

MYOFASCIAL PAIN SYNDROME AND FIBROMYALGIA: DIAGNOSIS AND MANAGEMENT

Hy Dubo, MD, Andrew A. Fischer, MD, PhD, Bryan J. O'Young, MD, Marta Imamura, MD, PhD, and David A. Cassius, MD

> *The phenomena of pain belong to that borderland between the body and soul about which it is so delightful to speculate from the comfort of an armchair but which offers such formidable obstacles to scientific inquiry.*
> —J.H. Kellgren, 1948

MYOFASCIAL PAIN SYNDROME

1. **Define myofascial pain syndrome (MPS).**
   MPS is a condition characterized by local and referred pain and the sensory, motor, and autonomic symptoms; and signs that are caused by one or more myofascial trigger points.

2. **Describe the main components of myofascial pain: trigger points, tender spots, taut bands, and muscle spasm.**
   - **Myofascial trigger points (MTrPs)** are small exquisitely tender areas, within palpable taut bands of muscle fibers that spontaneously, on compression or with needle penetration, cause pain in a distant region, called the referred pain zone (RPZ).
   - **Tender spots (TSs)**, in contrast to TrPs, induce pain locally without referral.
   - **Taut bands (TBs)** consist of a group of tense muscle fibers that are tender and demonstrate hard consistency on palpation. TrPs or TSs represent the most tender, pressure-sensitive area within the TBs.
   - **Muscle spasm (Msp)** is diagnosed by tenderness and hard consistency extending over an entire muscle, not limited to selected fibers, as in taut bands. Msp is an involuntary, usually painful, muscle contraction/shortening. The spasm may be initiated by MTrPs within the same muscle and can be part of **spinal segmental sensitization (SSS)** caused by nociceptive input of other tissues (muscles or joints) within the spinal segment.

3. **How do you diagnose MTrPs?**
   By careful history assessment and skillful, specific physical exam.
   - **Pain diagram** completed by the patient assists in identifying the pain distribution and RPZ. Precise pattern and area of most intense pain described by the patient is *the* most valuable clue as to the **location of MTrPs**. Use of pain referral diagrams with MTrP sites (Travell and Simons) and dermatomal charts assist in locating and diagnosing MTrPs in single or regional muscle groups.
   - Diagnosis of specific SSS by physical exam quickly determines which muscles within the sensitized myotome(s) need to be examined for MTrPs (*see* Chapter 71).
   - **Palpate the muscle(s)** by flat or pincer palpation to identify TBs. Press over the maximum tender spot/trigger point to produce local pain and **jump sign**. Irritate further to produce TrP **referred pain**. Ask the patient if this reproduces his/her usual pain complaint(s).

- **Elicit local twitch response** by snapping palpation across the TB in accessible muscles.
- Examine for **painful restricted stretch range** of muscles harboring MTrPs.
- **Muscle weakness** without atrophy may be present.

Simons D, Travell J, Simons L (eds): General overview. In Myofascial Pain and Dysfunction: The Trigger Point Manual, vol. 1: Upper Half of Body, 2nd ed. Baltimore, Williams & Wilkins, 1999, pp 31–35.

4. **Name the two most reliable criteria for the diagnosis of MTrPs.**
   - **Point** (focal) **tenderness**
   - **Reproduction** (recognition) of **symptoms** on compression of the point of maximum tenderness

   Gerwin R, Shannon S, Hong CZ, et al: Interrater reliability in myofascial trigger point examination. Pain 69:65–73, 1997.

5. **How is tenderness (degree of sensitization) of a TS or MTrP quantified?**
   Tenderness is quantified by an algometer. A **pressure algometer** is a pocket-sized force gauge fitted with a disc-shaped plunger with a 1 cm^2 surface. Applied over the maximum tender spot, the pain pressure threshold (PPT) is established (i.e., the minimum force that induces pain). An abnormal degree of tenderness consists of a PPT that is lower by 2 kg/cm^2 relative to a normosensitive control point. Algometry procedures have been determined to be valid and reliable.

   Fischer AA: Algometry in diagnosis of musculoskeletal pain and evaluation of treatment outcome: An update. In Fischer AA (ed): Muscle Pain Syndrome and Fibromyalgia. New York, Haworth Medical, 1998, pp 5–32.

6. **What are central and attachment MTrPs?**
   - **Central MTrP** is located near the center of muscle fibers and is closely associated with dysfunctional motor endplates (*see* question 10).
   - **Attachment MTrP** is located at the musculo-tendinous junction and/or attachment site of muscle taut bands against bone. It can be recognized as enthesopathy with tenderness and thickening at the attachment site. Such changes may be facilitated by the development of sensitized sclerotome as a component of SSS.

7. **What are primary and secondary MTrPs?**
   - **Primary MTrP** is a central TrP caused by direct trauma, acute or chronic overload, or repetitive use of the muscle in which it occurs.
   - **Secondary MTrP** develops in a synergist or antagonist of the muscle harboring the primary TrP. Secondary MTrP also arises from irritative foci in sclerotomal ligaments, joints, bursae, tendons, discs, as well as radicular or visceral tissue. Peripheral nociceptor sensitization with subsequent development of central sensitization and SSS causes secondary MTrPs within the myotome of the involved sensitized spinal segment.

8. **What is the difference between an active and a latent MTrP?**
   An **active trigger point** causes a clinical pain complaint spontaneously or during movement. A **latent trigger point** is clinically quiescent with no spontaneous pain or pain on movement. Latent TrPs are tender on compression and manifest all findings characteristic of active TrPs, including their location within a TB. Latent TrPs can be activated by compression, overuse of the muscle, or by prolonged immobilization of a muscle in a shortened position. The development of central sensitization can convert latent MTrPs into symptomatic active MTrPs within muscles of the sensitized myotome.

9. **List perpetuating factors of MPS.**
   - **Mechanical stresses** include skeletal asymmetry and disproportion (e.g., short leg, hemipelvis), poor posture, and overuse of muscles.

- **Nutritional inadequacies** include low "normal" levels of vitamins B_1, B_6, B_{12}, and folic acid and low calcium, potassium, iron, and hemoglobin levels.
- **Metabolic and endocrine disorders** include hypometabolism due to suboptimal thyroid function, hyperuricemia, and hypoglycemia.
- **Psychological factors** include depression, anxiety, and post-traumatic stress disorder.
- **Chronic infection, allergies,** and **sleep disorders** have all been cited as perpetuating factors.
- **Articular, radicular,** and **visceral disorders** and **fibromyalgia** may perpetuate MTrPs due to the process of central sensitization and SSS.

10. **Describe the pathophysiologic changes leading to the formation of MTrPs and peripheral sensitization.**

The integrated hypothesis of Simons regarding TrP formation emphasizes tissue damage, release of sensitizing substances, motor endplate dysfunction with excessive release of acetylcholine, and increased electrical endplate noise causing sustained sarcomere contraction with resultant contraction knots and taut bands. An energy crisis develops due to increased metabolic demand and hypoxia, causing enhanced release of activating and sensitizing substances leading to peripheral sensitization.

Microanalytical techniques of recording chemical sensitizing milieu from human muscle fibers in an active MTrP region show significantly increased prostaglandins, bradykinin, serotonin, norepinephrine, tumor necrosis factor–α (TNF-α), interleukin 1 β, calcitonin gene-related peptide (CGRP), substance P, and decreased pH compared to latent TrPs and normal control sites. CGRP is known to increase release of acetylcholine in the endplate region.

Active MTrPs are dynamic irritative foci of peripheral nociceptor sensitization that can initiate, amplify, and maintain central sensitization.

Gerwin R, Dommerholt J, Shah J: An expansion of Simons' integrated hypothesis of trigger point formation. Current Pain Headache Rep 8:468–475, 2004.

Shah J, Phillips T, Danoff J, Gerber L: An in-vivo microanalytical technique for measuring the local biochemical milieu of human skeletal muscle. J Appl Physiol 99(5):1977–1984, 2005.

11. **What is central sensitization? Explain its role in chronicity.**

Peripheral sensitization causes afferent nociceptive discharge from muscle or any other peripheral tissue pain generator to bombard the dorsal horn of the spinal cord via C and A delta nerve fibers. This leads to central nervous system (CNS) **sensitization** as a result of pathophysiologic, chemical, molecular, and immunologic processes that lead to functional and structural changes **(neuroplasticity)** of the spinal cord. These changes induce a state of sensitization within the spinal segment that manifests clinically as hyperalgesia, allodynia, referred pain, motor dysfunction, and autonomic dysfunction. Allodynia develops due to opening of "silent" nociceptors via A beta fibers, which emerge because of phenotype switch from A beta mechanoreceptor to C fiber-type functional nociceptor. Dorsal horn bombardment via A beta fibers now leads to amplification and maintenance of central sensitization, whereby light touch and low-pressure stimuli become painful. Peripheral sensitization initiates and drives central sensitization and, once established, becomes self-perpetuating because of synaptic and functional changes within the spinal cord. The transition from acute to chronic pain is a direct result of peripheral sensitization causing central sensitization and neuroplasticity of the CNS, rather than a factor of time alone. Central sensitization may occur within hours after the onset of peripheral sensitization, but the development of neuroplastic functional and structural CNS changes requires much longer and, once established, becomes much more difficult to eradicate.

A major cause of chronic MPS is failure to treat effectively and eradicate MTrPs before central neuroplastic changes develop.

Rygh LJ, Svendsen F, Fiska A, et al: Long-term potentiation in spinal nociceptive systems—how acute pain may become chronic. Psychoneuroendocrinology 30:959–964, 2005.

Woolf CJ: Pain: Moving from symptom control toward mechanism-specific pharmacologic management. Ann Intern Med 140:441–451, 2004.

Woolf CJ, Salter MW: Neuronal plasticity: increasing the gain in pain. Science 288:1765–1769, 2000.

12. **Define SSS and its relationship to peripheral and central sensitization.**

    SSS is a hyperactive facilitated state of the spinal cord that develops in reaction to an irritative focus originating in peripheral sensitized tissues. Hyperexcitability spreads from sensory to motor components of the spinal segment, inducing hypertonicity, muscle spasm/shortening, and initiating or activating MTrPs within a myotomal pattern. In the thoracic region, spread to intermediolateral column leads to viscero-somatic and somato-visceral interrelationships, because of convergence of somatic and visceral afferents at the same spinal segmental level in the dorsal horn (lamina I and V).

    The clinical manifestation of central sensitization and SSS involves five functional components of the spinal segment: **dermatome, sclerotome, myotome, viscerotome** (in the thoracic region), and **segmental sympathetic** overactivity. A vicious cycle develops between SSS and peripheral irritative foci, each increasing the sensitization of the other.

    With chronicity, a single SSS may sensitize other adjacent spinal segments, leading to multiple levels of SSS with **myotomal spread of MTrPs** to distant sites and development of widespread pain.

    Fischer AA: Functional diagnosis of musculoskeletal pain and evaluation of treatment results by quantitative and objective techniques. In Rachlin E, Rachlin I (eds): Myofascial Pain and Fibromyalgia, 2nd ed. St. Louis, Mosby, 2002, pp 145–174.

13. **What is the relationship between musculoskeletal (MSK) pain and SSS?**

    SSS can be diagnosed by objective examination techniques in the vast majority of patients with musculoskeletal pain. Therefore, SSS should be identified or ruled out, no matter which peripheral tissue pain generator is present. Although TSs/TrPs are irritative foci sending nociceptive signals to the spinal segment, the SSS can antidromically induce sensitization in the periphery (peripheral nervous system and local tissues), causing TSs/TrPs, Msp, and tenderness within the myotome. SSS may also activate previously latent MTrPs or amplify and maintain active trigger points. This dysfunctional pain processing in the CNS is considered the essential mechanism in chronic MSK pain conditions, including MPS and fibromyalgia (FM). Failure to recognize, clinically diagnose, and treat SSS in early stage leads to amplification, persistence, and more widespread pain symptoms. Treatment methods that do not dampen or eliminate the SSS often lead to failure to eradicate MTrPs by physical therapy and/or TrP injection procedures targeted at the peripheral TrPs alone. This may lead to transient benefit with recurrence of TrP symptoms and dysfunction, rather than long-term relief.

    The clinical significance of SSS is that it is consistently associated with musculoskeletal pain and desensitization of the involved segment(s) alleviates the symptoms (*see* Chapter 71).

14. **How is MTrP deactivated on a peripheral level?**

    MPS due to TrPs is often unrecognized, misdiagnosed, and mistreated, causing unnecessary pain, dysfunction, suffering, and disability. Accurate diagnosis is essential. Understand pain mechanisms and target management at those mechanisms to inactivate or eradicate TrPs/TS/TB/sensitized nociceptors. Table 74-1 summarizes therapeutic techniques targeted at peripheral pain mechanisms.

    The goal of TrP release and stretch techniques is to disrupt the contracture of sarcomeres in the contraction knot of MTrP, with release of taut bands to relieve pain, regain full stretch of muscle fibers, and restore function.

    Steroids provide no added benefit, are myotoxic, and have systemic side effects with multiple injections. Needling is the effective treatment regardless of solution injected, but local anesthetic has the advantage of decreasing post-injection soreness and allows for more extensive, less painful needling. Botox is expensive, not proven to be more effective

TABLE 74-1. THERAPEUTIC TECHNIQUES TARGETED AT PERIPHERAL PAIN MECHANISMS

Manual TrP Release Techniques	Injection/Needling Techniques of MTrPs	Augmentation Maneuvers
Vapocoolant spray and passive stretch or active limbering, relaxation exercises	Injection—deposited in one location as bulk	Directed eye movements
Intermittent ice and stretch	Infiltration—depositing small amount over multiple spots	Coordinated breathing—slow exhalation
TrP pressure release and stretch	Dry needling—repetitive insertion and withdrawal to mechanically break up and disrupt abnormal tissue	PIR
Deep stroking massage of TrP/TB	PIB (Fig. 74-1)	Reciprocal inhibition
Augmentation maneuvers	N&I (Fig. 74-2)	RAA
	Augmentation maneuvers after N&I	One or more maneuvers can be used in combination with manual TrP release or post–TrP injection/needling techniques to enhance relaxation and to achieve more effective muscle stretch.

N&I = needling and infiltration, PIB = preinjection block, PIR = postisometric relaxation, RAA = relaxation by activation of antagonist, TB = taut bands, TrP = trigger point.

than injection with local anesthetic or normal saline, and is not indicated as a first-line treatment.

Fischer A: New injection techniques for treatment of musculoskeletal pain. In Rachlin E, Rachlin I (eds): Myofascial Pain and Fibromyalgia, 2nd ed. St. Louis, Mosby 2002, pp 403–419.

Rachlin E, Rachlin I: Trigger point management. In Rachlin E, Rachlin I (eds): Myofascial Pain and Fibromyalgia, 2nd ed. St. Louis, Mosby, 2002, pp 231–251.

Simons D, Travell J, Simons L: Myofascial Pain and Dysfunction, Vol. 1: Upper Half of Body, 2nd ed. Baltimore, Williams & Wilkins, 1999, pp 126–166.

15. **Name three therapeutic techniques that deactivate MTrPs using the central pain pathways.**
    - **Paraspinous block** (PSB) with 1% lidocaine (Fischer; *see* Chapter 71): PSB blocks afferent nociceptive input to the dorsal horn from the periphery. This immediately desensitizes the hyperalgesic components of the spinal segment (e.g., dermatome, sclerotome, myotome) and deactivates the MTrPs within the myotome.
    - **Intramuscular stimulation** (IMS) (Gunn): Dry acupuncture needling provides stimulation of deep paraspinal muscles. This results in relaxation of shortened muscles and desensitizes hyperalgesic dysfunction of the other components of the spinal segment.
    - **Manual spinal manipulative/mobilizing techniques** (Maigne): Manual spinal techniques are aimed at pain of spinal origin with segmental effects involving dermatome, sclerotome, and myotome.

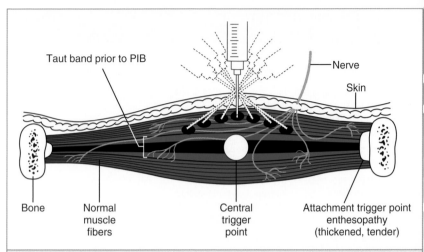

Figure 74-1. The technique of preinjection block (PIB) is illustrated. Penetrate next to the point of maximum tenderness of the trigger point (TrP)/tender spots (TS) into normal tissue where 0.1–0.5 mL of 1% lidocaine is infiltrated at one stop. Then withdraw needle to subcutaneous level, redirect to next stop, and repeat multiple stops as per black circles in the diagram. Spread the anesthetic in this way along the normal tissue side of the taut band (TB), which will be needled and infiltrated post-PIB. This blocks pain nociceptor afferents from reaching the dorsal horn and allows pain-free, more extensive needling of the TrP/TS/TB without amplification of central sensitization. (Adapted from Fischer A: New injection techniques for treatment of musculoskeletal pain. In Rachlin E, Rachlin I [eds]: Myofascial Pain and Fibromyalgia, 2nd ed. St. Louis, Mosby, 2002, pp 403–419.)

Beneficial effects of all three methods can be observed immediately. Long-term effects require eradication of peripheral irritative foci (i.e., ligamentous and MTrPs) causing or perpetuating the SSS.

Fischer A: New injection techniques for treatment of musculoskeletal pain. In Rachlin E, Rachlin I (eds): Myofascial Pain and Fibromyalgia, 2nd ed. St. Louis, Mosby 2002, pp 403–419.

Gunn CC: The Gunn Approach to the Treatment of Chronic Pain: Intramuscular Stimulation for Myofascial Pain of Radiculopathic Origin, 2nd ed. New York, Churchill Livingstone, 1996.

Maigne R: Segmental vertebral cellulotenoperiosteomyalgic syndrome. In Diagnosis and Treatment of Pain of Vertebral Origin: A Manual Medicine Approach, 2nd ed. Florence, KY, Taylor & Francis, 2006, pp 103–112.

16. **What management techniques can be targeted at central and peripheral mechanisms combined?**
    1. **Segmental neuromyotherapy** systematic approach (*see* Chapter 71)
       - Diagnose level of SSS (e.g., C5 or L5).
       - PSB with 1% lidocaine to desensitize the SSS immediately.
       - Needling and infiltration (N&I) of supraspinous/interspinous ligament TrP.
       - Preinjection block to anesthetize the painful sensitive area for N&I (*see* Fig. 74-1).
       - N&I of MTrPs/TS and TBs is necessary for long-term relief (*see* Fig. 74-2).
    2. **Postinjection segmental physical therapy** (Box 74-1).
       Treatment targeted at pain mechanisms should address both central and peripheral sensitization in order to prevent or reverse long-term pain and dysfunction.
       After dampening or elimination of the SSS and eradication of the peripheral pain generators, begin an exercise program of strengthening and aerobic conditioning. Premature emphasis

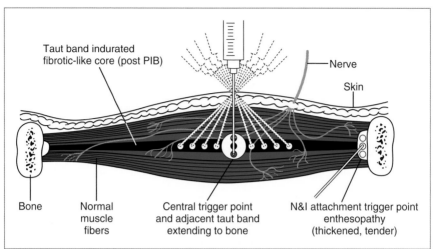

Figure 74-2. The effect of preinjection block (PIB) and technique of N&I of the trigger point (TrP)/taut band (TB) are shown. PIB relieves neurogenic muscle fiber contraction and shrinks the TB to about 20% of its original thickness (width). The remaining fibers (solid black) demonstrate very hard linear, fibrotic-like resistance on palpation and needling penetration. Needling and infiltration (N&I) consists of repetitive needling and infiltration of the central TrP with 1% lidocaine, fanning out along both sides of the TB with N&I (fast in and fast out) at multiple stops (white circles in diagram). Needling of the TB elicits local twitch response. Attachment TrPs (enthesopathy) should also have N&I where the TB attaches to bone. N&I is aimed primarily at disrupting the central TrP contraction knots/sensitized nociceptor mechanism as well as mechanically breaking up the indurated fibrotic-like core of the TB. (Adapted from Fischer A: New injection techniques for treatment of musculoskeletal pain. In Rachlin E, Rachlin I [eds]: Myofascial Pain and Fibromyalgia, 2nd ed. St. Louis, Mosby, 2002, 403–419.)

BOX 74-1. POSTINJECTION SEGMENTAL PHYSICAL THERAPY

Immediate therapy
- Moist heat
- Spray and passive stretch or
- Spray and active limbering, relaxation exercises
- Eyes down, exhale, and relaxation by activation of antagonist(s) with stretch specific for muscles of the involved myotome
- Electrical stimulation of treated muscle (tetanizing and sinusoid surging currents)

Subsequent therapy
- Home program of relaxation and self-stretching exercises
- Postural correction and elimination of perpetuating factors (*see* question 9)
- Strengthening and aerobic conditioning

---

on strengthening and work hardening leads to acute flare-ups of pain, muscle shortening/spasm, muscle weakness, and incoordination with functional deterioration.

Fischer AA: New injection techniques for treatment of musculoskeletal pain. In Rachlin E, Rachlin I (eds): Myofascial Pain and Fibromyalgia, 2nd ed. St. Louis, Mosby, 2002, pp 403–419.
Fischer AA: Treatment of myofascial pain. J Musculoskel Pain 7:131–142, 1999.

17. **What is the role of acupuncture in the management of MTrPs?**
Acupuncture plays an important role in the deactivation of TrPs. From a physiologic viewpoint, the needling effects of acupuncture on the TrP stimulates the A delta fibers. At the dorsal horn, the A delta fibers block the pain-producing activity of the C fibers arising from the peripheral nociceptors. This mechanism also reduces or prevents the sensitization of the spinal cord by suppressing the peripheral nociceptive input.

From a biomechanical viewpoint, the solid needle tip of the acupuncture minimizes tissue damage when compared to the shear effects of the sharp, bevelled, and cutting tip of the hypodermic needle.

Baldry PE: The deactivation of trigger points: In Baldry PE (ed): Acupuncture, Trigger Points and Musculoskeletal Pain, 2nd ed. New York, Churchill Livingstone, 1998, pp 101–108.

FIBROMYALGIA

18. **Define FM.**
FM is a clinical disorder in which there is central neuromodulatory dysregulation with amplification of sensory impulses due to sensitization of the CNS. The clinical manifestations include chronic widespread pain with tenderness at anatomically defined tender points, sleep disturbance, severe fatigue, and postexertional pain.

Price DD, Stoud R: Neurobiology of fibromyalgia syndrome. J Rheum 32(Suppl 74):22–28, 2005.

19. **List the diagnostic criteria for FM.**
1. Widespread pain of greater than 3 months duration, extending above and below the waist, to the right and left side of body, and axially.
2. Tenderness over at least 11 of the following 18 specified **tender points** (9 bilateral, 9 symmetrical):
   a. Occipital: at suboccipital muscle insertions
   b. Low cervical: at anterior aspects of the intertransverse spaces C5–C7
   c. Trapezius: at midpoint of the upper border
   d. Supraspinatus: at origins, above the scapula spine near the medial border
   e. Second rib: at the second costochondral junctions lateral to junctions on upper surfaces
   f. Lateral epicondyle: 2 cm distal to the epicondyle of humerus
   g. Gluteal: in upper outer quadrants of buttocks and anterior fold of muscle
   h. Greater-trochanter: posterior to the trochanteric prominence
   i. Knee: at the medial fat pad proximal to the joint line
   Critical pressure pain threshold over the tender points as quantified by algometer is 4 kg or less. The combination of criteria 1 + 2 yields a sensitivity of 88.4% and a specificity of 81.1%.

Wolfe F, Smythe HA, Yunus MB, et al: The American College of Rheumatology 1990 Criteria for the Classification of Fibromyalgia. Arthritis Rheum 33: 160–172, 1990.

20. **What comorbid, concomitant, and other disorders may be associated with FM? Why is it important to identify them?**
The physician should search for comorbid, concomitant, and associated disorders (Box 74-2), because treatment strategies are specific and different from those required for FM alone. The presence of a second clinical disorder does not exclude the diagnosis of FM.

Bennett R: Fibromyalgia: Present to future. Curr Pain Headache Rep 8:379–384, 2004.
Yunus MB: Central sensitivity syndromes. JIRA 8:27–33, 2001.

21. **Are there any precipitating or "triggering" factors in the development of FM?**
There is increasing evidence that FM is one of many overlapping clinical sensitization syndromes capable of being "triggered" when an individual is exposed to one of the following stressors:

BOX 74-2. COMORBID, CONCOMITANT, AND OTHER DISORDERS ASSOCIATED WITH FIBROMYALGIA

Comorbid Central Sensitivity Syndromes
Chronic fatigue syndrome
Migraine/tension headaches
Irritable bowel syndrome
Regional soft tissue/MPS
TMJ and myofascial dysfunction
Primary dysmenorrhea
Interstitial cystitis
Restless legs syndrome
Concomitant Rheumatic Disorders
RA
OA
SLE
Sjögren's syndrome
AS
Other Associated Disorders
Lyme disease
HIV
Hepatitis C
Hypothyroidism
Hypoestrogenism
Hypermobility
Multiple region MTrPs
Arnold Chiari syndrome

AS = ankylosing spondylitis, HIV = human immunodeficiency virus, MPS = myofascial pain syndrome, MTrPs = myofascial trigger points, TMJ = temporomandibular joint, OA = osteoarthritis, RA = rheumatoid arthritis, SLE = systemic lupus erythematosus.

- Physical trauma (e.g., motor vehicle collision)
- Surgical procedure
- Acute infection
- Emotional distress or catastrophic event
- Autoimmune disease or other pain syndrome that can lead to central sensitization

Stressors such as these have been shown to be temporally associated with the development of FM, and the symptoms and signs of FM continue well after the "stressor" has abated. Evidence in the medical literature suggests that motor vehicle collision (MVC) trauma or other stressors in concert with genetic factors may lead to the development of FM.

McLean SA, Williams DA, Clauw DJ: Fibromyalgia after motor vehicle collision: Evidence and implications. Traff Inj Prevent 6:97–104, 2005.

22. **How do imaging, laboratory, and electrodiagnostic tests contribute to the diagnosis of FM and MPS?**

They are useful for diagnosing or excluding other conditions that might be associated with, or perpetuating, both syndromes. The presence of pathology on imaging tests does not exclude the presence of FM, MPS, or both. There are no diagnostic gold standard tests. Diagnosis of FM (*see* question 19) and MPS (*see* question 3) require careful history assessment and skillful physical examination.

KEY POINTS: MYOFASCIAL PAIN SYNDROME AND FIBROMYALGIA

1. The precise pattern of pain described by the patient is the most valuable clue to the location of myofascial trigger points (MTrPs) causing the symptoms.

2. The clinical manifestation of central sensitization includes hyperalgesia of the dermatome, sclerotome, and MTrPs within the myotome of the territory of the sensitized spinal segment (SSS).

3. The clinical significance of SSS is that it is consistently associated with musculoskeletal pain.

4. Treatment to desensitize the involved spinal segment can alleviate pain due to MTrPs within the myotome.

5. Fibromyalgia requires an integrated pharmacologic and nonpharmacologic approach to treatment.

23. **What common peripheral pain generators should you look for in FM?**

A skilled search for nociceptive pain generators is essential, because treatment can decrease the total pain by eliminating regional sources of pain as well as decreasing the perpetuation and amplification of central sensitization. Some common peripheral pain generators include MTrPs, enthesopathies, bursitis, tendonitis, degenerative and inflammatory joint disease, radiculopathies, visceral pain, and dysfunction.

Borg-Stein J: Management of peripheral pain generators in fibromyalgia. Rheum Dis Clin North Am 28:305–317, 2002.

24. **What are the main differences between MPS and FM?**

See Table 74-2.

25. **What is FM/MPS complex?**

FM and MPS can coexist in the same patient and may interact with one another. MTrPs can be found in over 70% of patients with FM if searched for by skilled palpation. A patient with widespread pain and tender points at classic sites for FM may have one of the three following clinical diagnoses:
- FM alone
- FM/MPS complex
- MPS multiple region—mimicking FM

Accurate diagnosis and differentiation among the three possible diagnoses are important because strategies for treatment are different.

TABLE 74-2. DIFFERENTIATION BETWEEN MYOFASCIAL PAIN SYNDROME AND FIBROMYALGIA

	Myofascial Pain Syndrome	Fibromyalgia
Pain	Pain caused by trigger points in taut bands of muscle that can be identified by palpation Activation by compression reproduces patient's local and/or referred pain complaint	Pain diffuse and not limited to taut band Pain on compression of tender points Pain complaint not reproducible by activation of a tender point and no referral pattern
Gender	Equal	Mostly female (8:1 ratio)
Critical level of tenderness	2 kg/cm^2 lower than normosensitive opposite side or surrounding area	4 kg pressure or less (thumb nail blanch) algometer more reliable
Symmetry	Asymmetric	Symmetric
Pain distribution	Usually limited to 1 region, but may involve multiple regions	Widespread sites: right and left sides, above and below waist and axial
Tissues involved	MTrPs limited to muscle tissue only MTrPs initiate sensitized spinal segment with resultant allodynia/hyperalgesia of dermatome, sclerotome, and MTrPs within muscles of the involved myotome	Muscular tender points in upper trapezius, supraspinatus, and gluteus; tender points in other tissue sites such as medial knee fat pad, humeral epicondyles, insertion of muscles in occiput, costochondral junction, greater trochanter
Pathophysiologic basis	Local dysfunction in part of involved muscle with MTrP formation and peripheral nociceptive sensitization (*see* question 10)	Diffuse CNS sensitization and dysfunction related to sensory *processing* and autonomic and neuroendocrine regulation
Mode of onset	Frequently, acute muscle strain or overuse of a specific group of muscles	Usually insidious leading to chronic generalized pain and fatigue Cause unknown, but one-third result in onset following a triggering event (*see* question 21)
Response to treatment	Immediate relief of pain by needling of TrPs and/or infiltration with local anesthetic Manual TrP release techniques may be effective (*see* question 14)	Local injection of anesthetic does not relieve diffuse tenderness and pain MTrPs present in FM/MPS complex can be treated by TrP therapy, but needling is more painful, post-needling soreness is increased, and shorter duration of relief

FM = fibromyalgia, MPS = myofascial pain syndrome, MTrPs = myofascial trigger points.

TABLE 74-3.	MEDICATIONS FOR TREATING FIBROMYALGIA
Medications	Comments
Antidepressants	
Tricyclics (low dose)	Most commonly used; significant improvement in pain, sleep, mood, and fatigue in multiple randomized controlled trials (RCTs) versus placebo. (Muscle relaxant similar to tricyclics in chemical structure.)
Amitriptyline	
Doxepin	
Cyclobenzaprine	
Selective serotonin reuptake inhibitors (SSRIs)	More effective than placebo; SSRIs may improve mood and fatigue but have little effect on pain when given alone.
Fluoxetine *plus*	
Amitriptyline or	
Cyclobenzaprine	
Serotonin/norepinephrine-reuptake inhibitors	Action like tricyclics but fewer side effects. Significant decrease in pain, depression, and anxiety versus placebo in RCTs.
Duloxetine	
Venlafaxine	
Milnacipran	
Anti-epileptic drugs	
Gabapentin	Improved pain, sleep, fatigue, and quality of life in multicenter RCT versus placebo.
Pregabalin	
Selective hypnotics	
Zopiclone	Improve sleep and fatigue but not pain versus placebo
Zolpidem	
NMDA receptor antagonists	
Ketamine	Effective for pain relief but cognitive side effects limit use.
5-HT3 receptor antagonists	
Tropisetron	Significant efficacy for pain and other symptoms versus placebo. Experimental and not yet clinically available.

Data from Baker K, Barkhuizen A: Pharmacologic treatment of fibromyalgia. Curr Pain Headache Rep 9: 301–306, 2005; and Mease P: Fibromyalgia syndrome: Review of clinical presentation, pathogenesis, outcome measures and treatment. J Rheum 32(Suppl 75):6–21, 2005.

26. **How would you treat a patient with FM?**
FM requires both **pharmacologic and nonpharmacologic** treatment in an integrated approach. Targeted pharmacologic intervention aimed at central and peripheral pain mechanisms dampens CNS sensitization and enhances analgesia. Strategies for managing dysfunctional sleep, fatigue, emotional stress, mood disorders, cognitive dysfunction, as well as FM comorbid and associated disorders are required. Education programs should explain that the illness is real, regardless of unrevealing laboratory and imaging tests. Instruction in relaxation techniques and self-efficacy are recommended. Individualized aerobic fitness programs have been shown to improve cardiovascular fitness and deconditioning. Transcutaneous electrical nerve stimulation (TENS) and acupuncture benefits are less well-documented. Treatment of concomitant MTrPs as well as other peripheral pain generators

(see question 22) can improve overall symptoms of FM. Because of the complex nature and heterogeneity of FM, there is no clear consensus on the treatment of choice for any single type of intervention. Optimal FM management requires a combination of nonmedicinal and pharmacologic therapies best arrived at when patients and health care professionals work as a team.

Goldenberg DJ, Burkhardt C, Crofford L: Management of fibromyalgia syndrome. JAMA 292:2388–2395, 2004.

Lemstra M, Olszynski WP: The effectiveness of multidisciplinary rehabilitation in the treatment of fibromyalgia: A randomized controlled trial. Clin J Pain 21(2):166–174, 2005.

Morris CR, Bowen L, Morris AJ: Integrative therapy for fibromyalgia: Possible strategies for an individualized treatment program. South Med J 98:177–184, 2005.

27. **What medications have proven to be efficacious in the treatment of FM?**
    Simple analgesics and anti-inflammatory drugs are of limited benefit, acting at peripheral pain mechanisms only. Tramadol, acting centrally, has been shown to decrease pain in FM. Opioids also act centrally but should be avoided because of risk of tolerance, addiction, and adverse effects. They can be used judiciously as in any other chronic pain state but not as a first-line medication. Other medications directed at central mechanisms are listed in Table 74-3.

WEBSITES

1. http://arthritis-research.com/content/8/3/208

2. www.emedicine.com/pmr/topic84.htm

3. www.nlm.nih.gov/medlineplus/fibromyalgia.html

CHAPTER 75

COMPLEX REGIONAL PAIN SYNDROME: ASSESSMENT AND MANAGEMENT

Bryan J. O'Young, MD, Nathan J. Rudin, MD, MA, Warren Slaten, MD, and Ninghua Wang, MD, PhD

Pain...seems to me an insufficient reason not to embrace life. Being dead is quite painless. Pain, like time, is going to come on regardless. Question is, what glorious moments can you win from life in addition to the pain?

—Barrayar, Lois McMaster Bujold (1949–)

CLINICAL PRESENTATION/DIAGNOSIS

1. **What are some common descriptive terms for neuropathic pain?**
   - **Allodynia:** Pain from a stimulus that is normally nonpainful.
   - **Hyperalgesia:** Increased pain from a stimulus that is normally less painful.
   - **Hyperesthesia:** Stronger than normal sensation elicited by a given stimulus.
   - **Hyperpathia:** Prolonged sensation of pain that persists after repetitive stimulation (e.g., tapping).
   - **Summation:** Increasing sensation of pain with repetitive stimulation.

2. **What is complex regional pain syndrome (CRPS)?**
   CRPS is a syndrome characterized by continuous and severe pain in a region of the body, usually a limb. The current (1993) diagnostic criteria are:
   - The presence of an initiating noxious event or a cause of immobilization *(optional)*
   - Continuing pain, allodynia, or hyperalgesia with pain disproportionate to any inciting event
   - Evidence of edema *at some time,* changes in skin blood flow, or abnormal sweating in the region of pain

   This diagnosis is excluded by the existence of conditions that would otherwise account for the degree of pain and dysfunction. Other features not covered in the criteria may include weakness; dystonia, often with contracture; increased nail growth; increased or decreased hair growth; and osteoporosis (in advanced stages).

   CRPS was previously known as *reflex sympathetic dystrophy (RSD),* a term still in colloquial use.

   Merskey H, Bodguk N (eds): Classification of Chronic Pain, Descriptions of Chronic Pain Syndromes, and Definition of Pain Terms, 2nd ed. Seattle, IASP Press, 1994.

3. **How does CRPS type I differ from CRPS type II?**
   In **type I,** *no specific nerve injury* has been identified. There is an initiating noxious event or cause of immobilization without presence of a known nerve injury. In **type II,** there is a *known injury to a specific nerve,* although the signs and symptoms may not be limited to the distribution of the injured nerve. Type I was previously known as RSD and type II as *causalgia.*

4. **Why were the names RSD and causalgia changed to CRPS?**
   The term CRPS has been used since 1993 because the International Association for the Study of Pain (IASP) felt that the terms RSD and causalgia were inadequate to represent the full spectrum of signs and symptoms. The diagnostic criterion for CRPS is based on descriptive terms, rather than the poorly understood pathophysiology of the condition. The term "complex" was included to convey the reality that RSD and causalgia express varied signs and symptoms.

5. **Besides RSD and causalgia, what were some of the other terms used to denote CRPS?**
   - Sympathetically maintained pain syndrome
   - Algodystrophy
   - Shoulder-hand syndrome
   - Sympathalgia
   - Sudek's atrophy
   - Post-traumatic osteoporosis
   - Traumatic vasospasm

6. **What is sympathetically maintained pain (SMP)?**
   Pain maintained by sympathetic efferent innervation or by circulating catecholamines. SMP is diagnosed by performing a sympathetic block, either by anesthetizing the local sympathetic ganglion or infusing sympatholytic medications (phentolamine, guanethidine, and others). If sympathetic block produces significant pain relief, the condition can be categorized as SMP. If the block produces no relief, the condition is categorized as *sympathetically independent pain* (SIP). However, sympathetic blocks have systemic effects, and the injectate can anesthetize nerve root and peripheral nerve fibers; therefore, a positive response needs to be interpreted cautiously.

7. **What is the difference between CRPS and SMP?**
   CRPS is a clinical diagnosis, whereas SMP refers to a pain mechanism. A patient with CRPS may or may not have SMP. CRPS patients with SMP or SIP may appear clinically identical. Besides CRPS, SMP may contribute to other pain syndromes, including peripheral neuropathies, postherpetic neuralgia, and phantom limb pain.

   CRPS patients should be evaluated with sympathetic block because patients with SMP may respond to treatments that might not otherwise be effective, such as clonidine, repeated sympathetic blocks, or others (Table 75-1).

8. **Explain the known mechanisms of CRPS and SMP.**
   The precise mechanisms for the unique pathophysiology of CRPS are unknown. Many theories have been proposed to explain the mechanisms of SMP that may be involved in CRPS. These mechanisms are classified into central and peripheral processes.

   Theories related to **central processes** include the following:
   - **Gate control theory:** Input from large-diameter fibers inhibits input from small, unmyelinated pain fibers, preventing central processing of the pain input. In SMP, it is believed that the large fibers are injured, with relative sparing of the small unmyelinated nociceptive fibers, so the pain input from the smaller fibers is unmodulated.
   - **Turbulence theory:** Nerve injury causes formation of altered nerve input, creating "turbulence," which modifies the brain's perception of normal cutaneous afferent activity.
   - **Central sensitization:** The ongoing "nociceptive barrage" from hypersensitized pain afferents causes chemical and structural changes in the dorsal horn of the spinal cord. Wide-dynamic-range neurons in the dorsal horn develop a lower firing threshold and respond to a broader range of stimuli. They are sensitized during trauma by type-C unmyelinated fibers. The afferent fibers are excited by sympathetic activity and then induce more pain. As a result, the painful area becomes larger and still more sensitive, leading to hyperalgesia and allodynia.

   Theories related to **peripheral processes** include the following:
   - **Artificial synapse theory:** At the site of nerve discontinuity, sympathetic efferent fibers propagate impulses to the somatic sensory afferents. This depolarization results in a

TABLE 75-1. MEDICATIONS USED TO TREAT COMPLEX REGIONAL PAIN SYNDROME

Symptoms	Medications
Recent-onset CRPS	Short "pulse" of oral steroid (prednisone, methylprednisolone)
Pain associated with inflammation, persistent myofascial pain	NSAIDs (ibuprofen, naproxen, nabumetone, others), COX-2 inhibitors (celecoxib), tramadol
Profound allodynia, hyperalgesia, burning pain	Topical lidocaine patch, topical capsaicin, mexiletine, intravenous lidocaine infusion, anticonvulsants
Sympathetically maintained pain	Clonidine (oral or patch), nifedipine, phentolamine infusion, phenoxybenzamine, local anesthetics (sympathetic ganglion block)
Constant pain with/without sleep disturbance, especially if accompanied by depression	Sedating tricyclic antidepressants (amitriptyline, desipramine, nortriptyline, others), SNRI antidepressants (venlafaxine, duloxetine)
Constant burning and/or lancinating pain	Anticonvulsants (gabapentin, pregabalin, carbamazepine, lamotrigine, levetiracetam, zonisamide, others)
Muscle spasm/cramp, myofascial pain	Antispasticity agents (baclofen, tizanidine), "muscle relaxants" (cyclobenzaprine, metaxalone, others)
Refractory and/or widespread pain	Oral or transdermal opioids, calcitonin, bisphosphonates (pamidronate, alendronate, others), ziconotide (intrathecal only)
Dystonia	Botulinum toxin

COX-2 = cyclo-oxygenase-2, NSAIDS = nonsteroidal anti-inflammatory drugs, SNRI = seratonin-norepinephrine reuptake inhibitor. Adapted from Harden RN: Pharmacotherapy of complex regional pain syndrome. Am J Phys Med Rehabil 84:S17–S28, 2005.

perception of pain centrally and causes a release of pain-sensitizing substances peripherally.

- **Spontaneous discharge theory:** After nerve injury, regenerating axons results in excessive numbers of sodium and calcium channels and α-adrenergic receptors. These channels discharge spontaneously, and circulating catecholamines augment this activity, resulting in hyperalgesia and abnormal chemosensitivity.

Birklein F: Complex regional pain syndrome. J Neurol 252:131–138, 2005.

Harden RN, Rudin NJ, Bruehl S, et al: Elevated systemic catecholamines in complex regional pain syndrome and relationship to psychological factors: A pilot study. Anesth Analg 99:1478–1485, 2004.

9. **What events can trigger CRPS?**
CRPS commonly occurs after localized trauma, such as fractures, sprains, or crush injuries. However, it can also develop following immobilization (e.g., prolonged casting or bracing), surgery (especially arthroscopy), peripheral nerve injury, stroke, or brain trauma.

10. What are the clinical features of CRPS?

The initial and primary complaint is described as severe, constant burning and/or deep, aching pain, usually in a limb. Allodynia is usually present; hyperpathia and summation may be present. Any stimulation of the skin is perceived as excruciatingly painful. The pain is most often diffuse and nondermatomal. Initially localized to the site of injury, the symptoms tend to become more diffuse with time, usually spreading distal to proximal.

The staging of CRPS (Box 75-1) is a concept that is gradually growing out of favor. The course of the disease appears to be so unpredictable among various patients that staging is not helpful in the treatment of CRPS. The clinical features listed for each stage may not all be present. The rate of progression varies greatly from one individual to another. In addition, symptoms from stages I and II may fade as the disease progresses to stage III.

Bruehl S, Harden RN, Galer BS, et al.: Complex regional pain syndrome: Are there distinct subtypes and sequential stages of the syndrome? Pain 95:119–124, 2002.

Harden RN, Bruehl S, Galer BS, et al: Complex regional pain syndrome: Are the IASP diagnostic criteria valid and sufficiently comprehensive? Pain 83:211–219, 1999.

11. How is the pain described in CRPS?

The pain is best described as out of proportion to that expected from the initial injury. The initial and primary complaint in one or more extremities is described as severe, constant,

---

BOX 75-1. STAGES OF COMPLEX REGIONAL PAIN SYNDROME

Stage I (acute to subacute stage)

- Severe pain develops at the site of injury and the immediate surrounding area.
- Skin becomes exquisitely painful to touch and light pressure (allodynia).
- Localized swelling may develop.
- Muscle cramps, joint stiffness, spasm and/or dystonia may develop. There is often subjective weakness.
- Skin may become warm, red, and dry, then becomes cold, cyanotic, and sweaty.
- Patients tend to guard the affected limb from contact, leading to myofascial pain in the injured region and along the limb's kinetic chain.
- Stage I CRPS may resolve spontaneously, respond to treatment and resolve, remain at this stage, or progress to Stage II. The likelihood of treatment response or resolution decreases with subsequent stages.

Stage II (dystrophic stage)

- Pain becomes more severe and more diffuse.
- Swelling may spread and may change from soft to hard (brawny).
- Hair may become coarse, then scant.
- Nails may grow faster, then grow slower and become brittle, cracked, and heavily grooved.
- Tendinitis, contracture, and tissue atrophy (including muscle wasting) develop.
- Juxta-articular osteoporosis (demonstrable on x-ray) can occur early, but in this stage, it becomes severe and diffuse.

Stage III (atrophic stage)

- Marked tissue atrophy and contracture eventually become irreversible.
- Allodynia may spread to involve the entire limb.
- "Spread" of CRPS to other limbs is very rare but may occur.

burning, or deep aching pain. Any tactile stimuli of the skin may be perceived as painful (allodynia). There may be prolonged sensation of pain (hyperpathia) after repetitive stimuli such as tapping. Although the pain may radiate in a dermatomal or nerve distribution, it is more often diffuse and nondermatomal. The pain is generally localized to the site of injury, and the pain and symptoms tend to become more diffuse with time. The pain usually starts in the extremity and, with progression, spreads proximally.

12. **How do the clinical presentation and course of CRPS differ in children?**
The biggest difference between CRPS in children and adults is that with appropriate treatment, the prognosis in children is generally favorable. Children often have complete or near-complete recovery using physical therapy and cognitive-behavioral treatment, with little or no use of nerve blocks and analgesics. This suggests that pediatric and adult CRPS may be quite different disorders. In addition, often there is no preceding neurologic or traumatic event, and the lower extremity is affected more often. Bone scan results are more variable and, when positive, show decreased rather than increased uptake. Osteoporosis is rare. Individual and family psychological issues can be key elements in the maintenance of pediatric CRPS. Careful attention to these issues is required and may be essential to treatment success.

Berde CB, Lebel A: Complex regional pain syndromes in children and adolescents. Anesthesiology 102:252–255, 2005.
Logan DE, Guite JW, Sherry DD, Rose JB: Adolescent–parent relationships in the context of adolescent chronic pain conditions. Clin J Pain 22(6):576–583, 2006.

13. **Is there a gender difference in how men and women experience CRPS?**
Like most forms of pain, CRPS affects men and women differently. Women exhibit greater coping skills, but they have a greater sensitivity to painful stimuli. Women over the age of 50 are likely to exhibit worse manifestations of the disease and progress more rapidly. Women with CRPS (in contrast to men) are more proactive about their disease and are more likely to seek early intervention when symptoms evolve. Allodynia is more flagrant in women than men.

14. **What is shoulder-hand syndrome?**
Shoulder-hand syndrome has been used to describe any CRPS condition affecting those areas. However, the classically described shoulder-hand syndrome is a variant of CRPS found in the weakened upper limb in patients with hemiplegic or hemiparetic stroke. There is pain and limited motion in the affected shoulder, wrist, and hand. Shoulder-hand syndrome may respond to early treatment with moderate doses of oral steroid, combined with aggressive range of motion (ROM) and edema control.

DIAGNOSTIC STUDIES

15. **Which diagnostic tests can help to diagnose CRPS?**
As the diagnostic criteria suggest, CRPS is diagnosed by *history and physical examination*. X-rays, triple-phase bone scan, sympathetic blockade, infrared thermography, and electromyography/nerve conduction studies may be helpful but cannot prove or disprove the diagnosis.

Birklein F: Complex regional pain syndrome. J Neurol 252:131–138, 2005.

16. **What x-ray findings are typical in CRPS?**
Early in the course, x-rays may be normal. Periarticular osteoporosis may develop later.

KEY POINTS: DIAGNOSTIC CRITERIA FOR CRPS

1. Continuing pain, allodynia, or hyperalgesia with pain disproportionate to any inciting event is present.

2. There is evidence at some time of edema, changes in skin blood flow, or abnormal sweating in the region of pain.

3. An initiating noxious event or cause of immobilization *(optional)* is present.

4. No other diagnosis satisfactorily explains the degree of pain and dysfunction.

5. In type I CRPS, there is no defined nerve injury. In type II CRPS, there is a defined nerve injury.

6. CRPS is best diagnosed by history and physical examination and is neither proven nor disproven by diagnostic studies such as x-ray and bone scan.

17. **What are the typical findings in the triple-phase bone scan in patients with CRPS?**
The blood flow and blood pool phases may show asymmetric uptake between limbs, whereas the static phase (most sensitive) shows increased periarticular uptake. The sensitivity and specificity of the bone scan for CRPS are low, limiting its clinical usefulness.

18. **Are there specific abnormal laboratory findings in CRPS?**
No. All are within normal limits, including calcium, phosphorus, and alkaline phosphatase.

19. **Is there one test or a combination of diagnostic tests that definitively establishes the diagnosis of CRPS?**
No. Laboratory tests, x-rays, and triple-phase bone scan are helpful, but the diagnosis is established on clinical grounds.

20. **What other disorders should be considered in the differential diagnosis of CRPS?**
   - Systemic lupus erythematosus
   - Radiculopathy
   - Infectious arthritis
   - Muscle or tendon impingement or tear
   - Scleroderma
   - Peripheral nerve entrapment
   - Rheumatoid arthritis
   - Paraneoplastic syndrome
   - Peripheral neuropathy
   - Inflammatory arthritis
   - Factitious or conversion disorders

MANAGEMENT

21. **What are the basic principles for treating CRPS?**
    1. **Early diagnosis and treatment** lead to better outcome.
    2. **Immediate and aggressive pain control** is essential to improve comfort, reduce suffering, and help re-establish normal limb use. Pain should be sufficiently controlled to permit rehabilitation.
    3. **Rehabilitation** (physical and/or occupational therapy) is required to encourage normal use of the limb, prevent or treat contracture, prevent or control edema, and restore strength and motion.
    4. **Psychological support** is vital, including pain management skills training, relaxation exercises, patient and family education, and psychotherapy for comorbid depression and/or anxiety.

22. **Which drugs can be used to treat CRPS?**
    Medications commonly used to treat CRPS are based on the type and characteristics of pain (*see* Table 75-1). Different classes of medications may be combined for added effect, keeping potential drug interactions firmly in mind. The majority of drugs are used "off-label" (no specific FDA indication is available for CRPS).

23. **Which physical modalities are used to treat CRPS?**
    - **Transcutaneous electrical nerve stimulation (TENS)** may provide some pain relief by modulating afferent input to the dorsal horn.
    - **Contrast baths** (alternating cold and hot water) for the affected extremity may help to reduce the patient's vasomotor symptoms.
    - **Edema control** measures, including massage, elevation, and graded compression, can help maintain or increase motion and function.
    - **Desensitization techniques** may increase the patient's tolerance of normal sensory input and decrease allodynia and hyperalgesia.
    - **Ultrasound** may provide pain relief and promote increased motion in patients with secondary myofascial pain and contracture.

24. **Does amputation relieve the pain of CRPS?**
    No. Amputation of the painful limb almost always results in severe phantom pain, often with development of CRPS in the residual limb. Pain prevents most CRPS amputees from using a prosthesis.

    Dielissen PW, Claassen AT, Veldman PH, et al: Amputation for reflex sympathetic dystrophy. J Bone Joint Surg Br 77:270–273, 1995.

25. **What injection techniques are used to treat the patient with RSD CRPS?**
    - **Upper extremities:** Bier block and stellate ganglion blocks
    - **Lower extremities:** Bier blocks, sympathetic ganglion blocks (stellate or lumbar), epidural injections (intralaminar or transforaminal), plexus blocks, peripheral nerve blocks, and trigger point injections (for myofascial pain)

26. **What is a Bier block?**
    In this technique, sympatholytic agents (guanethidine, reserpine) are infused intravenously into the affected limb. Circulation in the limb is restricted by a tourniquet, creating a high concentration of drug in the limb, followed by a pressure tourniquet around the affected limb at 100 mmHg above systolic blood pressure. These agents, which decrease sympathetic activity, are then allowed to circulate in a high concentration in the affected limb, until the tourniquet pressure is decreased.

KEY POINTS: MANAGEMENT OF CRPS

1. If CRPS is suspected, start aggressive treatment quickly.

2. The best treatment for CRPS is a combination of pain control with medications and sympathetic blockade, rehabilitation, and psychotherapy.

---

27. **How is a stellate ganglion block performed?**

Stellate sympathetic ganglion block is performed in patients with CRPS of the upper limb. The stellate ganglion lies medial to the vertebral artery at the level of the C6 vertebra, in close proximity to the recurrent laryngeal nerve. Fluoroscopic guidance is recommended for this procedure given the risk of intravascular, intrathecal, or intrapleural injection. Recurrent laryngeal nerve block is a frequent complication.

With the patient in the supine position and the neck extended, direct the needle toward the tubercle of the C6 vertebral body (Chassaignac's tubercle). Once the needle comes into contact with the bone, withdraw it a few millimeters. Aspirate the syringe to rule out intravascular or intradural position. Administer a 1-mL test dose of local anesthetic. If the patient tolerates the test dose without difficulty, slowly administer the remainder of the solution with periodic syringe aspirations. Anesthetic type and dose are described in the references.

A more recently described technique involves using fluoroscopy to localize the C7 or C6 uncinate process. With a cephalad medial oblique approach, the anesthetic is instilled at the base of the uncinate process along the sympathetic chain.

Lennard TA (ed): Pain Procedures in Clinical Practice, 2nd ed. Philadelphia, Hanley & Belfus, 2000.

Saini BS, Abdi S, Stauss T, et al: Improving safety and effectiveness: A novel technique for stellate ganglion block. ISIS Scientific Newsletter 4(3):8–10, 2002.

28. **What signs and symptoms suggest an effective stellate ganglion block?**

Pain relief, Horner's syndrome (miosis, ptosis, nasal congestion, and anhidrosis), and an increase in skin temperature of the extremity. The patient needs to know that benefit from the injection is often short-lived (24–48 hours). For subsequent injections, greater relief and longer duration of relief are the criteria to justify continuing this treatment.

29. **After comprehensive conservative care, including medications and physical therapy and the use of sympathetic blocks, are there other treatment options for CRPS?**

Yes. These include dorsal column (spinal cord) stimulation, intrathecal medication delivery, and surgical or radiofrequency paravertebral sympathectomy. These treatments are reserved for intractable CRPS, and their success rates are variable.

30. **What are the indications for surgical paravertebral sympathectomy?**

After four to six stellate ganglion injections, if the patient is still getting significant relief from injections but the relief is not lasting, then he or she may benefit from surgical sympathectomy. If injections no longer have even a temporary effect, then benefit from surgery is less likely. The chance of benefit is greater with a shorter interval between injury and sympathectomy.

With surgery, risks include return of pain; the possibility of sympathalgia, a painful condition of muscle fatigue and pain that is usually temporary; and Horner's syndrome, which may be permanent. Compensatory sweating may occur at other sites. Presently, dorsal column stimulation is preferred over sympathectomy.

> Schwartzman RJ, Liu JE, Smullens SN, et al: Long-term outcome following sympathectomy for complex regional pain syndrome type 1 (RSD). J Neurol Sci 150:149–152, 1997.

31. What is the prognosis for adults with CRPS?
Guarded. Early diagnosis and treatment improve the prognosis, but there is no definitive treatment at this time.

> Pittman D, Belgrade M: Complex regional pain syndrome. Am Fam Physician 56:2265–2275, 1997.

WEBSITES

1. eMedicine.com: Complex Regional Pain Syndromes
   www.emedicine.com/pmr/topic123.htm

2. National Institute of Neurological Disorders and Stroke: CRPS Reference Page
   www.ninds.nih.gov/disorders/reflex_sympathetic_dystrophy/reflex_
   sympathetic_dystrophy.htm

3. Reflex Sympathetic Dystrophy Syndrome Association:
   www.rsds.org

BIBLIOGRAPHY

1. Babur H: Reflex sympathetic dystrophy. J Neurol Orthop Med Surg 12:46–59, 1991.
2. Bonica J: Causalgia and other reflex sympathetic dystrophies. Postgrad Med 53:143–148, 1983.
3. Bonica J: The Management of Pain, 2nd ed. Philadelphia, Lea & Febiger, 1990.
4. Kirkpatrick A: Reflex Sympathetic Dystrophy/Complex Regional Pain Syndrome. Clinical Practice Guidelines, 2nd ed. Reflex Sympathetic Dystrophy Syndrome Association of America, 2000: www.rsds.org/cpgeng.htm
5. Merskey H, Bodguk N (eds): Classification of Chronic Pain, Descriptions of Chronic Pain Syndromes, and Definition of Pain Terms, 2nd ed. Seattle, IASP Press, 1994.
6. Pittman D, Belgrade M: Complex regional pain syndrome. Am Fam Physician 56:2265–2275, 1997.
7. Raj P, Kelly J, Cannella S, McConn K: Multidisciplinary management of reflex sympathetic dystrophy. Pain Digest 2:267–273, 1992.
8. Schwartzman R, McLellan T: Reflex sympathetic dystrophy: A review. Arch Neurol 44:555–561, 1987.
9. Young MA, Baar K: Women and Pain. Why It Hurts and What You Can Do. New York, Hyperion Publishers, 2001.

GENERAL CONCEPTS OF PEDIATRIC REHABILITATION

Frank S. Pidcock, MD, James R. Christensen, MD, and Melissa K. Trovato, MD

CHAPTER 76

One of the essential qualities of the clinician is interest in humanity, for the secret of the care of the patient is in caring for the patient.

−Frances Weld Peabody (1881−1927)

1. **Why are the neonatal reflexes an important part of the examination of infants suspected of having neurologic disorders?**

   The neonatal or primitive reflexes are part of the bundled software included with the newborn brain that provides a temporary set of automatic instructions for protection against the hostile extrauterine world. They include the Moro reflex, asymmetric tonic neck reflex, tonic labyrinthine reflex, positive supporting, rooting, palmar grasp, plantar grasp, automatic neonatal walking, and placing. If the neonatal reflexes persist beyond 4–6 months of age, or manifest themselves in a mandatory fashion that "locks" the child in specific positions, they become chains that bind, rather than rails to guide the child on the path to independent movement. Their presence in a persistent or obligatory fashion is one of the earliest clues of impairment to the motor control centers of the nervous system.

2. **How do the asymmetric and symmetric tonic neck reflexes differ?**

   - The asymmetric tonic neck reflex **(ATNR)** is one of the classic neonatal reflexes that gradually fade away by age 6 months to allow independent reaching and head turning. It is a fencer's pose with head turned toward the opponent with rapier extended and opposite arm flexed at the elbow.
   - In contrast, symmetric tonic neck reflex (the **STNR**) is the only reflex that is not present at birth and that is also absent at the child's first birthday. It provides postural stability as the child makes the precarious transition from crawling to standing. It is reminiscent of Aesop's fables. When the child's neck is flexed, the arms flex and the hips extend, recalling the fable about the "dog and the bone." If the neck extends, the arms extend and the hips flex, a perfect position for steadying oneself before attempting to pull up to stand, reminiscent of the fable about the "fox and the grapes."

3. **What is the earliest age at which a child can learn to operate an electric wheelchair safely?**

   Children attain the cognitive and perceptual skills required to safely drive a motorized wheelchair between 3 and 4 years of age. Because exploration of surroundings through movement is one of the chief means of learning in early life, introduction of an alternative to ambulation for children for whom mobility is severely limited is desirable as early as possible. Don't forget that a child in a wheelchair requires the same vigilant supervision as any other rambunctious preschooler.

4. **Should you be concerned if a newborn presents with an isolated Klumpke's palsy?**

   Yes! Dr. Eng taught that she never observed an isolated Klumpke's palsy secondary to birth trauma (and she saw many, having published several articles on the subject, including two reviews comprised of 321 children). Although the lower plexus may be involved, it is essentially always seen in conjunction with upper plexus injury. If a true isolated lower plexus injury is observed in a neonate, one must rule out other causes such as spinal cord injury, outlet tumors (rare), and anomalous brachial plexus (very rare).

Eng GD, Binder H, Getson P, O'Donnell R: Obstetrical brachial plexus palsy (OBPP) outcome with conservative management. Muscle Nerve 19:884–891,1996.

5. Why do more infants have flattened skulls? What can be done about it?
One of the surprising effects of the "Back to Sleep" campaign, which has reduced the incidence of sudden infant death syndrome by more than 50% since 1992, has been the increase in incidence of babies with flat heads. Positional plagiocephaly is the term used to describe an asymmetrically shaped head that is deformational and not related to premature closure of the cranial sutures. When identified early, the asymmetry is treated with repositioning and supervised "tummy" time. More severe plagiocephaly may be treated with a cranial orthosis to assist with reshaping. Orthotic treatment may be initiated as early as 3 months and as late as 18 months to 2 years.

Littlefield TL, Reiff JL, Rekate HL: Diagnosis and management of deformational plagiocephaly. BNI Quarterly 17(4):1–8, 2001.

6. Does infantile torticollis go away?
Congenital muscular torticollis (CMT) should be treated conservatively at first with physical therapy for passive stretching. In most cases, early intervention will prevent the need for a surgical procedure and spare the child from the potential consequences that include craniofacial asymmetry, intermittent head tilt, and scoliosis. If it does not disappear, nonmuscular problems such as benign paroxysmal torticollis, Klippel-Feil syndrome, hemivertebrae, and congenital absence of one of the cervical muscles should be considered. An appropriate evaluation would include x-rays of the cervical spine and a neurology consultation. Reappearance of torticollis may occur after appropriate treatment. These episodes are usually brief and may be associated with episodes of illness and fatigue or during a growth spurt.

Binder H, Eng GD, Gaiser JF, Koch B: Congenital muscular torticollis: Results of conservative management with long-term follow-up in 85 cases. Arch Phys Med Rehabil 68:222–225, 1987.

7. Do Apgar scores predict cerebral palsy or mental retardation?
The Apgar score was developed to quickly identify the newborn infant in need of resuscitation. It has little predictive significance for the development of neurologic problems under 15–20 minutes after birth. In a large multicenter collaborative project, 4.8% of surviving infants had Apgar scores of <3 out of 10 at 1 minute postbirth. In this group the risk of cerebral palsy was only 1.7%. However, 15% of infants who had 5-minute Apgar scores of <3 had cerebral palsy. A score of <3 at 15 minutes was associated with mortality in approximately 53% of cases, with a risk for cerebral palsy of 36% in survivors.

8. How do brain magnetic resonance imaging (MRI) scans correlate with gestational age and type of cerebral palsy?
Most children with cerebral palsy who were born prematurely show evidence of periventricular leukomalacia (PVL) on brain MRI. A second but much less common finding is posthemorrhagic porencephaly. Abnormalities seen at term or near term in children with cerebral palsy are border zone infarcts, bilateral basal ganglia–thalamic lesions, subcortical leukomalacia, and multicystic encephalomalacia. Diffusion tensor imaging of PVL suggests that the motor impairments in some children with cerebral palsy may be caused by disruptions of sensory connections outside of the usually implicated corticospinal pathways.

Hoon AH, Lawrie WT, Melhem ER, et al: Diffusion tensor imaging of periventricular leukomalacia shows affected sensory cortex white matter pathways. Neurology 59:752–756, 2002.
Okumura A, Hayakawa F, Kato T, et al: MRI findings in patients with spastic cerebral palsy. Dev Med Child Neurol 39:363–372, 1997.

9. **Is cerebral palsy caused by obstetrical misadventure?**
    Unfortunately, the perception that cerebral palsy is caused by something that went wrong
    at birth has been a part of popular folklore since its initial description by William John Little
    in 1868. This issue has since been scrutinized carefully by many epidemiologists. An
    association between asphyxia at birth and the development of cerebral palsy was detected in
    only 3–13% of cases.

10. **Does it make sense to limit movement of the more functional upper extremity
    in a child with congenital hemiplegic cerebral palsy?**
    Constraint-induced movement therapy is a technique that uses limb restraint combined with an
    enriched program of stimulation for a set period. Trained therapists engage the child in
    developmentally appropriate tasks that are usually embedded in play activities. The techniques
    include repetitive practice and a behavioral approach known as "shaping" that addresses a
    specific task in small, intermediate steps that are made more challenging as the child
    accomplishes them. The age of initiating this type of treatment varies, as does the type of
    constraint (e.g., casts, bivalve cast splints, mitts, slings) and duration of treatment.

    Gordon AM, Charles J, Wolf SL: Methods of constraint-induced movement therapy for children with
    hemiplegic cerebral palsy: Development of a child-friendly intervention for improving upper extremity
    function. Arch Phys Med Rehabil 86:837–844, 2005.

11. **Should strengthening exercises be prescribed for children with cerebral palsy?**
    Adults with cerebral palsy report that *fatigue* is the major reason for not walking or a decrease
    in the distance of walking as they age. This has major repercussions for young adults with
    cerebral palsy who would like to transition to community-based living arrangements where they
    must be able to function over longer distances than in a household or school environment.
    Children with cerebral palsy are at increased risk for decreased bone density, stiff muscles, and
    selective muscle atrophy. Six weeks of strength training in children with spastic diplegia and
    hemiplegia has been shown to increase gait velocity through increasing cadence without
    increasing energy expenditure.

    Bottos M, Feliciangeli A, Sciuto L, et al: Functional status of adults with cerebral palsy and implications for
    treatment of children. Dev Med Child Neurol 43(8):516–528, 2001.
    Damiano D, Abel M: Functional outcomes of strength training in spastic cerebral palsy. Arch Phys Rehabil
    79:119–125, 1998.

12. **What are the earliest signs of Duchenne's muscular dystrophy (DMD)?**
    The early developmental history of children with DMD is normal with age-appropriate
    achievement of milestones, such as raising head from prone and sitting independently. In
    retrospect, there is often a history of difficulty in arising from the floor, frequent falls, or an
    abnormally loud "thud" when walking. Neck flexor muscles are involved early, and these
    children have a characteristic difficulty in raising their heads when supine. At approximately
    3–6 years of age, the lag in motor development becomes inescapable. The child shows difficulty
    with climbing stairs, develops a waddling gait to compensate for proximal weakness with
    lordosis, and develops toe-walking to maintain the center of gravity over the feet and prevent
    collapse at the knees.

13. **When should one worry about idiopathic adolescent scoliosis?**
    Other causes of adolescent-onset idiopathic scoliosis include relatively minor problems such as
    a leg-length discrepancy or poor posture, as well as serious conditions such as vertebral and
    spinal cord tumors, osteoid osteomas, and spondylolisthesis. Muscle spasms and hysteria
    are other conditions that may present as a scoliosis. Because idiopathic scoliosis is generally a
    painless condition, a report of **pain,** especially at the convexity of the scoliotic curve, must
    be taken seriously, and further evaluations to determine an etiology are mandatory. Other red

flags that signal the need to evaluate a child in greater detail are **onset before puberty** and presentation in a **male**.

14. **How do pulmonary function tests help in the management of scoliosis in DMD?**
Forced vital capacity (FVC) increases during the first decade of life in children with DMD, plateaus in the early part of the second decade, and then gradually declines between ages 10 and 20. Plateau values of less than 1200 mL are associated with severe progressive scoliosis. The least severe forms of DMD have plateau FVC values of more than 1700 mL. Patients with higher peak FVC values also have slower progression of restrictive lung disease. Because an FVC value of less than 40% increases perioperative morbidity irrespective of the severity of scoliosis, frequent clinical examination and spine x-rays are indicated during the adolescent growth spurt so that rapid progression of spinal scoliosis can be detected before the surgical "window of opportunity" for correction closes.

McDonald CM, Abresch RT, Carter GT, et al: Profiles of neuromuscular diseases: Duchenne muscular dystrophy. Am J Phys Med Rehabil 74(Suppl 5):S93–S103, 1995.

15. **Who was Gavriil Ilizarov? What was he doing in Siberia in the 1950s?**
In 1951, Professor Ilizarov was in Siberia developing a surgical procedure for lengthening limbs. His method was to create an osteotomy followed by application of an external fixator to apply controlled osseous distraction. The gap caused by slow separation of the ends of the bone is filled in with new bone tissue. The rate of lengthening is approximately 1 mm/day. In general, the femur is not be lengthened more than 6–10 cm at one time. Upper limits for lengthening in other bones are: tibia, 10–15 cm; humerus, 10–15 cm; and forearm, 5–10 cm. Postprocedure, intensive therapy for stretching soft tissue and muscle to accommodate the lengthening bone is essential to the success of the procedure.

Paley D, Kovelman HF, Herzenberg JE: Ilizarov technology. Adv Oper Orthop 1:243–287, 1993.

16. **Are acquired spinal cord injuries (SCIs) more common in children than adults?**
No. The incidence of all new SCIs is 10,000 per year in the United States, but only 3–5% of those occur in children under 15 years of age. If a child acquires an SCI, he or she is more likely to develop tetraplegia (56% of cases in children) than an adult. This increased susceptibility to cervical injuries can be explained in part by more ligamentous laxity, shallow angulation of the facet joints, incomplete ossification of vertebral bodies, and relative underdevelopment of neck muscles for a relatively large, heavy head. There are also pediatric disorders predisposing to SCI such as Down syndrome, juvenile rheumatoid arthritis, and skeletal dysplasias.

17. **Are there signs that help distinguish fractures resulting from child abuse versus accidental trauma?**
A high index of suspicion, backed up by appropriate medical findings, is the key to identifying nonaccidental childhood trauma. Fractures suggestive of abuse include multiple fractures in various stages of healing, such as growth plate fracture; transverse metaphyseal fracture ("bucket-handle" fracture) near the growth plate of femur, tibia, and humerus; spiral fractures of long bones; and unusual locations of fracture (posterior rib, sternum, scapula). Nonskeletal associated findings include retinal hemorrhages and subdural hemorrhages, especially when multiple and appearing at different ages. Reporting suspected child abuse is required by law. If you're wrong, the result of the investigation is inconvenience and ruffled feathers. If you're right, the result may well save a life.

18. **What is the WeeFIM?**
Developed in 1987, the WeeFIM is a measure of functional abilities and need for assistance associated with disability in children ages 6 months to 7 years. It can be used after the age of 7 as long as the child has delays in functional abilities. There are six subdomains that include 18 items rated on a 7-point ordinal scale (from dependence to independence).

19. **What is the COAT?**

COAT stands for Children's Orientation and Amnesia Test. It is a 16-item test of orientation and memory designed for children recovering from traumatic brain injury (TBI). It assesses general orientation, temporal orientation, and memory. On the COAT, a score within 2 standard deviations (SD) of the mean for age defines the end of post-traumatic amnesia (PTA), the period after injury during which the brain is unable to store and recall new events or information. The duration of PTA is important to define, especially in someone assumed to have a more minor TBI, because it correlates strongly with long-term cognitive and memory outcome. In pediatrics, many clinicians use ≥ 7 days of PTA as a marker for severe TBI. More than 50% of children who meet this criterion have persistent behavioral and/or psychiatric problems.

Brown G, Chadwick O, Shaffer D, et al: A prospective study of children with head injuries. III. Psychiatric sequelae. Psychol Med 11:63–78, 1981.

20. **Does outcome after TBI follow the general pediatric brain injury rule that "outcome is better with earlier insults" (because of plasticity of the developing central nervous system)?**

Unfortunately, for younger children this is not the case. Although some studies using narrower age ranges have shown no significant differences with age, others have shown that older children and adolescents do better than younger children. Plasticity, which is so important in recovery from focal brain injuries such as infantile strokes, may be at a disadvantage because of the diffuse nature of the injuries. The physical and neurochemical properties of the younger brain may make it more susceptible to injury. Also, because *new* learning is affected after TBI, development of the younger child is much more compromised.

21. **What injury prevention strategies are most effective?**

The main principles of brain injury prevention include decreasing the amount and rate of energy transfer, using "passive" or automatic strategies rather than strategies based solely on behavioral change, and using focused and specific recommendations. Don't say "be careful"; instead, say "use a car seat," "buy and use a bike helmet," and "throw out the baby walker"! Prevention needs to be approached from multiple simultaneous angles, including passive strategies, education, financial incentives (e.g., bicycle helmet coupons/subsidies), and "mandatory use" legislation. The first step is for all professionals working with children to remember the need for and importance of prevention.

KEY POINTS: STRATEGIES FOR PREVENTING BRAIN INJURY

1. Decrease the amount of energy transfer.

2. Use passive or "automatic" strategies (e.g., seat belts).

3. Be specific with recommendations.

4. Always think about prevention.

22. **Is there such a thing as executive function in children?**

The executive system describes those mental processes necessary for formulating goals, planning how to achieve them, and carrying out the plans effectively. Executive function can also be thought of as those processes that allow mental flexibility—the ability to mentally initiate and sustain thoughts and plans appropriately, inhibit unwanted thoughts and actions, and yet mentally "shift gears" when appropriate. Remember the mnemonic **ISIS**—**i**nitiate, **s**ustain, **i**nhibit, **s**hift.

23. **Describe executive dysfunction in children with brain injury.**
Executive dysfunction in children after closed head injury is related in part to the frontal lobe injuries. Failure to develop higher-level executive functions in these children may be misinterpreted as the development of new deficits. This often manifests itself when students are expected, based on normal development, to have reached a stage of increased independence. A common example of this is when children go from elementary to middle school. Elementary school is a highly structured environment that does not expect the student to independently organize his or her day, whereas middle school expects the student to independently organize many diverse activities and responsibilities (multiple classrooms, multiple teachers, increased homework, lockers, etc.).

24. **Will children return to their pretrauma abilities after sustaining a moderate TBI?**
Although children with moderate TBI can be expected to score within the normal range on neuropsychological and behavioral tests, their performance will be less than their predicted pretrauma abilities level, based on very closely matched controls. These persisting deficits impact on real-life functioning as evidenced by school achievement tests and grades, after *both* moderate and severe TBI. Of course, there is a strong correlation between severity and neurobehavioral outcome within the moderate and severe range.

WEBSITES

1. www.hemikids.org

2. www.wemove.org

CHAPTER 77

DEVELOPMENTAL MILESTONES: A HEAD-TO-TOE CONTINUUM

Scott E. Benjamin, MD, Melissa K. Trovato, MD, Beth A. Stiens, MEd, and Edward A. Hurvitz, MD

The aim of life is self-development. To realize one's nature perfectly—that is what each of us is here for.

—Oscar Wilde (1854–1900)

1. **How can one understand developmental milestones instead of just memorizing the events and ages at which they take place?**

   It is actually a fairly logical progression. Think of development as a continuum with one function building on top of another. Development proceeds in a head-to-toe direction as follows: head control, then trunk control, followed by rolling (which includes head, trunk, and some limb control), then sitting, crawling, pulling to stand, cruising with hand-held assistance or along furniture, then independent walking, running, etc.

   In addition, think of mass activity replaced by individual, specific actions. Infants react to a stimulating toy with their whole body, whereas an older child will reach, crawl, or walk toward the toy.

2. **How does muscle tone differ between premature and term infants?**

   The muscle tone of an infant born at 28 weeks' gestation is completely hypotonic. Muscle tone increases first caudally, beginning with flexion of the thigh at the hip at approximately 30 weeks' gestation and progresses cephalad. Flexion of the four limbs appears at 36 weeks. In the full-term newborn, flexor tone predominates.

3. **What are handy mobility milestones to remember?**
   - **Rolling (first prone to supine, then reversed):** 4–5 months
   - **Sitting independently:** 6–7 months
   - **Walking:** 1 year
   - **Running:** 2 years
   - **Stairs (adult style):** 4 years
   - **Skipping:** 5 years (boys later than girls)

4. **What are handy fine motor milestones to remember?**
   - **Grasping items:** 4–5 months
   - **Hand-to-hand transfers:** 6 months
   - **Pincer:** 10–11 months
   - **Feeding with spoon:** 18 months
   - **Scribbling:** 18 months
   - **Copying circle:** 3 years
   - **Copying cross:** 4 years
   - **Copying triangle:** 5 years

5. **What are handy language milestones to remember?**
   - **Babbling:** 7–8 months
   - **Single words:** 1 year

- **Body parts:** 18 months
- **Short sentences:** 2 years
- **Full sentences:** 3 years
- **Paragraphs:** 4 years
- **Knowing colors:** 5 years

6. **What are handy social skill milestones to remember?**
   - **Interactive games (pat-a-cake):** 9 months
   - **Taking off clothes (shoes):** 15 months
   - **Copying housekeeping:** 18 months
   - **Parallel play:** 3 years
   - **Social interaction:** 4 years

7. **What are some critical milestones to remember by age?**
   Table 77-1 is a guideline. Use it for a rough estimate, not for diagnostic purposes
   (*see* question 15). These are 50th percentiles.

   www.aap.org/healthtopics/stages.cfm

8. **At what age do 50% of children walk independently?**
   Most children can walk with one hand held at 12 months. If a child has not passed this milestone
   by 13 months of age, there may be a need for closer monitoring of the child's progress in
   attaining other milestones.

9. **How do you approach the child with persistent toe-walking that lasts more
   than 3–6 months beyond the initiation of independent walking?**
   Persistent toe-walking may not be associated with any orthopedic or neurologic problems in
   7–24% of the normal childhood population. This is generally referred to as idiopathic or
   idiosyncratic toe-walking. The differential diagnoses should include mild cerebral palsy spastic
   diplegia, transient focal dystonia of infancy, hereditary spastic paraparesis, and congenital short

TABLE 77-1. CRITICAL MILESTONES BY AGE

Age	Gross Motor	Fine Motor	Language	Social
6 months	Sitting	Hand to hand, palmar grasp	Makes sounds	
1 year	Cruising (walks by holding on), early walking	Pincer grasp	"Mama," "Dada," one or two other words	Interactive game
18 months	Walks up stairs with help	Scribbling	10 words, body parts	Takes off clothes, feeds self, copies housekeeping
2 years	Running	Circular scribbling	Short sentences	
3 years	Stands on one foot, rides tricycle	Copies circle	Full sentences	Parallel play
4 years	Up stairs adult style	Copies cross	Speaks in paragraphs	Social interaction
5 years	Skips (boys later)	Copies triangle	Knows colors	

tendocalcaneus. Toe-walking has also been associated with mental retardation, autism, and childhood schizophrenia. Evaluation should consist of a thorough birth history (e.g., prematurity, complications at birth), family history of toe-walkers or other neurologic problems (e.g., hereditary spastic paraparesis), developmental history, physical exam for gait, spasticity/dystonic findings, and range of motion (ROM). Electromyography has been used to rule out spasticity during gait. Close monitoring over several months to years will either demonstrate spontaneous resolution of the toe-walking over time or more apparent persistence of increased tone or mild to moderate developmental issues. Treatment of idiopathic toe-walking includes monitoring, ROM, and gait training. If not recognized or treated, contracture can develop, leading to bracing, serial casting, and, potentially, soft tissue release.

Caselli M, Rzonca E, Lue B: Habitual toe-walking: Evaluation and approach to treatment. Clin Podiatr Med Surg 5(3):547–549, 1988.

Sobel E, Caselli M, Velez Z: Effect of persistent toe walking on ankle equinus. J Am Podiatr Assoc 87(1):17–22, 1997.

10. **At what ages do children typically begin to go up and down stairs, alternating their feet?**
Children typically begin going *up* stairs with alternating feet at 3 years of age; they typically begin going *down* stairs with alternating feet at 4 years of age.

11. **At what age is hand dominance usually established?**
Usually by 2 years of age. Early hand dominance may be a sign of a neurologic deficit, such as weakness caused by hemiplegic cerebral palsy, with resultant decreased use of the affected side.

12. **What do the words *squeeze, palmar, scissor, chuck,* and *pincer* have in common?**
They are different types of grasp through which an infant progresses, beginning at approximately 4 months of age. The squeeze grasp is first achieved, with progression through the other grasp types until a fine pincer grasp is achieved at approximately 10–11 months of age.

13. **What do I do if language development is delayed?**
Order an **audiology evaluation** to check for hearing and make sure that the child is in an environment that stimulates language. It is important to start speech and language intervention as early as possible.

14. **Why have you not mentioned toilet training?**
Toilet training varies by culture and by family. It generally starts at approximately 18 months and is usually completed by 3 years. There is a wide variance, especially with overnight continence. Suffice it to say that children should be dry all day by age 3. Children with disabilities will often toilet train later, because of cognitive, mobility, sensory, or other problems relating to their diagnoses.

15. **How do I use developmental milestones in practice?**
One has to approach the child with disability with an understanding of normal development in order to use adaptive equipment to assist the child in gaining increased interaction with the environment. For example, for a child with spina bifida, one might consider the following:
- **3–8 months:** Use tumble form chair to allow the child to visually inspect the environment.
- **8–14 months:** Place child in a 90-degree seat to allow bimanual interaction with the environment, sitting experience, and exploration. Also, use sitting cart to allow exploration.
- **14–25 months:** Place child in standing frame to provide standing experience and weight-bearing for developing bones and muscles.

16. **How can development be assessed more formally?**
    Some of the more popular assessments are described in Table 77-2.

TABLE 77-2.   ASSESSMENTS OF DEVELOPMENTAL MILESTONES

Tool	Assessment
DDST—Denver Development Screening Test PEDS—Pediatric Evaluation of Development ASQ—Ages and Stages Questionnaire CDI—Child Development Inventory	Screening tools that can be administered in the office Administration requires anywhere from 2 to 15 minutes Some are just questions, some (e.g., DDST) involve small items to test specific tasks
Bayley Infant Neurodevelopmental Screen	Full developmental test to assess risk for infants aged 3–24 months
Peabody Developmental Test of Motor Proficiency	An assessment of gross and fine motor skills from birth to 83 months
B & O—Bruininks-Oseretsky	A scale of motor proficiency for children aged 4.5–14.5 years

17. **What if a child has poor motor development in the absence of any neuromuscular pathology?**
    Developmental coordination disorder (DCD) has been defined as "an impairment of both functional performance and quality of movement that is not explicable by age, intellect, or other diagnosable conditions." This syndrome has many names, including developmental dyspraxia and "the clumsy child." Idiopathic toe-walking (*see* question 9) and the sensory integration syndrome may be a part of this same clinical picture. DCD is a diagnosis of exclusion and is treated through a variety of therapy approaches.

    www.canchild.ca

18. **What are the asymmetric tonic neck and Moro reflexes? What are their significance developmentally?**
    These are primitive reflexes that should appear and disappear in sequence during certain stages in development. Their persistence may indicate central nervous system (CNS) or other nervous system dysfunction. Both reflexes should disappear at approximately 6–7 months, although they may be prolonged in the premature infant.
    - **Asymmetric tonic neck reflex:** Turning the head to the side elicits ipsilateral arm extension and contralateral flexion and should dampen with repetition. (Fencer's posture as an obligatory response is abnormal at any age.)
    - **Moro reflex:** Placing the baby in a semiupright posture, allowing initial neck extension and then release, causes initial abduction and extension of arms, and flexion of thumbs, followed by adduction and flexion of the upper extremities. Asymmetry is abnormal and may reflect brachial plexus, other limb injury, or CNS injury.

19. **What is the parachute response?**
    The infant is held in prone vertical suspension and then suddenly thrust downward by the examiner. The infant's upper and lower extremities extend and reach for support to protect from falling. These postural responses appear at 6–7 months. They are not suppressed

and persist for life. The postural responses, if delayed or absent, may indicate CNS dysfunction, immaturity, or motor neuron disease.

20. **When does "stranger anxiety" appear?**
Beginning at 5 months, the infant starts the process of operation and individuation differentiating between the mother and self. Eventually, the infant develops a sense of belonging to a central person, and by 7–8 months, behavior toward strangers differs from that with familiar people. This behavior, termed "stranger anxiety," is manifested by crying or a look of wariness when handled by strangers.

21. **How is the hip examination important in the evaluation of children in a physiatry practice? What is Galeazzi's or Allis sign?**
The hip examination is essential in the assessment of newborns, infants, and children who are either nonambulatory or have abnormal muscle tone. As a physiatrist, one may encounter children with hip problems caused by diagnoses such as cerebral palsy, spinal cord injury, or spina bifida. These conditions may carry an increased risk of hip subluxation or dislocation. In older infants and children with conditions such as these, hip ROM and knee height difference should be evaluated. **Galeazzi's** or **Allis sign** refers to the comparison of knee height, making note of a discrepancy between height of both knees. A discrepancy may be a positive sign of hip subluxation.

22. **Name and explain three theories of childhood development.**
   - **Neuromaturational theory:** Motor development takes place in a cephalocaudal direction, from proximal to distal.
   - **Dynamic systems theory:** Motor development occurs as the end product of multiple internal and external components or subsystems.
   - **Neuronal group selection theory:** The interaction of genetics and environment (nature–nuture) leads to a dynamic regulation of neural networks by cell migration and neuronal growth.

   Helders P, Engelbert R, Custers J, et al: Creating and being created: The changing panorama of pediatric rehabilitation. Pediatr Rehabil 6(1):5–12, 2003.

KEY POINTS: MOST USEFUL DEVELOPMENTAL MILESTONES

1. Gross motor: Cruising/walking (12 months)

2. Fine motor: Pincer grasp (10–12 months)

3. Speech: 10 words/body parts (18 months)

4. Social: Social interaction (4 years)

BIBLIOGRAPHY

1. Behrman RE: Nelson's Pediatrics, 17th ed. Philadelphia, W.B. Saunders, 2004.

2. Carpenter DL, Batley RJ, Johnson EW: Developmental evaluation of infants and children. Phys Med Rehabil Clin North Am 7:561–582, 1996.

3. Illingworth RS: The Development of the Infant and Young Child, 9th ed. New York, Churchill Livingstone, 1989.

4. Molnar GE, Alexander MA (eds): Pediatric Rehabilitation, 3rd ed. Philadelphia, Hanley & Belfus, 1999.

CHAPTER 78

CEREBRAL PALSY: DIAGNOSIS AND TREATMENT

Edward A. Hurvitz, MD, Rita N. Ayyangar, MD, and Mindy Aisen, MD

There are only two lasting bequests we can hope to give our children. One is roots; the other, wings.

–Hodding Carter (1907–1972)

1. **What is cerebral palsy (CP)?**

   In 2005, the following definition of cerebral palsy was published by an international working group on the topic: CP describes a group of disorders of the development of **movement and posture,** which cause activity limitation, that are attributed to **nonprogressive** disturbances in the **fetal** or **infant brain.** The motor disorders of CP are often accompanied by disturbances of sensation, cognition, communication, perception, and/or behavior and/or by a seizure disorder.

   "Fetal or infant" allows some latitude as to the upper limit of age of diagnosis. It is generally accepted that the onset occurs before the age of 2 or 3 years, and practically speaking, the disturbance has occurred before the affected function has developed (e.g., walking or talking). It is also important to note that the lesion resulting in CP is static. Some children with progressive neurologic disorders may be misdiagnosed as having CP before evidence of progressive neurologic impairment is apparent. However, as children grow and age, their muscles may become tighter, and as they age, they may have increasing functional deficits, generally as secondary effects of spasticity and other primary problems.

   Bax M, Goldstein M, Rosenbaum P, et al: Executive Committee for the Definition of Cerebral Palsy. Proposed definition and classification of cerebral palsy. Dev Med Child Neurol 47:571–576, 2005.

2. **What causes CP?**

   Cerebral palsy is a heterogeneous condition in terms of etiology. The principal distinction of CP from other phenotypically similar disorders is the time of onset of the damage to the nervous system—the damage has occurred before the affected function has developed. Although low birth weight and prematurity greatly increase the risk of CP, in most cases the cause of the damage is unknown. Neuroimaging may show periventricular leukomalacia, intraventricular hemorrhage, or congenital brain malformations. Other causes of early nervous system damage can include exposure to lead or mercury, kernicterus, placental inflammation (possibly caused by prenatal maternal infection), head trauma (shaken baby syndrome), encephalitis, and meningitis.

3. **How is cerebral palsy diagnosed?**

   Clinical diagnosis based on the definition in question 1 is the most common way. In less severe cases, developmental delays and the manifestations of spasticity may not be present for up to a year. Patients may, in fact, initially be floppy. The common complaints are developmental delay, trouble with feeding, drooling, and the arms and/or legs feel stiff with the legs often crossing over each other (scissoring). Sometimes, cerebral palsy can "go away," especially if the diagnosis is made in the first year of life. The most important thing to determine is that there is **no loss of milestones,** which would indicate a neurodegenerative disorder, hydrocephalus, or even a tumor. Metabolic testing to rule out other diagnoses is often indicated. A magnetic resonance imaging (MRI) or brain computed tomographic scan (CT) will demonstrate the findings noted above.

Part of the diagnosis is a description of the clinical manifestations; individuals with **spastic diplegia** have legs that are more involved than arms, those with **spastic quadriplegia** have total body involvement, and those with **spastic hemiplegia** have only one side involved, with the arm usually affected more than the leg. Some children may have dystonia, chorea, athetosis, or ataxia, often in addition to spasticity. Pure ataxia is rare and is usually associated with a problem in the posterior fossa.

4. **What is the GMFCS?**

The Gross Motor Function Classification System is used to classify the mobility of people with CP and allows a more universal language for discussing function of people with cerebral palsy. Interrater reliability is highest when the GMFCS is used to classify the gross motor function of children aged 2–12. This is a **five-level classification** with best function at I and least capability at V.

- **Level I**: Ambulatory with no assistive device, indoors and out
- **Level II**: Upright ambulatory in home but has impaired balance for outdoors
- **Level III**: Standing ineffective for distance ambulation; requires wheelchair in home and in community
- **Level IV**: Requires wheelchair for household mobility
- **Level V**: Very limited movement, even with the use of an adaptively controlled power wheelchair

Palisano R, Rosenbaum P, Walter S, et al: Development and reliability of a system to classify gross motor function in children with cerebral palsy. Develop Med Child Neurol 39:214–223, 1997.

5. **Will the child walk?**

The best indicator of how children are going to develop is how they are currently doing. **Head control** by 9 months and **sitting balance** at age 2 are indicators of future walking. Bleck listed seven **primitive reflexes** and found that a child whose response was abnormal for two of these reflexes by age 12 months had a poor prognosis for walking. These were:

Should be absent	Should be present
Asymmetric tonic neck reflex	Parachute reaction
Symmetric tonic neck reflex	Foot placement
Moro response	
Neck-righting reflex	

Walking in these studies includes use of a walker or crutches.

Bleck EE: Orthopedic Management of Cerebral Palsy. London, Mac Keith Press,1987.

6. **What does the gait look like?**

Children with hemiplegia will **toe-walk** with plantar flexion and excess knee flexion on the involved side, and their involved arm is held in flexion synergy. Diplegic children often have bilateral **equinovarus** deformity, **knees that are flexed and in valgus,** and "**scissoring**" (the feet crossing in front of each other with each step). Rotational problems, including **femoral anteversion** and **tibial torsion,** often cause internal rotation of the feet.

7. **Is cerebral palsy associated with mental impairment?**

Not necessarily. CP covers a wide spectrum of clinical presentations. Many children have normal to above-normal cognition, whereas others are severely impaired. Mental deficiency is noted in approximately 50–75% of children with CP. Only approximately one third of diplegic children have some degree of mental impairment, but many have perceptual-motor deficits. Learning disorders, attentional difficulties, and psychiatric impairments are more common in children with cerebral palsy and should be addressed to promote academic and emotional/behavioral development.

8. **How can the schools help?**
The parents should obtain early intervention services for the child. The law requires that every state provide education for every child, with appropriate services for children with special needs. The parents should contact their local school district, inform them that they have a child with special needs, and have the child evaluated. The family will have an **IFSP** (Individual Family Service Plan) or, if the child is older than 3, an **IEPC** (Individual Education Planning Committee) with the school staff to determine the child's service eligibility. Children under 3 generally receive physical or occupational therapy once or twice a week.

9. **Should you worry about seizures?**
Many children with CP have seizures. Children with spastic quadriplegia are most prone, followed by those with spastic hemiplegia. There is no need for a baseline electroencephalography (EEG); evaluation and management can wait until symptoms are present.

10. **What about sleep?**
Sleep disturbances are common in children with CP. Compared to age-matched controls, children with severe CP had more apneas and hypopneas per hour of sleep, resulting from problems such as fewer body position changes, macroglossia, glossoptosis, and aspiration from gastroesophageal reflux. There may also be a primary disturbance in sleep organization caused by brain stem dysfunction. Sleep logs and actigraphy may be helpful in those with sleep-onset insomnia and circadian rhythm abnormalities. Melatonin (1–3 mg) given 30–60 min before bedtime may be very useful in conjunction with an established calming bedtime routine. Nocturnal polysomnography is critical to the evaluation of sleep maintenance difficulties, and the EEG segment can help distinguish epileptic and nonepileptic arousals.

Kotagal S, Gibbons VP, Stith JA: Sleep abnormalities in patients with severe cerebral palsy. Dev Med Child Neurol 36:304–311, 1994.

Stores G, Wiggs L (eds): Sleep disturbance in children and adolescents with disorders of development: Its significance and management. Clin Dev Med 155: 2001 [entire issue].

11. **What kinds of visual problems occur?**
Strabismus is a common problem in those with cerebral palsy, resulting from an imbalance in the eye musculature. It is often treated with ophthalmologic surgery. **Hemianopsia** may be present with dense hemiplegia with a middle cerebral artery lesion.

12. **What kind of problems does hypertonicity cause?**
Spasticity is defined as a velocity-dependent resistance to stretch. It is a common manifestation of the upper motor neuron syndrome (decreased dexterity, hyperreflexia, spasticity, paralysis). **Dystonia** is a movement disorder in which involuntary sustained or intermittent muscle contractions cause twisting and repetitive movement, abnormal postures, or both. The most prominent findings in both are hypertonicity of the musculature and impaired motor control. (Reducing spasticity improves motor control, but of course does not normalize it—other factors such as weakness, impaired coordination, and impaired sensation also play a role.) Spasticity can cause **contractures** secondary to muscle tightness, especially in the gastrocnemius–soleus group, hamstrings, adductors, hip flexors, biceps, wrist flexors, and opponens pollicis. **Hip dislocation** can occur as a result of tight adductors (*see* question 13). **Scoliosis** or **lordosis** from spasticity and weakness is another frequently noted problem that may worsen rapidly as the child goes through a growth spurt (*see* question 14). Spasticity can also cause difficulty with seating and interfere with caretakers' ability to perform transfers and other aspects of care.

Sanger TD, Delgado MR, Gaebler-Spira D, et. al: Classification and definition of disorders causing hypertonia in childhood. Task Force on Childhood Motor Disorders. Pediatrics 111:e89–e97, 2003.

13. **What should be done about the hips?**

In children with tight hip musculature, especially the adductors, the hips should be followed with plain x-rays on a regular basis (every 12–18 months), because hip dislocation can affect up to 30% of the children. Orthopedic procedures such as **adductor tenotomies** or **derotational osteotomies** help prevent dislocation. Surgical reduction of a dislocated hip is indicated for ambulatory children or for nonambulatory children with pain or seating difficulties. In younger children, hip dislocation can lead to improper development of the hip joint and painful arthritis in young adulthood. In spastic quadriplegic children with very high tone, hip dislocation is very common. Unfortunately, results of surgical repair have been variable in this group, and surgery may not be indicated.

14. **What should be done about the spine?**

The incidence of scoliosis increases with greater neurologic involvement, with an incidence of 60% in children with spastic quadriplegia. Scoliosis in CP progresses more rapidly and produces different curve patterns than idiopathic scoliosis. Hip dislocation and pelvic obliquity can contribute to worsening curves. Seating problems, pressure sores, and cardiopulmonary compromise are potential complications. Ambulatory children are managed with bracing and surgery (fusion, rod placement). Nonambulatory children are often best managed with molded seating but may need other interventions as well.

15. **What should be done about the other limbs and joints?**

Spasticity often leads to contracture, especially in muscles that cross two joints. Contractures worsen with growth, because bones grow faster than muscles. The main joints at risk are the ankles (plantar flexion) and flexion contractures at the knees, hips, elbows, and wrists. The first-line treatment is repeated, gradual, sustained **stretching. Serial casting** and **orthoses** are used, especially for the ankles, knees, and elbows. Casting can be combined with blocks (*see* question 17). If these methods fail, **orthopedic surgery** is indicated for muscle and tendon lengthening. Muscles that are lengthened will lose almost a grade of strength. As children grow, these interventions (including surgery) will need to be repeated.

16. **When should antispasticity medications be used?**

Oral antispasticity medications (diazepam, baclofen, dantrolene, tizanidine, etc.) are indicated for the treatment of **generalized spasticity.** They are useful in severely involved children to aid with hygiene and prevent mass extensor spasm. They are less commonly used in more functional children because of adverse effects. They may be used if the child might be a candidate for a rhizotomy or other more extensive interventions. Each drug has its own complications; diazepam, tizanidine, and baclofen are sedatives, baclofen and dantrolene sodium cause hepatic problems (liver functions must be monitored), and baclofen can lower the seizure threshold.

17. **What are nerve/motor point blocks?**

Nerve/motor point blocks are indicated for **spasticity affecting specific muscle groups.** They are commonly done to decrease scissoring caused by adductor spasticity, equinovarus foot deformity during gait, and hamstring, elbow flexor, or wrist/finger flexor tightness.

Botulinum toxin injections lead to presynaptic inhibition of motor nerve function. Tone reduction peaks 2–4 weeks after injection, and effects can last 3–6 months. A variety of injection techniques are used, with some practitioners using electromyograph (EMG) guidance and others visually locating motor points. The child's skin is commonly treated with Emla cream or ethyl chloride spray for local anesthesia. Sedation or general anesthesia is used for younger children or more involved blocks.

Phenol and, less commonly, **alcohol** are neurolytic, and are effective for 3–6 months. The injection needle is used as a cathode for nerve stimulation and amperage is reduced for precise localization. An aggressive stretching and motor reeducation program are indicated after block procedures.

18. **When is a rhizotomy indicated? What can it do?**

The selective dorsal rootlet rhizotomy is a neurosurgical procedure designed to decrease the excitatory input to the motor neuron, thereby decreasing spasticity. The procedure consists of a laminectomy and exposure of the cauda equina. The dorsal roots are electrically stimulated, and various criteria are used for determining which parts of the root contain more fibers involved with abnormal reflexes. These rootlets are than severed. This technique allows for decreased tone without sacrificing significant sensation.

The ideal patient is a **young child (ages 3–8) with spastic diplegia who is ambulatory with a spastic gait.** Generally, any child who could make significant functional gains if his or her spasticity was reduced could benefit, as well as children with significant seating problems. Children with poor head and trunk control, and children who use spasticity for functional purposes (e.g., extensor spasms to stand) are poor candidates for the procedure. After surgery, the children require an extensive physical and occupational therapy program to recover from postoperative weakness and to maximize functional gains.

www.med.nyu.edu/rusk/services/pediatrics/rhizotomy.html

19. **When is the intrathecal baclofen pump best used in patients with CP?**

The **intrathecal baclofen** (ITB) pump is an electronic programmable pump device that is implanted under the skin and connected to a catheter, with its tip usually at T12 or higher so that it releases baclofen directly into the cerebrospinal fluid (CSF). ITB therapy is indicated in children with CP who have moderate to severe generalized spasticity and/or dystonia. It may be used in nonambulatory or ambulatory children weighing more than 28 lb, who have enough torso room for the pump and can follow through with maintenance and refill needs. In general, acceptance has been high in patients with CP despite the relatively high maintenance required for regular refills, reprogramming of the pump, and management of complications. Common complications include CSF leaks, catheter kinks or breaks, infections (such as pump pocket infections and meningitis), pump programming errors that lead to drug overdosage or underdosage, and pump malfunction.

www.medtronics.com

KEY POINTS: TREATMENT OF HYPERTONIA

1. Generalized tone: Medications, comprehensive therapy program, seating system

2. Regional tone: Rhizotomy, baclofen pump, multistage orthopedic surgery, therapy

3. Focal tone: Range of motion, casting, splinting, injection therapy

20. **When should I consult orthopedics? Neurosurgery?**

The rhizotomy and baclofen pump **decrease spasticity** but have no effect on shortened, contracted muscles. Orthopedic surgery can **lengthen muscles** and change the biomechanics of gait through tendon transfers, but it does not change the basic neurology. A combination of techniques is often required to gain greatest improvement in gait. Gait laboratory analysis is useful in many cases for determining the appropriate interventions.

Sussman MD (ed): The Diplegic Child: Evaluation and Management. Rosemont, IL, American Academy of Orthopedic Surgeons, 1992.

21. **Who were Karel and Berta Bobath? What is the Bobath treatment program?**
Karel and Berta Bobath began treating children with CP in the 1940s. He was a neurologist and she was a physical therapist. The Bobath treatment program is based on normalizing movement patterns and inhibiting abnormal reflexes. Most therapists incorporate some of these techniques in treatment, along with a **neurodevelopmental therapy** (NDT) approach that encourages children to sit correctly before they crawl, crawl correctly before they stand, etc.

    www.bobath.org.uk/

22. **What's new in therapy for cerebral palsy?**
It was once thought that strengthening was bad for spastic musculature. It was thought that it would increase spasticity and abnormal reflexes. Recently, benefits of strengthening have been reported. **Resistive exercises** have led to increased strength and improved gait pattern. Several new programs and treatment philosophies have emerged based on increased intensity of therapy. Some, like **conductive education,** require a short-term but very intensive commitment by the family. The effectiveness of these programs is being researched. **Hippotherapy** uses a horse as a tool in physical therapy; several beneficial effects have been suggested, and the programs are fun and motivating for the children.

    Recently, there has been a greater focus on therapy for the upper extremity. Several centers are now using **constraint-induced therapy (CIT)** techniques to improve upper extremity function, particularly in children with hemiplegia. CIT, first used in adult stroke patients, involves restraining the less involved extremity with a cast or splint and **mass practice** for the more involved side through an intensive therapy/activity program. Early trials have been successful, although the degree of success in the long term is unknown. it is not known how much carryover there is over the long term.

    Conductive education: www.aquinas.edu/clc/
    Damiano DL, Dodd K, Taylor NF: Should we be testing and training muscle strength in cerebral palsy? Develop Med Child Neurol 44:68–72, 2002.
    Taub E, Ramey SL, DeLuca S, Echols K: Efficacy of constraint-induced movement therapy for children with cerebral palsy with asymmetric motor impairment. Pediatrics 113(2):305–312, 2004.

23. **What are AFOs?**
Ankle-foot orthoses (AFOs) aid in gait by controlling the equinus or equinovarus deformity. Articulated AFOs have an ankle joint and are capable of dorsiflexion. Some braces, called **ground reaction AFOs,** are designed to prevent crouching by producing a knee-extension moment with anterior shin pressure during stance phase. They are effective only in the absence of significant knee or hip flexion contractures. For children with spasticity, AFOs are designed with features to decrease abnormal reflexes, including a footplate that extends past the toe to discourage toe flexion and a metatarsal support to discourage stimulation to a particularly reflexogenic area of the foot. Nonambulatory children wear AFOs to prevent contracture and during supported standing.

24. **What are some of the seating issues in cerebral palsy?**
The goals of seating are **proper postural alignment, comfort,** and **mobility.** Positioning should protect the joints and skin, support the trunk and pelvis to prevent deformity, and discourage abnormal reflexes. Extensor reflexes can be inhibited by keeping the hips, knees, and ankles at **at least 90 degree angles.** Head support can discourage the asymmetric tonic neck reflex. Power chairs are important mobility devices for many children.

25. **What kind of oropharyngeal problems and swallowing difficulties are seen with cerebral palsy?**
Children with CP may have difficulty with swallowing, speech, and drooling because of oral motor control problems. **Dysphagia** can lead to difficulty with adequate nutrition or aspiration. **Fiberoptic endoscopic evaluation of swallowing** (FEES) is a direct visualization technique

that gives a better view of the sequence and timing of swallowing, as well as the amount of residual food left with each swallow. Interventions include positioning, such as chin tuck, or using the wheelchair head rest to control the head position and dietary changes, usually involving soft foods over liquids and full solids. Swallowing evaluations are helpful to resolve conflicts between families and the school about safety and appropriateness of oral feeding. With severe aspiration or caloric need problems, a gastrostomy tube is indicated. If the aspiration is asymptomatic, placement of a G-tube is somewhat controversial, and less of an absolute indication. Significant drooling problems are managed with glycopyrrolate, scopolamine patches, and, in severe cases, surgery (realignment of the salivary ducts). Botulinum toxin injections into the salivary glands utilizing ultrasound guidance are showing promise as a safe alternative in the management of severe drooling. The effect can last up to 24 weeks.

Jongerius PH, Rotteveel JJ, van Limbeek J, et al: Botulinum toxin effect on salivary flow rate in children with cerebral palsy. Neurology 63(8):1371–1375, 2004.

26. **What are some of the growth and physical development problems that children with CP face?**
Children with spastic quadriplegic CP are at high risk for poor growth and **undernutrition**. However, ambulatory children with CP face problems with **obesity**. Children with cerebral palsy are at higher risk for **osteopenia** as a result of poor oral intake, limited exposure to sunlight, and the concurrent use of antiseizure medications (all of which interfere with absorption and metabolism of **calcium** and **vitamin D**).

27. **How do I help children who have communication problems?**
Speech problems are often accompanied by spasticity, decreased coordination, and choreoathetosis. Augmentative communication devices must compensate for lack of speed and accuracy. Special switches have been developed to improve access to technology, as well as software that allows for greater options with fewer demands for accurate keyboard use.

28. **What other equipment should I consider?**
Various activities of daily living may require specialized seating. There are **feeder seats, car seats, corner seats,** and **bath seats. Prone or supine standers** are used to encourage weight-bearing and standing activities. If children have difficulty sleeping at night, **supine liers** can position them more comfortably. Computers are important for school and recreation. An assisted-technology assessment can aid with access problems. Specialty equipment may be commercially available or custom modified.

29. **Describe some of the adapted recreational options for children with cerebral palsy.**
Most recreational activities can be adapted, depending on the resources and willingness of the community. The **Special Olympics** offers the child a chance to participate in peer-level athletic competition. There are many adapted **horseback-riding programs.** Horseback riding can be recreational as well as therapeutic. **Computers** can open up many recreational opportunities. In today's world, a child who is severely impaired can interact on an even plane with others through the Internet.

30. **What are some of the critical psychosocial issues to address?**
Children with cerebral palsy are at high risk for development of psychological and behavioral problems. Like other children with disabilities, they often have difficulties with peer interaction and other issues of social competence. Higher functioning kids will have more awareness of disability with resultant adjustment issues. Vocational issues, long-term care concerns, advocacy training, and access to proper resources are all factors to be considered when managing a family with a child who has CP.

31. **What is the best thing I can say to this family?**
A family needs to hear that there will be support for them from their doctor and from their community. The physician should demonstrate this by listening to the family's concerns, providing medical information, and providing access to resources. They also need to know that cerebral palsy has a wide spectrum of clinical presentations and functional prognoses and that the effort they put in can make a positive difference in the final outcome.

WEBSITES

1. www.Aacpdm.org (go to resources, then library)

2. www.UCP.org

BIBLIOGRAPHY

1. Gormley ME Jr: Management of spasticity in children (Pts. 1 & 2). J Head Trauma Rehabil 14:207–209, 1999.
2. Molnar GE: Cerebral palsy. In Molnar GE (ed): Pediatric Rehabilitation. Baltimore, Williams & Wilkins, 1992, pp 481–533.

CHAPTER 79

NEURAL TUBE DEFECTS: ANATOMY, ASSOCIATED DEFICITS, AND REHABILITATION

Sam S.H. Wu, MD, MPH, MBA, Jeffrey M. Cohen, MD, Valerie S. Bodeau, MD, Steven A. Stiens, MD, MS

The farther back you can look, the farther forward you are likely to see.
—Winston Churchill (1874–1965)

1. **What are neural tube defects (NTDs)? How are they categorized?**
   Neural tube defects **(myelodysplasia)** result from aberrations in neural tube closure (neurulation). The neural tube closes in a zipper-like fashion between the 23rd and 28th day after conception. There are three major types of NTDs:
   - **Anencephaly** is a failure of closure of the anterior neuropore, resulting in variable loss of cranial structures, and is almost universally lethal.
   - An **encephalocele** is a cystic structure that forms at the craniocervical junction. The degree of impairment ranges from mild to severe, depending on cyst contents.
   - **Spina bifida** is a general term used to describe a group of NTDs with failure of the vertebrae to fuse posteriorly.

2. **What are the three subtypes of spina bifida?**
   - **Spina bifida occulta:** The most common type is present in up to 10% of the population. Although the posterior vertebral structures do not form normally, the spinal cord and the meninges are not involved, and the individual is usually asymptomatic. The bony defect can usually be seen on plain radiographs. There may be cutaneous manifestations overlying the defect, such as a hairy tuft, dimples, or hemangioma.
   - **Meningocele:** A cystic structure that contains the meninges and cerebrospinal fluid (CSF) protrudes through the open vertebral defect, but the spinal cord is not involved. This defect is usually repaired at birth. There is usually no or mild involvement of the underlying nervous system.
   - **Myelomeningocele (MMC):** This is herniation of the spinal cord and the meninges through the vertebral defect. This can occur at any point along the vertebral axis, but the lumbosacral junction is the most common site. Neural deficits can involve neurogenic bowel and bladder, motor and sensory involvement, hydrocephalus, and Chiari malformations. The precise deficits depend on the level of the herniation.

3. **What are the etiology and incidence of NTDs?**
   The etiology of NTDs is multifactorial. There appears to be a genetic predisposition combined with a geographic or environmental factor. Ireland and England have the highest incidence at 3–4 per 1000 live births. The United States has an incidence of 0.6 per 1000 live births. NTDs are very rare in Asian and Pacific Islander populations. Environmental factors associated with NTDs include maternal hyperthermia, parental exposure to Agent Orange, low socioeconomic status, and use of medications, particularly anticonvulsants. Folic acid supplementation, taken prenatally and during the first trimester, reduces the incidence of NTDs by 70%.

   Agent Orange exposure: www.va.gov/hac/forbeneficiaries/spina/spina.asp

Cornel MC, de Smit DJ, de Jong-van den Berg LTW: Folic acid: The scientific debate as a base for public health policy. Reprod Toxicol 20:411–415, 2005.

Detrait ER, George TM, Etchevers HC, et al: Human neural tube defects: Developmental biology, epidemiology, and genetics. Neurotoxicol Teratol 27:515–524, 2005.

4. **What testing is available for prenatal detection of NTDs?**
An association between elevated alpha fetoprotein (AFP) levels and pregnancies with an NTD has been known since the early 1970s. Routine prenatal care now includes testing of maternal serum analytes between pregnancy weeks 15 and 22 (the triple or quadruple screen) for NTDs, Down syndrome, and trisomy 18. If an elevated AFP level is found, and other factors such as gestational dates, twins, ethnicity/race, and maternal diabetes have been considered, further work-up such as a level II ultrasound can be done. Invasive testing such as amniocentesis or chorionic villus sampling is being increasingly reserved for high-risk pregnancies, or when noninvasive testing provides ambiguous results.

Bubb JA, Matthews AL: What's new in prenatal screening and diagnosis? Prim Care Clin Office Pract 31:561–582, 2004.

5. **What are the leading factors affecting morbidity and mortality in individuals with MMC?**
See Table 79-1.

TABLE 79-1. FACTORS AFFECTING MORBIDITY AND MORTALITY IN MENINGOMYELOCELE (MMC)

Leading Factors	Morbidity and Mortality
Hydrocephalus	May occur in 95% of all children with MMC and requires shunt placement in up to 85%.
Renal failure	May lead to death in patients with MMC. Reflux, hydronephrosis, and recurrent infection are the primary causes of renal failure.
Pressure ulcers	A major cause of morbidity in these adolescents and adults.
Tethered cord	A defect caused by the abnormal attachment of the spinal cord at its distal end (filum terminale), which prevents the normal ascension of the conus medullaris from its earlier distal position to the L1–L2 vertebral level. This defect can occur in 11–15% of children after MMC repair. The average age at diagnosis is 6 years. Signs and symptoms can include recent changes in lower-extremity motor strength or sensation; recent changes in functional mobility; and new onset of spasticity, back pain, scoliosis, or bowel or bladder incontinence.
Hydromyelia	A cavitation in the spinal canal, which can present as neck rigidity, pain, weakness, or spasticity in the upper or lower extremities, rapidly progressive scoliosis, or worsening in bowel or bladder function.
Obesity	A frequent problem in individuals with MMC. Their reduced daily energy expenditure is caused by paralysis, lack of muscle mass, and decreased physical activity.
Latex hypersensitivity	Develops over time and can occur in up to 80% of patients with spina bifida. A negative diagnostic test does not rule out future sensitization. Therefore, these patients should avoid all exposure to latex-containing material, including catheters and other medical and nonmedical equipment.

6. **Are other central nervous system (CNS) complications associated with neural tube defects?**
   A Chiari II malformation (herniation of cerebellar tonsil through the foramen magnum) is the most common complication, followed by hydrocephalus (both congenital and acquired), tethered cord syndrome, and syringomyelia.

   McLone DG, Dias MS: The Chiari II malformation: Cause and impact. Childs Nerv Syst 19(7–8):540–550, 2003.

   Piatt JH Jr: Syringomyelia complicating myelomeningocele: Review of the evidence. J Neurosurg 100(2 Suppl Pediatrics):101–109, 2004.

7. **What are the cognitive deficits in patients with MMC?**
   - **General intelligence:** Low IQ scores are associated with higher-level lesions. IQ scores are adversely affected by CNS infections and shunt malfunctions.
   - **Higher-order cognitive functions:** Regardless of IQ, many have significant impairments in problem-solving, conceptualization, efficiency of processing, and mental flexibility. Verbal performance is often better than quantitative. Therefore, neuropsychological testing is particularly valuable for quantification and remediation of these deficits.

   Dise JE, Lohr ME: Examination of deficits in conceptual reasoning abilities associated with spina bifida. Am J Phys Med Rehabil 77:247–251, 1998.

8. **What are the bowel and bladder deficits associated with MMC?**
   - **Neurogenic bowel dysfunction** can involve dyssynergy of intestinal peristalsis, total or partial absence of rectal fullness sensation, or a lack of anorectal sphincter control. More than 80% of children with myelomeningocele have neurogenic bowel dysfunction.
   - **Neurogenic bladder dysfunction** affects >80% of those with MMC. They may have partial or complete denervation of the bladder with poor compliance and poor contractility. In the vast majority (86%), the internal sphincter is incompetent. In a third, there is detrusor–sphincter dyssynergia, resulting from a partially functional external sphincter.

KEY POINTS: NEURAL TUBE DEFECTS

1. Neurogenic bowel and bladder are present in all but the lowest sacral lesions.
2. The higher the lesion, the greater the likelihood of cognitive impairment.
3. Children born today with a neural tube defect have a near normal life span.
4. Mobility is dependent on the level of the lesion.
5. Folic acid supplementation greatly reduces the risk of neural tube defects.

---

9. **What are the major factors determining ambulation potential in individuals with myelomeningocele?**
   The degree of ambulation is dependent on multiple factors, including cognitive function, level of neurologic lesion, musculoskeletal complications, obesity, motivation, and age. Table 79-2 lists the motor strengths associated with ambulation potential.

   McDonald C, Jaffe K, Mosca V, Shurtleff D: Ambulatory outcome of children with myelomeningocele: Effect of lower extremity muscle strength. Dev Med Child Neurol 33:482–490, 1991.

10. **Describe the orthopedic deficits associated with MMC.**
    See Table 79-3.

TABLE 79-2. FACTORS DETERMINING AMBULATION POTENTIAL IN MMC

Ambulation Potential	Associated Motor Strength
Community ambulation without assistive devices	Grade 4–5 gluteal and tibialis anterior function
No complete reliance on wheelchair use; majority are community ambulators	Grade 4–5 iliopsoas and quadriceps function
Partial or complete reliance on wheelchair use	Grade 0–3 iliopsoas function

MMC = meningomyelocele.

TABLE 79-3. ORTHOPEDIC DEFICITS ASSOCIATED WITH MMC

Level of Spinal Involvement	Musculoskeletal Deficits and Complications
T6–T12	Kyphosis, scoliosis, hip and knee flexion contractures, and equinus foot
L1–L3	Scoliosis, hip flexion and adduction contractures, hip dislocation, knee flexion contractures, and equinus foot
L4–L5	Scoliosis, lordosis, hip and knee flexion contractures, hip dislocation, knee extension contractures, and calcaneovarus or calcaneus foot
S1–S4	Cavus foot

MMC = meningomyelocele.

11. **What orthotic choices are available to improve ambulation in individuals with MMC?**
See Table 79-4.

12. **What about surgery for MMC?**
The goals of early surgery are prevention of infection and preservation of neurologic function. Adhesions between the arachnoid and dura are cut. Anomalous roots are identified, and any ending blindly are excised. A water-tight closure of the dura is made, leaving maximal space for the enclosed spinal cord.

WEBSITES

1. Evidence-based practice in spina bifida: Developing a research agenda
www.sbaa.org/site/DocServer/01intro.pdf?docID=1521

2. Medline Plus
www.nlm.nih.gov/medlineplus/neuraltubedefects.html

3. National Center on Birth Defects and Developmental Disabilities
www.cdc.gov/ncbddd

4. Spina Bifida Association of America
www.sbaa.org

TABLE 79-4. ORTHOSES TO IMPROVE AMBULATION IN MMC

Level of Injury	Orthotics	Description
Midthoracic		Therapeutic ambulation in early age, but later requiring wheelchair.
	Parapodium	Provides structural support from the midthoracic level to the feet and allows for both standing and sitting. Children can ambulate therapeutically with a swing-through gait, using a walker or crutches. However, as the child grows, the base plate of the parapodium needs to be enlarged to maintain stability; ambulation thus becomes more difficult in older children.
	Swivel walker	A modification of the parapodium with a footplate attachment that translates lateral trunk movement to forward propulsion. It has increased ambulation efficiency over the parapodium.
Low thoracic/ high lumbar		Household-level ambulation
	Reciprocal gait orthosis	Composed of bilateral hip-knee-ankle-foot orthoses with an elaborate cable system that links hip flexion in each hip with the contralateral hip extension. Energy expenditure for ambulation with this orthosis approaches that of wheelchair locomotion.
Midlumbar		Limited community ambulation.
	Hip-knee-ankle-foot orthosis	May be needed for ambulation in presence of hip instability.
	Knee-ankle-foot orthosis	Correct or prevent knee deformity.
	Ankle-foot orthosis	May be adequate when knee extension strength is >3/5.
Low lumbar/ sacral		Community ambulation.
	Floor reaction orthosis	For nonfixed calcaneal foot deformity, to increase knee extension moment.
	Ankle orthosis	For ankle stabilization.
	Shoe modifications	For foot deformities.

MMC = meningomyelocele.

BIBLIOGRAPHY

1. Diamond M, Armento M: Children with disabilities. In DeLisa JA (ed): Physical Medicine and Rehabilitation: Principles and Practice. Philadelphia, Lippincott Williams & Wilkins, 2005, pp 1493–1517.

2. Hays RM, Massagli TL: Rehabilitation concepts in myelomeningocele. In Braddom RL (ed): Physical Medicine and Rehabilitation. Philadelphia, W.B. Saunders, 2000, pp 1213–1229.

3. Molnar GE, Murphy KP: Spina bifida. In Molnar GE, Alexander MA (eds): Pediatric Rehabilitation, 3rd ed. Philadelphia, Hanley & Belfus, 1999, pp 219–244.

4. Woodhouse CR: Myelomeningocele in young adults. BJU Int 95(2):223–230, 2005.

REHABILITATION OF THE PERFORMING ARTIST: FUNDAMENTALS

CHAPTER 80

Scott E. Brown, MD

Great art is as irrational as great music. It is made with its own loveliness.
—George Jean Nathan (1882–1958)

1. **Are performing artists *really* injured in the line of duty? How many artists are injured by performing their art? What is the rate of injury for performing artists in music and in dance?**
   In a survey of the members of the International Conference of Symphony and Opera Musicians, 76% reported having had at least one medical problem severe enough to interfere with performance, and 36% reported four severe problems. The annual incidence of injury in student musicians is 5.7% of male conservatory students and 11.5% of female conservatory students. In some studies, injuries have affected as many as 90% of dancers.

2. **What are the special considerations in the physical examination of a musician?**
   Injured musicians often expect a greater level of expertise from their doctors in specificity of diagnosis and treatment. If possible, musicians should be examined while playing their instrument. Although most patients will be able to bring their instruments to the examination, a piano is needed in the office for pianists. Problems with embouchure (the position of the lips and mouth in playing a wind or brass instrument), focal dystonia, and ergonomic and other technical problems will be missed if the musician is not examined while playing. Videotaping in the office as well as during rehearsal and performance can be a helpful adjunct.
   A thorough but directed musculoskeletal and neurologic exam should be undertaken. Underlying medical problems may present earlier in musicians, who are more sensitive to the functional effects of minor impairment early in the course of disease. A careful search for tendon anomalies should be done, especially in string and wind instrument players. A common problem that can cause difficulties in the left hand of violin players and the right hand of clarinet players is the conjoined flexor sublimis tendons of the small and ring fingers. Other specific problems for which to examine include hypermobility, hand span, dycoordination and uneven playing, muscle tension, and excessive gripping or pressure on the instrument.

3. **What areas should be included in the physical examination for dancers?**
   For dancers, a complete lower-extremity biomechanical evaluation must be done that includes the following:
   - Lumbar range of motion (ROM)
   - Pelvic tilt
   - Hip joint internal and external rotation with the hip in neutral (0 degrees flexion or extension)
   - Femoral anteversion or retroversion
   - Hamstring flexibility
   - Q angle
   - Tibial torsion
   - Toe out
   - Ankle ROM
   - Foot pronation
   - First metatarsophalangeal (MTP) joint ROM

As with musicians, it may be helpful to see the performer dancing. The pointe position can only be assessed with the patient wearing toe shoes.

4. **What are the common nerve entrapments seen in musicians?**
The most common symptom complex is numbness and tingling in the medial forearm and the small and ring fingers and is usually attributed to thoracic outlet syndrome. As in the general population, the neurologic examination and electrodiagnostic studies usually appear normal. Given the absence of objective findings, this has been called **"functional"** or **"symptomatic" thoracic outlet syndrome**. Most instruments are held or played in front of the body, potentially tightens the anterior chest and neck muscles. The resulting symptoms, suggestive of **medial cord entrapment,** may involve some nonaxonotmetic process or may only be a referred symptom. Management relies on stretching, posture, instrument modification, and proper pacing. **Carpal tunnel** and **cubital tunnel syndromes** are seen with almost equal frequency. If a focal dystonia is diagnosed, a thorough search for **entrapment neuropathy** should be undertaken.

5. **What are the most and least dangerous instruments?**
Highest injury rates in university-level student musicians are seen with piano, guitar, and harp. Intermediate risk includes the bowed strings, percussion, clarinet, saxophone, flute, and organ. Lower risk appears to include all brass instruments, the oboe, and the bassoon.

6. **What is meant by "overuse" in performing artists?**
Overuse practice is an activity in which anatomically normal structures have been used in a so-called normal manner, but to a degree that has exceeded their biologic limits. The pathologic changes that may result from overuse practices (the overuse syndromes) depend on the tissues affected and the degree and type of damage (i.e., inflammation, fatigue, structural change). Many of the commonly used synonyms for overuse (i.e., repetitive stress injury) combine cause and effect into a single entity rather than considering them as separate events, which in turn reduces diagnostic precision.

7. **What are the goals of dance screening?**
Dance screening is the preparticipation physical assessment of prospective dancers. The process has also been used for follow-up assessment after rehabilitation from an injury. The key objectives of a dance screening program are to:
- Establish normative data
- Uncover pathology
- Quantify risk factors
- Develop characteristics for a given level of performance
- Establish baseline data to set educational, training, or rehabilitative goals
- Determine if an individual dancer possesses attributes necessary for participation in that form of dance (controversial)

There is no universally agreed on protocol for dance screening.

8. **What is turnout?**
Turnout refers to the total amount of external rotation of both lower extremities. Ideally, most of a dancer's turnout should come from true external rotation at the hip joint. The ideal classical ballet aesthetic stresses 180 degrees of turnout, which would require the dancer to have 90 degrees at each hip. This rarely occurs, and in order to meet expectations of teachers and company directors in attaining the 180 degrees, the dancer has to cheat biomechanically.

9. **How is the female athletic triad relevant to dancers?**
The Task Force on Women's Issues of the American College of Sports Medicine met in 1992 and outlined a position stand on the female athletic triad: **disordered eating, amenorrhea,**

and **osteoporosis.** The Task Force found that the triad occurred not only in elite athletes but also in dancers. Disordered eating is a common response to the pressures of meeting an aesthetic ideal of thinness. Exercise and anorexia produce a state of hypothalamic hypogonadism. Decreased ovarian hormone production and hypoestrogenemia result from hypothalamic amenorrhea, which ultimately produces osteoporosis. The Task Force found that the triad is often denied, especially in the dance world. If even one component of the triad is detected, the Task Force encourages a high index of suspicion for osteoporosis and other less obvious medical sequelae, such as arrhythmias, depression, and stress fractures.

KEY POINTS: REHABILITATION OF THE PERFORMING ARTIST

1. The greatest number of "performing arts injuries" among university-level student musicians are seen among piano, guitar, and harp players.

2. The female athlete triad includes disordered eating, amenorrhea, and osteoporosis.

10. **Who is Pilates?**
Joseph Pilates was a German athlete who initially developed a philosophy of physical conditioning as he helped to rehabilitate German soldiers shortly after World War I. His approach not only incorporated physical exercise but also stressed the mind–body interaction. After coming to the United States in the 1920s, he opened a studio that quickly became popular with dancers. His progam allowed various jumping and other analogous dance activities to be performed supine (gravity eliminated). This program continues to be popular in the dance world for cross-training and injury rehabilitation.

11. **What is the differential diagnosis of groin pain in a dancer?**
A clunk or pop, often described as a feeling of the hip joint coming out of place, occurs when the **iliopsoas** snaps across the **iliopectineal** eminence, especially when the flexed, abducted, externally rotated hip returns to the neutral position. Other causes of hip/groin pain include a torn acetabular labrum, femoral neck stress fracture, adductor sprain, and rectus femoris tendinitis and myofascial pain (especially in a poorly trained dancer who incorrectly uses this muscle to raise the leg forward).

12. **A ballet dancer successfully rehabilitates a "groin pull" (adductor sprain) but continues to have difficulty with pirouette turns. Why might this be?**
The pirouette turn is a fundamental movement in ballet that requires a series of rotational momentum transfers. To turn to the right, the front-facing dancer extends one leg in front of the body, then rotates that leg in the horizontal plane around the side until it reaches its physiologic ROM limit. The momentum of the elevated leg is then transmitted back to the body to provide the angular force necessary to complete the turn while the right foot is brought back to the supporting left leg's knee. The momentum transfer is accomplished by the adductor muscles of the right leg slowing its rotation by eccentric contraction as it reaches its ROM limit. The adductors may be stretched uncomfortably because the rotating right leg may continue to carry significant momentum as the end range is reached. Any reduction in the range of the rotating leg shortens the time that it can build momentum. Less momentum will ultimately be transferred back to the body, and the movement will have a jerky appearance or the turn will be incomplete.
    Treatment must focus on fully rehabilitating the adductor muscles through their full length–tension curves for both concentric and eccentric contraction.

13. **In dance, what harm can come from a bad attitude?**
Attitude is a routine classical ballet position in which the gesture leg is held extended at the hip behind the body. The increased lumbar lordosis required for this maneuver subsequently increases spinal posterior element overuse stress. Facet pain and spondylolysis can result when the hyperlordosis is intensified by additional biomechanical factors such as femoral anteversion, psoas tightness, thoracolumbar fascia shortening, thoracic kyphosis, genu recurvatum, weak abdominal muscles, and volitional hyperlordosis while cheating turnout.

WEBSITES

1. www.artsmed.org

2. www.iadms.org

BIBLIOGRAPHY

1. Brandfonbrener AG: Joint laxity and arm pain in musicians. Med Probl Perform Art 15:72–74, 2000.

2. Brown SE: Workers' Compensation and performance injuries. Med Prob! Perform Art 11:111–115, 1996.

3. Dawson WJ, Charness M, Goode DJ, et al: What's in a name? Terminologic issues in performing arts medicine. Med Probl Perform Art 13:45–50, 1998.

4. Laws K: Momentum transfers in dance movement. Med Probl Perform Art 13:136–145, 1998.

5. Liederbach M: Screening for functional capacity in dancers: Designing standardized, dance-specific injury prevention screening tools. J Dance Med Sci 1:93–106, 1997.

6. Novella TM: Pointe shoes: Fitting and selection criteria. J. Dance Med Sci 4:73–77, 2000.

7. Otis CL, Drinkwater B, Johnson M, et al: The female athletic triad. Med Sci Sports Exerc 29(5):i–ix, 1997.

8. Robson BE: The female athletic triad. J Dance Med Sci 2:42–44, 1998.

9. Ryan AJ, Stephens RE: Dance Medicine: A Comprehensive Guide. Pluribus Press, Chicago, 1987.

10. Sataloff RT, Brandfonbrener AG, Lederman RJ (eds): Textbook of Performing Arts Medicine, 2nd ed. San Diego, Singular Publishing Group, 1997.

SPORTS MEDICINE: FUNCTIONAL DIAGNOSIS, FOCAL INTERVENTIONS, AND REHABILITATION FOR PREVENTION

CHAPTER 81

Stuart Willick, MD, Eva Young, MD, and Joel M. Press, MD

Success is how high you bounce when you hit bottom.

—General George Patton (1923–2004)

1. What is PASSOR?

The Physiatric Association for Spine, Sports, and Occupational Rehabilitation (PASSOR) is a section of the American Academy of Physical Medicine and Rehabilitation formed "to foster the growth of the specialty of physiatry in research, education, and the physiatric practice of musculoskeletal medicine with a special emphasis upon spine, sports, and occupational rehabilitation."

www.aapmr.org/passor.htm

2. What are the key questions to ask when discussing an injury with an athlete?

- What was the **mechanism** of injury? (What happened?)
- Is this a **recurrent injury,** a **repetitive overload** injury, or a new, acute traumatic event? If the athlete has been previously injured in the same area, it implies either inadequate rehabilitation or the progression of chronic microtraumatic injury.
- Where else has the patient been injured? A **kinetic chain analysis** of injuries often reveals events proximal or distal to the site of acute injury, which has rendered the new site more vulnerable to overload.
- What **treatment** has the patient received? An alarming number of musculoskeletal injuries do not receive adequate attention and proper rehabilitation.
- What **other medical conditions** does the patient have? Do not assume that the patient is healthy just because he or she is an athlete. Many individuals with asthma, cardiac conditions, and metabolic and hormonal disorders are active participants in sports. Treatment regimens need to take this information into account.

3. What is involved in the preparticipation history and examination?

The history needs to include a review of previous neurologic and musculoskeletal **injuries** and their rehabilitation, a thorough family and personal **cardiovascular and respiratory disease** inquiry, review of **thermoregulatory and endocrine dysfunction,** and evaluation for the presence or absence of unpaired organs.

The preparticipation history and examination is used to:
- Detect conditions that will restrict athletic participation, predispose to injury, or limit the level of performance
- Evaluate level of fitness and maturity
- Determine general health
- Establish an open physician–athlete relationship for maximal health education
- Fulfill medical–legal requirements

www.physsportsmed.com/issues/1999/08_99/glover.htm

4. **What is a musculoskeletal examination?**

In a complete musculoskeletal examination, the examiner notes **biomechanical deficits** such as inflexibilities and motion restrictions at the level of the joints, connective tissue, muscle, and fascia. **Strength** and dynamic and **proprioceptive ability** are also assessed. These findings, along with the neurologic exam, give a more complete diagnosis from an anatomic and functional standpoint. Biomechanical deficits and imbalances can be determined that may be important in prescribing a comprehensive rehabilitation program.

5. **What are the most common sports injuries?**

This depends on the sport (Table 81-1). Athletes involved in high-impact sports that require jumping and landing on hard surfaces (e.g., basketball, volleyball) are at risk for injuries in the knee and ankle, such as anterior cruciate ligament tears, meniscal tears, and inversion ankle sprains. Activities involving more upper-extremity movement (e.g., tennis, baseball, racquetball) may cause injury to the rotator cuff and elbow. Sports such as cheerleading, volleyball, gymnastics, and weight-lifting may predispose to back injuries resulting from hyperextension and repetitive extension.

TABLE 81-1. COMMON SPORTS INJURIES CAUSED BY MUSCULOTENDINOUS OVERLOAD

Injuries	Sport(s)
Acromioclavicular ligament sprain	Weight lifting, gymnastics
Rotator cuff tendinitis	Baseball, tennis, swimming
Medial epicondylitis	Golf, baseball (pitching), tennis (forehand)
Lateral epicondylitis	Tennis (backhand)
de Quervain's tenosynovitis	Rowing, golf
Spondylolysis, lumbar spine	Gymnastics
Trochanteric bursitis	Running
Adductor tendinitis	Hockey, soccer
Iliotibial band friction syndrome	Running
Patellofemoral pain	Basketball, cycling, running, soccer, weight lifting
Achilles tendinitis	Running, basketball
Ankle sprains	Baseball, basketball, soccer, volleyball
Plantar fasciitis	Running, soccer, tennis
Flexor hallucis tendinitis	Dance

6. **What is a "stinger" or "burner"?**

These are traction or compression injuries to the brachial plexus, probably at the root level. These typically occur in the upper roots and are more common in contact sports, such as football, where head and neck contact may result in nerve root compression or stretch with upper plexus tension. Sharp, burning pain is experienced down the arm and generally lasts from seconds to minutes. Persistent neurologic findings and recurrent stingers require a comprehensive evaluation.

http://sportsmedicine.about.com/cs/neck/a/neck3.htm

7. **What injuries are associated with running?**
Most running-related injuries occur in the lower extremities. Forces up to three times the body's weight are placed on the lower limb joints during running. In particular, injuries include plantar fasciitis, medial tibial stress syndrome, Achilles tendinitis, patellofemoral pain syndrome, and iliotibial band friction syndrome. Stress fractures commonly occur in the tibia, metatarsals, and fibula and less commonly in the femur and pelvis.

   http://orthopedics.about.com/cs/sportsmedicine/a/runninginjury.htm

KEY POINTS: PLANTAR FASCIITIS

1. Plantar fasciitis is a common cause of heel pain in adults.

2. It is caused by overload of the plantar fascia and volar foot muscles.

3. It is commonly found in runners as a result of overuse.

4. A classic sign is worse pain with the first few steps in the morning.

5. Treatment includes relative rest, correction of biomechanical factors, a stretching and strengthening program, and night splints and orthotics.

6. It is usually self-limiting, and time until resolution is often 6–18 months.

7. For more information, consult www.aafp.org/afp/20010201/467.html.

8. **What causes shin splints?**
A shin splint, or **medial tibial stress syndrome (MTSS),** is caused by an overload of structures in the posteromedial leg. MTSS is a continuum of pathology that may include posterior tibial tendinitis, medial soleus enthesitis, tibial periostitis, tibial stress responses, and tibial stress fracture.

   www.wheelessonline.com/ortho/shin_splints_medial_tibial_stress_syndrome

9. **In addition to shin splints, what is another cause of anterior leg pain?**
Chronic exertional compartment syndrome is a common cause of anterior leg pain. It manifests as pain, swelling, and, sometimes, weakness and paresthesias of the leg, with activity. These symptoms are the result of **intercompartmental swelling** of the muscles of the anterior compartment of the leg with exercise and always subside with rest. Compartment syndrome may also occur, though less commonly, in the deep posterior and lateral compartments of the leg. Diagnosis is made by measuring intercompartmental pressures before and after exercise. If symptoms persist despite conservative treatment (correcting biomechanical abnormalities, modifying training regimen), then fasciotomy is recommended.

   www.physsportsmed.com/issues/1996/04_96/edwards.htm

10. **What is a common cause of low back pain in young athletes?**
Spondylolysis, which is a defect in the pars interarticularis, is a common injury found in many athletes (e.g., gymnasts, dancers, football players, and wrestlers) who are subject to twisting and hyperextension loading of the lumbar spine. The defect most commonly occurs at L5, and is best seen on single positron emission computed tomography (SPECT) scan, because plain radiographs may often be negative. Treatment remains controversial, with some authors recommending rigid bracing for varying durations. However, the vast majority of patients seem to do well with conservative care and can return to play with few or no symptoms.

Baker RJ, Patel D: Lower back pain in the athlete: Common conditions and treatment. Prim Care 32(1):201–229, 2005.

Herman MJ, Pizzutillo PD, Cavalier R: Spondylolysis and spondylolisthesis in the child and adolescent athlete. Orthop Clin North Am 34(3):vii, 461–467, 2003.

Standaert C: Spondylolysis in the adolescent athlete. Clin J Sport Med 12(2):119–122, 2002.

11. **What is the female athlete triad?**
    The female athlete triad is defined as the combination of **disordered eating, amenorrhea, and osteoporosis.** This disorder often goes unrecognized and is the result of maladaptive patterns of diet and exercise adopted in order to improve body image or performance. The consequences can be devastating, from osteoporotic fractures to death. Early recognition of the female athlete triad can be accomplished through risk factor assessment and screening questionnaires. Treatment involves a multidisciplinary approach involving the primary care physician, nutritionist, and psychologist. Preventive measures of female athlete triad starts with educating parents, coaches, and athletes in the health risks of the disorder.

    www.physsportsmed.com/issues/1996/07_96/smith.htm
    www.aafp.org/afp/20000601/3357.html

12. **What is "skier's thumb"?**
    Skier's thumb is instability of the metacarpophalangeal (MCP) joint of the thumb caused by tearing of the ulnar collateral ligament (Fig. 81-1). The most common mechanism of injury is a skier landing with his or her hand on a ski pole, causing a valgus force on the thumb. Partial tears may be treated conservatively with a molded spica splint. Surgery is indicated for complete rupture of the ligament resulting from development of chronic instability of the MCP joint.

    www.hughston.com/hha/a_14_1_2.htm

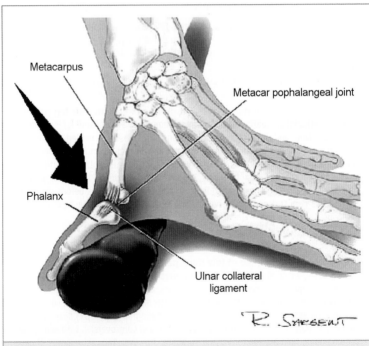

Metacarpus

Metacar pophalangeal joint

Phalanx

Ulnar collateral
ligament

R. SARGENT

Figure 81-1. Skier's thumb.

13. **Is surgery necessary for a meniscal tear of the knee?**

    Not always. Meniscal injuries associated with mechanical locking, loss of full range of motion, and persistent pain that limits daily activity will probably require surgical treatment. However, because of the good vascular supply to the peripheral one third of the menisci, there is potential for healing. Many meniscal injuries that minimally affect daily activities during the first few weeks after injury can be cautiously watched for symptomatic improvement and possible resolution of symptoms. If symptoms persist after 6–8 weeks (depending on the demands of the athlete), magnetic resonance imaging (MRI) and surgical consultation are typically indicated.

    www.sportsinjurybulletin.com/archive/meniscal-tears.html

14. **What is a hip pointer?**

    A hip pointer is a contusion to the iliac crest with subperiosteal hematoma, usually the result of direct trauma. The injured athlete has difficulty walking and standing upright because of the pain and muscular tightening in that area. The true hip joint is unaffected.

    www.emedx.com/emedx/diagnosis_information/hip_pelvis_disorders/hip_pointer_outline.htm
    http://orthopedics.about.com/cs/hipsurgery/g/hippointer.htm

15. **Is it possible to participate in sports without surgical repair of a torn anterior cruciate ligament (ACL)?**

    Sometimes. The ACL provides the majority of rotatory stability at the knee. If it is torn, stability during lateral and twisting movements is lost. Most high-level athletes and young recreational athletes who wish to return to the same level of sports competition need surgical repair. Reconstructive surgery reestablishes some of the restraint to rotatory and anterior instability. After ACL reconstruction, an aggressive rehabilitation program is required. Some patients will do well without surgery and can return to sports activities, particularly "straight-ahead" sports such as bicycling. Keys to both nonoperative and postoperative treatment include aggressive strengthening and proprioceptive training.

16. **What important considerations are involved in rehabilitation of patellofemoral pain syndrome?**

    Patellofemoral pain syndrome is often a result of poor tracking of the patella in the trochlear groove throughout the full range of flexion and extension. Emphasis needs to be placed on stretching posterior and lateral structures that may be tight (i.e., the iliotibial band, hamstrings, gastrocsoleus), strengthening structures that directly or indirectly move the patella medially (e.g., medial quads, hip external rotators), proprioceptive retraining of patellofemoral motion (e.g., taping), and strengthening exercises that do not increase patellofemoral joint reaction forces excessively.

    http://familydoctor.org/479.xml
    www.physsportsmed.com/issues/2004/0704/labotz.htm

17. **How does the iliotibial band (ITB) friction syndrome occur?**

    ITB syndrome is a lateral knee pain syndrome caused by overload of the ITB. Pain is produced as the ITB rubs over the lateral femoral condyle, typically between 20 degrees and 30 degrees of flexion. Pain may also occur near the insertion site of the ITB on the anterolateral tibia at Gerdy's tubercle. Causes include running on uneven surfaces, sudden increases in running mileage, and incorrect footwear in either pronators or supinators.

    www.aafp.org/afp/20050415/1545.html

18. **What is "turf toe"?**

    Turf toe refers to a sprain injury of the plantar capsule of the MTP joint of the great toe. It is generally caused by excessive forces placed on the MTP joint during push-off or running on hard surfaces (i.e., artificial turf in football and soccer). The athlete complains of pain and swelling of the first MTP joint, which worsens when attempting push-off. Splinting for 7–10 days and/or taping to limit dorsiflexion are necessary to prevent further injury.

    http://orthopedics.about.com/cs/toeproblems/a/toeproblems_5.htm

19. **Describe the important aspects of the rehabilitation of rotator cuff injuries.**
    Rehabilitation should include assessment of the entire kinetic chain (e.g., cervical, thoracic, and lumbar spine and upper and lower extremities). This is especially important in the overhead athlete. Muscles should be strengthened both concentrically and eccentrically, individually, and in groups. Progression should lead to sports-specific exercises to maximize the chances for successful return to sports. Rotator cuff rehabilitation must address the following:
    - **Flexibility deficits,** particularly in the external rotators and posterior capsule
    - **Joint motion restriction** within the sternoclavicular, acromioclavicular, scapulothoracic, and glenohumeral articulations
    - **Strength deficits,** particularly in the scapular stabilizers (rhomboids, lower and middle trapezius, and serratus anterior) as well as the cuff muscles

    http://familydoctor.org/268.xml

20. **How is tennis elbow treated?**
    Lateral epicondylitis, also known as tennis elbow, is the result of repetitive overload of the extensors and supinators of the wrist. Rehabilitation focuses on stretching tight wrist extensors, strengthening the wrist extensors, and avoiding aggravating factors. Limitations of motion at the shoulder, poor cervicothoracic posture, and poor kinetic chain mechanics must be corrected. Counterforce braces and occasionally corticosteroid injections can be helpful. (For more information on tennis elbow, see Chapters 41 and 42.)

    www.sportsinjuryclinic.net/cybertherapist/front/elbow/tenniselbow.htm

21. **What is "little league elbow"?**
    Little league elbow is the consequence of repeated valgus overload in the skeletally immature elbow. During late cocking and acceleration, medial structures are stretched while lateral structures are compressed. The distraction forces on the medial side may cause enlargement or avulsion of the medial epicondyle and osteochondritis dissecans, while the compressive lateral forces may induce radial head and capitellar growth disturbance, fractures, and articular cartilage breakdown.

    www.emoryhealthcare.org/HealthGate/11703.html

22. **What is biker's palsy?**
    Biker's palsy refers to an entrapment or pressure neuropathy of the ulnar nerve at the wrist within Guyon's canal. It may occur in distance cyclists because of direct pressure on the ulnar side of the hand with standard handlebars. Sensory and motor symptoms are confined to the ulnar-innervated structures distal to this area, with sparing of the flexor carpi ulnaris muscle and the dorsal ulnar cutaneous sensory patch. Methods of prevention include wearing padded bicycle gloves, changing hand position frequently, and the use of "aero-bars," which allow weight-bearing through the forearm. Carpal tunnel syndrome can also be seen in long-distance cyclists.

    http://ajsm.highwire.org/cgi/content/abstract/33/8/1224

23. **Why do gymnasts get low back pain?**
    Gymnastics, like other sports that require a lot of hyperextension of the spine, can place excessive loads on the posterior structures of the spine. In particular, loads are placed on the pars interarticularis (the site of spondylolysis) and on the facet joints. Other sports with a high incidence of low back pain are cheerleading, weight lifting, and football.

    www.ncbi.nlm.nih.gov/entrez/query.fcgi?cmd=Retrieve&db=PubMed&list_uids=12831692&dopt=Citation

24. **What is functional musculoskeletal rehabilitation?**
    Functional rehabilitation implies that the exercises performed by the patient for a specific musculoskeletal disorder are done in the planes of motion, with the types of contraction, and in a coordinated fashion similar to the sport or activity that the patient performs. A functional

rehabilitation program should "look like" the activity the patient performs on a daily basis with his or her specific sport. Straight-leg raises, for example, would be a means of strengthening lower-extremity musculature including the quadriceps muscle and hip flexors. However, there are very few "functional" activities that a person would do during the day that would simulate this motion. A more appropriate functional activity might be a partial squat or a step-up or step-down exercise to activate the quadriceps and hip flexor musculature.

25. What are open and closed chain exercises, and why are they used?
A **closed kinetic chain (CKC)** is operational when the distal segment of the motion chain is fixed in space and movement at one segment will move the other segments in a predictable pattern. An **open kinetic chain (OKC)** is operational when the distal segment moves freely. An example of a CKC movement is a simple squat, whereas an example of an OKC movement is throwing a baseball. Both types of exercises are used in sports injury rehabilitation depending on the type of motion that is being functionally addressed. Most running injuries involving the lower extremities will emphasize CKC activities, whereas rehabilitation of shoulder and elbow injuries in tennis and throwing sports may emphasize OKC exercises.

26. What does "rehabilitation beyond the resolution of symptoms" mean?
Many musculoskeletal injuries appear to resolve despite the treatment patients are given. After treatment of the acute inflammation, symptoms from many ailments disappear, and athletes mistakenly assume it is safe to return to sport. However, absence of pain does not always imply absence of pathology, and stopping rehabilitation at this point is inadequate. Most musculoskeletal injuries in sports are the result of chronic overload, in which biomechanical alterations have occurred and microtraumatic tissue injury has occurred. These biomechanical changes, consisting of muscle imbalances, inflexibilities, and weaknesses, need to be addressed to prevent recurrence of injury.

27. When should you use the philosophy "no pain, no gain"?
In most cases of rehabilitation of musculoskeletal and sports injuries, the patient needs to be careful not to push beyond the limits of pain when significant muscle, tendon, bone, or ligament injury has occurred. Pain often will be a guideline that is approached but not forced past. On the other hand, the healthy patient who wants to "get stronger" is expected to experience some soreness of muscles after lifting the necessary weights to obtain strength gains. The assumption is that in the latter case, muscle has been subjected to systematically applied overload and that adequate recovery time has been given so that full recovery between exercise sessions has been achieved.

BIBLIOGRAPHY

1. Bruckner P, Khan K: Clinical Sports Medicine. Sydney, McGraw-Hill, 1993.
2. Fu FH, Stone DA: Sports Injuries: Mechanisms, Prevention, Treatment. Baltimore, Williams & Wilkins, 1994.
3. Kibler WB, Herring SA, Press JM: Functional Rehabilitation of Sports and Musculoskeletal Injuries. Gaithersburg, MD, Aspen Publications, 1998.
4. Press JM (ed): Sports Medicine. Physical Medicine and Rehabilitation Clinics of North America. Vol 5, no 1. Philadelphia, W.B. Saunders, 1994.

COMPLEMENTARY MEDICINE: WHAT WORKS

David Kim, MD, Bryan J. O'Young, MD, Mark A. Young, MD, MBA, Marc S. Micozzi, MD, PhD, and Jeffrey Meyers, MD

CHAPTER 82

What works will no longer be called conventional or complementary medicine—it will just be called good medicine.
        –Former U.S. Surgeon General C. Everett Koop in Micozzi MS: *Fundamentals of Complementary and Integrative Medicine*

1. **What is complementary medicine (CM)?**
   CM is defined by the National Center for Complementary and Alternative Medicine of the National Institutes of Health (NIH) as a "group of diverse medical and health care systems, practices, and products that are not presently considered to be part of conventional medicine." CM continues to grow significantly in popularity. It offers a "healing-oriented" approach toward health that accentuates the important relationship between physician and patient. CM integrates the best of complementary and alternative medicine with the best of traditional conventional medicine.

   National Center for Complementary and Alternative Medicine of the NIH: http://nccam.nih.gov/

2. **How is complementary medicine different from conventional medicine?**
   The focus of CM is to improve the overall health and well-being of the patient, as opposed to the more specific condition-focused approach of conventional medicine, in continuity with managing specific medical conditions. By improving overall health, treatment of specific diseases is more effective and long-lasting. Complementary medicine can be used to help manage specific medical conditions and in most cases, works well with conventional medicine.

3. **What are some examples of CM?**
   Common examples of CM include acupuncture and traditional Chinese medicine, aromatherapy, Ayurveda, chiropractic therapy, use of dietary supplements, electromagnetic therapies, massage, homeopathy, naturopathy, osteopathy, chi gong, and Reiki.

   NCCAM Publication No. D156, May 2002.

4. **IS CM part of medical education?**
   Increasingly, CM is gaining attention in medical education institutions. Along with technologic advances in medicine, patients perceive many shortcomings in conventional medicine, including a breakdown in the physician–patient relationship and communication. CM, through its emphasis on healing-oriented medicine and optimization of doctor–patient communication, is earning a respected place in medical education.

   Bell IR, Caspi O, Schwartz GE, et al: Integrative medicine and systemic outcomes research: Issues in the emergence of a new model for primary health care. Arch Intern Med 162(2):133–140, 2002.
   Maizes V, Schneider C, Bell I, Weil A: Integrative medical education: Development and implementation of a comprehensive curriculum at the University of Arizona. Acad Med 77(9):861–863, 2002.

5. **How prevalent is the use of CM?**

A study in *JAMA* suggested a 47.3% overall increase in total visits to complementary medicine practitioners between 1990 and 1997. The number of visits to complementary medicine practitioners in 1990 was greater than to all primary care doctors. A total of 89% of the visits were not prescribed by a physician, and 72% of patients did not discuss them with their physician. The largest, most recent, and comprehensive survey of CM medicine by the U.S. Centers for Disease Control/National Center for Health Statistics showed that more than two thirds of Americans regularly use complementary medicine.

Barnes PM, Powell-Griner E, McFann K, Nahin RL: Complementary and alternative medicine use among adults: United States, 2002. Semin Integrat Med 2(2):54–71, 2004.

Eisenberg DM, Davis RB, Ettner SL, Appel S: Trends in alternative medicine use in the US, 1990–1997. JAMA 280:1569–1575, 1998.

6. **What are the most common uses of complementary therapies?**

CM therapies are commonly used to treat chronic conditions such as back problems, anxiety, depression, chronic pain, and headaches, as well as many functional disorders such as irritable bowel syndrome and premenstrual syndrome. CM is useful in rehabilitation, restoration of function, and management of pain following injury and medical procedures.

7. **Why do patients use CM?**

There is literature suggesting that patients may seek complementary practitioners because of dissatisfaction with conventional medicine. Most use CM not only because they may be dissatisfied with conventional medicine, but also because they find complementary therapies more acceptable and consistent with their lifestyles and attitudes toward health and life.

Austin JA: Why patients use alternative medicine. JAMA 279:1548–1553, 1998.

8. **What is mind–body medicine?**

Mind–body medicine is a general term for an approach to health that uses physical and nonphysical therapies that make use of the anatomic, biochemical, hormonal, and physiologic connections between the brain and the body.

9. **What are some of the nonphysical therapies?**

Examples include biofeedback, counseling, cognitive-behavioral therapy, homeopathy, and a variety of spiritual practices.

10. **What is psychoneuroimmunology?**

Psychoneuroimmunology is a branch of science that studies how the mind (psycho), brain and nervous system (neuro), and immune system (immunology) interact with each other to produce physiologic effects and influence healing.

11. **What is the effect of stress on the immune system?**

The psychoneuroimmunology literature shows a number of physiologic changes caused by stress. It has been shown that death of a spouse results in immunosuppression for at least 2–6 weeks after the event. Examinations have shown depressed humoral immunity. Sleep deprivation inhibits neutrophil phagocytosis. Stress also increases muscle tone, cortisol, and adrenaline levels, which contribute to dysregulation of the "fight-or-flight" response.

12. **Can emotions affect health?**

There are many studies that show positive emotions correlate to better health. One such study showed that optimism was associated with higher levels of general health perceptions, vitality, mental health, and lower levels of pain.

Achat H. Kawachi I. Spiro A 3rd. et al: Optimism and depression as predictors of physical and mental health functioning: the Normative Aging Study. Ann Behav Med 22(2):127–130, 2000.

13. Can mind–body therapies enhance patient compliance?

Yes. A randomized, controlled study showed that elderly patients who had mind–body interventions and were involved in a 5-month walking program walked more frequently, for longer durations, and greater distances than the control group who did not receive intervention.

Luskin F, Newell K. Mind-body approaches to successful aging. From Watkins A. Mind Body Medicine. New York, Churchill Livingstone, 1997, pp 251–268.

14. Can mind–body therapies decrease chronic pain?

Many anecdotal case reports, several surveys, and controlled studies of large groups of patients show that mind–body therapies may decrease chronic pain. Stricter randomized controlled studies are being done to evaluate this finding in greater depth.

15. What is energy medicine?

Energy medicine encompasses a wide variety of noninvasive treatments, which include Reiki, healing touch, reflexology, and acupressure.

16. When is energy medicine used?

The primary uses have been acceleration of wound healing, pain relief, relaxation, improving overall health, assisting in the preparation and follow-up of medical procedures, enhancement of spiritual development, drug detoxification, and support in the dying process.

17. What does the literature say about energy medicine?

Energy medicine is not as well documented as other areas of CM. Energy medicine, as well as many complementary medicine therapies, presents special challenges to study in the confines of the present "gold standard" of double-blinded, randomized, placebo-controlled trials. It must be considered that the present-day research paradigm is designed and best suited to study drugs, not complex systems such as energy or mind–body medicine.

18. What is a chakra?

A chakra is a focal center of energy. There are several chakras located from the head to the feet. It is thought that bioenergy flows through these centers. When they are blocked, energy flow is constricted, resulting in disease. The number of chakras varies according to the philosophy of the treatment modality or healing tradition.

19. What is Reiki?

Reiki is a Japanese form of energy medicine developed in the mid-1800s. It postulates that energy is channeled from chakras of the practitioner to the patient. It does not use the energy of the practitioner, who serves mainly as a energy channel.

20. What is healing touch?

Healing or therapeutic touch is based on ancient hands-on healing techniques used in a modern setting. Practitioners use touch to balance energy in a client to promote physical, spiritual, and emotional healing.

21. What is homeopathy?

Homeopathy is the use of extremely diluted substances to cure illness and improve health by focusing on symptoms, not on pathologic diagnoses.

KEY POINTS: USES FOR COMPLEMENTARY MEDICINE

1. Mind–body techniques have been used to successfully treat chronic pain and other medical conditions, to provide supportive care to patients undergoing and recovering from medical procedures, and to improve health and wellness.

2. Meditation has been shown to be effective in treating a number of conditions, including chronic pain, anxiety, and depression, and to provide supportive care to patients undergoing and recovering from medical procedures.

3. Energy medicine techniques offer safe and noninvasive methods to provide supportive care to patients undergoing and recovering from medical procedures and to improve health and wellness.

4. Spiritual beliefs and practices can aid in healing, and discussion of them is desired by many patients.

22. How dilute are the solutions?
The actual substance can be diluted 1 trillion times.

23. What are the three principles of homeopathy?
- **Like cures like:** For example, if the symptoms of a cold are similar to poisoning by mercury, then mercury would be the homeopathic remedy.
- **Minimal does:** The remedy is taken in an extremely dilute form; normally 1 part of the remedy to around 1 trillion parts of water.
- **Use of the single best remedy for the individual:** No matter how many symptoms are experienced, only one remedy is taken, and that remedy will be aimed at alleviation of the entire symptom complex.

24. Do patients want to incorporate spirituality into treatment?
The majority do. In a major study, two thirds of pulmonary outpatients felt that they would trust their doctors more if they were to address spiritual beliefs. Ninety-four percent of patients who engaged in a spiritual practice wanted their doctor to address their beliefs. Even among those for whom spiritual practice was not important, half wanted their doctor to at least inquire about spirituality.

25. What is spirituality?
The official definition by the American Association of Medical Colleges (AAMC) is broad: "Spirituality is recognized as a factor that contributes to health in many persons. The concept of spirituality is found in all cultures and societies. It is expressed as an individual's search for ultimate meaning through participation in religion and/or belief in God, family, naturalism, rationalism, humanism, and the arts." All of these factors may influence how patients and health care professionals perceive health and illness and how they interact with one another.

26. What is the most common spiritual practice as it relates to medical therapy?
Studies by the American Pain Society show that prayer is the most commonly used nondrug method of controlling pain, and more than 75% of patients practice it.

McNeill JA, Sherwood GD, Starck PL, Thompson CJ: Assessing clinical outcomes: Patient satisfaction with pain management. J Pain Symp Manag. 16:29–40, 1998.

27. What are the health benefits of meditation?
Studies show that 10–20 minutes of meditation a day can benefit chronic pain, insomnia, hostility, depression, postmenopause syndrome, infertility, cancer, and AIDS.

Coker KH: Meditation and prostate cancer: integrating a mind/body intervention with traditional therapies. [Review]. Semin Urol Oncol 17(2):111–118, 1999.

Grossman P, Neilmann L, Schmidt S, Walach H: Mindfulness-based stress reduction and health benefits. A metaanalysis. Psychosom Res 57(1):35–43, 2004.

Sephton SE, Salmon P, Weissbecker I, et al: Mindfulness meditation alleviates depressive symptoms in women with fibromyalgia: results of a randomized clinical trial. Arth Rheum 57(1):77–85, 2007.

28. List a few pertinent questions for the health care provider to ask about CM.
- Is CM treatment safe?
- Does the CM therapy prevent the patient from receiving needed medical management?
- Can the CM therapy be continued in conjunction with conventional treatment?
- Is conventional medicine falling short in some way that might be addressed by CM?

29. List a few pertinent questions for the patient to ask the CM provider.
- Is there evidence of efficacy and safety of the treatment?
- What is the provider's experience with the CM treatment?
- How many treatments will be needed?
- What is a reasonable time frame for a "fair" trial of the treatment?
- What are the costs, and are they reimbursed by insurance?
- What are the toxicity and safety risks or adverse effects of the treatment?
- Will the CM provider communicate with the patient's conventional physician?

Chez R, Jonas W, Eisenberg D: The Physician and Complementary and Alternative Medicine Essentials of Complementary and Alternative Medicine. Philadelphia, Lippincott Williams & Wilkins, 1999, pp 31–45.

BIBLIOGRAPHY

1. Cassidy CM (ed): Contemporary Chinese Medicine and Acupuncture. New York, Churchill Livingstone, 2002.

2. Coughlin P (ed): Principles and Practice of Manual Therapeutics. New York, Churchill Livingstone, 2002.

3. Frishman WH, Weintraub FD, Micozzi MS (eds): Complementary and Integrative Therapies for Cardiovascular Disease. St. Louis, Elsevier-Mosby, 2005.

4. Leskowitz E (ed): Complementary and Alternative Medicine in Rehabilitation. St. Louis, Churchill Livingstone/ Elsevier Science, 2003.

5. Micozzi MS (ed): Fundamentals of Complementary and Integrative Medicine, 3rd ed. Philadelphia, Saunders/ Elsevier, 2006.

6. Standish LJ, Calabrese C, Galantino ML (eds): AIDS and Complementary and Alternative Medicine. Philadelphia, Churchill Livingstone, 2002.

7. Weintraub M (ed): Alternative and Complementary Treatment in Neurologic Illness. Philadelphia, Churchill Livingstone, 2001.

WEBSITES

1. National Center for Complementary and Alternative Medicine: National Institutes of Health
   http://nccam.nih.gov/

2. Medicine Plus: Alternative Medicine
   http://www.nlm.nih.gov/medlineplus/alternativemedicine.html

INTERNATIONAL REHABILITATION MEDICINE: MAXIMIZING ABILITY THROUGH GLOBAL SYNERGY AND COLLABORATION

Bryan J. O'Young, MD, Mark A. Young, MD, MBA, Steven A. Stiens, MD, MS, Mao Bin Wang, MD, Linamara Batistella, MD, PhD, Mathew Lee, MD, MPH, Jorge Lains, MD, Peter Lee, MD, and Haim Ring, MD, MSc PM&R

CHAPTER 83

The service we render to others is really the rent we pay for our room on this earth. It is obvious that man is himself a traveler; that the purpose of this world is not "to have and to hold" but "to give and serve."

—Sir William Grenfell, international diplomat (1867–1945)

1. What is international rehabilitation medicine?

Rehabilitation medicine has steadily gained international recognition because of its unique, important role in helping people with disabilities gain greater functional independence in the face of aging and disease. International rehabilitation involves synergistic exchange of ideas and resources among diverse nations and cultures. It focuses on strengthening scientific knowledge, increasing and disseminating research in rehabilitation, providing humanitarian rehabilitation assistance, and optimizing quality of life for people with disabilities.

Battistella, Linamara R., MD, PhD, President, International Society of Physical and Rehabilitation Medicine: www.isprm.org/

2. Are there international organizations representing international rehabilitation medicine?

The International Society of Physical and Rehabilitation Medicine (ISPRM) is the premier global organization representing the specialty of physical medicine and rehabilitation (PM&R) (known as PRM abroad, for physical and rehabilitation medicine). Recognized by the World Health Organization (WHO), ISPRM serves as a leader in international rehabilitation and is a staunch advocate for people with disabilities. ISPRM fulfills its vision through vital committee activity, biennial meetings, and humanistic outreach.

3. What are the goals of international rehabilitation medicine?

International rehabilitation medicine is essential for improving the quality of rehabilitation care for both developed and developing nations. The ISPRM accomplishes this noble mission by:

- Sharing knowledge in daily clinical practice with developing and industrialized nations
- Establishing cross-cultural, pan-international exchange programs for residents, educators, and researchers in order to improve global "sharing and caring" within the domain of teaching, patient care, and humanitarianism
- Developing a uniform, standardized international PM&R curriculum
- Sponsoring global workshops on residency education and training (the Prague Summit and the Brazilian Convocation)
- Working in conjunction with allied medical professions, such as physical therapists (PTs), occupational therapists (OTs), and speech language pathologists (SLPs), in developing global academic initiatives

- Providing assistance to international agencies, private agencies, or government-sponsored agencies for special programs, such as rehabilitation of mass disasters (e.g., tsunamis, earthquakes)

Ring H: International rehabilitation medicine: Closing the gaps and globalization of the profession. Am J Phys Med Rehabil 83(9):667–669, 2004 [invited editorial].

4. **Through rudimentary measures, how can PM&R be integrated into the medical care in developing countries?**
Use of public sanitation, immunization, and other simple protective measures are essential, because many rehabilitation conditions resulting in disability originate from preventable diseases. Low-technology forms of education such as local workshops and demonstration projects can enhance education and "disability literacy." Assistive devices can be fabricated from abundantly available materials and natural resources (i.e., bamboo canes and crutches).

5. **How has technology made the "global rehabilitation village" a smaller place?**
Technologic innovations including the web, internet, blogs, video teleconferencing, and voice-over-the-net telephony have dramatically united physiatrists throughout the world in the service of mankind. The web can be compared to a central communication center where physiatrists located in the far reaches of the globe are able to connect and interact seamlessly, spontaneously, and in real time. Although widespread computer access is still out of reach of many people, its availability is steadily growing. For many international citizens, technology has truly served the role of a great "equalizer," allowing physicians in developing nations the opportunity to access books, information, and resources. Free availability of fully featured Internet e-mail accounts (Gmail, Yahoo, Hotmail, MSN, AOL) has facilitated international humanitarian objectives in a technocentric fashion.

Recent telephonic technologic innovations such as VOIP or Internet telephone networks such as SKYPE have freely facilitated real-time voice and video communication with colleagues. Web-based collaborative word-processing programs such as WRITEBOARD allow authors, researchers, and collaborators all over the world to write, share, revise, and compare documents. International online web-based group chat utilities, such as CAMPFIRE, allow real-time chat for groups of 2–40 people. Computer-based videoconferencing capability can also play a role in residency education. Recent examples include a lecture and clinical bedside demonstration by an Indian physiatrist on peripheral neurologic manifestations of leprosy to a group of American physiatrists.

6. **In what global humanitarian initiatives have physiatrists participated?**
Operation Functional Recovery (OFR) is an international humanitarian initiative founded by rehabilitation professionals aimed at helping survivors of natural and man-made disasters by bringing together rehabilitation and professionals of all backgrounds, including physiatrists, podiatrists, physical therapists, occupational therapists, speech language pathologists, orthotists and prosthetists, nurses, and others to heighten awareness of disaster preparedness and to improve functional outcomes after disaster. Initially founded during the tumultuous days after Hurricane Katrina, OFR has successfully taken bold steps to mobilize the rehabilitation community for a greater good. Projects have included providing specialized rehabilitation wound care programming in the region as well arranging for delivery of orthopedic rehabilitation shoes and foot orthotics for people with diabetic foot ulcerations and peripheral neuropathies.

www.apta.org/AM/Template.cfm?Section=Archives2&Template=/Customsource/TaggedPage/PTIssue.cfm&Issue=11/11/2000
www.isprm-edu.org/human.html

7. **Provide a recent example of how the international rehabilitation community has united to help victims of natural disasters.**
Increasingly, PM&R has come to play an important role in the recovery effort of worldwide natural disasters. The world had barely been recovering from earlier natural disasters, such as

the tsunami in South Asia and East Africa, as well as the earthquakes in Turkey, Pakistan, and Indonesia, when Hurricane Katrina hit New Orleans, Mississippi, and the Gulf region. Physiatrists played an important role in the recovery effort through OFR, a physiatry-led humanitarian initiative.

KEY POINTS: INTERNATIONAL REHABILITATION MEDICINE

1. The International Society of Physical and Rehabilitation Medicine is recognized by the World Health Organization as the premier global organization representing the specialty of physical medicine and rehabilitation.

2. Operation Functional Recovery is an interdisciplinary international humanitarian initiative founded by rehabilitation professionals aimed at helping survivors of natural and man-made disasters.

3. Participation in global physiatric humanitarianism leads to a broader and more enlightened view of the world.

4. Through a delicate balance of disability advocacy, governmental diplomacy, and community outreach, global physiatric "ambassadors" can make the world a better place and create a better tomorrow.

8. Are there international learning opportunities in PM&R?

The ISPRM Faculty Student Educational Exchange Committee serves as a central clearinghouse for unique educational and learning opportunities in physical and rehabilitation medicine across all continents. The committee maintains a website at www.isprm-edu.org. The primary functions and responsibilities of the committee include:

- To serve as a central clearinghouse for international learning opportunities in rehabilitation
- To facilitate placement of medical students, residents, faculty physicians, and allied rehabilitation professionals in global voluntary didactic rotations
- To share information about global PR&M educational opportunities with the membership of the organization
- To track the outcomes, progress, and successes of the committee's educational initiatives
- To interface and network with other rehabilitation educational organizations in pursuit of international education and scholarship in the field
- To track the individual accomplishments and endeavors of the committee

9. Is there an international faculty for *PM&R Secrets*?

Yes. Throughout this book, there are authors from many different countries who have contributed generously to global education through authorship, coauthorship, and review of material contained herein. In addition, this chapter can be said to symbolically represent the collaborative efforts of the international rehabilitation community because the plenary membership of ISPRM input has been sought. Names of specific international *PM&R Secrets'* faculty are listed at www.pmrsecrets.com.

10. How does participation in international rehabilitation medicine improve local physiatric practice?

Participation in an international physiatric organization (Box 83-1) leads to a broader and more enlightened view of the world. The traveling physiatrist acquires a keen understanding of the world and develops a transcendent sense of caring by experiencing, learning, teaching, and sharing. Through a delicate blend of disability advocacy, governmental diplomacy (www.isprm-edu.org/ISPRM%20-%20PHOTOLITHUANIA.htm), and community outreach, global physiatric "ambassadors" can make the world a better place and create a better tomorrow.

BOX 83-1. LISTING OF NATIONAL PHYSIATRY ORGANIZATIONS BY CONTINENT

Australia
- Australasian Faculty of Rehabilitation Medicine

Europe
- Austrian Society of PM&R
- The Royal Belgian Society of PM&R
- British Society of Rehabilitation Medicine
- Cyprus Society of Physical Medicine and Rehabilitation
- Dutch Society of Physical Medicine and Rehabilitation
- German Society of Physical Medicine and Rehabilitation
- Hellenic Society of Physical Medicine & Rehabilitation
- Italian Society of Physical Medicine and Rehabilitation
- Polish Rehabilitation Society
- Portuguese Society of PM&R
- Romanian Society of Physical Medicine and Rehabilitation
- Slovenian Society of Physical & Rehabilitation Medicine
- Society for Physical Medicine & Rehabilitation of Serbia & Montenegro
- Spanish Society of Physical Medicine & Rehabilitation
- Turkish Society of PM&R

South America
- Argentinian Society of Physical Medicine & Rehabilitation
- Bolivian Society of Physical Medicine & Rehabilitation
- Brazilian Society of Physical Medicine & Rehabilitation
- Chilean Society of Physical Rehabilitation & Medicine
- Colombian Society of Physical & Rehabilitation Medicine
- Ecuadorian Society of Physical & Rehabilitation Medicine
- Peruvian Society of Physical Medicine & Rehabilitation
- Uruguayan Society of Physical Medicine
- Venezuelan Society of Physical Medicine & Rehabilitation

North America
- American Academy of PM&R
- Association of Academic Physiatrists
- American Congress of Rehabilitation Medicine
- Canadian Association of Physical Medicine & Rehabilitation
- Cuban Society of Physical Medicine & Rehabilitation
- Mexican Society of Physical Medicine & Rehabilitation
- Nicaraguan Society of Physical Medicine & Rehabilitation
- Panamian Society of Physical Medicine & Rehabilitation
- Puerto Rico Society of Physical Medicine and Rehabilitation

---

Continued

BOX 83-1. LISTING OF NATIONAL PHYSIATRY ORGANIZATIONS BY CONTINENT—CONT'D

Africa and the Middle East
- Egyptian Society for Rheumatology and Rehabilitation
- Israeli Association of Physical Medicine and Rehabilitation
- Kuwait Society of Physical Medicine and Rehabilitation
- Saudi Arabian Society for Physical & Rehabilitation Medicine
- Turkish Society of PMR
- Société Tunisienne de Médecine Physique, de Rééducation et de Réadaption Fonctionelles

Asia
- Bangladesh Association of PMR
- Chinese Association of Rehabilitation Medicine
- Chinese Society of PMR
- Chinese Taipei Society of PMR
- Hong Kong Association of Rehabilitation Medicine
- Iranian Society of Physical Medicine and Rehabilitation
- The Japanese Association of Rehabilitation Medicine
- Korean Academy of Rehabilitation Medicine
- Pakistan Society for the Rehabilitation of the Disabled
- Philippine Academy of Rehabilitation Medicine
- Thai Rehabilitation Association

WEBSITES

1. http://cirrie.buffalo.edu/journal/journals.html

2. www.isprm-edu.org/literature.htm

3. www.mja.com.au/public/issues/177_07_071002/cam10158_fm.html

4. www.monduzzi.com/proceedings/moreinfo/20030518.htm

5. www.unicef.org/

6. www.uwmedicine.org/Global/NewsAndEvents/PressReleases/2006/Gates+Gift+for+Global+Health+Institute.htm

BIBLIOGRAPHY

1. Banja JD: Ethics, values, and world cultures: The impact on rehabilitation. Disabil Rehabil 18:279–284, 1996.

2. Young MA, Disler P, O'Young B, et al: International rehabilitation education: A comparative analysis and panel discussion. Monduzzi Int Med J (Italy) 1:469–478, 2003.

3. Young MA, Disler P: Global physical medicine and rehabilitation education: The Prague 2003 Summit. Monduzzi Int Med J (Italy) 6:777–782, 2003.

CHAPTER 84

EPILOGUE: PHYSICAL MEDICINE AND REHABILITATION—OR IS IT PHYSICAL MEDICINE VERSUS REHABILITATION?

Randall L. Braddom, MD, MS

Perhaps, the field of physical medicine and rehabilitation (PM&R) should use the ampersand (&) as its symbol. In the early days of PM&R, there were actually two distinctly separate fields. One was physical medicine, led by Frank Krusen, MD (1898–1973), who penned the first textbook on the subject, *Physical Medicine*,[1] in 1941. He was assisted in this endeavor by Earl Elkins, MD (who became the first secretary of the American Board of PM&R) and by Robert Bennett, MD (the first PM&R resident). The textbook concerned the use of heat, light, electricity, mechanotherapy, and other developing aspects of "physical medicine." Although the book had eight full pages about the use of fever therapy for the treatment of gonorrhea, it said little or nothing about classical rehabilitation involving neurologic impairments such as stroke or spinal cord injury. For example, the word "paraplegia" does not even appear in the book.

The early practice of physical medicine centered on the use of exercise and physical modalities for the treatment of pain and physical impairments. Technologic advances in the 1930s and 1940s made possible the use of new modality devices, such as the ultrasound and short-wave diathermy machines. (Short-wave diathermy was actually an adaptation of the multicavity magnetron, the radar apparatus first used by allied forces near the end of World War II.) In the introduction to *Physical Medicine*, Krusen gave this definition: "Physical medicine or physical therapy may be defined as that science which deals with the management of disease by means of physical agents such as light, heat, cold, water, electricity and mechanical agents." He used the terms *physical therapy*, *physical medicine*, and *physiotherapy* interchangeably at that time.

The early organizations that fostered the development of the field also used *physical medicine* and *physical therapy* interchangeably. These included the Council of Physical Therapy of the American Medical Association; the American Congress of Physical Therapy (now the American Congress of Rehabilitation Medicine); the American Society of Physical Therapy Physicians; and the American Academy of Physical Medicine (now the American Academy of Physical Medicine and Rehabilitation). Later, after the growth of the field of physical therapy in the United States, Krusen realized that the field should no longer be called physical therapy, and also that its practitioners could no longer be referred to as physical therapy physicians. Consequently, he invented de novo the terms *physiatry* and *physiatrist*. A stimulating historical account of the early development of the field of PM&R is found in his Zeiter lecture in 1969.[2] A more in-depth description of the early history of the field has been published in a series of recent articles based on Krusen's diary.[3–6]

The rehabilitation side of the field was led by a number of individuals, especially Howard Rusk, MD (1901–1989). Rusk was an internist in St. Louis who left his practice in 1942 (at the age of 41) and joined the Army Air Corps. As chief of medical services at Jefferson Barracks in St. Louis, he noted that many of the soldiers being treated ended up back in the facility because they were not physically and mentally prepared to successfully return to active military duty. He designed physical and mental programs to assure that they could handle their military assignments, and, by doing so, cut the recidivism rate dramatically. This attracted the attention of military brass, and Rusk was summoned to Washington to a design a similar program for the entire Army Air Corps. It is estimated that his Convalescent Training Program saved more than 5 million man-hours during the war. It also gave countless disabled veterans the hope and the sense of purpose they needed to succeed in civilian life after the war. Rusk earned the Distinguished Service Medal for his work and eventually retired as a brigadier general in the U.S. Air Force Reserve.

After the war, Rusk decided not to return to practice in St. Louis, convincing the medical school at New York University to free some wards in Bellevue and Goldwater Hospitals in which to rehabilitate civilians. At first, his efforts were met with skepticism and ridicule by his fellow doctors, but he gained the support of several prominent individuals, including Bernard M. Baruch, Louis J. Horowitz, and Bernard and Alva Gimbel. He was able to raise funds and gain publicity for his work. At the same time, Arthur Hays Sulzberger, owner of *The New York Times*, hired Rusk to write a weekly column on health issues for the paper. Rusk continued to write the column until 1971. After tirelessly promoting rehabilitation for civilians, and with the help of his benefactors, Rusk founded the Institute of Physical Medicine and Rehabilitation, at New York University (NYU) Medical Center, which opened in 1950. The Institute was later renamed the Institute of Rehabilitation Medicine; in 1984, NYU honored Rusk by renaming the hospital the "Howard A. Rusk Institute of Rehabilitation Medicine."*

Rusk edited the book *Rehabilitation Medicine* in 1958. The book described in detail many of the rehabilitation techniques that we still use today for the disabling conditions, from stroke to spinal cord injury. By the third edition of this book, in 1971,[7] the amount of material on musculoskeletal subjects was still limited to only one chapter, and the space allotted specifically to back pain was less than eight pages. Rusk was a strong advocate of the *team approach* to the patient:

> We stressed, however, that over and above this group of patients are a number with severe disabilities—paraplegia, quadriplegia, severe hemiplegia with aphasia, the demyelinating diseases, and some of the other clinical problems—whose needs could not be met without a concentrated long-term program that included full utilization of the allied health disciplines and specialized rehabilitation technics. We noted that it was obvious that no medical practitioner, general or specialist, could have at his disposal for the care of his patients all of the varied facilities, equipment, specialized skills, and allied health professional personnel needed for the management of such patients.[8]

Physiatrists owe a great deal to both Krusen and Rusk, as well as to the other early pioneers of our field. Most of us can even trace our educational roots back to either Rusk or Krusen. For example, I consider myself a great-grandson of Krusen, because he trained Ralph Worden, MD, who trained Ernest W. Johnson, MD, who was responsible for my training.

The field of physical medicine and rehabilitation was officially recognized as a medical specialty in 1947, with the formation of the American Board of Physical Medicine. The first board examination was held in September of that year in Rochester, Minnesota. But it was not until 1949 that the word "rehabilitation" was added to the name, and it became the American Board of Physical Medicine and Rehabilitation. To a large extent the board represented the bonding together of two different fields. Both "physical medicine" and "rehabilitation" practitioners used similar principles to treat their patients (including a holistic approach), but the union between them has been in "marital counseling" ever since.

These two fields within PM&R have waxed and waned in popularity with physiatric practitioners, from the beginning of the field all the way to the present. For example, when I was a resident at The Ohio State University (1969–1972), we were taught both physical medicine

---

*This section has been adapted from the website of the Western Historical Manuscript Collection-Columbia of the University of Missouri and the State Historical Society of Missouri (www.umsystem.edu/whmc/invent/3981. html).

and rehabilitation, but the majority of us at that time were more interested in physical medicine (including electrodiagnosis). Many of us thought of ourselves to some extent as being like orthopedists who did not do surgery.

But times change. In 1983, Medicare switched its payment system for inpatient care from a cost reimbursement model to a prospective payment model (based on Diagnosis Related Groups, or DRGs). This system classified inpatient hospital cases into one of approximately 500 groups expected to have similar hospital resource use, including the likely complications or comorbidities. It was created by Robert Fetter and John Thompson at Yale University. Medicare realized that its new DRG system did not fit inpatient rehabilitation and exempted it, continuing to pay for inpatient rehabilitation using the cost-reimbursement model. With the advent of this new prospective payment system, hospitals suddenly changed from wanting to keep patients as long as possible to wanting to discharge them as soon as possible.

Hospital administrators and for-profit companies soon recognized that inpatient rehabilitation was one of the few inpatient areas exempt from the DRG system. This resulted in a decade or more of massive growth in inpatient "DRG-exempt" rehabilitation hospitals and units all across the United States. For example, when I was the chair of the Department of PM&R at Indiana University at that time, the number of DRG-exempt rehabilitation beds in Indiana went from less than a hundred to more than a thousand in just a few years. And all of these new facilities needed a physiatrists to medically direct them. This caused a dramatic increase in what physiatrists were being offered in compensation packages. At one point, my brand new graduating residents were making more money on their first day on the job as medical directors of these new facilities than I was making. The PM&R residents in the United States subsequently increased both in number and quality. The number of residency programs in the United States went from only 4 in 1945 to 62 in 1975, then jumped to 79 by 1995. The number of residency positions went gradually from 12 in 1945 to 464 in 1975, and jumped to a peak of 1356 by 1995. (The number was slightly down to 1236 by 2004.)

Dr. Ted Cole referred to this period of massive growth in inpatient rehabilitation in the decade or so after the onset of the Medicare DRG system as the "golden age" of rehabilitation medicine. Needless to say, the interest of the residents during this time shifted from physical medicine toward rehabilitation medicine.

But times change. In the early 1990s, many physiatrists began to get involved in various types of spinal injections and were more interested in the outpatient practice of physical medicine than in inpatient rehabilitation. This new trend caught on quickly, as mirrored by the formation of PASSOR as a Council of the AAPM&R. As the AAPM&R Website defines them: "The Physiatric Association of Spine, Sports and Occupational Rehabilitation (PASSOR) is the official musculoskeletal council of the American Academy of Physical Medicine and Rehabilitation representing more than 1,100 physical medicine and rehabilitation specialists. PASSOR represents the special needs of the musculoskeletal medical practitioner." There were 15 founding members of PASSOR, and their first president was Jeffrey A. Saal, MD, in 1993. At that time, I was on the board of directors of the AAPM&R and participated in some of the negotiations that resulted in the development of PASSOR as a "council." The physicians spearheading this movement were not happy with the focus of the AAPM&R at that time and felt that their needs were being largely ignored. They expressed a feeling that the AAPM&R's focus was almost exclusively on the rehabilitation side of the field, especially in its program offerings at the annual meeting. (This was due to some extent to the fact that the annual meeting at that time was run jointly by the AAPM&R and the American Congress of Rehabilitation Medicine, or ACRM).

In one meeting I attended, the representative of PASSOR stated that it was their intention to establish their own organization outside the AAPM&R unless changes were made in the focus of the organization. Responding to this expressed need, the Board of Directors of the AAPM&R included PASSOR as a council and began to try to better balance the annual meeting and other educational offerings between physical medicine and rehabilitation.

Informal musculoskeletal fellowships, most of which were really more like apprenticeships, sprang up around the country to teach spine injections and other spine procedural skills. These informal fellowships slowly evolved into formal fellowships, and official recognition with "added qualifications" became available under the rubric of "pain medicine." As stated in the ABPM&R Website: "In March 1998, The American Board of Physical Medicine and Rehabilitation (ABPMR) and The American Board of Psychiatry and Neurology (ABPN) joined the American Board of Anesthesiology (ABA) in recognition of Pain Management (Pain Medicine) as an interdisciplinary subspecialty. The respective Boards have agreed upon a single standard of certification."

One of the important things about this new trend was that it involved a new work activity for physiatrists, that of spinal procedures (from epidurals to percutaneous discectomies). While doing these procedures was a natural extension of what was already being done in physical medicine, this obviously represented some "field creep" into anesthesiology and neurosurgery. PM&R had experienced field creep before, as others have tried to creep (with variable success) into our field. Some past examples of this included the medical orthopedic movement, led by Inman and others; the interest of family medicine in spinal cord injury rehabilitation; the interest of neurologists in "neurorehabilitation"; the loss of ultraviolet therapy to the dermatologists; and the incursion into cardiac rehab by cardiologists. But this might have been the first time that we were the ones doing the creeping.

The ebb and flow of interest between physical medicine versus rehabilitation is now firmly in the physical medicine camp.

There has also been a change in "how" physiatrists join in practice. Physiatrists in the past practiced almost exclusively in physiatric groups, but now they are also joining orthopedic, neurology, anesthesiology, and multispecialty groups. The most recent Learner's Needs Assessment (LNA) survey of physiatrists done by the AAPM&R (1995) shows that 57% of the respondents stated their primary focus is musculoskeletal medicine, whereas 37% focused on rehabilitation medicine.

Regardless of the reasons for the recent increase in physical medicine and spinal procedures, we are now challenged to consider the outcome. It has many implications for our field, especially in regard to how we train residents. It is my feeling that the historic and ever-changing division of interest in physical medicine versus rehabilitation (including the current field creep) is good for the field, good for physiatrists, and more importantly, good for those we treat. Here are some of the reasons for this:

1. **The expanding field of PM&R allows physiatrists the freedom to choose from a remarkably wide choice of work activities.**
PM&R is not an organ-based field like cardiology or nephrology. Like family medicine, we reserve the right to treat the whole body. We are blessed to have expertise in *both* physical medicine and in rehabilitation. This gives the physiatrist almost unlimited latitude in choosing daily work activities. In my own case, I confess that I need to change my work activity from time to time, and PM&R has offered me a broad latitude to move around within the field. At different times in my life, I have done outpatient musculoskeletal medicine, outpatient electrodiagnostic practice, rehab inpatient medicine, worked with children and adults, been a medical director of both outpatient and inpatient programs, an academician, a private practitioner, and even the CEO of a hospital. I have been on the staff of every kind of hospital, from military to for-profit to not-for-profit to sectarian to nonsectarian to community to university to VA, etc. Try doing all that in an organ-based field! I am fond of telling medical students that there are so many different things to do in PM&R that you shouldn't ever get bored, and even if you eventually do, by then the field will have invented a whole new potential work activity for you.

Every field has to evolve over the course of time, especially because one of the few constants we have is constant change. For example, some rehabilitationists wondered if the field could survive after a cure for polio was found. Other fields have faced this as well, such as when some otolaryngologists wondered if their field would survive after antibiotics wiped out the need to do mastoidectomies. The new trend in our field to do spinal injections and procedures is merely part of this field evolution and further expands the breadth of the field.

2. **The ongoing tension between physical medicine and rehabilitation is beneficial and will continue to aid in the development of the field.**
It is my contention that the union of physical medicine and rehabilitation has been beneficial for both fields. For example, the rehabilitationists began using the physical techniques including heat, light, electricity, and mechanotherapy to help in the treatment of patients with severe impairments. Meanwhile, the physical medicine practitioners learned how to use a team approach and to treat the patient not just as a malfunctioning body part, but as a whole.

Although some physiatrists will continue to choose to subspecialize in a relatively circumscribed area of either physical medicine (e.g., pain medicine practice) or rehabilitation (e.g., traumatic brain injury in children), the truth is that most of us will continue to do a blended practice. The 2005 LNA survey of physiatrists indicates that most physiatrists are still involved (using percentage of time allocation) in practicing doing the whole field of PM&R (direct outpatient care, 50.1%; direct inpatient care, 23.1%; administration, 9.8%; academic activities, 4.4%; and research, 2.8%). More than 60% of physiatrists continue to do electrodiagnostic studies. If we were to construct an "average" physiatrist in terms of current work activity, he or she would probably start the day by making rounds at a hospital on an inpatient rehab unit, doing some inpatient consultations, perhaps visiting a subacute facility, and then going to an outpatient setting to see patients who need a wide range of services, from pain management to electrodiagnostic evaluation to follow-up from inpatient rehabilitation.

The great majority of physiatrists are still practicing the whole field. The historic tension between "physical medicine" and "rehabilitation" is clearly making both fields better, just as having a competitor can make a business better. In fact, the tension has been a large factor in making the field of physical medicine and rehabilitation so much more than just the arithmetic sum of its parts.

3. **Demographics continue to force us to maintain our skills in both physical medicine and rehabilitation.**
The development of the PM&R specialty has largely mirrored that of internal medicine (IM). Faced with internists subspecializing in the various organs, IM developed a fellowship system. Rather than fighting this trend to subspecialization, IM embraced and empowered it. IM almost went so far, however, as to disenfranchise the "general" internist. But when they came face to face with the demographics and practical realities of IM practice, as well as by the rising influence of family medicine, they quickly changed and began fostering again the field of general internal medicine. PM&R is now facing the same subspecialization tensions and has responded by providing opportunities to subspecialize in areas such as pediatrics, pain medicine, and spinal cord injury medicine. A trained physiatrist can evaluate and care for a very wide variety of patients. However, there is still a very strong role for the "undifferentiated physiatrist," as patient access to physiatry is still dependent on the distribution of the small number of trainees. As "baby boomers," the largest single demographic group in our society, reach retirement age, it is clear the variety of their potential needs will require general physiatry as well as the subspecialists.

4. **The broader the field of PM&R, the more effective it can be, both medically and economically.**
There is a measure of security in having the ability to do a broad range of things. Various imaging studies of the central and peripheral nervous system have threatened to make

electrodiagnosis obsolete over the last 30 years. Fortunately, electrodiagnosis is more developed and electromyography is still the best way to assess motor unit physiology. Long-term studies and outcomes of various patient groups receiving various musculoskeletal injections and procedures are yet to be completed. At the same time, the physiatrists are becoming involved in many new areas of patient care, such as transplant rehabilitation, burn rehabilitation, and management of surgically implanted pumps and nerve stimulators. Broad training allows for diversification of practice as clinical demands change and new opportunities emerge.

5. **We continue to be uniquely trained to use the holistic patient-centered team approach, which adds value to any of our work activities.**
Regardless of what direction "field creep" might take in the future of physiatric practice, we continue to have some training advantages. Physiatrists are trained to view the patient as a whole and not to reductionistically view the patient just as an abnormal lab test or as a disease. It also allows us to see the big picture of not just what the impairment is, but what the impairment means to the patient in every aspect of life—for example, from ambulation to ADL (activities of daily living) independence to sexual functioning to income maintenance. This "big picture" of the patient not only makes our practice more effective and efficient, but it is also of enormous benefit to the patient. It can truly focus the physiatrist on the knowledge, attitudes, and methods needed to add not just years to life, but life to years.*

Physiatrists also invented the team approach in medicine and used it years before anyone else even thought of it. It is amusing to me when I see an article in the newspaper about a physician in another specialty touting his or her new "team approach." The article invariably describes it as a new approach to patient care as if they had just invented it. Although this is new to other fields, it is not to us. We were doing a team approach to patient care before it was "cool." Being able to function as the leader of a team magnifies our ability to help our patient in an integrated and well-coordinated manner, and will be more and more essential to success in the future practice of medicine in general and in physiatry in particular.

This epilogue has discussed the obvious tensions that have historically existed between physical medicine and rehabilitation, as currently seen in the field creep of physiatrists into spinal injections and procedures. However, my overall message is that this tension has historically benefited both parts of the field, has made us all more effective in treating patients, and represents only the natural evolution and ebb and flow of practice activity in our field. Despite field creep and other changes that occur in our field, this tension is beneficial in that it will help keep us focused on maintaining the physiatric principles that are at the core of our being, including the holistic and team approaches to the patient.

But times change! And we are blessed to be in a field that has shown a remarkable and ongoing capacity to change with the times!

REFERENCES

1. Krusen FH: Physical Medicine. Philadelphia, W.B. Saunders, 1941.
2. Krusen FH: Historical development in physical medicine and rehabilitation during the last forty years. Walter J. Zeiter Lecture. Arch Phys Med Rehabil 50(1):1–5, 1969.
3. Opitz JL, Folz FJ, Gelfman R, Peters DJ: The history of physical medicine and rehabilitation as recorded in the diary of Dr. Frank Krusen: Part 1. Gathering momentum (the years before 1942). Arch Phys Med Rehabil 78(4):442–445, 1997.
4. Folz FJ, Opitz JL, Peters DJ, Gelfman R: The history of physical medicine and rehabilitation as recorded in the diary of Dr. Frank Krusen: Part 2. Forging ahead (1943–1947). Arch Phys Med Rehabil 78(4):446–450, 1997.

*The author of this phrase is unknown, but is believed to be Dr. George Morris Piersoll of the University of Pennsylvania, circa 1947. The original phrase was: "It is not enough that we, physicians, add years to life; we must also add life to years." Acknowledged in Flax HJ: Life to Years. Rockville, MD, self-published,1995.

5. Gelfman R, Peters DJ, Opitz JL, Folz FJ: The history of physical medicine and rehabilitation as recorded in the diary of Dr. Frank Krusen: Part 3. Consolidating the position (1948–1953). Arch Phys Med Rehabil 78(5):556–561, 1997.

6. Peters DJ, Gelfman R, Folz FJ, Opitz JL: The history of physical medicine and rehabilitation as recorded in the diary of Dr. Frank Krusen: Part 4. Triumph over adversity (1954–1969). Arch Phys Med Rehabil 78(5):562–565, 1997.

7. Rusk HA: Rehabilitation, 3rd ed. Mosby, St. Louis, 1971, p vii.

8. Rusk HA: Rehabilitation. Mosby, St. Louis, 1958.

INDEX

Page numbers in **boldface type** indicate complete chapters.